Early Language Intervention for Infants, Toddlers, and Preschoolers

Robert E. Owens, Jr.

College of Saint Rose

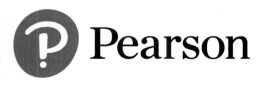

330 Hudson Street, NY 10013

To my grandson Dakota in his quest to communicate with us
Love from "Gran'pa Pie and Apple Bob"

and

*To all the dedicated speech-language pathologists
who work with young children.*

Editorial Director: *Kevin Davis*
Executive Portfolio Manager: *Julie Peters*
Content Producer: *Megan Moffo*
Portfolio Management Assistant: *Maria Feliberty*
Executive Product Marketing Manager: *Christopher Barry*
Executive Field Marketing Manager: *Krista Clark*
Procurement Specialist: *Deidra Smith*
Development Editor: *Jill Ross*
Cover Design: *Carie Keller, Cenveo*
Cover Art: *Halfpoint/Fotolia*
Media Producer: *Michael Goncalves*
Editorial Production and Composition Services: *Cenveo® Publisher Services*
Full-Service Project Manager: *Bonnie Boehme*
Text Font: *ITC Stone Serif Std*

Credits and acknowledgments for materials borrowed from other sources and reproduced, with permission, in this textbook appear on the appropriate page within the text.

Every effort has been made to provide accurate and current Internet information in this book. However, the Internet and information posted on it are constantly changing, so it is inevitable that some of the Internet addresses listed in this textbook will change.

Cataloging-in-Publication data is on file with the Library of Congress.

1   16

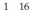
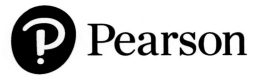

Student Edition
ISBN-10:   0-13-461890-4
ISBN-13: 978-0-13-461890-6

eText
ISBN-10:   0-13-453776-9
ISBN-13: 978-0-13-453776-4

eText Package
ISBN-10:   0-13-450968-4
ISBN-13: 978-0-13-450968-6

Contents

Preface

As a Ph.D. candidate, back when there were dinosaurs, I was summoned to the department chair's office because I had somehow "misdeclared" my field of study. In a gruff voice the chair, a women in her 70s, demanded to know in "what" I was getting my degree.

"Language disorders," I readily responded.

"Impossible!" came her immediate reply.

Somewhat confused and taken aback, I restated, "Language disorders."

"Speech or hearing?" she demanded.

"Language," I insisted somewhat hesitantly.

"Speech or hearing?" she again demanded.

"Then I guess 'speech,'" I sheepishly replied.

"Good," she huffed, and then added "We can't have people making up their own degrees," as she dismissed me with a wave.

It was the mid-1970s, and thankfully the times have changed. Not only is language a very viable part of communicative disorders and sciences, or what was back then called speech therapy, but we've added augmentative communication (AAC), work with nonsymbolic children and adults, and feeding and swallowing, to name a few.

Oh, don't get me wrong, I had training in some of those areas. Thanks to the forward-looking vision of Jim MacDonald, my adviser, we had plenty of coursework in intervention with nonsymbolic children. I even had a course in AAC, which we, the students, taught ourselves, given that none of the faculty had any expertise in that area. Despite the fact that we met in the back room of a bar for three or more hours every Thursday night and that we made up the course requirements and did all the teaching ourselves, it was one of the most rigorous courses in my Ph.D. program. I've kept my interest in working with nonsymbolic children ever since.

So you had a course or two, big deal, you might be thinking. What makes you think you know enough to write a text? Maybe I don't, but I've had lots of great research by others and my own experience to base it on. While at Ohio State University, I studied with Jim and worked in his Environmental Language Program as a language trainer for three years. That provided the base.

When, as a fresh Ph.D., I arrived at State University of New York at Geneseo to teach, I was the "new kid," so I got the supervision assignment no one else wanted: developmental centers where we warehoused children and adults with developmental disabilities. Talk about frustration!—frustration for all of us: the clients, students, and me, their supervisor. At the same time, I was asked to write a language intervention program for a preschool run by the local Association for Retarded Citizens. Out of these experiences came my graduate course called "Severe Communication Impairments" and *The Program for the Acquisition of Language with the Severely Impaired* (PALS) (Owens, 1982). Both were the result of a lot of designing and trial and error. PALS is out of print, but I'm happy to report that I have taught a nonverbal communication course every semester. Over time, it has morphed from intervention primarily with institutionalized adults to early communication intervention (ECI). Along the way, I've continued to consult with agencies serving young populations and to help students providing intervention for little ones. At the College of St. Rose, each semester I teach a graduate course in infant, toddler, and preschool language disorders.

My interest in ECI stems from two other sources. First, as a young child, I was very sickly. In fact, I have the distinction of having been declared dead by medical personnel twice before the age of 1. I know that on one of those occasions my father, a navy pharmacist mate, brought me back, and on the other my grandfather threatened to take out the entire medical staff at the hospital unless they saved me. Nothing like good old lower-class bravado to get some action!

My second reason for continued interest in this topic is my gran'kids. Sydney wasn't with us for long. A preemie, she died within six weeks. Her brother Dakota has both severe intellectual disability and severe cerebral palsy. Thanks to botox shots in his legs and lots of physical therapy, mostly at home, he can, at age 9, pull to a stand and cruise by holding onto furniture. He self-feeds too, but meaningful communication seems to elude us except on those rare occasions when he will produce a fully formed sentence. The youngest, Zavier, has no large motor difficulties and wants to communicate with everyone but was restricted by apraxia of speech that severely limited his intelligibility. That didn't keep him from trying. Now an overactive 8-year-old, he has intelligible speech and seems to be doing fine.

As a gran'pa, albeit one who lives almost 400 miles away, I continue to try to find novel ways to aid their communication. Ironically, both Dakota and "Zav" attended preschool in the same center and in the same classroom where I worked as a student language trainer approximately 40 years before.

About This Book

ECI is an important and growing area of interest in education. It is well documented that intervention efforts early in a child's life can have great benefits later for the child and family. In addition, early intervention of all types, not just ECI, can save taxpayers money later in the form of fewer special education services.

Although increasing numbers of speech-language pathologists are working in ECI, some graduate education programs have been slow to educate future practitioners in the specific needs of very young children. Few texts on the subject exist, which is why I wrote this book.

But why do we need a text that specifically targets very young children? As I tell my students, "We're not in Kansas anymore, Toto." The model for working with infants and toddlers is very different from that with older children. One size does not fit all.

Those who know my work will recognize my commitment to functional communication throughout this text. Functional communication intervention takes the teaching of language out of the realm of formal teaching and targets language as it is being used. With young children, this may mean creating both a need and a means to communicate. This entails bringing the family into intervention as full members of the intervention team. As Jim MacDonald was fond of saying, "You can't teach one person to communicate." Communication by its nature requires at least two partners. That's where the family comes in.

So relax. Snuggle up to the book. And be prepared for a different but extremely rewarding type of communication intervention. For those of you who love little children, I hope you will find the experience of learning about and later practicing in ECI a rewarding one.

The Enhanced eText

A digital version of this text is available in a package that may be adopted as a print plus digital package from Pearson. Students can register for use of the Enhanced eText, which contains links to videos that enhance the content and quizzes to self-check their understanding and reinforce knowledge and application.

Instructor Ancillaries for this Text

This text is accompanied by an Instructor's Manual and Test Bank and PowerPoint Slides. These resources are available free of charge and may be downloaded by adopting professors at pearsonhighered.com in the Instructor's Resource Center.

Acknowledgments

An African American friend of mine acknowledges his heritage by saying that he stands on the shoulders of giants. I feel equally humbled by the many men and women, some no longer with us, who have contributed directly or indirectly to the field of early communication intervention. My partial list, in no particular order, includes

- Jim McLean, Ph.D., and Lee Snyder McLean, Ph.D., for their early work with intellectual disability and with young children. There never was a more generous or gracious couple.
- Jim MacDonald, Ph.D., Ohio State University, with whom I had the privilege of being his student and a language trainer in his Environmental Language Program
- Barry Prizant, Ph.D., and Amy Wetherby, Ph.D., the dynamic duo of early intervention with children with autism spectrum disorder
- Louis Rossetti, Ph.D., who for so long was a voice in the wilderness of early intervention
- Ayala Manelson, Toronto, who had the vision and the foresight to establish and foster the Hanen Program and who can light up any space with her presence
- Luigi Girolametto, Ph.D., University of Toronto, who initially worked with Ayala and as a professor has contributed mightily to our understanding of working with parents
- David Yoder, Ph.D., and Jon Miller, Ph.D., University of Wisconsin, for their early work with intellectual disability
- Richard Schiefelbusch, Ph.D., for his early work with intellectual disability
- Stephen Calculator, University of New Hampshire, for his work with intellectual disability and augmentative communication
- Jean Wilcox, Ph.D., Arizona State University, who has shared so much of her knowledge and expertise with all of us
- Lyle Lloyd, Ph.D., Purdue University, for his work with intellectual disability
- Ann Kaiser
- Elizabeth Crais
- Cynthia Cress
- Janice Light and Kathryn Drager and their wonderful work with very young children and AAC
- Carol Goosens, who was working with individuals with intellectual disability long before many others
- Mary Ann Romski and Rose Sevcick, two towers of knowledge in AAC and wonderfully gracious individuals
- Catherine Lord
- Ivar Lovaas, the father of ABA
- Pat Mirenda
- Joe Reichle and his early work in AAC
- Leslie Rescorla
- Jeff Sigafoos
- Steve Warren, Paul Yoder, and the forward-thinking folks at Vanderbilt University

Several centers of higher education have also been incubators for innovative work in early communication intervention, including at the University of Washington, Pennsylvania State University, Vanderbilt University, and the University of North Carolina, Chapel Hill.

No doubt I have missed someone. My memory isn't always as sharp as it should be. If I have overlooked anyone, please know that it was not done purposefully and I apologize for the oversight. Let me know and I'll add you next time.

The professional assistance of several people has been a godsend, including that of my colleagues at The College of Saint Rose. Saint Rose has an environment that fosters collaboration and individual professional growth, and it's a wonderful place to work. I have been encouraged to continue my writing by the academic atmosphere established by President Carolyn Stafanco, Dean of Education Margaret McLane, and my department chair, James Feeney. Other great faculty in Communication Sciences and Disorders include Dave DeBonis, our resident audiologist and a warm friend; Jack Pickering, who runs our transgender voice clinic and teaches voice and co-teaches counseling with me; Anne Rowley, our other language person, who brings to the task a wealth of syntactic knowledge and empathy; Julia Unger, the world's sweetest person, director of the Council for Effective Communication, and our fluency expert; and fellow clinical faculty members, including Jackie Klein, Director of Clinical Education, and Elizabeth Baird, Marisa Bryant, Sarah Coons, Colleen Fluman, Elaine Galbraith, Julie Hart, Barbara Hoffman, Kate Lansing, Jessica Evans, Melissa Spring, Lynn Stephens, Robin Anderson, Lottie Dunbar, and Zhaleh Lavasani.. You have all made me feel welcomed and valued. Three clinical faculty and knowledgeable professionals, Barbara Hoffman, Elizabeth Baird, and Colleen Fluman, were especially helpful with preparation of Box 9.1 and Appendix A. I would be remiss if I didn't also acknowledge the fine students and graduate students at Saint Rose.

In addition, a special thanks to my former colleagues at SUNY Geneseo, for whom I have only the highest respect. Our program in communicative disorders and sciences may be gone, thanks to draconian budget cuts, but that does not detract from our accomplishments and from our being, by any objective measure, one of the finest educational programs in the country. We can all be proud of what we did for our field, the quality of the education our students received, and the speech, language, and hearing services we provided for over 60 years to the local community.

Many dear friends offered advice and their expertise to help me in assembling this tome. They include Dr. Addie Haas, a dear friend, traveling buddy, and all-around wonderful person; my colleagues at SUNY New Paltz; Dr. Brenda Louw, chairperson of the Department of Communication Disorders at East Tennessee State University; and Professor Omid Mohamadi, Department of Speech Therapy at Tabriz University of Medical Sciences and Health Services, who has published two books in Persian titled *Early Detection of Speech and Language Disorders in Children* and *Early Detection of Autism Spectrum Disorder in Children*, and helped with the writing of Chapter 6.

I can't claim the expertise to write this entire text, and I have had the good fortune to be able to rely on Dr. Jessica Kisenwether, assistant professor at Misericordia University, who contributed the pediatric feeding and swallowing chapter. She is an intelligent, energetic young professional with a bright future.

I would also like to thank the reviewers of this edition:

- Valerie E. Boyer, Southern Illinois University Carbondale
- Barbara Davis, University of Texas at Austin
- William Harn, Lamar University
- Megan Mahowald, Minnesota State University–Mankato

And finally, a huge thank-you to my partner, who daily offers encouragement and support. I'm thankful every day that we met.

Early Language Intervention for Infants, Toddlers, and Preschoolers

1

Components of Early Intervention

Of necessity, we need to begin with some background and the legal basis for early intervention. Then we'll look at the components of a thorough intervention program. If you have volunteered or are working in early intervention, then you may be familiar with at least some of these components.

When you have completed the chapter, you should be able to:

- List the elements of early intervention.
- Explain the guidelines for assembling an Individualized Family Service Plan.
- Describe the process of evaluating research.

Terms with which you should be familiar:

Cultural competence	Evidence-based practice (EBP)
Developmental disabilities	Handicap
Disability	Impairment
Early communication intervention	Individualized Family Service Plan (IFSP)
Early intervention	Transdisciplinary team

1

Sean was a beautiful baby, pink and plump. The first child of his young parents, he seemed to interact with them less than they expected, but they just attributed his behavior to his personality. They were a bit sad that Sean made little eye contact and smiled infrequently, but figured this would change.

Feeding seemed to be particularly troublesome, but Sean's parents were reassured that nursing would improve when he gained better motor control. When this did not occur, the physician counseled that his parents should relax. It was most likely, they were told, that their concern was being transmitted to Sean in some way and further discouraging typical feeding development. Otherwise Sean seemed to be developing normally. He continued to prefer aloneness rather than interacting with others.

Although Sean's motor behavior seemed to be developing typically, it became harder and harder for Sean's parents to overlook his lack of interaction. He mostly whined and cried and failed to develop gestures or vocalizations. It seemed difficult for Sean to focus on a single toy or person. Instead he interacted aimlessly with toys, going quickly from one to another. With other objects, such as a fuzzy sock, he seemed almost obsessive in his attention.

Finally, Sean's parents and even the physician became concerned. At 27 months of age Sean was evaluated by a team of specialists. Tentatively, he was diagnosed as having autism spectrum disorder (ASD). His parents began the long search for an appropriate early intervention program. And so shall we. Throughout this text, we'll explore early intervention options based on what we know from research and clinical practice.

Working in early intervention offers a special opportunity. As you move through your education and practicum and plan a career as a speech-language pathologist (SLP) or possibly a teacher, you may naturally gravitate to the "little folk." That translates into infants, toddlers, and preschoolers, the subject of this text.

I enjoy working with a variety of clients, but these three age groups own a warm spot in my heart. They'll make you laugh, and they'll test your problem-solving skills. Much of what you'll do in assessment and intervention will seem like play, because that's how we intervene with very young children. Working with young children can be rewarding, but it also requires you to be a skilled clinician.

We'll have an entire book to work on your skills, but first let's meet another friend of mine. Mikey, as his mom calls him, was born six weeks premature, the third child of his recently divorced, single mother to be a preemie. After his birth, Mikey spent six weeks in the neonatal intensive care unit (NICU). Mikey's mom is a smoker who drank, sometimes heavily, during her early pregnancy which may have contributed to his early birth and development.

At 13 months of age, Mikey was not babbling except for the occasional sound in isolation. He had poor eye contact with people and objects, and his interaction with objects, such as toys, was indiscriminate. Every object seemed to be treated in the same way. Mikey was in danger of falling behind. While life rarely offers guarantees, one way to help his development is through early intervention (EI).

Overview of EI

The term EI applies to an educational approach for young children, ages birth to 3 years, who have or are at risk of developing a disability that may affect their development. The purpose of EI is to provide both prevention of future difficulties and remediation of current ones. The focus is on both the child and the family and may be home, center, or hospital based, or any combination of these. Although intervention may begin at any time, it's best for a child to begin as early as possible given the rapid rate of human learning and development in the earliest years.

Because of Mikey's delays in developing speech and language, he'll need special help. When the primary focus of intervention is a young child's speech, language, communication, and/or feeding, we refer to the child's program as early communication intervention (ECI). Although I'll focus in this book on the linguistic aspects of ECI, it's impossible to isolate one aspect of ECI from the others. For example, although I may be pursuing augmentative and alternative communication (AAC) through the use of signing, the cause may be childhood apraxia of speech with accompanying feeding difficulties. These areas must also be addressed in a holistic approach.

The importance of early intervention, especially ECI, cannot be overstated. Maturational changes in the first three years may affect communication and other developmental areas throughout an individual's life. The early years can have a dramatic effect on a child's ability to increase her or his vocabulary, achieve reading comprehension, and increase social interaction (Calandrella & Wilcox, 2000). Building support for children's development in the early stages of life can help alleviate later childhood learning and behavioral problems.

As an SLP, you won't be expected to accomplish all this alone. You'll need allies and helpers, and that's where families and an intervention team come in. Most children reside in families of one shape or another, and that family has a huge influence on a child's development and learning. In ECI, we rely on family members to become the agents of change. Just the sheer amount of time families spend with their kids should be evidence of family members' potential as communication facilitating partners for those children.

If you are an SLP or a communication disorders student, this model of intervention may seem different from what you've learned in lectures or in practicum, especially in school settings. Working with young children, family members, and other professional care providers, such as teachers and aides, plus physical and occupational therapists within a team may take some adjustment on your part too. But all that can wait for a few chapters.

Right now, let's begin our exploration of all these topics with the legal basis for EI and some of the issues that flow from this legislation. EI isn't just a good idea. In the United States and other developed countries, it's mandated by law.

 Watch this video to see what parents and practitioners have to say about early intervention.
https://www.youtube.com/watch?v=8vhASm6qkZE

Legal Basis for Early Intervention

Getting government-mandated services for very young children wasn't an easy task. As a society, we have tended to view education as beginning at age 6 when a child goes to school.

The impetus for EI came from worldwide efforts, such as those of the World Health Organization (WHO, 1981). WHO's focus on health care for vulnerable groups, such as mothers and children, implies that disease and disabilities can best be prevented if women are educated before and during pregnancy and if the infant population is targeted for health and intervention services (Kritzinger, 2000). We'll discuss later the holistic model of intervention WHO has fostered and the family and community implications of these for EI.

Before we wade into legislation that outlines the shape of EI in the United States, we should briefly define three terms: *disability*, *impairment*, and *handicap*.

- Disability implies an inability or lack of ability to perform particular tasks, functions, or skills.
- Impairment refers to an abnormality in function or structure.
- Handicap refers to the social consequences of disability or impairment that prevent an individual from realizing her or his potential.

These terms are reflected in legislation and regulations governing EI. Although all three terms are used to refer to the affected individual, they affect the family and community as well. For example, handicaps may be preventable with inclusion and social adaptation.

EDUCATION OF THE HANDICAPPED ACT AMENDMENTS

Several laws establish the requirements for EI. Public law (PL) 99-457, passed in 1986 and called the *Education of the Handicapped Act Amendments*, mandated that states establish

FIGURE 1.1 **Definition of Developmental Disability**

Although PL 99-457 mandated comprehensive service for infants and toddlers with developmental disabilities (DD), it took 14 more years and the passage of PL 106-402 (2000) to get the current definition of developmental disability as a severe, chronic disability of an individual that

- Is attributable to mental or physical impairment or a combination of impairments;
- Is manifested before the age of 22 years;
- Is likely to continue indefinitely;
- Results in substantial functional limitations in three or more areas of life activity, such as self-care, receptive and expressive language, learning, mobility, self-direction, capacity for independent learning, and economic self-sufficiency; and
- Reflects the individual's need for a combination and sequence of special, interdisciplinary, or generic services, individualized supports, or other forms of assistance that are of lifelong or extended duration and are individually planned and coordinated. (ASHA, 2005b)

Despite the variety of disorders that fit under the DD rubric, children with DD generally share the common characteristic of severely impaired speech and language development (McLean, Brady, & McLean, 1996; Sigafoos & Pennell, 1995).

comprehensive service for infants and toddlers with developmental disabilities (DD) and for their families. See Figure 1.1 for a definition of DD. The term *developmental disability* refers to a number of specific conditions, such as intellectual disability, autism spectrum disorder, and cerebral palsy (Graziano, 2002). You may or may not be familiar with these terms. We'll clarify them in Chapter 2.

Prior to passage of PL 99-457, there had been no federal legal requirement to provide EI services. PL 99-457 required that qualified professionals complete an assessment of each child and that both assessment and intervention be provided by a multidisciplinary team. The purpose of the assessment is to confirm the presence and extent of disability and to identify

- A child's unique needs, accomplishments, and strengths,
- A family's strengths and needs as they relate to the child's development, and
- The nature and extent of early intervention services appropriate to the child and family.

Evaluation must describe a child's functioning in the areas of cognitive, physical, speech and language, and psychosocial development and in self-help skills. Even with the federal legislation, eligibility for services varies by state.

INDIVIDUALS WITH DISABILITIES EDUCATION ACT (IDEA)

Four years after 99-457, the U.S. Congress passed the *Individuals with Disabilities Education Act* of 1990 (IDEA). IDEA requires free, appropriate public education (FAPE) for children with disabilities. Part B of IDEA outlines programs for preschool children based on each child's Individualized Education Plan (IEP). Hopefully, you're already familiar with an IEP from other courses. Part C specifies programs for infants and toddlers as provided in an Individualized Family Service Plan (IFSP). Don't worry, we'll characterize an IFSP later.

The Individuals with Disabilities Education Act was reauthorized in 1997 in PL 105-17. Part C of PL 105-17 strengthens the requirement that services be provided within the context of the family. Family members are now part of the interdisciplinary team and also primary decision-makers in the collaborative effort.

INDIVIDUALS WITH DISABILITIES EDUCATION IMPROVEMENT ACT (IDEIA)

In 2004, IDEA was again reauthorized as the *Individuals with Disabilities Education Improvement Act* (IDEIA). Part C of this federal law addresses services for children with disabilities and significant developmental delays from birth through age 2 years with possible extension to age 6. The primary focus of Part C is on supporting a family's ability to meet the developmental needs of its infant or toddler. This includes the right to an individualized program developed by IFSP or IEP teams and offered in the natural environment or the least restrictive environment (LRE).

SUMMARY

Those are the pieces. Let's pull it all together. Several principles of intervention outlined in the legislation and in the regulations that followed are important in designing early intervention programs (ASHA, 2008a, 2008b, 2008c, 2008d). Taken together, they state that services should be

- Comprehensive, coordinated, team-based, and transdisciplinary in nature to optimize the participation of children and their families and integrated to meet the needs of children and their families;
- Family-centered and responsive to a family's priorities as well as the culture and values of the family, including each family's unique situation, culture, language(s), preferences, resource, and priorities;
- Individualized for a child and family;
- Developmentally supportive and promote a child's participation in his/her natural environment;
- Developmentally appropriate for a child's age, cognitive level, strengths, and family concerns and preferences;
- Provided in the least restrictive and most natural environment for a child and family; and
- Based on the highest quality and most recent research evidence on intervention effectiveness merged with professional expertise and family preferences.

These elements are also supported by the ECI guiding principles of the American Speech-Language-Hearing Association (ASHA, 2008b).

Elements of an Early Intervention Program

That was a lot to digest. Let's explore some of these elements of EI further. Specifically, we'll discuss the elements of a transdisciplinary team; the importance of families, especially the child and parents or caregivers; individualized assessment and intervention; the Individualized Family Service Plan; the importance of the natural environment; and the importance of evidence-based practice (EBP).

TRANSDISCIPLINARY TEAM

The team is responsible for providing the most appropriate service delivery based on the individualized needs of a child and family. Although IDEA 2004 uses the term *multidisciplinary teams*, team models vary depending on the needs of the child and family. As we will see, interdisciplinary and transdisciplinary are two other commonly used team models. These models differ in the amount of communication and coordination that exists among team members (Paul-Brown & Caperton, 2001). In each model, depending on the child, a variety of professional disciplines can be represented. How they are represented is the key.

In the center where I worked prior to becoming a professor, 22 distinct disciplines could potentially be involved. The actual number varied depending on the needs of the specific child and family. It may be helpful to imagine the three models along a continuum from minimally to maximally collaborative and cooperative. Let's discuss each briefly.

Team Models

Multidisciplinary team members, such as an SLP, evaluate a child separately and determine his or her needs independently. Each professional completes an evaluation, makes his or her own recommendations, and may provide services separate from other disciplines. Although each discipline's findings are usually pulled together by the service coordinator or team leader, there is little collaborative planning or implementation. As a result, there is the potential for gaps or overlaps in services.

Families may feel that their views are ignored because they are often not treated as full members of the multidisciplinary intervention team. Families report being overwhelmed by the number of individual professionals consulting with them and making recommendations. Difficulties reported by families of children with disabilities are often the result of poor coordination across services and professionals (Harbin et al., 2004).

In contrast, interdisciplinary teams have established lines of communication among the professionals, resulting in a greater degree of collaboration. Interdisciplinary teams place more emphasis on group discussions, shared responsibilities, and resource coordination. Assessments may be conducted either separately by each professional or by the team using an "arena" method of evaluation in which some or all team members are present. Members may consult with one another before, during, and after the evaluation to integrate assessment plans, findings, recommendations, and intervention goals.

The family is considered part of the interdisciplinary team and may either interact with the child during the assessment or observe and validate the information obtained by different professionals. Although a child still may be assessed by different disciplines independently, the team members consult to provide the family with a cohesive report. Disciplines may provide services separately, but they set goals and plan cooperatively and coordinate implementation of intervention services.

In a transdisciplinary team approach, professional boundaries are reduced even further and, ideally, collaboration is maximized. Parents and facilitators from multiple disciplines share responsibility for planning and implementing, while at the same time contributing their own unique expertise. The transdisciplinary approach is characterized by (Paul, Blosser, & Jakubowitz, 2006; Thomas, Correa, & Morsink, 2001)

- Flexible team roles;
- Modification of some traditional responsibilities;
- Inclusion of the family as a team member;
- Shared information and skills; and
- Continuing interaction, communication, and coordination during planning, assessment, and intervention.

Ideally, transdisciplinary teams fully integrate the family and different disciplines. All members of the team participate in the assessment. At the conclusion, the team develops an integrated service plan by consensus through collaboration with the family.

While participation in the EI team is a family decision, family members, in my experience, are usually open to the invitation, even if somewhat tentatively. Other potential team members might be extended family members and friends, as well as representatives of agencies currently serving or anticipated in the future to serve the child or family, such as a physical therapist from the United Cerebral Palsy (UCP) association or a neurologist (Polmanteer & Turbiville, 2000). Others, such as a babysitter or daycare provider, family doctor, or neighbor, may provide information while not being an actual member of the team. Because each member or informant brings a different perspective, his or her participation increases the chances of developing the most comprehensive and effective intervention possible for the child and the family.

The need for a transdisciplinary approach becomes very evident when we consider the gap that often exists between first concerns and the age at which a child is identified as needing intervention services (Kritzinger, Louw, & Rossetti, 2001). If team members have

TABLE 1.1 Transdisciplinary Framework for Early Identification of Risks for Communication Disorders

Developmental Period	Biological Risk Events	Early Identification and Family Support Opportunities
Preconception/ Conception	Possible genetic abnormalities based on family history of genetic disorder/disability	Risks assessment; informational counseling
	Genetic and chromosomal disorders or risk factors, such as drug use, teen pregnancy, or multiple fetuses	Informational counseling
Prenatal	Defective gene, uteroplacental abnormalities, or teratogens, such as maternal alcohol or drug use	Ultrasound, other diagnostic tests, parental education on risks
Perinatal	Prematurity, low birth weight, birth complications, feeding difficulties, severe weight loss	APGAR; hearing screening; parental education, guidance, and counseling; diagnostic assessment; possible SLP early involvement in NICU or SCN
Postnatal	Disease, recurring otitis media, illness, injuries, delayed communication and early social disorders, failure to thrive	Counseling; diagnostic assessment, recurring assessment, medical and developmental education, including ECI

Information from Kritzinger, Louw, & Rossetti, 2001.

been trained within a transdisciplinary team, they are mindful of the at-risk signs in several areas of development and can be alert for indicators of potential developmental problems, thus potentially closing this gap. Table 1.1 presents a transdisciplinary framework for early identification of risks for communication disorders.

While training programs can improve health care professionals' knowledge of other areas of development and concern, they may do little to change attitudes (Moodley, Louw, & Hugo, 2000). For example, although professionals may have a favorable impression of service teams, they may also have concerns about autonomy and a potential blurring of professional boundaries. One word of advice is to be sensitive to these potential concerns when working with other professionals and to proceed carefully.

For this model to work best, professionals need to trust each other and to share knowledge freely. Having worked in such a setting, I found that it was best for disciplines to learn about each other by assisting in both assessment and intervention. Although this approach is time consuming and the learning curve is very steep for new employees, it maximizes knowledge across disciplines. Such knowledge is crucial when you serve as team leader or primary service provider, as I've done on several occasions.

Primary Service Provider

One professional on the team, possibly the SLP, is designated as the primary service provider (PSP). The PSP usually provides direct cross-disciplinary services for the child and family while other professionals act in a consultative manner. Hopefully, this model will help to avoid fragmenting of services.

The majority of children who receive EI services have communication impairments (U.S. Department of Education, 2008). According to ASHA, when a child's primary needs are communication or feeding and swallowing, the PSP should be an SLP. As a result, speech-language pathologists are often the PSP for infants and toddlers with disabilities and for their families. In this capacity, SLPs are also highly involved in the transition of children from early intervention to preschool services.

In practical terms this means that you as PSP may be responsible for helping the family implement physical therapy or neurological recommendations as well as providing ECI. I told you ECI would be a challenge. But don't worry, no one will expect you to do this on the first day. You'll grow into the job. Nor will you be abandoned by the other team members. The key word here is *team*.

Regardless of your role, as an SLP you are integral to the EI team. Sometimes you'll function as the PSP, particularly when a child's main need is communication and/or feeding and swallowing. At other times, you'll play a support role to professionals in other disciplines.

THE IMPORTANCE OF FAMILIES

Effective early intervention is family centered. This model, based on research evidence, influences the roles assumed by all those involved in the intervention process. In family-centered intervention, parents are partners with professionals who help parents become invested in the process through positive assessment experiences and positive intervention outcomes.

Family involvement in early intervention can produce positive effects for a child's physical, cognitive, social, and language skills; foster a parent's sense of personal control and self-efficacy; and increase a parent's overall satisfaction with intervention services (Applequist & Bailey, 2000). That's a lot!

Families of young children with potentially handicapping conditions often cope with increased stress and feelings of disappointment or loss, social isolation, frustration, and helplessness. The stress of raising a child such as Sean or Mikey, mentioned earlier, may affect the family's well-being and in turn interfere with the child's development. If these issues are not addressed, they can, in extreme cases, lead to divorce, to parental or sibling emotional problems and even parent suicide, and to physical abuse of the child. In recognition of the unique position of the family and of the increased stressors, EI focuses on the entire constellation of the child, the family unit, and individual family members.

Despite potentially positive outcomes and the legal requirement for EI services to occur within the family unit, a gap remains between the expectations of service providers and family members (Blue-Banning, Summers, Frankland, Nelson, & Beegle, 2004). Some professionals still have difficulty moving to a truly family service model. When professionals maintain control, parents are not treated as equal partners (Blue-Banning, Turnbull, & Pereira, 2000).

Family-centered intervention is premised on the assumption that families should have a large input in identifying their concerns and hoped-for outcomes of intervention. The more a family is involved as an equal partner, the more enabling and empowering the process becomes. As a part of this cooperative effort, families should be offered a choice of the level of participation they desire. Nearly all caregivers will need some direction and guidance to maximize their participation.

Successful early intervention also depends on quality relationships between all parties: children, parents, and intervention facilitators. These relationships have a direct impact on the parent-child relationship. As ECI service providers, SLPs are in a unique position to help parents appreciate the importance of their interactions with their child.

Interacting with Families

The family is a constant in a child's life. It is important to view a child with special needs and her or his family from a strengths perspective by considering what each party brings to intervention. Ideally, family-centered practitioners recognize this and

■ Collaborate with the family in all aspects of service delivery;
■ Exchange information freely, completely, and in an unbiased manner;
■ Honor a family's cultural diversity;

- Understand that families have different coping mechanisms; and
- Facilitate networking between families.

If these things are addressed, it will ensure that intervention services are provided in a responsive and flexible manner.

Once professionals begin to view the family as the service delivery unit, several principles of family-centered practice should follow (Rossetti, 2001), including

- Individualizing service delivery based on recognition of a family's strengths,
- Responding to family-identified priorities and to changes in family priorities over time, and
- Supporting family and cultural lifestyles and values.

Families vary tremendously in the characteristics of individual family members. In addition to the individual characteristics of each child, there are varying family histories, current circumstances, and the family's reasons for seeking services. For example, I have worked with parents who had been ordered by family court, because of a past history of abuse, either to participate in their child's intervention or go to prison, pay a fine, and/or lose custody of their child. As you can imagine, in such a situation, motivation to participate may be very different from that found among other parents who do not have this history. One of your first tasks may be to educate parents in the importance of early intervention and of their involvement and expertise.

EI programs also differ tremendously in their target populations, if any, such as that of UCP; governing agencies; mission; personnel; and service model and histories. I've worked with programs run by school systems, servicing agencies, hospitals, and SLPs in private practice. As you can image, there is no one-size-fits-all model of ECI to be applied in the same way in every setting with every family. Early intervention specialists need to recognize these differences and adapt their practices accordingly. You'll find as we progress through this text that flexibility will be one of your greatest assets.

Overcoming Potential Barriers

According to professionals, the most frequent barriers to working with families are clinician factors, such as caseload size and lack of time, and family factors, such as lack of interest, lack of education, and cultural or value differences. To these, we might also add a lack of experience and training by some professionals.

The problem does not totally reside with professionals. Families often fail to implement or to sustain agreed-upon intervention plans. In part, this failure to conform to professional recommendations occurs because intervention plans and the family's values are at odds or because plans do not fit the family's daily routines. In a truly ecological model of EI intervention, the family's lifestyle is central to constructing intervention plans (Dunst, 2002).

By definition, early intervention is based on a partnership. Ideally, families and professionals work together to devise plans and implement intervention (Dunst, 2002). As a professional in such a partnership, you'll impart information, skills, and knowledge to the families who are then free to make informed decisions based on your input.

Young children whose parents participate in communication intervention activities make more language gains than children whose parents are not involved in intervention (Chao, Bryan, Burstein, & Cevriye, 2006). Working collaboratively, SLPs and families can identify goals and typical daily routines within which these goals might be addressed. Through parent-professional collaboration, parents can be empowered to (Chao, Bryan, Burstein, & Cevriye, 2006)

- Establish the desired performance of their child,
- Determine the characteristics and severity of a problem, and
- Select appropriate intervention strategies based on an individual child's unique needs.

Professionals can implement parent training through regular child-centered parent meetings, individual center-based services, scheduled SLP visits to the home, or a combination of these.

To be successful, you'll need to strive to develop a sensitive and trusting parent-professional relationship and to respond to a family's priorities and concerns. The key to being effective is helping the parents to be in control of important decisions and actions in relation to their child and EI services. This is accomplished by supporting and strengthening the competence they already possess.

CULTURAL CONSIDERATIONS

The population of the United States is changing. If present trends continue, the current white non-Latino majority will be the largest minority within a few decades. It is increasingly evident that to be effective, SLPs and other professionals must learn to deliver services to families that differ in background from themselves.

According to PL 99-457, early intervention must by its nature reflect respect for individuality and for racial, ethnic, cultural and other differences found across diverse family backgrounds and be responsive to each family's needs. At the very least, materials distributed to caregivers should be in the native language, procedures should be nondiscriminatory and in the language to which the infant has been most exposed, and multiple methods of assessment should be employed.

SLPs should be mindful that much of what we think we know about caregiver-infant interactions comes from American majority culture. Even such seemingly beneficial intervention techniques as expansion or providing feedback in a more mature form ("Yes, the doggie is eating") following a child's utterance ("Doggie eat") may represent a behavior not found in parent-child interactions in other cultures.

Cultural self-awareness is the first step in your becoming a culturally competent SLP. **Cultural competence** is a dynamic, ongoing process of attaining knowledge, skills, attitudes, behaviors, and practices that enable you, as a professional, to work effectively in cross-cultural settings. In doing so, an SLP honors and respects the beliefs, behaviors, language, and interpersonal and parenting styles of clients. Ideally, cultural competence operates at an individual, agency, and system level and includes everything from the manner in which clients are addressed to the art that covers the walls of the agency or school and the use of translators when needed.

Cultural competence is not an end point or the result of attending one workshop on the topic of diversity and inclusion. It's a process. I've been learning about different cultures all my life, and my cultural competence is still evolving and most likely will always be so. I'm still a work in progress, I hope.

The process begins by recognizing your own culture-based beliefs, behaviors, and customs. Most SLPs are part of the mainstream culture, a majority that in many ways is blissfully unaware of the effects of majority culture on its own thoughts and actions. Awareness alone is not enough, but it's a place to begin your exploration.

Like all children, a child with developmental disability is part of an ecology that includes parents, siblings, extended family members, friends, neighbors, and community. The family is embedded within broader cultural contexts. Ethnic and cultural groups can vary significantly in their beliefs about disability, the nature of family and community supports, medical practices, and use of professional services.

Of course, needs vary according to individual family circumstances. Some of the most often cited needs of parents from other than the majority culture are

- ▪ Needing information about their child's condition,
- ▪ Exploring ways of interacting with and teaching their child,
- ▪ Explaining their child's condition to others,
- ▪ Finding respite or child care and community supports, and
- ▪ Identifying specialized professional services.

The type and amount of perceived support from formal and informal sources correlate highly with successful coping by the family. Many Latino families rely heavily on extended family members and religious organizations as important sources of support. As much as possible, these resources should be included in the intervention process.

Parents with greater English language proficiency report higher levels of support and fewer needs. In contrast, low English proficiency is associated with higher needs for support and lower support from family and friends. Language barriers and the physical or social isolation of a family may significantly affect informal support networks and the needs those networks fulfill more than they affect access to the formal service system.

Latino Families

In the United States, Latinos represent the largest identifiable ethnic group and include individuals of all races, comprising approximately 13 to 14 percent of the total population. Although most Latinos share a common language and perhaps some broad cultural traits, they differ in many ways from one another with respect to sociocultural and immigration histories, social class, education, dialect, occupation, familiarity with the majority culture, and place of origin.

Latino families living in the United States are at risk for reduced access to health and other community support services for children with disabilities. Several factors, including language barriers, limited knowledge of systems and services, unfamiliarity with acceptable help-seeking behavior, possible distrust of the professional service system, and perceived discrimination by agencies or service providers, contribute to this situation. These factors, especially if they occur in combination with poverty, divorce, low education, and social isolation, may contribute to increased need for and reduced access to services.

Throughout this text and in accordance with EI principles, I'll urge that ECI programs teach parents to serve as the primary intervention agents for their children. Parental involvement is fundamental in the early intervention model in order to generalize therapy strategies and communicative gains to the home and other settings (Wolery & Bailey, 2002). It is important that such communication-based interventions embody the socialization practices and communicative preferences of parents from diverse cultural groups. For example, language socialization practices among some Latino families may include the following behaviors (Delgado-Gaitan, 2004):

- Adults do not always use words to describe actions,
- Adults do not consider children equal conversational partners,
- Adults do not consider play routines to be significant,
- Children are cautioned not to interrupt adults or older siblings, and
- Children do not typically retell understood events.

It's important to stress that these behaviors are generalizations, and not all members of a particular linguistic or cultural group adhere to the same beliefs. Like Asians and Asian Americans, Latinos in the United States represent many different cultural beliefs.

On face value, the practices mentioned seem to be in opposition to what the majority culture, represented by many professionals, believes to be the best practices. The key is for professionals to learn to work within differing cultural confines and not dictate a one-size-fits-all approach. SLPs and other professionals need to explore the beliefs and practices of each individual family and adapt intervention accordingly.

To increase parental participation and provide more appropriate ECI services, SLPs can interview parents and observe interactions to ascertain the value of talk and status relative to communication, and to discern beliefs related to language facilitation routines. For example, Mexican American mothers in one study did not believe their children exhibited a communicative disorder even while acknowledging their children's limited verbal skills. They expected that their children would not speak or comprehend until 3 years of age (Mendez-Perez, 1998). Nor did the mothers understand the need for or the methods of intervention being provided.

In contrast, another study of Mexican immigrant mothers with lower socioeconomic status (low-SES) backgrounds, whose children were receiving center-based early intervention services, perceived their children as exhibiting a communication delay and were able to explain possible causal factors (Kummerer, Lopez-Reyna, & Tejero Hughes, 2007). The mothers focused primarily on their children's speech intelligibility and/or expressive language. To promote more culturally responsive intervention, mothers recommended that professionals speak Spanish and provide a rationale for and information about the therapy process.

Bilingual Development

The United States is extremely linguistically diverse. At this time, more than 300 languages are spoken within its borders, and nearly one in five residents over the age of 5 speaks a language other than or in addition to English (U.S. Census Bureau, 2010). These figures reflect immigration patterns (Portes & Hao, 1998; Wong-Fillmore, 2000). The language of a family is part of its cultural identity and a venue for transmitting cultural values and for fostering attachment and intimacy.

Sadly, some SLPs are still recommending that parents not talk to their children in their native or heritage language. As a result, some non-English-speaking parents reportedly cease talking with their child. This is the exact opposite of what the child requires (Ijalba, Jeffers-Pena, & Giraldo, 2013). Let's sort this out.

While it may, on the surface, seem logical that a child with a communication impairment (CI) should be limited to input in only one language and that for a child with CI growing up in an English-speaking country the language should be English, the entire notion flies in the face of everything research has shown. Children with communication deficits can develop bilingually and need parental input in the language of the home. English input will occur through the media and school.

A family's decision about the use of heritage languages is complex and includes consideration of cultural traditions and beliefs, as well as the family's aspirations. There are also practical concerns, such as schooling and daycare.

Several studies have shown that typically developing (TD) monolingual and bilingual children are similar in the sequence, rate, and quality of their linguistic development (Hamers & Blanc, 2000; Petitto & Holowka, 2002). In addition, bilinguals demonstrate advantages in certain areas of metacognition and metalinguistics (Bialystok, 2001; Bialystok & Craik, 2010).

Both bilingual and monolingual children with a range of disorders, such as specific language impairment (SLI), Down syndrome, and autism spectrum disorder (ASD), have patterns of development similar to those of TD children (Gutiérrez-Clellen, Simon-Cereijido, & Wagner, 2008; Håkansson, Salameh, & Nettelbladt, 2003; Kay-Raining Bird et al., 2005; Paradis, Crago, Genesee, & Rice, 2003). Further, bilingual children with LI have been shown to use skills developed in one language to facilitate learning in another (Hua, 2008; Seung, Siddiqi, & Elder, 2006).

Advising parents to speak only English with their children is contrary to the recommendations of the American Speech-Language-Hearing Association (ASHA, 2004c, 2005a, 2011). Language use between parents and children is complex and unique to each family. SLPs are advised to support parents in their decisions about language use within the family. These guidelines are consistent with those from other professionals (Artiles & Ortiz, 2002; Bialystok, 2001).

If, as we have mentioned, communication intervention is to be provided by the family in consultation with an SLP, then SLPs need to support the development of the language spoken in the home. This seems especially important in ECI. The home language provides a means of communication while the child learns English (Gutiérrez-Clellen, 1999; Kohnert, Yim, Nett, Kan, & Duran, 2005).

PARENTS/CAREGIVERS*

The parent-child or caregiver-child interactional dyad is an especially powerful context for ECI, providing an opportunity to support and extend the experiences of both members. Some EI programs still view the parent-child relationship as an add-on to intervention and continue to focus all their resources on the child, rather than recognizing and enhancing the parent-child interactional process as an avenue through which we can influence a child's environment and ultimately the child's development (McCollum, Gooler, Appl, & Yates, 2001).

It's essential that, as an SLP, you pay attention to interactions between a parent and child. This dyad is the filter through which all intervention will pass, whether we choose to recognize it or not. The results of a meta-analysis of language intervention with

---

* Throughout the text, I shall use the term *parent* to refer to a child's biological or adopted parent and the more generic term *caregiver* to refer to parents or other care providers such as classroom teachers.

preschool children have found parent-implemented approaches to be effective (Roberts & Kaiser, 2011). Parent-implemented language interventions can have a significant, positive impact on both the receptive and expressive language skills of children.

The importance of working with caregivers, especially mothers, is evident when we look at caregiver behavior. One study of the language used by mothers from low-SES and rural backgrounds with their infants at ages 6 and 15 months of age found that maternal language use at 6 months significantly predicted later maternal language use (Abraham, Crais, Vernon-Feagans, & the Family Life Project Phase 1 Key Investigators, 2013). In other words, mothers who use fewer language strategies at the earlier time are likely to use fewer later. If we hope to enrich maternal language to young children, we need to begin in infancy, promoting varied and increased maternal language use.

Although a family-centered approach that emphasizes the parent-child interaction may appear to be a logical approach, the very personal nature of the relationship and the importance of that relationship in forming a parent's self-worth makes parent-child interactions a sensitive arena of intervention requiring a good deal of professional skill and tact. I know one young mother who does not follow professional guidance because she feels that professionals talk down to her. Rather than dismissing these concerns as those of an oversensitive mother, we as professionals need to do everything possible to prevent and address such feelings.

Evidence tells us that parent-child interaction patterns reflect cultural belief systems. Although Part C of the *Individuals with Disabilities Education Improvement Act* of 2004 requires that professionals respect the diversity of families, culturally and linguistically appropriate EI programs have not been routinely implemented (Kalyanpur, Harry, & Skrtic, 2000; Madding, 2000). To improve participation, collaboration, and service delivery with families from diverse backgrounds, SLPs need to understand and respect culturally specific beliefs and values (Garcia, Mendez-Perez, & Ortiz, 2000; Rodriguez & Olswang, 2003; Salas-Provance, Erickson, & Reed, 2002).

One way for SLPs to help parents alter their own behavior so that it matches and supports that of their child is to help parents see the world from their child's perspective (McCollum, 2001). Rather than focusing on educating parents about general development, you can help parents understand the development of their own individual child. Through this process, parents can become more sensitive and responsive to their child's behavior and needs.

Understanding can be aided with guided observation and conversation ("Did you notice how your daughter . . . I think she's trying to . . .") in which an SLP helps a parent observe and interpret the child's development. In similar fashion, an SLP can observe and interpret the parent-child interaction with the goal of identifying appropriate and inappropriate parent behaviors and making suggestions that expand and enhance the parent-child interaction. "Inappropriate" does not mean when compared to some general norm. Is the behavior appropriate in response to the child's behavior or level of functioning? For example, you might say, "I liked how you talked about the 'doggie'; it might help your son focus if you also pointed." To be effective, this SLP-parent conversation must be accomplished in an atmosphere that is responsive to and respectful of parents.

SLPs can explore with parents the family's beliefs and knowledge about (Kummerer et al., 2007)

- Their child's speech and/or language disabilities,
- The difference between and importance of both receptive and expressive language,
- Why intervention is recommended,
- The role of speech-language therapy and the speech-language pathologist,
- Why it is important for parents to participate in ECI,
- How clinicians will interact with the child and the family,
- How the clinician and family can work collaboratively,
- The amount of time and effort needed to remediate the child's difficulties, and
- How the family can generalize strategies to the home setting.

These topics are important because uninformed or discouraged parents may be less effective as agents of change. Such exploration is not a singular event. Parents need to be informed at each step in the ECI process.

INDIVIDUALIZED FOR EACH CHILD

As with any good intervention, SLP services in ECI must be tailored to the individual child. This requires thorough and ongoing assessment and monitoring of a child's communication behavior and accurate record keeping. Flexibility is the key as a young child develops and new opportunities to intervene become available.

Although federal law requires identification of young children with disabilities, professionals have yet to identify a reliable, valid, and inexpensive screening tool for language delay in children under age 2. Most testing and sampling methods are time consuming and difficult to use solely as screening devices. In contrast, parent report measures offer some hope as screening instruments because they are inexpensive to distribute and administer.

Several variables interact when we look at intervention with young children. As a group, children who begin receiving intervention services at a younger age require fewer intervention visits than those who begin later, regardless of the type of disorder (Jacoby, Lee, & Kummer, 2002). Most professionals would agree that intervention needs to start early in life for the greatest potential impact. That being said, children with associated developmental disabilities, such as cerebral palsy or intellectual disability, frequently require more intervention to demonstrate improvement than children with no associated conditions.

NATURAL ENVIRONMENT

In 2001, the World Health Organization (WHO) endorsed a new model of disability that considers health and disability in relation to each other and to participation in daily life activities (World Health Assembly, 2001). In other words, disability is not viewed as a function of the person. Instead, disability is considered to be the outcome of the interaction of health conditions and an individual's context. The degree of disability is measured in terms of the extent to which an individual's impairment creates challenges for participation in typical activities or routines in that individual's environment. In order to provide the most appropriate and effective intervention, an SLP, in collaboration with a child's caregivers, needs to understand the ways in which a child's communication abilities facilitate or hinder participation in a range of daily activities and routines.

The Individuals with Disabilities Education Improvement Act, Part C (IDEIA, 2004) uses the term *natural environments* to refer to settings that are typical for infants and toddlers. Natural environments include family homes, early care and educational settings, and other community settings where the family spends the majority of its time with the children. It's in these natural environments that the child participates in the typical activities and routines envisioned in the WHO model. The most frequent natural environment for intervention services is the family home.

IDEIA requires that individualized programs be offered in a child's natural environment or in the least restrictive environment (LRE). Providing early intervention services in settings other than the home or community settings is allowed only if it can be justified because it cannot be done satisfactorily in a natural environment. When EI services are provided in a less natural environment, the IFSP must include a justification. As a child reaches the age of eligibility for preschool services, the IDEIA similarly requires these services to be provided in the LRE, which may be a preschool classroom. One goal of IDEIA is to prevent families from having to receive intervention in multiple locations in a nontransdisciplinary manner.

Intervention may occur both in individual or group sessions as long as services are individualized for the child and family. Hybrid models are common. For example, group sessions can provide an adjunct to individual intervention services, with each supporting the other.

In developing countries, where SLPs may be in short supply and there may be multicultural and multilingual low-income populations, community-based intervention provided by local clinics affiliated with regional hospitals may be best (Fair & Louw, 1999). In this environment, local community workers can provide limited communication intervention and parent training under the direction of an SLP.

Although center-based or group EI has the potential, if not handled sensitively, to be threatening to some parents, it also offers an opportunity for children and parents to interact with other children and parents. When carefully guided, these interactions can be an enjoyable way for parents to observe other parent-child interactions and to enhance parent interactional skills as an adjunct to home-based services.

The most common argument for not providing services in the natural environment is the cost, primarily in time and travel by the PSP and other professionals. Note that this argument is made from the perspective of service providers and not that of the family. Children and families are typically better served in their homes, daycare centers, or play groups than they are in clinical or segregated disability-focused facilities.

Daily Routines and Activities

Home-based intervention involves more than just a location for services. The context of a family's daily routines and activities offers an opportunity for a child to learn and develop within events occurring naturally in the home environment. Parents naturally use daily routines and activities as opportunities for teaching. A child's activities, such as eating and being bathed, are an integral part of everyday life and a familiar part of a family's day. These activities have a profound impact on the cognitive and communicative functions children develop and offer meaningful and functional opportunities for learning communication. SLPs, working in partnership with families, can coach parents on the ECI methods for including individualized communication activities throughout the day.

Use of the term *natural environment* signals a shift in the focus of the intervention process as well as the location. Intervention becomes centered on the authentic interactions of everyday activities and meaningful experiences that a child has with his or her family and caregivers. By maximizing learning opportunities within daily routines and activities, caregivers increase intervention throughout the day in meaningful ways. As a consequence, families are not required to set aside special time for intervention in an already busy day. Intervention is accomplished within the preexisting schedule of family life.

Daily activities and routines offer learning opportunities for the development of communication and other important skills. Think of ECI services as being focused on a child's participation in his or her unique natural communication environments (Campbell, 2004; Campbell & Sawyer, 2007; McWilliam, 2010). Restricted participation results in missed opportunities to learn and grow. When participation in an activity or routine is limited, that event becomes a restrictive context in which learning new skills is constrained. In contrast, when participation is enabled or enhanced, a young child can acquire new skills by participating with family members and other caregivers. Thus, the focus of intervention is improving participation. Here's where you come in. Participation is enhanced by communication, which in turn, facilitates learning of other important developmental skills.

The ECI service structure will vary depending on many factors, including the individual family, funding agency, and the population served. Continued research is needed to address the validity of different models of intervention with particular families and contexts. Only then can we provide truly evidence-based intervention services.

Unfortunately, ECI outcomes identified on IFSPs are not always associated with participation in activities and routines in the natural environment. IFSPs need to address both (Wilcox & Woods, 2011)

- A child's performance abilities and disabilities, and
- A child's use of those abilities for participation in the activities and routines that constitute his/her natural environments.

Within this environmental model, it is easy to see, for example, that teaching a child AAC without related changes in the child's environment to embrace AAC does the child and family a huge disservice. Similarly, teaching a child to request without teaching others in the child's environment to respond also fails to address communication development and use.

Inclusion

To the maximum extent appropriate, when young children with disabilities are educated in infant and toddler programs, these children should be integrated with children who do not require intervention services. Special classes, separate schooling, or removal from the general education environment should occur only when the nature or severity of the disorder is such that the child may not be able to achieve academically in general education classes even with supplementary aides and services.

Several researchers have reported the positive impact of natural, inclusive settings on the developmental, academic, adaptive, and social progress of young children with disabilities (Holahan & Costenbader, 2000; Odom, 2000; Vakil, Freeman, & Swim, 2003). Such gains, however, do not occur automatically. They require that inclusion be carefully and thoughtfully planned, instituted, and carried out. Important factors contributing to successful outcomes for children are (Cross, Traub, Hutter-Pishgahi, & Shelton, 2004)

- ■ Positive teacher/staff attitudes,
- ■ Individualized professional relationships with parents,
- ■ Individualized interventions that reflect the child's needs, and
- ■ Environmental adaptations that are child specific.

If these factors are not present, then children such as my grandson, sitting quietly to the side in his wheelchair, are ignored.

Inclusive placement can be promoted in several ways, including (Etscheidt, 2006)

- ■ Expanding professional development for EI providers,
- ■ Coordinating and increasing exploration of environments, and
- ■ Improving the "readiness" of inclusive placements

Let's explore each briefly.

Professional development. Service providers may not be prepared to meet the legal requirements of IDEA and IDEIA, including providing services in natural environments and LREs (Bruder & Dunst, 2005). Novice professionals, such as you when you begin your working career, may have difficulty understanding, adapting, and using natural environmental practices or may believe special service or center-based models are preferable (Campbell & Halbert, 2002; Raab & Dunst, 2004; Summers et al., 2001). To counter these difficulties, professional development can focus on helping staff to (Cross et al., 2004)

- ■ Embed engaging learning opportunities into activities in inclusive settings, and
- ■ Integrate individualized intervention within natural environments.

Professional development offers a cost-effective way to improve services, particularly for children with more severe disabilities (Campbell & Milbourne, 2005).

Coordination. IFSP and IEP teams need to consider a full continuum of natural and inclusive placements. Service coordination among early childhood agencies is essential (Soodak et al., 2002). Conflicts arise when service providers have different expectations, especially concerning the nature and degree of family involvement (Rosenkoetter, Whaley, Hains, & Pierce, 2001). The need for coordination is especially acute as a child transitions from IFSP services to preschool IEP services. Although the IDEIA provides a uniform process to help young children and their families transition successfully, in actual practice there is service disruption, disorganization among preschool providers, and stress for parents (Hanson et al., 2000).

Improved readiness. Childcare providers and teachers in natural environments or LREs can plan for and provide appropriate supports for children with disabilities. It's important to remember that the law requires "Programs, not children, . . . to be ready for inclusion" (Odom, 2000, p. 25). Within inclusive preschool settings, individualized teaching strategies can address the learning and development of each child. This ensures that instruction matches the child's readiness, preferences, and interests (Tomlinson, 2004; Vakil et al., 2003).

Although a child's social or academic readiness must be considered in placement decisions, behavioral needs are often used to justify a child's placement in a more restrictive setting. Although research confirms that between 10 and 15 percent of all preschool-age children exhibit moderate to severe levels of problem behaviors, preschool teachers view disruptive behavior problems as their most significant challenge (Joseph & Strain, 2003; Kupersmidt, Bryant, & Willoughby, 2000).

Challenging behaviors, such as screaming or hitting, are particularly evident for young children with autism spectrum disorder (ASD) and often lead to removal from natural or inclusive settings (Horner, Carr, Strain, Todd, & Reed, 2002; Smith & Daunic, 2004). The IDEIA clearly requires educators to address behavioral challenges through the use of positive behavioral supports, discussed later in this text, designed to foster increased participation by children with disabilities in regular education environments or other LREs.

Individualized Family Service Plan (IFSP)

As mentioned, legislation has moved the focus of EI from the child with disabilities to the child as part of a family unit. The primary example of that change is the use of the Individualized Family Service Plan (IFSP). Based on the earlier Individualized Educational Plan (IEP) for school-age children, the IFSP addresses both child and family needs that affect a child's development.

At the very least an IFSP should include

- The child and family's current status,
- The recommended services and expected outcomes, and
- A projection of the duration of service delivery.

It's essential that the family understand the contents and feel some ownership of the plan through participation in the process. The plan should be reviewed periodically and updated as needed to accommodate the child's and the family's changing needs.

One key person in the process of drafting and implementing the IFSP is the service coordinator, or primary service provider (PSP), because IDEA (1997) states that the coordinator should be the service provider most knowledgeable of the child's disability. The task of the service coordinator is to assist with the identification, implementation, and coordination of services for both the child and the family. In this role, the service coordinator is the link between multiple agencies and the family and child. As such, it is the coordinator's responsibility to ensure that

- The family's priorities drive the service system,
- The collaborative intent of the legislation is realized between and among providers and the family, and
- The early intervention experience is perceived positively by the family.

Traditionally, the IFSP has been developed by the child's mother or parents, the PSP, and other team members. This can be extremely intimidating and uncomfortable for a parent who may wonder if her or his priorities and concerns will be honored and considered seriously. Unfortunately, one study found that as few as 40 percent of IFSPs were reviewed by other family members, extended family members, or friends (Boone & Coulter, 1995).

FAMILY AS TEAM MEMBERS

The IFSP is a collaborative document. For example, family members should participate in the assessment of the child's strengths and needs, and the IFSP should reflect this collaboration between families and providers in its description of a child's levels of functioning. Families are included in the planning of the evaluation and alerted about what to expect. Naturally, families will have questions for service providers, and the honest answering of these can go a long way toward building the desired collaborative relationship.

Families can be encouraged to discuss their concerns and priorities, and their resources for promoting the development of their child. In addition, the family may elect to include these in the IFSP. In either case, professionals can listen to the family and honestly address these issues. For example, even though most families feel that receiving services from multiple agencies is more responsive to their needs than is single agency service delivery, many IFSPs include only a single service provider. The PSP in consultation with the family can insure that a variety of appropriate agencies, groups, and organizations are included in the IFSP if that is the family's wish.

OUTCOME STATEMENTS

One important aspect of the IFSP is the outcome statement of the changes the family wants for itself and/or the child. At the very least, one child outcome must be on the IFSP.

Family outcomes are changes that family members identify as being beneficial to them. These changes may be either directly related to the child, such as "We want to try to take Maria to the church play group so that she'll have more playmates," or not related, such as "We want to find another place to live so that we'll be closer to the bus line." Note that the outcomes are written with a "so that" clause to provide both a rationale and a measure for success. If, for example, the family has moved but is not closer to public transportation, then they have not fulfilled this outcome.

Both child and family outcomes should reflect the family's concerns, priorities, and resources and be written in language the family understands. Families feel ownership of the IFSP when it's written in their words and with their priorities.

According to parents, the use of jargon by service providers is a major stumbling block in the IFSP process that can interfere with the establishment of a family–service provider collaborative partnership (Turnbull, Turbiville, & Turnbull, 2000). A child outcome, for example, might read, "Shelley needs to talk in single words so she can tell us what she wants." For a student who may have struggled to learn to write IEP behavioral goals, this IFSP plain language may come as a shock to you.

IFSP outcome statements are very different from the goal and objective statements you may have learned for a school-age child's IEP. The difference reflects the *service plan* rather than *treatment plan* format of the IFSP. Not only is an IFSP more flexible than an IEP, but as mentioned, it can address issues beyond those related only to the child. Once the IFSP has identified services needed to achieve the outcomes identified by the family and other team members, it's up to the team to make a plan for those services in which they include goals and objectives more like those in an IEP.

Reportedly, early intervention service providers find it more difficult to include family outcomes than child ones. Family outcomes may require accessing resources that are not as familiar to providers, and some family issues, such as housing needs or the need to stop smoking, may be uncomfortable for or outside the expertise of many professionals. As a consequence, the overwhelming majority of outcomes tend to be child oriented.

Before we discuss some guidelines for SLPs, take a look at what a practicing speech-language pathologist at Cincinnati Children's Hospital says about the importance of EI.
https://www.youtube.com/watch?v=qnVUVw7kFjM

GUIDELINES FOR SLPS

IFSP guidelines for SLPs serving as PSPs or service coordinators are as follows:

■ *Discuss the family's goals and expectations for the child and their perception of his or her development.* Although often omitted, the family visit is a part of the IFSP development that families say is the most important to them as an opportunity for service providers to know them as families.

■ *Discuss what parents want as outcomes of intervention.* What does the family want the child to be able to do?

■ *Review these outcomes with the family, discussing consistency across all interactional environments.* This information is especially important for an SLP who must know the environments of the child and family and also how those environments work for them. A child's home is not always the best location for services, especially if the family finds visits intrusive and prefers that services be provided in some other natural environment, such as a daycare center.

■ *Include in reports and in the IFSP the family's assessment of their child's skills.* We'll discuss caregiver input later, but let's note that it can be a valid source of information when families have direction and guidance.

■ *Include other people in the child's environment in the IFSP process.* This can provide the SLP with information about the child's communication in a variety of settings, and thus facilitates the implementation of intervention strategies.

■ *Avoid jargon, and write reports in the words of the family.* It's important here to use the family's words so they know they were heard and to avoid professional jargon that may have little meaning for the family.

■ *Assist other team members to access input from the family in the IFSP process.* (Polmanteer & Turbiville, 2000)

I've included a sample IFSP in Appendix A. The length precludes presenting it within this chapter. Other samples are available at websites listed in the appendix.

The Need for Evidence-Based Practice

As clinicians, we all strive to provide the best, most well-grounded intervention for our clients as is humanly possible. In other words, we try to use methods that have been shown to work or are effective. Discerning efficacy is a portion of something called evidence-based practice (EBP). In EBP, clinical decision-making is informed by a combination of scientific evidence, clinical experience, and client needs.

Evidence-based practice is based on two assumptions (Bernstein Ratner, 2006):

■ Clinical skills should grow from the current research, not simply from experience, and

■ The expert SLP should continually seek new therapeutic research to improve treatment efficacy.

In the field of speech-language pathology, interest in EBP is relatively new and there are few guidelines on providing services.

As noted in ASHA's *Roles and Responsibilities of Speech-Language Pathologists in Early Intervention: Guidelines* (2008b), there are few areas in ECI in which clear, unequivocal answers emerge from empirical research. That does not relieve us of the responsibility to provide the best, most efficacious assessment and intervention possible. Until such time as guidelines do exist, SLPs need to base decisions on the best available evidence. I have tried to provide such evidence throughout this text.

Research-based considerations are derived from study and evaluation of empirical evidence. Unfortunately, not all research findings are created equal, and an SLP must consider the certainty of a range of evidence. This range may include the following (Schlosser & Sigafoos, 2002):

■ *Inconclusive*: Despite establishing that certain outcomes are *not* plausible, the design flaws in the study preclude conclusions that outcomes are related to actions by the investigators.

■ *Suggestive*: Serious design flaws still exist even though certain outcomes are plausible and are within the realm of possibility.

■ *Preponderant*: Although minor design flaws exist, certain outcomes are not only possible but were made more likely because of the actions of the investigators.

■ *Conclusive*: Given the strong research design, certain outcomes are undoubtedly the result of the actions by the investigators.

While space precludes a more detailed description, each clinically certified SLP has taken a research course that ideally enables him or her to evaluate research objectively.

EVALUATING RESEARCH

Let's assume that we wish to know if training a child in joint or shared attending results in improvement in communication. A possible model for evaluating assessment and intervention services in light of clinical research would consist of the following steps (Schlosser, 2003):

- *Develop a well-built question.* The nature of the question will determine the search for answers and highlight the relevant underlying issues. A well-built question would honestly describe a child and his or her capabilities relevant to a clinical issue, explain the child's environment and caregivers and their relevance, explicitly describe the clinical problem, and specify expected outcomes (Sackett, Richardson, Rosenberg, & Haynes, 1997; Schlosser, 2003). A question is based on the best clinical data available relevant to the child and caregivers.

- *Select evidence sources.* Database searches will yield the most recent evidence. Unfortunately, the value of this evidence is only as good as the database itself. Much evidence is unfiltered in terms of quality. Professional journals, either electronic or paper, such as the *Journal of Speech, Language, and Hearing Research*, are a better source. Information available from online websites such as *Wikipedia* is often outdated or biased, is not peer reviewed to assure quality, and must be treated with a critical eye. I'll make the blanket statement that if you're basing your intervention on sites such as *Wikipedia*, you're doing your clients and yourself a disservice. Part of being a professional is having a strong base for what you do clinically.

- *Execute a search strategy.* The next step is to identify keywords and keyword combinations that will yield the desired evidence efficiently. Many search engines, such as ERIC (Education Resources Information Center) have a thesaurus to aid in selecting search terms. It's usually best to begin by targeting research syntheses such as *meta-analyses* based on rigorous and systematic search and synthesis of the available evidence. Although growth has been steady, only limited meta-analyses are available at present. In this case, SLPs will need to consult individual studies. Anecdotal information, claiming results with only limited or no research findings, should be avoided or examined with great caution.

- *Examine and synthesize the evidence.* All evidence should be evaluated for internal, external, and social validity. Internal validity is related to the design and implementation of the study and to the checks included within it, including the agreement of observers on the implementation and results (Schlosser, 2002). The brevity of our present discussion precludes a thorough exploration of this topic. External validity is the extent to which the findings can be generalized beyond the participants or conditions of a study, or more specifically, generalized to your specific question. Here clinical/educational expertise is important in evaluating the applicability of the findings to your individual client. Finally, social validity is the degree to which clients and caregivers find the published intervention outcomes, methods, and goals to be socially significant for them. For example, a study finding that the use of AAC benefits a child's communication development may not be relevant if the family is strongly opposed to even discussing AAC. On the other hand, these data may be helpful in persuading this or another family that AAC is worth considering.

- *Apply the evidence.* Findings are discussed with the family to obtain their viewpoints, preferences, concerns, or expectations. For example, as mentioned, a family may have strong reservations about the impact of AAC on their child, despite research findings, or may prefer to try an intervention method that the research evidence indicates is invalid. In either case, the SLP will have been correct to share the scientific evidence so that caregivers can make an informed decision. Remember that no decision is carved in stone and that education of the SLP and the child and family should be ongoing.

- *Evaluate the application of the EBP evidence.* This is a two-step process of evaluation and revision. In addition to efficacy measurement, the SLP engages in the social validation of the outcomes through the family. The big question is, of course, whether the intervention really works. Measures of change should be objective, observable, and measureable. Lack of change after reasonable time and effort should lead to revision of the method. Keep valid data on your own intervention methods. You may have the nascent steps in a future research study.

Research-based evidence in ECI is still emerging and sometimes seems confusing or contradictory (ASHA, 2008b). Studies vary in their focus, which may include the parent or caregiver, the child, the parent-child interaction, the intervention environment, or combinations of these. The agent of change may be an SLP or other team member, a family member or peer, or a combination. Intervention may occur in groups or individually and may be massed or distributed throughout the day. To add to this variability, much of the empirical data comes from preschoolers rather than infants and toddlers. This said, there is research evidence—some strong, some not so strong—to support various intervention approaches and strategies, and it is these methods that we shall weave throughout this text.

On a final note, fields of study such as communication disorders are constantly evolving. This means that new methods, materials, and applications are continually being presented. As professionals, we will always be faced with research findings that vary from highly effective to ineffective. This is the nature of an innovative profession, and thankfully it leaves room for your creativity, intuition, and good clinical judgment.

Conclusion

Developmental delays in infants and toddlers are significantly under-identified. Data indicate the ongoing need for improved early identification of infants and toddlers with developmental disabilities. In addition, the American Speech-Language-Hearing Association is firmly on record against the "wait and see if the child develops functional speech" approach to infant and toddler communication impairment (ASHA, 2005b).

Some people, maybe even you—although I hope to change that through this text—view EI as a nice idea but fail to understand its benefits. Research evidence gathered over almost 50 years indicates that EI

- Increases developmental and educational gains for the child,
- Improves the functioning of the family, and
- Results in long-term social and economic benefits for society.

Compared to special needs children who do not receive EI services, children who do

- Need fewer special education and other habilitative services later in life;
- Score higher on mathematics, reading, and language achievement tests at all grade levels; and
- Show fewer antisocial or delinquent behaviors.

In addition, money invested in EI services is more than balanced by savings in later special education and by the child's potential for lifetime income, which results in higher taxes being paid back to state and local governments that provide these services. Various studies have estimated that every dollar invested in EI saves from four to seven dollars in school-age special education services.

According to the 30th Annual Report to Congress (U.S. Department of Education, 2008), 9.1 percent of all school children and adolescents and 5.8 percent of preschool children receive special education services. In contrast, only 3.9 percent of infants and toddlers receive early intervention services. Stated another way, only 43 percent of children who would qualify for special education by school age are identified and receive early intervention at or before age 3. As you can see, there's a huge need for early identification and intervention that is not being met.

SLPs, administrators, and teachers face significant challenges in their attempts to obtain funding for very young children who have communication disorders. This may be even more difficult with children who have complex communication needs requiring more costly intensive speech and language services and potentially costly AAC technologies. Justification of ECI services is the key and strengthens the case for the need for EBP and demographic information.

A family-centered perspective, emphasizing both partnership and collaboration with families, is a cornerstone of early intervention. Intervention centered on the priorities and needs of individual families is generally more acceptable to families than are other approaches and has the additional advantage of strengthening and building family confidence and competence even beyond the intervention task. Competence and confidence flow from successful interactions with their child.

With this as our background and justification, let's begin to examine the pieces of ECI. In the next chapters, we'll describe the children serviced in EI programs and models for ECI assessment and intervention.

✅ Click here to gauge your understanding of the concepts in this chapter.

2

Early Communication Impairment

When you have completed this chapter, you should be able to:

- Explain late language emergence.
- Describe four types of established-risk infants served by early intervention (EI) programs.
- Describe four types of at-risk infants served by EI programs.
- List early identification signs and behaviors.

Terms with which you should be familiar:

Anemia
Apgar score
Apnea
At-risk
Autism spectrum disorder (ASD)
Bronchopulmonary dysplasia (BPD)
Cerebral palsy (CP)
Communication impairment (CI)
Continuous positive airway pressure (CPAP)
Deafness
Established risk
Fetal alcohol spectrum disorder (FASD)
Intellectual disability (ID)

Intraventricular hemorrhage (IVH)
Jaundice
Legal blindness
Low birth weight
Maltreatment
Morbidity
Necrotizing enterocolitis (NEC)
Neglect
Patent ductus arteriosis (PDA)
Preterm
Respiratory distress syndrome (RDS)
Retinopathy of prematurity (ROP)
Total blindness
Total parenteral nutrition (TPN)

Kimberly was adopted from China when she was 5 months old. Shortly after she arrived in the United States, she experienced her first seizure. Although her seizures are now controlled by medication, she continues to lag behind other children in motor, social, and communication milestones. A diagnosis by a neurologist when she was 22 months old found that Kimberly had cerebral palsy and severe developmental delays. In the United States, 15 percent of all children 3 to 17 years of age have a developmental disability (Centers for Disease Control and Prevention [CDC], 2016). Like Kimberly, more than 500,000 of these children below 36 months of age are eligible for EI services as mandated by Part C of the Individuals with Disabilities Education Improvement Act, 2004 (Rosenberg, Zhang, & Robinson, 2008).

Communication delays and feeding and swallowing problems are the most prevalent symptoms in these young children with developmental disabilities (DD). Communication deficits may include reduced or atypical babbling or interacting, limited use of communicative gestures and development of intent, or slow growth of or regression in vocabulary and word combining (American Speech-Language-Hearing Association [ASHA], 2008b).

Approximately 10 to 20 percent of toddlers and young preschoolers are late talkers (Rescorla & Achenbach, 2002; Rescorla & Alley, 2001). A recent study of 24-month-old single-born children found 13.4 percent showed late language emergence (LLE) (Zubrick, Taylor, Rice, & Slegers, 2007). Luckily, most late-talking toddlers mature out of their difficulties (Rescorla, Dahlsgaard, & Roberts, 2000). Those that do not may have a communication impairment (CI).

Communication impairment (CI) is a significant disability in young children and is characterized by difficulty receiving, sending, processing, and comprehending concepts or verbal and nonverbal communication. Ranging in severity from mild to profound, CI may be evidenced in any or all modes of communication and social interaction (ASHA, 1997–2015). CI is associated with several known disorders. To this I would add that feeding and swallowing, while not strictly communication, could also qualify as communication impairments because they can impede interaction and can signify other disorders, such as cerebral palsy or oral apraxia, that may impair communication.

As you might guess, CI affects many aspects of a child's development. For example, toddlers with language delays appear to show more social withdrawal relative to typically developing (TD) toddlers (Horwitz et al., 2003; Irwin, Carter, & Briggs-Gowan, 2002; Rescorla, Ross, & McClure, 2007). Delays in language may cause toddlers to be less likely to join social interactions or to be sought out by other toddlers. Similar outcomes are found among preschool children with other language difficulties.

The more limited a child's communication behavior, the more difficult it is for that child to learn the link between communication behavior and results. For example, within the first few months of life, TD children learn that their behavior can affect other people in their environment. Making this connection is a vital first link in developing communication intent which is, in turn, crucial to language development.

There is also a relationship between the presence of CI and behavioral problems. Language problems in preschool may lead to behavioral/emotional disorders later. As a speech-language pathologist (SLP), you'll find that about half of all children with CI that you serve, whether in clinics or schools, also have a behavioral or emotional problem (Cohen, 2001). The relationship between communication and behavioral difficulties among 18- to 35-month-old children is strongest in children with neurodevelopmental delays (ND), such as low intellectual abilities or neurological insult, including traumatic brain injury (TBI), and in those with autism spectrum disorder (ASD) (Rescorla & Achenbach, 2002; Rescorla & Alley, 2001; Rescorla, Ross, & McClure, 2007). These conditions will be described in more detail later.

Late Language Emergence

Several factors can contribute to CI. Among these are low birth weight and premature birth. Both of these significantly predict *late language emergence* (LLE), a hallmark characteristic of children with language impairment (LI) and often the first diagnostic symptom of a larger language problem. Children who are less than 85 percent of their optimum birth weight, born earlier than 37 weeks, or both are at almost twice the risk for LLE as optimal birth weight, full-term infants (Zubrick, Taylor, Rice, & Slegers, 2007). Interestingly, late talkers do not have elevated rates of either fetal or birth complications, two factors that might lead to later developmental problems.

Other significant factors in LLE include a family history of LLE, male gender, and early neurobiological growth. Factors such as parental educational levels, socioeconomic resources, parental mental health, parenting practices, and family functioning are less significant. Predictors among 24-month-olds of later language impairment included problems in gross and fine motor development, poor adaptive and psychosocial development, and negative temperament or mood quality.

The proportion of late talkers is much higher for boys than for girls (Horwitz et al., 2003; Paul, 2000; Rescorla, 2002; Rescorla & Achenbach, 2002; Rescorla & Alley, 2001). Male children are at almost three times the risk for LLE compared with female children (Zubrick, Taylor, Rice, & Slegers, 2007). These differences may reflect underlying biological differences in children's gender. John Locke in his "Duels and Duets" (2011) suggests that males and females are born prewired to engage with others in very different ways that reflect gender and may influence language development. Interestingly, the gender effect is much less significant, or in some cases nonsignificant, if we look at the language abilities of all children and not just those who exhibit LLE (Feldman et al., 2000; Pan, Rowe, Singer, & Snow, 2005; Rescorla & Achenbach, 2002).

Although a mother's educational level is positively associated with a number of language indices in the first 3 years and maternal and paternal education is reported to be a predictor of language impairment in school-age children, this factor may be less important with very young children. For example, the amount of maternal talkativeness, a variable often associated with educational level, does not seem to be related to growth in children's vocabulary production in the 24- to 36-month period (Pan et al., 2005). In contrast, the type and quality of maternal input may be a very significant factor.

The relation between psychosocial development and LLE is unclear and does not show the somewhat more straightforward relationship of other variables such as gender and maternal education. For example, assessments of early psychosocial development often contain language-related questions. A child may be considered to have psychosocial developmental problems based on the amount of talking with other children. This clearly presupposes the language skills to do so. In other words, psychosocial differences may be a consequence of limited language ability, not a cause of it (Redmond & Rice, 2002).

Interestingly, mothers of children with LLE are more likely to use dysfunctional parenting practices (Zubrick, Taylor, Rice, & Slegers, 2007). Thus, the psychosocial profiles of late talkers often include problematic child temperament, abnormal child behavior, and dysfunctional parenting. We have to be cautious because these data are correlational, meaning two things change together, and do not imply cause in either direction.

Risk of Communication Impairment

A significant delay often exists before communication impairments are recognized. Although most children develop their first words between 12 and 15 months of age, it is common for health professionals to wait until a child is 24 to 30 months of age before referring a child for an evaluation. So much variability exists in the developmental pace of TD children that criteria for identifying children with problems have been difficult to establish. This is further complicated because many children who are late talkers catch up on their own.

You can see why it is doubly important that child specialists be able to identify children with CI earlier in the child's life and with greater accuracy. Given these difficulties, professionals often discuss young children with the potential for communication difficulties in terms of a child's *risk* of developing such impairments.

Risk could be broadly defined as exposure to biological and environmental conditions that can increase the likelihood of negative developmental outcomes. Early risk factors are considered to be particularly important because an infant is believed to be especially vulnerable. Biological risk factors include genetic or gestational disorders, prematurity,

TABLE 2.1 Examples of Established Risks

CATEGORIES	EXAMPLES
Chromosomal and genetic disorders	Down syndrome, fragile X syndrome
Nervous system/neurological disorders	Cerebral palsy
Developmental disorders	Autism spectrum disorder (ASD)
Gestational malformations	Spina bifida, craniofacial anomalies
Metabolic conditions	Tay-Sachs disorder
Sensory disorders	Deafness, blindness

These classifications change as we learn more about etiology. For example, there is increasing evidence that ASD has a genetic/biological basis.

and low birth weight, and may result from prenatal (prior to birth), perinatal (at birth and shortly thereafter), and postnatal (beginning at about 1 month of age) causes. You may be surprised to learn that CI often runs in families, indicating a genetic factor. Approximately half of the families of children with CI have at least another affected family member.

Environmental risk factors reside outside the infant and include such factors as low socioeconomic status (low SES) and parental psychopathology (Laucht et al., 2000). Environmental variables may include poor nutrition, poor or nonexistent health services, and abuse. Sadly, all children with disabilities are at increased risk for maltreatment in the home, which, of course, may compound other factors (Sullivan & Knutson, 2000).

A wide variety of etiologies and conditions characterize the EI population. Although there is some overlap in the following statistics, these disorders include

- Neurological dysfunction: 50 to 70 percent of premature and low birth weight infants (Aylward, 2005; Reichman, 2005)
- Intellectual disability: 1 percent or more (Maulik, Mascarenhas, Mathers, Dua, & Saxena, 2011)
- Cerebral palsy: 6 to 25 percent of high-risk infants (Aylward, 2005)
- Autism spectrum disorder: 1 in every 68 children (CDC, 2014)

PL 99-457 outlines two broad categories of children served by EI programs: those with established risk, such as those with Down syndrome, or those in at-risk categories, such as preterm or low birth weight infants. In established risk, presented in Table 2.1, there is a strong existing relationship between the condition and developmental difficulties. For example, most boys with fragile X syndrome experience educational and communicative challenges.

Children considered to be at-risk *may* experience significant developmental delay. At-risk factors include anything with the potential to interfere with a child's ability to interact in a typical way with the environment and to develop typically. At-risk factors may be both biological and environmental in nature and may include, but are not limited to, the following:

- Preterm birth,
- Low birth weight,
- Physical abuse,
- Severe, chronic caregiver or child illness,
- Lack of or limited prenatal care,
- Chronic or acute caregiver mental illness or DD, and
- Caregiver alcohol or substance dependence.

Let's look at each type of risk briefly and then spend a little time with neonatal concerns. We'll discuss each broad risk category and several examples of each. Most of you are already familiar with some of these risk factors from earlier communication impairment courses and texts. I'll make some assumptions and cover what I believe to be more familiar conditions in less detail.

Established Risk

As a group, established risks are easier to identify and have a strong link with developmental difficulties. Although space precludes discussing all of the disorders in this category, let's examine a few of the more common ones in order to understand each one's relationship to development of communication, speech, and language. These include intellectual disability (ID), autism spectrum disorder (ASD), cerebral palsy (CP), deafness and deaf-blindness, and cleft palate. We'll spend a little more time with ASD, given the recent increase in the number of children identified with the disorder and the current educational emphasis on these children.

Many young children with intellectual disability, limitation in muscle control or sensory ability, or the presence of disorders such as ASD communicate primarily by presymbolic or nonsymbolic means, using individualistic gestures, vocalizations, and other behaviors, including problematic or challenging ones (Wetherby, Prizant, & Schuler, 2000). These children may or may not

- Be intentional in their communication,
- Be difficult to understand, or
- Communicate in ways unique to their interactions with parents and care providers.

A child's intent may be unclear or inconsistent, especially to strangers or those less familiar with the child. It may also be unclear how much communication the child comprehends outside of routine contexts such as feeding or dressing.

INTELLECTUAL DISABILITY (ID)

First, let's deal with terminology. As you sit reading this book, a relatively new term, intellectual disability (ID), is replacing an older one, *mental retardation* (Schalock et al., 2007). Intellect is our ability to think, reason, and learn; it's our capacity for knowledge and understanding. Individuals with ID have a deficit in general intellectual functioning.

The phrase *mental retardation* is a diagnostic term. Originally, it was meant as a more acceptable substitute for some rather pejorative words used by professionals and the public alike, such as *imbecile*. Unfortunately, over time, *mental retardation* itself has acquired some negative and shame-causing connotations, such as calling someone a "retard" as an insult or use of the shortened version, *'tard*. These usages contributed to the need to replace *mental retardation* with *mentally challenged* or *intellectual disability*.

Within the medical and education fields, there is a long history of changing nomenclature for various populations based on updated information, needs to be more sensitive, and political pressure. Several years ago, for example, in an effort to stress the person rather than the disability, ASHA decided on a person-first policy in all ASHA journals, resulting in "individuals with intellectual disabilities" rather than "intellectually disabled individuals."

In the United States, mental retardation (now called ID) is part of a broader category called *developmental disability* (DD) that includes autism, cerebral palsy, and other disorders that appear during the developmental period or prior to age 22. The presence of intellectual limitations is the distinctive feature of intellectual disability/mental retardation within the broader category of developmental disability.

In the broadest sense and in the larger rehabilitation community, "intellectual disability" is a category that can include individuals with disorders such as mental retardation, traumatic brain injury (TBI), and Alzheimer's disease (AD). Obviously, not all of these disorders or diseases are developmental in nature. They would not be development disabilities. For example, AD occurs primarily in the elderly.

FIGURE 2.1 **Relationship of Developmental Disabilities, Intellectual Disability, and Mental Retardation**

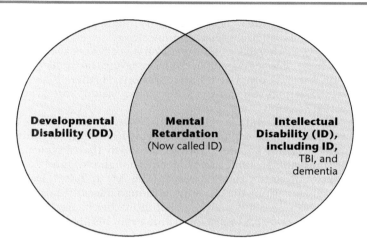

This sometimes confusing jumble of names is illustrated in Figure 2.1. These distinctions are further delineated in actual use. Many educators use ID to refer exclusively to what was previously called mental retardation. For example, in 2006, the American Association on Mental Retardation, the professional group working with this population, voted to change its name to the American Association on Intellectual and Developmental Disabilities (AAIDD). Throughout this text, I will follow this convention, with *ID* replacing *MR*. I apologize, but I didn't say this would be easy to follow.

Characteristics and Causes

Intelligence is one measure of general mental capability. Although not a perfect measure, intelligence quotient, or IQ, is frequently used to describe intelligence. As a rough measure, intellectual disability or limitations in general intellectual functioning are thought to be present if an individual has an IQ of approximately 70 or below accompanied by deficits in adaptive behaviors, such as self-help skills or speech and language. Given the imperfect nature of describing human behavior with a score or number, there has been a recent movement to look instead at the impact of ID on three domains related to everyday tasks (American Psychiatric Association, 2013):

- The conceptual domain, including language, reading, writing, math, reasoning, knowledge, and memory;
- The social domain, including empathy, social judgment, interpersonal communication skills, making and retaining friendships, and similar abilities; and
- The practical domain, or self-management, including personal care, job responsibilities, money management, recreation, and organizing tasks.

Rather than thinking about ID being across the board, it would be more accurate to consider disability within the context of an individual's environment and the need of that person for individualized supports in various contexts—in other words, how the individual functions within daily contexts. As you may recall from the first chapter, the World Health Organization (WHO) has proposed a different way of looking at disability that is based on an individual's ability to participate in his or her environment. This has led to a classification system, used more widely in other parts of the world and increasingly in the United States, called the International Classification of Functioning, Disability and Health, or ICF—a classification of health and health-related domains that includes an individual's body, and both individual and societal perspectives. In this system, body functions and structure are assessed across various activities and levels of participation. Thus, severity, not just of ID but of all disorders, is based on ability to participate and the level of support needed to do so.

Intellectual disabilities will vary in degree and effect across individuals. Any determination of ID must consider the typical community, linguistic diversity, and cultural differences in the way individuals and groups communicate.

Persons who have intellectual disability may have other coexisting conditions, such as cerebral palsy or hearing loss. In general, the more severe the intellectual disability, the more likely a person is to have other disabling conditions. Further discussion can be found at the AAIDD website, which you can access by typing "aaidd" into your search engine. Click on "Intellectual Disability" at the top.

Although almost every child is able to learn, develop, and become a participating member of the community, the cognitive functioning limitations of individuals with ID will result in a child's learning and developing more slowly than a typical child. Different severities of ID are presented in Table 2.2. Moderate though profound mental retardation is nearly always apparent within the first years of life. My grandson Dakota, mentioned previously, most likely functions in this range, although administering definitive testing is extremely difficult because of his multiple disabilities. In practical terms, it means that he will most likely require care and assistance throughout his life.

Although severity is often represented by categories, as in Table 2.2, the severity of any disability may be more accurately described as a continuum. In fact, a single dimension such as severity may give us little useful or practical information. A multidimensional descriptive approach might be more accurate, especially in an assessment. For our general purposes, however, categorical classification has the advantage of simplicity.

In general, when we speak of ID, we are referring to a slower overall rate of development, especially intellectually, lower intelligence, possible need for environmental supports, and possible multiple handicaps, such as seizure activity, cerebral palsy, and/or ASD. In most cases, communication is also impaired, as a result of delayed language development, poor motor control of speech, or both. Adults and children with ID may have difficulties with problem-solving and learning social interactional behaviors.

The causes of ID are many and varied, as you can see from the list in Table 2.3. In fact, it has been estimated that there are over 500 known causes. Many, such as genetic syndromes, are obvious at birth and are established risk factors. Others are more subtle and may be environmental in nature. For an excellent reference, see Shprintzen (1999).

Most likely, you've encountered ID in introductory courses. Let's look at just three common syndromes of ID.

Fragile X Syndrome (FXS)

Young male toddlers, preschoolers, and early school-age children with fragile X syndrome (FXS), the leading biological cause of ID in males, show significant communication delays, although substantial individual variability exists (Roberts, Mirrett, Anderson, Burchinal, & Neebe, 2002). Their relative strengths in verbal and vocal communication are balanced by deficits in gesture use, reciprocity, and symbolic play skills.

For those not familiar with FXS, it is a genetic disorder caused by a mutation in a gene on the X chromosome responsible for a key protein important in brain function. The gene that causes FXS is called the *Fragile X Mental Retardation 1* (FMR1) gene. Although females can also have FXS, the symptoms are usually not as severe as in males. The majority of males with FXS have mild to moderate mental retardation and other physical and behavioral manifestations, such as social withdrawal, limited attention span, hyperactivity, social deficits, and communication difficulties.

What we know from TD children can also be important for children with FXS. Maternal use of gestures at 24–36 months is positively related to the expressive language of children with FXS at early school age (Hahn et al., 2014). More specifically, maternal pointing to close entities while talking with toddlers evokes more speech responses from children with FXS during these interactions, especially when pointing is combined with *wh-* questions. These data lend additional support to the potential benefits of ECI.

TABLE 2.2 **Comparison of Severity Classifications of Intellectual Disability**

			OLDER MEASURES	APA*	AAIDD**	OTHER DISORDERS***
Severity	IQ	% of ID Population	Adaptive Function	Level of Support	Characteristics	
Mild	52–68	85	Many can achieve some success at elementary academic levels or beyond with sufficient supports; mostly self-sufficient with supports; can live independently with a minimal level of additional supports.	Intermittent	May only require additional supports during times of transition, uncertainty, or stress.	Fewer
Moderate	36–51	10	Adequate but limited communication skills; social cues, social judgment, and social decisions regularly need support; most self-care activities can be performed but may require extensive instruction and support; limited independent employment and living with additional moderate supports such as in group homes.	Limited	Can increase conceptual skills, social skills, and practical skills with additional training; may still require additional support to navigate everyday situations.	
Severe	20–35	3–4	Communication skills very basic; self-care requires assistance; may require safety supervision and supportive assistance; residence in supported housing usually.	Extensive	Have some basic communication skills and can complete some self-care tasks; usually require daily support.	
Profound	0–19	1–2	Dependent on others for all aspects of daily care, usually 24/7; communication skills limited; usually have co-occurring sensory or physical limitations.	Pervasive	Need daily interventions for individual function supervision to ensure health and safety; lifelong support for nearly every aspect of individual's routine.	Possibly Multiple

*American Psychiatric Association (*DSM-5*) (APA, 2013).
** American Association on Intellectual and Developmental Disabilities.
*** Most frequently cerebral palsy and seizure activity.

TABLE 2.3 **Causes of Intellectual Disability**

TYPE	EXAMPLES
Prenatal	
Chromosomal	
Errors in number	Down syndrome
	Klinefelter syndrome
Chromosome deletion	Cri du chat syndrome
Chromosomal defects	Fragile X syndrome
Single Gene Disorders and Genetic Abnormalities	
Metabolic disorders	Phenylketonuria (PKU)
	Tay-Sachs disease
Neuro-cutaneous syndromes	Tuberous sclerosis
Brain malformations	Hydrocephalus
	Microcephalus
	Cerebral malformation
	Craniofacial anomalies
Maternal Infectious Processes	Maternal rubella
	Congenital syphilis
Maternal Toxins & Chemical Agents	Fetal alcohol syndrome
	Drug-exposed fetus
Maternal Nutrition	Severe malnutrition during pregnancy
	Various amino-deficiencies
Trauma	Intracranial hemorrhage in fetus
Perinatal	
Third Trimester Problems	Complications of pregnancy
	Diseases in mother such as heart and kidney
	Disease and diabetes
	Placental dysfunction
Labor and Delivery Problems	Extreme prematurity and/or low birth weight
	Birth asphyxia
	Difficult and/or complicated delivery
	Birth trauma
Neonatal Problems	Severe, prolonged jaundice
Postnatal	
Brain Infections	Encephalitis
	Bacterial meningitis
Head Injury	Traumatic brain injury (TBI)
Toxins	Chronic lead exposure
Nutritional Issues	Severe and prolonged malnutrition
Gross Brain Disease	Tumors
	Huntington disease

TABLE 2.3 **Causes of Intellectual Disability** (*continued*)

TYPE	EXAMPLES
Psychosocial Disadvantage	Subnormal intellectual functioning in immediate family and/or impoverished environment
Sensory Deprivation	Maternal deprivation
	Prolonged isolation
Unknown	Perhaps the largest category of causes

Causes are not mutually exclusive, and a child may have more than one or mixed causes.

Sources:

Luckasson, R., Borthwick-Duffy, S., Buntinx, W. H., Coulter, D. L., Craig, E. M., Reeve, A., Schalock, R. L., Snell, M. E., Spitalnik, D. M., Spreat, S., & Tasse, M. J. (2002). *Mental retardation: Definition, classification, and systems of supports* (10th ed.). Washington DC: American Association on Mental Retardation.

U.S. National Library of Medicine. (2010, December 15). *Mental retardation.* U.S. Department of Health and Human Services, National Institutes of Health. Retrieved January 2, 2011, from http://www.nlm.nih.gov/medlineplus/ency/article/001523.htm

World Health Organization. (2010). *Mental retardation: From knowledge to action.* Retrieved January 2, 2011, from http://www.searo.who.int/en/Section1174/Section1199/Section1567/Section1825_8090.htm

Down Syndrome

Down syndrome (DS), another genetic disorder, is characterized by extra genetic material in chromosome 21. Children with DS have a characteristic delay in their language development, beyond what would be predicted by their general cognitive delay. This said, language and communication skills, including gestural development and use, follow the same course and sequence as that of TD children but at a slower rate (Chan & Iacono, 2001).

When compared with TD children, those with DS receive significantly less verbal input from parents measured by number of words spoken and rate of verbal behaviors (Thiemann-Bourque, Warren, Brady, Gilkerson, & Richards, 2014). In addition, the parental input to children with DS remains low after 24 months, rather than increasing as the children's language matures. These are parental behaviors that can be altered through ECI.

 If you've never worked with a child with Down syndrome, or even if you have, you might want to watch this video.

Prader–Willi Syndrome

Prader–Willi syndrome (PWS) is a rare genetic disorder caused by the deletion of genes on chromosome 15. The incidence of PWS is between 1 in 15,000 and 1 in 25,000 live births (NIH, 2014). Characteristics of PWS include low muscle tone, short stature, cognitive disabilities, problem behaviors, incomplete sexual development, and chronic feelings of hunger that can lead to excessive eating and morbid obesity. Although found all along the intelligence spectrum, the majority exhibit ID; approximately 40 percent of all those with PWS are considered to have mild ID.

Although there is great variability, the speech and language skills of individuals with PWS are generally below expectations based on intellectual levels. Poor speech sound development is attributed to poor oral motor skills. Almost all children with PWS demonstrate oral motor difficulties, including poor tongue mobility, short palates, and articulatory incoordination (Lewis, Freebairn, Heeger, & Cassidy, 2002). In addition, individuals with PWS have poor phonological skills indicative of a more general language deficit (Akefeldt, Akefeldt, & Gillberg, 1997; Dyson & Lombardino, 1989). Most children have delayed speech and poor receptive and expressive language. Cognitive deficits that may contribute to language problems include problems with auditory short-term memory and auditory verbal processing (Curfs, Wiegers, Sommers, Borghgraef, & Fryns, 1991; Dykens, Hodapp, Walsh, & Nash, 1992). Pragmatic difficulties include problems with maintaining topics and turn-taking (Downey & Knutson, 1995). Children with PWS often have delayed language, shorter utterances than TD children, and difficulty with narrative production, which may result from linear sequencing difficulties (Lewis et al., 2002).

AUTISM SPECTRUM DISORDER (ASD)

Autism spectrum disorder (ASD) is comprised of a set of heterogeneous disorders with a common core of symptoms caused by neurogenic deficits and characterized by severe and pervasive impairments in several areas of development (Matson & Boisjoli, 2008; Matson & Wilkins, 2008; Rutter, 2005). ASD refers to a continuum of disorders that also includes Asperger and Rett syndromes (American Psychiatric Association, 2013).

The fifth edition of the *Diagnostic and Statistical Manual* (DSM-V) of the American Psychiatric Association (2013) has very specific criteria for defining ASD. For a child to be diagnosed as having ASD, he or she must exhibit:

- Persistent deficits in social communication and interaction across different contexts. These may include deficits in social-emotional reciprocity, nonverbal communication, and developing and maintaining developmentally appropriate relationships.
- Restricted, repetitive patterns of behavior, interests, or activities. Of interest to SLPs, these may be manifested in stereotyped or repetitive speech and ritualized patterns of verbal or nonverbal behavior. Other examples include stereotyped or repetitive motor movements or use of objects; excessive adherence to routines; and excessive resistance to change. Individuals with ASD may also exhibit highly restricted, fixated interests of an abnormal intensity or focus; hyper- or hypo-reactivity to sensory input; or unusual interest in sensory stimuli.

Although the behaviors may be present in early childhood, they may not be fully manifested until later when social demands exceed a child's abilities. In either case, these behaviors limit and impair a child's everyday functioning

Even though I softened the medical language a bit, the definition is, by design, somewhat clinical. From a communication point of view, many, but not all, children with ASD exhibit

- Abnormal social interactions and difficulty adjusting to different social situations;
- Abnormal reaction to and difficulty integrating sensory information such as verbal and nonverbal aspects of communication;
- Difficulty with the give-and-take of conversation; and
- Poorly integrated verbal and nonverbal communication, including poor eye contact and body language, echolalia or repetition of others' speech, and repetition of certain expressions.

In general, as you might expect, the more severe the symptoms, the poorer language and overall development (Pry et al., 2005).

Associated characteristics that frequently co-occur with ASD include problems in sensory processing, motor planning, emotional regulation and arousal, and behavioral organization and control (Anzalone & Williamson, 2000; Prizant, Schuler, Wetherby, & Rydell, 1997). Children with ASD also have gross and fine motor skills below that of TD children (Provost, Lopez, & Heimerl, 2007). Evidence suggests that poor early oral and manual motor skills are one of the early distinguishing features of ASD (Gernsbacher, Sauer, Geye, Schweigert, & Goldsmith, 2008).

In general, children with ASD have relative strengths in knowledge of objects, rote memory, and visual-spatial processing. Deficits include weaknesses in social knowledge, semantic and conceptual memory, communication, and abstract problem-solving (Wetherby, Prizant, & Schuler, 1997).

Motor patterns of behavior may include rocking and a fascination with lights or spinning objects. In addition, a child may have an insistence on certain routines or a preoccupation with specific objects, foods, or clothing. Paired with these preferences, a child with ASD may have an adverse reaction to other sounds or textures. One child I knew would only eat foods that were the texture of well-blended mashed potatoes, no lumps allowed. Another child arrived at camp with ten outfits, one for each day, all the same.

ASD is much more common than previously believed. In 2014, after a national survey, the U.S. Centers for Disease Control (CDC) announced that

- The prevalence of ASD among children is 1 in 68;
- Boys are more likely to display ASD characteristics by 5 to 1; and
- Most children with ASD have IQs above 70 (above the general cutoff for ID).

ASD occurs in all racial, ethnic, and socioeconomic groups.

Although, as mentioned, most children with ASD have IQs above 70, that still leaves approximately 25 percent of children with ASD also exhibiting ID (Chakrabarti & Fombonne, 2001; Fombonne, 2003a, 2003b). It's worth emphasizing that in the past, untestable children were simply assumed to have severe or profound ID. Low expectations can become self-fulfilling. In nonverbal measures of intelligence, most individuals with ASD score in the normal and above normal ranges of intelligence (Dawson, Soulèires, Gernsbacher, & Mottron, 2007). It's important to remember that labels such as "intellectual disability" often refer to an individual's scores on a cognitive test and may say little about a child's potential to learn or to function day to day.

Early Identification

Some children who will eventually be diagnosed as having ASD manifest symptoms during infancy, while others display symptoms later in early childhood (Zwaigenbaum et al., 2007). Children with milder forms of ASD may not be diagnosed until early adolescence.

At present, many researchers are trying to identify the early signs of ASD. Early identification can lead to early intervention. The Autism Spectrum Disorder Foundation website, accessed by typing "myasdf" into your online search engine, provides some possible early warning signs. Click on "About Autism" and then "Identifying the Disorder."

A few studies have found that 12-month-old children with ASD can be distinguished from their TD peers and those with ID based on several behaviors. In general, 1-year-olds with ASD tend to exhibit (Zwaigenbaum et al., 2005)

- Excessive mouthing of objects,
- Aversion to touch,
- Extreme irritability,
- Fixation on objects,
- Lack of facial expression,
- Less eye contact with people, and
- Less orientation when name is called.

In addition, at 1 year of age, children who will later be diagnosed with ASD show a different pattern of crying compared to TD children and those with developmental delays.

More specifically, the cries of children with ASD have less variation and more dysphonation (Esposito & Venuti, 2009). Typical infant vocalizations are mostly composed of vowels, which make the vocal spectrum periodic. In contrast, dysphonic sounds have more random spectrums. Maternal reactions to the crying of infants later diagnosed with ASD are also qualitatively different, with less touching and rocking and more spoken language.

Parents often report concern about behaviors around 18 months, especially if a child is not talking. Other concerns are a child's not attending to the caregiver, poor socialization, lack of eye contact, and stereotypic behaviors. In general, however, it's rare for children below age 3 to display some of the behaviors characteristic of ASD, such as stereotyped or repetitive actions and sound-making, preoccupation with certain activities and actions, and resistance to change (Young, Brewer, & Pattison, 2003).

 Many SLPs and future SLPs have a great interest in ASD, in part because it seems so unfathomable. Early assessment is an area of intense study. This video focuses on the early signs of ASD.
https://www.youtube.com/watch?v=BEqrlbzskp4

Communication Development

Lack of communication skill is the greatest cause of concern for parents of children with ASD, and communication is often these children's primary intervention goal. Children with ASD are almost always delayed in speech and language acquisition and in communication in general (Tager-Flusberg, Paul, & Lord, 2005).

Most children with ASD have a language age well below both their nonverbal mental age and their chronological age. Although older research indicated that approximately half of young children with ASD failed to acquire speech as their primary mode of communication, some newer data suggest that, thanks to EI, only 20 to 30 percent do not develop usable spoken communication (Rogers, 2006; Stevens et al., 2000). Of course, this figure is still a high percentage.

Many characteristics common in children with ASD may impede interactions with adults central to development of intentional communication. These characteristics are as follows:

- Attention deficits, including minimal joint attention,
- Deficits in eye contact and gaze,
- Lack of meaningful play and symbolic play,
- Resistance to change,
- Abnormal sensory responsiveness,
- Restricted or obsessive interests,
- Self-stimulatory and/or self-injurious behaviors, and
- Heightened activity levels (Colgan et al., 2006; Paparella, Goods, Freeman, & Kasari, 2011; Sheinkopf, Mundy, Oller, & Steffens, 2000; Schopler, Reichler, & Renner, 2010; Spiker, Lin, Van Dyke, & Wood, 2012).

As a result, children with severe ASD may have difficulty learning within naturally occurring social interactions. The trick is to make those situations more instructional while retaining their basic social nature.

Parents may lack the knowledge and skills to support the communication efforts of children with ASD. The result of repeated unsuccessful experiences is these children may find social interactions to be overwhelming, confusing, and stressful. As a result, they may have limited engagement in social interactions and low motivation to participate. If you suddenly found yourself in a situation in which you did not know the language and the rules for interacting, you might, after repeated failure, respond in a similar manner.

We're unsure why some children with ASD learn to talk and others do not. We do know that early language ability and social competence are related to positive long-term outcomes and that verbal skills are the strongest predictors of later functioning (Howlin, 2005; Howlin, Mahood, & Rutter, 2000; Liss et al., 2001; Lord, Risi, & Pickles, 2004; Mawhood, Howlin, & Rutter, 2000; Stone & Yoder, 2001). Among preschool and early school-age children, the level of gestural attainment, rate of communication, and parent responsiveness are also significant predictors of language outcome (Brady, Marquis, Fleming, & McLean, 2004).

As you know, early gestural and interactive skills of TD children are important for initial symbolic communication and for transforming speech into conversation (Newson, 2001). Most gestures used by children with ASD are for behavior regulation. A limited number are related to social interaction, and few if any are for establishing joint attention. A limited use of joint attention gestures early in life may predict later diagnosis of ASD or another developmental disorder.

The transition from contact to distal gestures and the developmental hierarchy of gestures are important developmental markers. Some young children with ASD will show an overall deficit in early means of communication, such as eye gaze or early gestures, although they use means that are typical of later development, such as taking someone's hand to lead a person to a desired object. In addition, children with ASD are less likely than TD peers to coordinate gaze with other behaviors when requesting.

Many children with ASD, in the presence of communication deficits, develop idiosyncratic or individualistic communication means of meeting their needs. These include challenging behaviors. For example, children later diagnosed with ASD exhibit significantly more spinning and rotating of objects and unusual visual exploration of objects than TD children (Ozonoff et al., 2008).

Although more research is needed into the mechanisms of learning and ASD, one study reported that the most consistent predictor of vocabulary size for toddlers with ASD is word length measured in number of phonemes (Kover & Ellis Weismer, 2013). In turn, the number of spoken words at 18 months seems to be the best predictor of expressive language at 36 months (Westerlund, Berglund, & Eriksson, 2006). These and other language measures at age 2 are a significant predictor of vocabulary, grammar, verbal memory, and reading comprehension at age 13 (Rescorla, 2005). There is almost a cascade effect here in which language predicts more language. For me, this highlights the crucial need for ECI services.

Causes of ASD

The causes of ASD seem to be many and varied, although it is generally conceded that a strong genetic or biological basis exists, most likely on the X chromosome. The brains of many individuals with ASD differ in development both anatomically and physiologically from the brains of typical individuals. Neurological functioning differences may be related to neurotransmitters, such as an excess of serotonin and other natural opioids.

Although these symptoms can change over time, the disorder nearly always spans the life of the individual. Advances in early identification and the generally good response of children to early intervention have led to a call for even earlier assessment and intervention.

You may have heard that some parent groups blame infant vaccinations for causing ASD in children. Several government-sponsored studies in different countries around the globe have failed so far to find a link.

Whatever the root cause(s), there has been an explosion worldwide in the number of children identified as having ASD. Although there may be a myriad of reasons for the increase, it is at least in part the result of better identification, especially of mild ASD; less reluctance to use the term *autism*; and recent broadening of the term.

Regressive ASD

A significant percentage of young children with ASD, possibly as high as 50 percent, develop typically for approximately the first year and a half of life, followed by rapid and pronounced deterioration and challenging behaviors, psychopathology, seizures, and other roadblocks to development (Dhossche & Rout, 2006; Fombonne & Chakrabarti, 2001; Lingam et al., 2003). The mean age of regression is approximately 28 months and typically occurs over a 3-month period of time with a steep decline in communication and social behavior (Matson, Wilkins, & Fodstad, 2010).

Although it is unclear if children who regress demonstrate subtle behavioral differences prior to their regression, after regression they have greater impairment on core symptoms of ASD, co-occurring psychopathology, challenging behaviors, cognitive development delays, and poor social skills (Matson, Wilkins, & Fodstad, 2010; Moretti et al., 2008; Ozonoff, Williams, & Landa, 2005). In addition, children who regress have fewer interactions and poorer receptive language skills than children with ASD of a nonregressive type (Takarae, Luna, Minshew, & Sweeney, 2008).

The regression may be related to accelerated brain growth in the first year of life. Although the exact cause of regression is unknown, one study found that more than 60 percent of those who regress also exhibit seizures (Oslejsková et al., 2008), often accompanied by intellectual disability. These findings have not been replicated in other studies.

Parental Search for Answers

When a child is diagnosed with ASD, parents experience a range of feelings. Some will be relieved to finally have a name for their child's behavior, while others will have great difficulty accepting the diagnosis. In general, mothers who are more resolved emotionally to their child's condition (Wachtel & Carter, 2008) exhibit

- More cognitive and supportive engagement in play interactions,
- Greater verbal and nonverbal commenting that enhances their child's play and attending, and
- Greater reciprocity between mother and child and seeming mutual enjoyment.

This information highlights the importance of considering a mother's acceptance of her child's diagnosis and her own adjustment to this information.

Because intervention progress for children with ASD may be slow and intense, parental interest in alternative theories of causation and novel treatments is high. Families are seeking answers that provide hope or definitive promise of a cure. For our part, SLPs are prohibited by our code of ethics from promising a cure for any communication disorder.

In their search for answers, families may pursue alternative biologic and nonbiologic interventions to complement more standard ones. One study of 121 families working closely with intervention teams found that 56 percent of these families also had used some form of sensory integration therapy, 50 percent had tried elimination diets, and 61 percent had tried vitamin supplements (Smith, Groen, & Wynn, 2000).

Biologic treatments can be either bought over the counter or administered by a physician and include vitamin supplements and medication. Nonharmful vitamins and vitamin preparations, while they may have some short-term benefits, cannot substantiate claims of behavioral improvement. Other medical or quasi-medical alternatives include antibiotics and antifungal medications, diet and food additive approaches, and chelation/mercury or heavy metal detoxification. Detoxification approaches are related to the long-simmering controversy over the supposed link between vaccines and ASD.

Nonbiological alternative interventions might include facilitated communication, auditory integration training, and craniosacral manipulation, to name a few. In the early 1990s, some professionals were reporting remarkable success using facilitated communication—the use of a communication device, such as a computer keyboard, with physical guidance. Children who had never used words to communicate suddenly began to type messages. Later examination determined that success was, in part, the result of manipulation, whether conscious or unconscious, by the adult facilitator, discrediting facilitated communication as a method of intervention.

In auditory integration, the goal is to systematically reduce sensitivity to sound by exposure to altered music. Craniosacral manipulation by chiropractors, physical therapists, and occupational therapists attempts to alter the flow of cerebrospinal fluid and to change behavior through skull massage. Both auditory integration and craniosacral manipulation report some positive change although there is no credible scientific data. The difficulty in assessing alternative approaches is that some small aspect of an intervention may be effective for one aspect of ASD in a small number of individuals, but that's not enough to support wholesale adoption of that methodology.

Families' primary source of information on alternative interventions is other parents. With increasingly rapid access to information, especially on the Internet, families may be exposed to possible interventions that are neither evidence based nor recommended by knowledgeable professionals. Reported success is usually based on anecdotal reports or subjective case studies; few alternative interventions and treatments have been subjected to unbiased scientific study.

Some professionals have argued that families should be supported in their quest for more effective intervention methods as a way to assist them in learning about potential harm as well as benefits (Levy & Hyman, 2002). As an SLP, you may be called upon to educate families in critically reviewing the promised claims of alternative cures or interventions. In this capacity, you can help parents become informed consumers who can critically review the validity of proposed interventions and promised cures. This requires that you be knowledgeable about available intervention options. At the very least, promising alternatives should be evaluated for

■ Scientific evidence-based benefits,
■ Potential health risk,
■ Financial cost, and
■ Time commitment.

Of course, parents may elect to use an alternative intervention approach not recommended by the intervention team. In this case, you should remain alert to subtle behavioral changes and unwanted side effects and assist parents in assessing the results using objective data whenever possible (Levy & Hyman, 2002). As professionals, team members have an obligation to counsel families and recommend timely medical consultation.

CEREBRAL PALSY

Cerebral palsy (CP) is a group of chronic brain disorders that affect movement, muscle tone, and muscle coordination in approximately half a million people in the United States, including my grandson Dakota. Damage to one or more motor areas of the brain disrupts the brain's ability to control movement and posture because of the faulty signals sent to the muscles. The degree of severity depends on where and to what extent the brain is damaged. CP is characterized by spasticity or muscle tightness, involuntary movement, disturbance in mobility, difficulty in swallowing, and problems with both speech and language. It is reported that approximately 70 percent of people with CP also have some intellectual disability, although this percentage may reflect our inability to properly assess intellectual functioning in this population because of the motor impairment.

Approximately 70 percent of the cases of all types of neonatal brain injury are attributed to events occurring before labor begins. Estimates of the prevalence of CP are approximately 2 per 1,000 live births. Approximately 8,000 babies and infants are diagnosed with CP annually, with another 1,500 identified during the preschool years.

Cerebral palsy is not a disease, it doesn't worsen with time, and it is not contagious. Risk factors for CP include low birth weight, preterm birth, placental disorders, rubella or other infections of the mother during pregnancy, Rh or other blood incompatibility factors, prolonged loss of oxygen, and stroke or bleeding in the infant's brain.

The three main types of CP are spastic, athetoid, and ataxic. These are rarely seen in their pure form, and many individuals have mixed CP.

Many children with CP exhibit what is termed flaccid or hypotonic CP, characterized by poor muscle tone and a floppy posture. In contrast, some infants will exhibit rigidity or fluctuate between flaccidity and rigidity. The majority of these children will manifest one of the other forms of CP as they mature. My grandson Dakota began life as a flaccid child with an especially strong startle response. As he matured, his involuntary movements did not decrease and he developed mixed CP, primarily athetoid in nature.

▶ Although we've mentioned a child with flaccid muscle tone, it may be difficult to imagine a little person with this condition. You can watch an infant with flaccid muscle tone and listen to an explanation in this video.
https://www.youtube.com/watch?v=a_KyFpi0zcE

Spasticity, one of the three general types of CP, affects 70 to 80 percent of individuals with CP and is characterized by muscle stiffness and extreme difficulty moving. Opposing

TABLE 2.4 **Characteristics and Causes of Cerebral Palsy**

Type of Cerebral Palsy	Characteristics	Area of Brain Affected
Spastic	Spasticity, increased muscle tone in and/or opposing muscle groups	Motor cortex Pyramidal tract
	Rigidity and exaggerated stretch reflex	
	Jerky, labored, and slow movements	
	Infantile reflex patterns	
Athetoid	Slow, involuntary writhing	Extrapyramidal tract, basal ganglia
	Disorganized and uncoordinated volitional movement	
	Movements occur accompanying volitional movement	
Ataxic	Uncoordinated movement	Cerebellum
	Poor balance	
	Movements lack direction, force, and control	

muscle groups contract simultaneously making movement jerky and the body rigid. Athetoid or dyskinetic CP, found in approximately 10 to 20 percent of the people with cerebral palsy, is characterized by uncontrolled, slow writhing movements affecting primarily the limbs but also the face and tongue. Finally, ataxia, affecting less than 10 percent of the population with CP, affects balance and depth perception, leading to poor coordination, unsteady walking, and tremors accompanying voluntary movement. CP can affect one or both upper or lower limbs, one side of the body, or the entire body. Characteristics of the types and causes of cerebral palsy are presented in Table 2.4.

An early sign of CP is often failure to develop motor skills similar to other children. At age 2, my grandson Dakota moved about by either rolling or "combat crawling"—dragging himself along—on his stomach, and although he could get to his knees, he seemed incapable of crawling independently.

As you might imagine, lack of muscle control can severely hamper the coordination needed for speech, gesturing, signing, and even making eye contact. In addition to motor impairments, children with severe physical disabilities may be medically fragile and have sensory impairments including hyper/hyposensitivity, cognitive delays or disorders, and social impairments. These may be accompanied by seizure disorders or feeding difficulties. This condition is further complicated by the large percentage of individuals with cerebral palsy who also have intellectual deficits. Because most CP cases are diagnosed during infancy, these children will be prime candidates for EI.

Before we move on, we should at least mention a few other causes of neuromuscular limitations—dysarthria, of which CP is but one example, and childhood apraxia of speech (CAS). Dysarthria is a group of motor speech disorders resulting from neuromuscular dysfunction that may affect one, several, or all major components of speech production. Among infants and toddlers, dysarthria is frequently associated with either cerebral palsy or progressive neurological disease (Marquardt, 2000). In addition to a child's language production, major concerns are motor timing and muscle tone, persistent presence of reflexes, and poor speech production related to vocal fold irregularities, inadequate intra-oral pressure, imprecise consonant production, and persistent speech sound distortions (Leddy, Rosin, & Miller, 2003).

In contrast, CAS is an inability or difficulty with carrying out purposeful, voluntary movements for speech as a result of motor programming or planning difficulties. Characteristics frequently include inconsistent phoneme errors, especially on longer words or phrases, simplified syllable structure, word and bound morpheme omissions, trial-and-error speech behavior, slow rate of speech, and inappropriate or longer pauses. At age 2, my youngest grandson Zavier, who was later diagnosed with CAS, frequently only said the first syllable of a word, often simplifying it to a consonant-vowel or vowel-consonant structure.

DEAFNESS AND DEAF-BLINDNESS

Hearing impairment occurs when there is a full or partial decrease in the ability to detect or understand sounds. Those without the ability to use hearing for everyday purposes are said to have deafness. Young children with major impairments in both auditory and visual abilities are identified as having deafness and blindness or deaf-blindness. Each child will have unique communication, developmental, emotional, and educational needs. In general, as you might imagine, sensory deficits can lead to communication impairment and frequently to behavioral challenges.

Deafness

The degree of hearing impairment can be viewed as a continuum from typical hearing through degrees of loss to profound hearing loss or deafness. The severity of the loss is measured by the degree of loudness or the *intensity level* measured in decibels that a sound must attain before being detectible to an individual. A profound hearing loss is a 90 decibel (dB) threshold or greater. This means that sounds that are quieter than 90 dB are not detectable. The typically hearing person can hear sounds at 20 dB or less.

While the above definition of deafness is technically correct, it may be more appropriate to think of deafness in more practical terms. For example, the ability to benefit from auditory information is situationally dependent on the type of sound, interfering noise, and the context. In addition, we might think of deafness in terms of individual functioning. By this definition, a person is said to have *functional deafness* if she or he relies primarily on vision for environmental information and for learning language. Going a step further, we could state that a person with functional deafness would not access or develop the auditory centers of the brain in the same way as a typically hearing person.

The prevalence of profound hearing loss (90 dB or greater) in newborns in the United States is approximately 1–2 per 1,000 live births. Another 6–8 per 1,000 have severe loss of 70–90 dB (Cunningham & Cox, 2003; Kemper & Downs, 2000). Most children with hearing loss are born to parents with typical hearing, have hearing impairment at birth, and are potentially identifiable by mandatory neonatal hearing screening, although some types of degenerative hearing loss may not become evident until later (Task Force on Newborn and Infant Hearing, 1999).

The most common cause is genetic, the result of a recessive gene carried in the general population. Other causes of deafness may be maternal or infant disease or trauma.

Communication development. The age at which the hearing impairment develops is crucial to spoken language acquisition. Development of hearing loss either prenatally or during infancy can interfere with both social development and the development of spoken language, because a child is unable to access audible spoken communication from the outset.

It is worth noting that children born into families that sign usually have no delay in development of language and communication, although speech may be considerable impaired. As mentioned, most early hearing impairment occurs in children born to typically hearing parents, and these families often have neither the expectation of deafness nor prior experience with deafness and signing.

In general, language development in children with deafness is significantly and positively affected by early identification of hearing loss and early initiation of intervention services (Yoshinaga-Itano, 2003). Among children receiving EI services, those whose hearing loss is identified by 6 months of age demonstrate significantly better language than children identified later.

SLPs will need to provide more intense services to those who (Paul & Roth, 2011a)

- Begin treatment after their first birthday,
- Have higher PTAs after implantation or amplification, and
- Demonstrate lower nonverbal cognitive performance.

Children who receive cochlear implants at an early age are increasingly receiving ECI services that are not exclusively focused on deafness.

Assistive devices. Although hearing aids can amplify incoming sound, their use with infants can be problematic and the amplification may be insufficient for learning speech by children with profound hearing loss. Increasingly, infants are receiving cochlear implants (CIs), which provide stimulation to the surviving neural fibers of the cochlea through electrically generated impulses in response to sound. The majority of children with CIs show significantly better outcomes in oral language development, speech perception, and speech production than children with hearing aid amplification (Kirk et al., 2002; Svirsky, Robbins, Kirk, Pisoni, & Miyamoto, 2000).

The percentage of infants receiving cochlear implants differs across the country and is influenced by factors as varied as the presence of a regional implantation center, health insurance coverage, eligibility criteria at the specific implant center, and the size and political influence of the local Deaf community, which may oppose CIs, although this attitude is changing slowly. Important factors are an early age of implantation, lower pure tone average (PTA) thresholds when implanted, and higher nonverbal IQ (ASHA, 2004; Geers, Tobey, Moog, & Brenner, 2008). Children with CIs have similar rates of language learning to their TD hearing peers (Svirsky et al., 2000).

Blindness

Governments variously define legal blindness. In the United States, Canada, and most of Europe, legal blindness is defined by a visual acuity with the best possible correction of 20/200 or less in the better eye, as compared to 20/20 without correction for typical vision. The 20/200 value means that a person standing 20 feet from an object would see it with the same degree of clarity as a typically sighted person at 200 feet. In addition to visual acuity, many jurisdictions also consider visual field in the definition of legal blindness. The typical person can see about 180 degrees of field. Some of those who are legally blind have a visual field of less than 20 degrees.

A complete lack of form and visual light perception is called total blindness. A child described as having only "light perception" can distinguish light from dark but no more. Only approximately 10 percent of those deemed legally blind have no usable vision. My grandson Dakota was born without an occipital lobe and cannot process most visual information, although he does respond to light-dark contrasts and is able to use vision for some tasks, such as self-feeding.

Deaf-Blindness

Young children with major impairments in both auditory and visual abilities are identified as having deafness and blindness or *deaf-blindness*. Their dual sensory impairment can lead to unique communication, developmental, emotional, and educational needs. Sensory deficits can lead to communication impairment and frequently lead to behavioral challenges.

Usher syndrome (UD) is the most common disorder that affects both senses of hearing and vision. Characterized by hearing loss and an eye disorder called retinitis pigmentosa (RP), a degeneration of the retina, UD is a recessive genetic disorder. Children with the most severe form of UD may also have balance impairment. Approximately 3 to 6 percent of children with deafness and 3 to 6 percent of children with hearing impairment have UD. The prevalence in developed countries such as the United States is approximately 4 babies in every 100,000 births (National Institute on Deafness and Other Communication Disorders, 2014). Most children with UD are born to parents with typical hearing and vision.

Having a child with a dual sensory impairment or with other multiple impairments, such as a child with deafness, visual impairment, and cerebral palsy, can create emotional and financial stress on a family. If we consider the family as a unit, then having a child with deaf-blindness or other multiple handicapping conditions is likely to alter most areas of family functioning. Both family adjustment and interaction may be affected by the presence of a child with deaf-blindness because of the chronic stress associated with raising such a child, although parents of these children do not show evidence of greater psychopathology or personality disorders than the general population.

My grandson Dakota has ID, CP, and blindness. The severity of his condition makes definitive diagnosis difficult. Even with help from the state and the local school district, the financial burden is overwhelming and is only shouldered by the entire extended family contributing both time and money.

One potential family stress factor is disruption of *circadian* or biological rhythms tuned to the light-dark pattern of the 24-hour solar day. This rhythm is reflected not only in sleep-wake patterns but in a range of biological processes, including body temperature and hormonal circulation, controlled by the suprachiasmatic nucleus located bilaterally in the hypothalamus of the brain. For a child born with total blindness, the absence of cycled light results in a sort of freewheeling circadian rhythm that is not light dependent. In other words, the child's rhythm is not synchronized with that of the family, resulting in a sleep-wake cycle that is not consistent with that of family members (Rivkees, 2001). This mismatch can pose a major challenge to efforts to meet the child's needs and can cause considerable frustration and stress. In addition, the child's hearing impairment eliminates cyclical acoustic information that could potentially reduce the effects of blindness on the child's circadian rhythm.

Discipline and communication are areas of particular concern for parents. Although there is little research on children who have deaf-blindness, there is reason to believe that, similar to hearing parents of children with deafness, parents of children with deafness and blindness are more likely to use directing and controlling behaviors and to rely more on physical discipline than do parents of hearing children. Parents will require strong assistance in meeting the day-to-day behavioral needs of their child, especially if communication intervention is to center on family interactions as I suggested in Chapter 1.

The key to success for these children is the development of strong communication, social, and behavioral skills. Experts from several fields concur that early education and training for infants who have deafness and blindness should address development of strong communication skills first (Holte et al., 2006). Outcomes for a child who has deaf-blindness are optimized by an interdisciplinary team approach. Of course, the involvement of the family as members of the intervention team is vital.

CLEFT PALATE

Cleft palate and lip are congenital malformations resulting from the failure of oral structures at the midline to fuse during the first trimester of pregnancy. Surgery for cleft lip generally occurs at about 10 weeks of age while repair of a cleft palate, a more extensive surgical procedure, is usually done at 9 to 18 months of age. Although approximately 80 percent of infants born with palatal clefts develop normal speech with speech intervention following surgery, these same children may be at increased risk for cognitive impairment associated with the disorder and for resultant language impairment. In addition, submucus clefts are commonly associated with syndromes that may have their own associated patterns of development.

Of particular interest in the assessment of an infant with cleft palate are the infant's medical history, hearing status, feeding difficulties, language production, and speech sound inventory. Feeding and swallowing with be discussed in Chapter 10. The specific assessment and intervention techniques required to compensate for any velopharyngeal insufficiency are beyond the scope of this text.

At-Risk Children

Unlike children in established risk categories in which there is a strong link between their condition and developmental disability, those in at-risk categories may or may not experience developmental difficulties, although the possibility exists. At a practical level, this means that professionals, such as an SLP, must justify qualification of an at-risk child for EI. The criteria for qualification vary by state in the United States. In the following sections, we'll discuss some of the more common at-risk categories, including international adoption, low socioeconomic status, maltreatment/neglect, fetal alcohol spectrum disorder, drug-affected infants, premature birth, and low birth weight.

INTERNATIONAL ADOPTIONS

In 2012, approximately 9,000 children were adopted from other countries. Nearly two-thirds of these children came from China, Ethiopia, Russia, and South Korea (U.S. Department of State, 2012). Infants and toddlers adopted from countries with a different language and culture undergo a unique language learning experience and may be predisposed to language impairment. If you want to pursue this unique language acquisition process further, I recommend the excellent review by Glennen (2002).

Complicating language acquisition is the fact that 88 percent of all international adoptees are initially raised in institutional orphanages (Johnson, 2000). In addition, many of the countries from which they come have low personal income, poor nutrition, and limited access to health care. These risk factors create a less than optimal environment for early health and development.

Although institutional care varies from country to country and by region, delays in growth and development are strongly related to orphanage care. It is estimated that children raised in orphanages lose 1 month of linear growth for every 3–5 months in an orphanage (Johnson, 2000; Miller & Hendric, 2000). Although specific figures vary, at the time of adoption, a significant percentage of children (18–51%) are at least two standard deviations below average for height, weight, and head circumference (Johnson, 2000; Miller & Hendric, 2000; Rutter, 1998). Given the importance of early development, this lack of growth is a concern.

The heightened prevalence of several conditions and diseases, such as fetal alcohol spectrum disorder (FASD), iodine insufficiency, hepatitis B and C, tuberculosis, and intestinal parasites, among international adoptees may also adversely affect development of these children (Johnson, 2000; Miller & Hendric, 2000). Other factors include poor maternal health care, high-risk pregnancy or delivery, and premature birth.

Communication Development

Despite all the factors mentioned, most international adoptees develop normal language abilities in American English. Some will have a very rocky start.

Although a high prevalence of speech and language impairment, ranging from 30 to 69 percent, has been reported for international adoptees, much of this information is based on limited surveys (Krakow, Mastriano, & Reese, 2005; Miller & Hendric, 2000). Higher percentages may represent children raised in overseas orphanage environments who are at a higher risk for developmental language delays. Whatever the actual figures may be, adoptive parents' concerns are high, and 57 percent of internationally adopted children are seen by SLPs (Pollak & Bechner, 2000).

Communication development of international adoptees is unique. Development in the birth language is arrested and replaced by development of the adopted language, because adoptive families usually are unable to maintain the birth language (Glennen & Masters, 2002). Although preschool children adopted internationally have more difficulty than nonadopted TD children in identifying facial expression of emotions, those with stronger English language ability tend to be more accurate (Hwa-Froelich, Matsuo, & Becker, 2014).

LOW SOCIOECONOMIC STATUS

The risk of communication impairment is also associated with socioeconomic factors such as economic deprivation. Many children with LI come from homes lacking in stable and continuous childcare, adequate nutrition, and even rudimentary medical care. The combination of these factors constitutes a level of environmental stress that is detrimental in a number of developmental areas, including language.

Children in poverty are exposed to a substantially greater number of risk factors than are their middle-income peers (Evans & English, 2002). Beginning at conception, poverty significantly heightens a child's risk for (Halpern, 2000)

■ Birth complications such as fetal alcohol spectrum disorder,
■ Physical health problems such as asthma and malnutrition,

- Mental health problems,
- Inattentive or erratic parental care,
- Neglect and abuse,
- Removal from the home and placement in foster care, and
- Deficits in cognitive development and achievement.

Not only are there more risks, but the consequences of these risk factors can be more severe. In addition, children in poor families may be exposed to multiple risk factors.

Communication Development

The cumulative effect of biological and environmental factors can have a strong influence on poor children's cognitive and language development, increasing the already negative effects of poverty (Stanton-Chapman, Chapman, Kaiser, & Hancock, 2004). As the number of risk factors increases, the language ability of preschool children in poverty decreases.

Factors that seem most predictive of LI for children in low-income families are higher birth order, low maternal education, and single-parent homes. The cumulative effect of these and other risk factors accounts for the developmental delays seen in many of these children. Other possible social and family risk factors for LI may include

- Maternal anxiety and mental health problems,
- Maternal authoritarian childrearing practices,
- Poor mother-child interactions,
- Lack of maternal education,
- Head of the household's semiskilled or unskilled occupation,
- Minority ethnic status,
- Absent father,
- Stressful life events, and
- Large family size.

It should be obvious to you that some factors, such as education and occupation, are related. These factors, plus low socioeconomic status (LSES), can result in poor language development.

In general, children from LSES families hear and use less language than their middle-SES (MSES) peers. By the time children begin school, the child from an LSES family has heard only one-fourth the words of the MSES child. Children living in homeless shelters hear even fewer. As you know from your language development course, quality input is vital.

Early identification is important to ensure that these children are placed in appropriate EI programs to minimize or eliminate the effects of accumulated risk. Given the strong effect of these environmental factors, intervention focused on the child within her or his family is crucial to improving both the life conditions and educational and communicative outcomes for children in poverty.

MALTREATMENT/NEGLECT, FETAL ALCOHOL SPECTRUM DISORDER, AND PRENATAL COCAINE EXPOSURE

There is a clear interaction between language delays and the factors of caregiver maltreatment/neglect or fetal alcohol spectrum disorder (FASD) and early drug exposure (Hernandez, 2004; Hooper, Roberts, Zeisel, & Poe, 2003). As a result, SLPs are working with an increasing population of young children who have experienced maltreatment/neglect, FASD, drug exposure, or all three (Sokol, Delaney-Black, & Nordstrom, 2003). Language development is the primary EI concern with these children (Rogers-Adkinson & Rinaldi, 2006).

Maltreatment/Neglect

Maltreatment is "the physical and mental injury, sexual abuse, negligent treatment, or maltreatment of a child under the age of 18 . . . perpetrated by a person who is responsible for the child's welfare under circumstances which indicate that the child's health or welfare is harmed or threatened" (Keeping Children and Families Safe Act of 2003,

P.L. 108-36). Childhood neglect is a failure to provide for the basic needs of a child. Parental substance abuse is a contributing factor in a third to two-thirds of substantiated reports of child maltreatment and neglect.

Although the United States spends more money fighting child abuse than any other country, it has the highest rate of child abuse in the industrialized world (Lindsey, 2003). Legislation on the issue includes the following:

■ Child Abuse Prevention and Treatment Act (CAPTA) of 1974 mandated reporting of abuse and neglect and broadened focus of the child welfare system to include financial support for children in poverty and training and services for families to prevent further abuse or neglect.

■ Child Abuse Prevention and Enforcement Act (CAPEA, 2000) strengthened the public response to child maltreatment through child protection systems.

■ Keeping Children and Families Safe Act of 2003, P.L. 108-36 reauthorized, amended, and improved CAPTA. The law places greater emphasis on infants who experience abuse and neglect, are infected with or exposed to human immunodeficiency virus (HIV), have a life-threatening illness, or have been perinatally exposed to a dangerous drug.

Children in immigrant families are more than twice as likely as those from native-born families to experience multiple risk factors critical to their development, including exposure to violence and neglect (Jaycox, Zoellner, & Foa, 2002). In these families, maltreatment and neglect may stem from poverty, stress, and cultural differences. Childrearing practices are culturally based, and families may have varying views regarding the use and extent of punishment.

Communication development. A meta-analysis found that maltreated children exhibit consistently poorer language skills in receptive vocabulary and both receptive and expressive language (Lum, Powell, Timms, & Snow, 2015). There is a direct relationship between the amount of language input a child receives and the amount of language a child produces. Very socially depriving circumstances will affect language development negatively. In addition, some children who experience extreme deprivation show behaviors, such as rocking, self-injury, and atypical sensory interests, that are more characteristic of ASD although the underlying causes are distinctly dissimilar (Beckett et al., 2002; Fombonne, 2003a; Rutter, Kreppner, & O'Connor, 2001). For some children who have experienced extreme mistreatment or neglect, these behaviors may serve a self-soothing or adaptation function.

In some cases child protective proceedings (CPPs) may be brought by a state or local government agency to protect an allegedly abused or neglected dependent child. Families may temporarily lose parental rights, and the child may be placed in foster care or some other alternative setting. In these cases, the court typically sets conditions for eventual reunification. Permanent foster care or adoption is the least preferred option by the courts.

Although young children raised in a severely depriving environment have poor language skills, placement in an environmentally richer foster care situation has a positive effect on both their expressive and receptive language skills (Windsor, Glaze, & Koga, 2007). Even much of the delay associated with early institutionalization can be resolved when the environmental circumstances are altered. Change in children is not immediate, and even those in foster care for 12 months or more have smaller core vocabularies and shorter utterances at 30 months of age than their TD peers living with biological parents (Devescovi et al., 2005; Marchman, Martínez-Sussmann, & Dale, 2004).

Fetal Alcohol Spectrum Disorder

For some children, maltreatment begins in utero when they are exposed to the negative impact of maternal alcohol use. In these cases, a child may experience fetal alcohol spectrum disorder (FASD), a condition resulting from prenatal exposure to alcohol because of maternal alcoholism or heavy drinking, including episodic or "binge" drinking during pregnancy.

FASD includes a range of disorders that can occur in an infant whose mother drank alcohol during pregnancy, including fetal alcohol effects (FAE), alcohol-related neurodevelopmental disorder, alcohol-related birth defects, and the more severe fetal alcohol syndrome (FAS) (Wattendorf & Muenke, 2005). Each year, approximately 40,000 infants are born with FASD, costing the United States approximately $6 billion (U.S. Department of Health and Human Services, 2008). At least 2,000 of these children experience severe medical concerns (Braillion & DuBois, 2005). The sad fact is that these problems are preventable.

Diagnosis of FASD is based on

- Growth retardation below the 10th percentile for weight, height, or head circumference;
- Facial characteristics, including absent or indistinct philtrum (groove in the upper lip), thinned upper lip, and shortened eye openings or increased space between the eyes;
- Damage to the central nervous system (CNS), manifested as DD, ID, cognitive or behavioral problems, or a combination; and
- Evidence of maternal drinking during pregnancy.

Children with severe cases of FASD may be identified at birth if they experience alcohol withdrawal or if they have pronounced facial distortion and microcephaly, a small head circumference indicating a small brain (Chen, Maier, Parnell, & West, 2004).

Early intervention is key to reducing the impact of FASD (Loocke, Conry, Cook, Chudley, & Rosales, 2005). Unfortunately, children born with less apparent cases of FASD may not be identified until they attend school.

Prenatal Cocaine Exposure

Children with prenatal cocaine exposure (PCE) are often exposed to multiple drugs in utero, including alcohol, tobacco, and marijuana. PCE disrupts those regions of the brain associated with dopamine responses, adversely affecting cognitive processes such as sustained attention and auditory processing skills (Harvey, 2004). In addition, children with PCE have a decrease in the volume of white and gray matter, which also affects brain function (Dow-Edwards et al., 2006). Many PCE infants are preterm or have low birth weight.

Mothers who use drugs may not provide adequate stimulation to their infant (Mansoor et al., 2012; Minnes, Singer, Arendt, Farkas, & Kirchner, 2005; Siefer et al., 2004; Uhlhorn, Messinger, & Bauer, 2005). In addition to a mother's drug-seeking lifestyle, other adverse factors affecting language development may include low education level, poor verbal skills, depression, psychosocial distress, and single parenting. A variety of factors associated with poverty, such as environmental toxins, homelessness, and violence, also may negatively affect a child's development of language (Singer et al., 2008).

The effects of PCE on language development vary with age because of changing language demands. In infancy, PCE seems to have a direct effect on sensorineural processing (Anday, Cohen, Kelley, & Leitner, 1989). Infants with PCE overreact to stimuli, startle more with auditory stimuli, and habituate more slowly than infants with no cocaine exposure (NCE) (Potter, Zelazo, Stack, & Papageorgiou, 2000). PCE appears to have a direct effect on sensorineural processing by decreasing the speed of processing of auditory information (Anday et al., 1989).

At age one, children with PCE exhibit lower auditory comprehension than their peers with NCE (Singer et al., 2001). Studies with preschool children have reported mixed results, with some finding no LI while others report both receptive and expressive deficits. The majority of studies, however, found that PCE adversely affected language development. These negative effects seem to be stable across the preschool and early school-age years (Lewis et al., 2007; Morrow et al., 2003). All aspects of language may be affected (Bland-Stewart, Seymour, Beeghly, &. Frank, 1998; Madison, Johnson, Seikel, Arnold, & Schultheis, 1998; Malakoff, Mayes, Schottenfeld, & Howell, 1999; Mentis & Lundgren, 1995). Because this text deals with young children, we won't discuss the studies of older children except to say that LI and poor language abilities persist through childhood but vary with age, birth weight, gender, and amount of exposure in utero (Bandstra et al., 2011; Beeghly et al., 2006; Lewis et al., 2011; Lewis et al., 2013). Deficits in sustained attention and behavioral self-regulation persist (Ackerman, Riggins, & Black, 2010).

PRETERM AND LOW BIRTH WEIGHT INFANTS

Many of you were preterm or low birth weight. Like you, most very premature infants grow up to be normal, healthy children and adults. That said, they represent a significant portion of at-risk infants and toddlers as well.

Preterm Birth

The rate of preterm births in the United States is a growing public health problem that has significant consequences for families and costs U.S. society at least $26 billion a year (Tanne, 2006). Most neonatal or newborn deaths occur among preterm infants. In addition, preterm birth is an important risk factor for neurological impairment and disability (Tucker & McGuire, 2004).

Although treatment of preterm infants in a neonatal intensive care unit (NICU) or special care nursery (SCN) can greatly improve their survival, these infants remain vulnerable to many complications, including possible death. Long-term problems may include cerebral palsy, intellectual disabilities, visual and hearing impairments, behavior and social-emotional problems, learning difficulties, and poor health and growth.

In general, the more immature a preterm infant, the greater the need for life support, the longer the stay in a NICU/SCN, and the more likely the infant is to require rehospitalization. It is estimated that the economic burden associated with preterm birth in the United States is approximately $51,600 per infant (National Academy of Sciences, 2013). Nearly two-thirds of this cost, or $33,200 per preterm infant, is for medical care. In addition, maternal delivery costs are approximately $3,800 per preterm birth, and initial early intervention services costs are estimated to be $1,200 per infant annually. Special education services add another $2,200 annually to the cost of educating a child. Finally, the annual lost household and labor market productivity associated with preterm birth disabilities are estimated to be $11,200 per family with a preterm infant (National Academy of Sciences, 2013).

Most pregnancies last 37 to 42 weeks, and babies born during this window are called full term. Preterm labor refers to contractions that begin to open the cervix, the muscular ring closing off the uterus, before week 37. Preterm birth is the delivery of a baby before 37 completed weeks of gestation. Eighty-four percent of preterm infants are born between 32 and 37 weeks of gestation. About 10 percent are born between 28 and 31 weeks and are labeled very preterm, while only 6 percent, called extremely premature, are born prior to 28 weeks of gestation.

Most mortality and morbidity affects very preterm and extremely preterm infants. Morbidity is illness or disability. Although all preterm babies are at risk for health problems, those born before 32 weeks of gestation face the highest risk. These infants are very small, and their organs are very immature. Fortunately, advances in obstetrics and neonatology, the branch of pediatrics concerned with newborns, have improved the chances of survival.

The age of viability, or the age at which a fetus can survive outside the womb, varies internationally and changes with medical advances but at present is somewhere around 21–22 weeks in the United States. Although survival is possible for babies born as early as 22 to 27 weeks, most likely these children will face a lifetime of health problems.

Premature infants are often small and medically fragile. Usually, they are minimally responsive and require long periods of rest.

> Children born extremely preterm require a herculean medical effort to survive. As you can imagine, this effort takes an emotional toll on the family. To investigate further, you might wish to watch this video.
> https://www.youtube.com/watch?v=qwYmCm7Qnek

Prevalence. Over the past 20–30 years, the prevalence of preterm birth in most developed countries has been about 5 to 7 percent of live births (Tucker & McGuire, 2004). Until recently, the incidence in the United States has been about 11 to 12 percent (Figure 2.2). Although the overall rate of premature birth has increased by more than 30 percent since

FIGURE 2.2 **Preterm Births as a Percentage of Live Births in the United States, 1990–2014.**

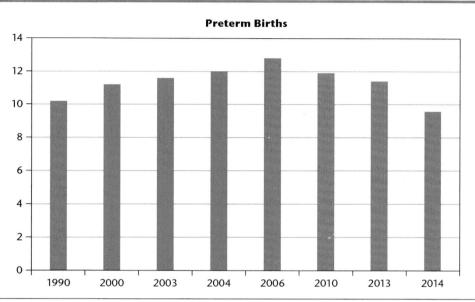

Source: Information from childstats.gov, 2015.

1981, the rate of birth before 32 weeks' gestation has remained almost unchanged. (See Table 2.5)

Several factors have contributed to the overall rise in the prevalence of preterm birth in the United States. These include increasing rates of multiple births; greater use of assisted reproduction techniques, such as in vitro fertilization; and more obstetric intervention, such as the increased use of caesarian section (Tucker & McGuire, 2004). In part, the rise may also reflect two other factors. First, ultrasonography, rather than the previously used date of the last menstrual period, is increasingly used to estimate gestational age more accurately. Second, the low gestational age cutoff, or the age used to distinguish preterm birth from spontaneous abortion, has varied by country and changed over time, making accurate comparisons difficult.

In the United States, the highest rates for preterm births are among African American women, and the lowest are among Asian or Pacific Islanders (National Academy of Sciences,

TABLE 2.5 **Percentage of Preterm Births in United States**

		GESTATIONAL AGE		
YEAR	OVERALL	34–36 WEEKS	32–33 WEEKS	LESS THAN 32 WEEKS
1990	10.62	7.3	1.4	1.92
1995	10.49	7.68	1.42	1.84
2000	11.64	8.22	1.49	1.93
2006	12.81	9.15	1.62	2.04
2012	11.54	8.13	1.49	1.92

Source: U.S. Department of Health and Human Services, Health Resources and Services Administration, Maternal and Child Health Bureau. (2013). *Child Health USA 2013.* Rockville, MD: U.S. Department of Health and Human Services.

2013). For example, in 2013, the rate for African American women was 17.8 percent, while the rates were 10.5 and 11.5 percent for Asian/Pacific Islander women and white women, respectively. These disparities cannot be fully explained by differences in socioeconomic conditions.

Infants who are the most preterm generally require the greatest attention. Many families find the experience to be an emotional roller coaster that is extremely difficult for parents.

A stay in the NICU/SCN. Initially, a preterm infant is kept in the NICU/SCN on an open warmer, a bed that keeps the baby warm by heating the surrounding air. Open warmers are used for infants who need a lot of care so that they can be reached more easily. Once the infant's breathing rate is stabilized, the infant is usually placed in an isolette, an enclosed plastic incubator with controlled air temperature. In general, infants grow faster if they are kept warm because they use less energy in *homeostasis*, or regulation of body temperature. When the infant weighs about 4 pounds and if there are no serious complicating factors, he or she is placed in an open crib.

All infants are attached to a heart and respiratory monitor. An alarm sounds if there is a significant change in the baby's heart or breathing rate. A pulse oximeter records the oxygen level in the infant's blood. The preterm infant's world, as illustrated in Figure 2.3, is not a pretty one.

Caring for a preterm neonate is a team effort. Team members may include the following:

- Neonatologist, a pediatrician specialized in the care of preterm infants
- Nurses who deliver most of the hands-on care

FIGURE 2.3 **Preterm Infant's World**

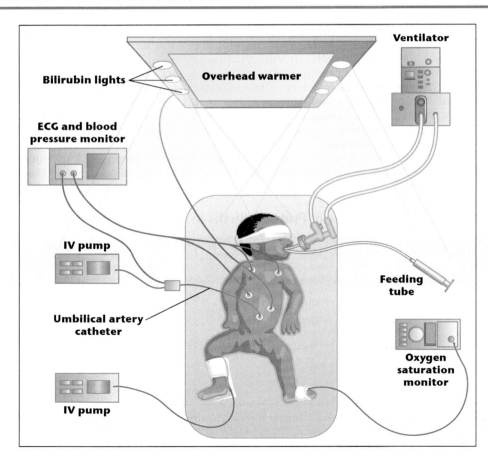

- Respiratory therapist who oversees the breathing needs of infants who receive oxygen or are on ventilators
- Occupational or physical therapist who evaluates the infant's developmental progress and plans a motor development program
- SLP who helps with early parent-child interaction and helps the family transition to home, where the SLP may be the primary contact person
- Social worker who helps families deal with the emotional stress

Low Birth Weight Infants

Although birth weight and gestational age are positively related, they are not interchangeable. The categories for low birth weight (LBW) are:

- Low birth weight: below 2,500 gm or 5.5 lb
- Very low birth weight: below 1,500 gm or 3.3 lb
- Extremely low birth weight: below 500 gm or 1.1 lb

According to the United Nations Children's Fund and World Health Organization (2004), 15.5 percent of all live births are of children with some type of LBW. In general, the prevalence of low birth weight is much higher in developing countries (16%) than in developed countries (7%). I was a low birth weight infant. Maybe you were too.

Approximately two-thirds of low birth weight infants are also preterm. Full-term infants may be of low birth weight or "small for gestational age," usually defined as below the 10th percentile, or among the lowest 1 in 10 babies by birth weight. Average weights and lengths for infants are presented in Table 2.6. Infants may also be small for gestational age as a result of *intrauterine growth restriction* (IUGR). Neonatal problems related to IUGR include

- Fetal distress;
- Meconium aspiration syndrome, or taking a stool into the lungs while in utero or during birthing;
- Hypoglycemia, or low blood sugar;
- Polycythemia, or overproduction of red blood cells, which can lead to coronary problems and blood clots;
- Hyperviscosity, or an increase in blood serum, which can lead to spontaneous bleeding;
- Hypothermia, or low body temperature; and
- Perinatal death.

Fetal growth restriction is the second leading cause of perinatal morbidity and mortality, with prematurity being the first. The prevalence of IUGR is estimated to be approximately 5 percent in infants.

There are two types of IUGR: asymmetric, in which the head develops at a typical pace; and symmetric, in which all parts of the fetus are restricted in growth. Symmetrical IUGR is the more serious condition because of the effect on the developing brain.

TABLE 2.6 **Newborn Infants' Weight and Length (Average)**

Age in Weeks	Length (cm)	Weight (Kg)	Head Circumference (cm)
Birth	50	3.5	34
10	55	4.5	38
20	63	6	41
30	70	7.5	45

Causes of Preterm Birth

Approximately 70 percent of preterm births are a result of spontaneous labor, either by itself or following spontaneous premature rupture of the membranes (PROM) of the amniotic sac in which the fetus resides while in utero (Goldenberg, Culhane, Iams, & Romero, 2008). PROM may be triggered by the mother's body's natural response to certain infections of the amniotic fluid and fetal membranes. The mother's use of tobacco also appears to be a factor in increased risk of PROM (Mercer et al., 2000).

The remaining 30 percent of preterm births result from early induction of labor or cesarean delivery because of pregnancy complications or health problems in the mother or the fetus (Iams, 2003). In most of these cases, early delivery is probably the safest approach for both mother and baby. Risk of neonatal death, defined as death at birth or within the first 27 days, is significantly reduced for infants delivered through cesarean section at 22 to 25 weeks of gestation compared to those delivered naturally (Malloy, 2008).

Preterm labor is now thought to be initiated by multiple mechanisms. Causes of early delivery may be spontaneous, related to multiple births, or caused by other conditions such as preterm rupture of the membrane holding the fetus, cervical difficulties, or high blood pressure associated with pregnancy. Early labor may also be induced or result from cesarean section in cases of concern for maternal or fetal health. In about 40 percent of all cases of preterm birth, the cause is unknown. The most important predictors of spontaneous preterm delivery are poor socioeconomic status and a history of preterm birth. The risk in women with a previous preterm delivery ranges from 15 percent to greater than 50 percent, and risk increases with the number of previous preterm births, especially when the gestational age of previous deliveries is low (Mercer et al., 1999). Women with previous preterm deliveries have a 2.5 times greater risk of a premature birth in their next pregnancy.

Any woman can deliver prematurely, but as noted previously, some women are at greater risk than others. In the United States, African American women are three to four times more likely to have a very early preterm birth than women from other racial or ethnic groups.

Lifestyle factors also may put a woman at greater risk for preterm labor (March of Dimes, 2007; National Academy of Sciences, 2013). These include

- Late or no prenatal care
- Smoking, drinking alcohol, or using illegal drugs. Tobacco use doubles the risk of preterm birth (Goldenberg, Culhane, Iams, & Romero, 2008). Both nicotine and carbon monoxide are associated with placental damage and decreased uteroplacental blood flow.
- Low (teen pregnancy) and high maternal ages
- Single marital status
- Domestic violence (including physical, sexual, or emotional abuse) or extremely high levels of stress, especially during pregnancy
- Lack of social support
- Long working hours with long periods of standing. Working long hours and undertaking hard physical labor under stressful conditions are probably associated with an increase in preterm birth among women from low socioeconomic groups.
- Low socioeconomic status (Smith, Draper, Manktelow, Dorling, & Field, 2007; Thompson, Irgens, Rasmussen, & Daltveit, 2006)

The relationship between these maternal demographic characteristics and preterm birth are unknown, although several of the factors may overlap. For example, poor women are more likely to lack good prenatal care and to work long hours. In the United States prior to the Affordable Care Act (also known as Obamacare), lack of health insurance was also a factor.

In addition, medical and health conditions during pregnancy also may increase preterm labor and delivery (March of Dimes, 2007; National Academy of Sciences, 2013); see Figure 2.4. However, women with one or more of these risk factors do not always have preterm infants. Conversely, only half the women who have preterm labor have a known risk factor.

FIGURE 2.4 **Medical and Health Conditions during Pregnancy That May Increase Preterm Labor and Delivery**

Persistent or recurrent intrauterine infections (including urinary tract, vaginal, sexually transmitted, and possibly other infections) account for 25 to 40 of preterm births and probably account for many repetitive incidents (Goldenberg et al., 2006; Goldenberg, Hauth, & Andrews, 2000).

Preexisting or pregnancy-related high blood pressure

Diabetes

Blood clotting disorders (thrombophilia)

Being underweight before pregnancy

Being greatly overweight. Obese women are more likely to develop *preeclampsia* and diabetes and to have infants with congenital anomalies (Goldenberg, Culhane, Iams, & Romero, 2008). Preeclampsia is maternal high blood pressure during pregnancy.

Short time period between pregnancies (less than six to nine months between birth and the beginning of the next pregnancy). It may take time for the uterus to return to its normal state. In addition, the mother may experience depletion of essential vitamins, minerals, and amino acids needed during pregnancy because of the short interval available to replenish these nutrients (Conde-Agudelo, Rosas-Bermudez, & Kafury-Goeta, 2006; Goldenberg, Culhane, Iams, & Romero, 2008).

Being pregnant with a single fetus after in vitro fertilization (Jackson, Gibson, Wu, & Croughan, 2004)

Multifetal pregnancy. Although multiple gestations account for only 2 to 3 percent of infants, they account for 15 to 25 percent of all preterm births. Nearly all higher multiple gestations will result in preterm delivery. Uterine overdistension is believed to be the cause (Romero, Espinoza, & Kusanovic, 2006). The incidence of multiple pregnancies in developed countries has increased over the past 30 years due primarily to increased use of assisted reproduction techniques, such as drugs that induce ovulation and in vitro fertilization. In the United States, the birth rate of twins has increased by 55 percent since 1980 while the rate of higher order multiple births increased fourfold, although this rate has decreased considerably since 1998.

Birth defects in the infant

Vaginal bleeding. The principal causes are either *placental abruption*, in which the placental lining separates from the uterine wall, or *placenta previa*, in which the placenta has attached to the uterine wall close to or covering the cervix, the narrow opening between the uterus to the vagina.

Sources: March of Dimes, 2007; National Academy of Sciences, 2013.

The interaction of factors that contribute to preterm birth is complicated. For example, mothers who smoke cigarettes are twice as likely as nonsmoking mothers to deliver before 32 weeks of gestation. Although prenatal smoking cessation programs can lower the prevalence of preterm birth, women from poorer socioeconomic backgrounds are least likely to stop smoking during pregnancy, further increasing their already elevated risk of preterm delivery. Interestingly, other interventions, such as better prenatal care, dietary advice, or increased social support during pregnancy, do not improve perinatal or postdelivery outcomes or reduce the social inequalities in the prevalence of preterm delivery.

Reducing the Risk

A woman may be able to reduce her risk for preterm delivery by receiving early and regular prenatal care. A preconception visit is especially important for women with chronic disorders, such as diabetes and high blood pressure. When potential problems are identified early and treated, it helps to reduce the risk for preterm birth. In addition, a woman can reduce her risk by reaching a healthy weight before becoming pregnant and by gaining only the recommended amount of weight (25 to 35 pounds) during pregnancy (American College of Obstetricians and Gynecologists, 2005).

Other possible ways to nurture a healthy, full-term pregnancy include (National Academy of Sciences, 2013):

- Eating healthy foods with increased amounts of folic acid, calcium, iron, protein, and other essential nutrients
- Managing chronic conditions such as diabetes and high blood pressure
- Following guidelines for healthy activity
- Avoiding smoking, alcohol, and recreational drugs, as well as some over-the-counter medications
- Avoiding sexual activity if there are complications, such as vaginal bleeding or problems with your cervix or placenta
- Limiting stress
- Taking care of your teeth, because gum disease may be associated with preterm birth

Physicians may also prescribe progesterone to reduce the risk of a subsequent preterm delivery in women who have previously had a premature baby and are currently pregnant with a single fetus (Meis et al., 2003). In addition, when a doctor suspects that a woman may deliver preterm, he or she may suggest treatment with corticosteroid drugs to speed maturation of fetal lungs and significantly reduce the risk of related neonatal complications, necrotizing enterocolitis (explained later), infection, and infant death (Roberts & Dalziel, 2006). Treatment is most effective when administered at least 24 hours before delivery.

Neonatal Complications

A number of complications are more likely in premature than full-term babies, especially during the first weeks. These complications include respiratory, circulatory, immunological, and feeding and digestive problems and range from mild to severe (Bromberger & Permanente, 2004; March of Dimes, 2007). Let's look briefly at each.

Respiratory problems. Approximately 70 percent of babies born before 34 weeks of gestation have some type of respiratory difficulty. The primary respiratory complications are neonatal respiratory distress syndrome (RDS), apnea, and chronic lung disease, called bronchopulmonary dysplasia (BPD). Each will be discussed in the following paragraphs.

Respiratory Distress Syndrome. About 23,000 babies a year, primarily those born before the 28th week of gestation, suffer from neonatal RDS (Martin et al., 2003). Neonatal RDS occurs in infants whose lungs are not yet fully developed and is primarily caused by lack of surfactant, a slippery substance that keeps the air sacs from collapsing and helps the lungs inflate as the chest cavity expands. You'll remember from your anatomy and physiology classes that the lungs are not connected to the chest cavity but are kept in contact through the surfactant.

Although the symptoms of RDS usually appear within minutes of birth, in some infants they may not occur for several hours. Symptoms may include a bluish color to the skin and mucus membranes, brief stoppage of breathing, and struggling breathing. For children with darker skin tone, the bluish tint may be evident in the palms, soles of the feet, flesh below the finger- or toenails, or the oral cavity. If a physician suspects that an infant has RDS, he or she will request a lung x-ray and blood tests to confirm the diagnosis.

Treatment usually includes delivering artificial surfactant directly to the infant's lungs and giving the infant warm, moist oxygen. A technique called continuous positive airway pressure (CPAP) delivers slightly pressurized air through the nose and can help keep the airways open. Although CPAP helps an infant breathe, it does not breathe for the child. In the most severe cases, infants may temporarily need the help of a respirator. Infants with RDS also need careful fluid management and monitoring to reduce the chances of infections.

The infant's condition often worsens for two to four days and then slowly improves. Complications may include

- Bleeding in the brain, called intraventricular hemorrhage,
- Bronchopulmonary dysplasia,
- Retinopathy and blindness,
- Blood clots, and
- Developmental delays and disorders.

Long-term complications may occur as a result of

- Oxygen toxicity,
- High-pressured oxygen being delivered to the lungs,
- Severity of the RDS, and
- Oxygen deprivation to the brain and other organs.

A small number of children may experience chronic bronchiolar inflammation, which can lead to collapse of the trachea. In these cases, the child may need a *tracheostomy*. Other infants with airway obstructions may also require this procedure. A tracheostomy is a surgically created opening through anterior portion of the neck into the trachea to enable direct access. A tube is then placed through this opening to provide an airway for breathing. Even in cases in which the tube is later removed and breathing is restored, problems in sound production may persist, delaying the onset of spoken language.

Apnea. When an infant stops breathing for 20 seconds or more, he or she may have apnea, the most common problem in premature neonates (Finer, Higgins, Kattwinkel, & Martin, 2006). The more immature the infant, the higher is the risk. While 25 percent of neonates weighing less than 2,500 grams, or 5.5 pounds, at birth experience some apnea, the condition is found in 84 percent of neonates weighing less than 1,000 grams or 2.2 pounds.

Apnea results from immaturity and/or depression of the central respiratory drive in the brain, located in the medulla and adjacent areas in the brainstem (Darnall, Ariagno, & Kinney, 2006). Infants with apnea have immature brainstem function, characterized by incompletely organized and interconnected respiratory neurons.

The diagnosis for apnea is one of exclusion because many diseases mirror the symptoms. When the other diseases have been ruled out, the physician is left with a diagnosis of apnea. A physical examination includes

- Monitoring the infant's cardiac, neurologic, and respiratory status,
- Observing the infant for signs of breathing difficulty, and
- Measuring heart rate, blood pressure, and pulse pressure for characteristic changes during an apneic episode.

If a related cause can be identified, such as either bacterial infection, called *sepsis*, or seizures, then medical treatment addresses the cause.

A variety of medications may be used to stimulate breathing efforts. In addition, either a device called a nasal cannula or CPAP may be used to provide extra oxygen and stimulate breathing. Sometimes an infant is placed on a respirator temporarily. During an apneic episode, a nurse in the NICU/SCN may stimulate breathing by patting the infant or touching the soles of her or his feet. Tactile stimulation is usually sufficient to terminate an isolated apneic event.

Bronchopulmonary Dysplasia. Many very preterm infants develop chronic lung disease, or bronchopulmonary dysplasia (BPD). BPD is clinically defined as oxygen dependence involving abnormal development of lung tissue—more specifically, inflammation and scarring in the lungs. Along with asthma and cystic fibrosis, BPD is one of the most common chronic lung diseases in children. Somewhere between 5,000 and 10,000 cases of BPD occur annually in the United States.

As you might have guessed, children with extremely low birth weight or extreme prematurity are most at risk. Most cases occur in preterm infants, usually those born at

30 weeks gestation or before and weighing less than 3.3 lb or 1,500 gm. Among premature and low birth weight infants, white males seem to be at greatest risk for developing BPD.

As the survival rate for RDS has improved, there has been a corresponding increase in the prevalence of BPD. You'll recall that one intervention for RDS is CPAP, which supplies necessary oxygen under pressure to the lungs of preterm infants. Sometimes, in order for these infants to survive, the amount of oxygen given must be at a higher concentration than in the air we breathe. Over time, the pressure from the ventilation and excess oxygen intake can injure a new-born's lungs. If symptoms of RDS persist to 28 postnatal days, then the condition will be considered BPD. The scarring and lung damage characteristic of BPD can be seen on an x-ray. BPD can also arise from other conditions, such as lung trauma, pneumonia, and other infections.

Although most infants eventually outgrow the more serious symptoms, BPD, in combination with other complications, can result in death. Infants with severe BPD remain at high risk for pulmonary infections and asthma during the first two years of life, requiring medical intervention. Advances in technology, such as use of prenatal glucocorticosteroids, early surfactant therapy, and gentler ventilation for infants with RDS, along with improved understanding of neonatal physiology, have lessened the overall impact of BPD among preterm infants.

Treatment attempts to support the breathing and oxygen needs, to help infants heal, and to enable them to develop in as typical a manner as possible. No current medical treatment can immediately cure BPD.

Circulatory problems. Preterm or low birth weight neonatal circulatory problems may include intraventricular hemorrhage (IVH), patent ductus arteriosis (PDA), retinopathy of prematurity (ROP), anemia, and jaundice.

Intraventricular Hemorrhage. IVH is the most common variety of neonatal intracranial or brain hemorrhage. Bleeding may occur anywhere in the brain, and most episodes are mild and resolve themselves with no or few lasting problems. In severe IVH, the fluid-filled structures in the brain called ventricles expand rapidly, causing pressure on the brain that can lead to brain damage. Fortunately, the prevalence of IVH has declined and the number of premature infants who survive IVH has increased because of improvements in obstetric care and in neonatal respiratory and fluid management, but long-term problems may persist for the child.

The bleeding usually occurs in the first three days of life. Fifty percent of IVHs occur in first 24 hours, and 90 percent in the first 72 hours. The prevalence of IVH in very low birth weight infants (<1,500 gm) or infants of less than 35 weeks' gestation is approximately 12 to 18 percent.

Diagnosis is confirmed using cranial sonography, CT scan, or some other imaging technique. The American Academy of Neurology suggests that all infants younger than 30 weeks gestational age be screened by cranial sonography at 7–14 days of postnatal life. If bleeding occurs, ultrasounds or sonographs are used to identify signs of possible complications. Consequences of IVH may include hydrocephalus from fluid in the ventricles, cerebral palsy, seizures, and developmental disability.

Medical care for IVH includes treating the underlying related factors as well as cardiovascular, respiratory, and neurological support. For fluid in the ventricles, surgeons may insert a tube, called a *shunt*, into the brain to drain the fluid, reducing the risk of brain damage. In milder cases, drugs sometimes can reduce fluid buildup.

Patent Ductus Arteriosis. Patent ductus arteriosis (PDA) is a congenital heart defect common in premature infants. In PDA, there is an abnormal circulation of blood between two major arteries near the heart. Because the fetus gets its oxygen through the placenta while in utero, a large arterial opening called the ductus arteriosus allows blood to bypass the lungs.

As a typical infant begins to breathe, the lungs release bradykinin, a chemical that constricts the ductus arteriosus until it closes, beginning within a few hours after birth and usually complete within the first few weeks of life. The closing of the ductus arteriosus enables blood to travel from the right side of the heart to the lungs via the pulmonary artery, pick up oxygen, return to the heart's left side, and pass into the rest of the circulatory system, much of it passing through the aorta. Premature children are more likely to be *hypoxic*, meaning too little oxygen reaches the lungs to produce sufficient levels of bradykinin to close the ductus arteriosis.

When the ductus arteriosus remains open (patent), blood flows directly from the aorta into the pulmonary artery, putting a strain on the heart and increasing the blood

FIGURE 2.5 **Typical Cardiac Blood Flow Compared to Patent Ductus Arteriosus (PDA)**

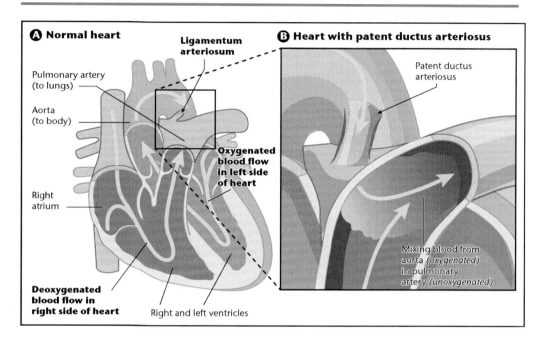

pressure in the lung arteries. Figure 2.5 presents typical blood flow and the flow associated with PDA.

The symptoms of a PDA depend on the size of the opening and the health of the infant's heart. The typical child with PDA is asymptomatic. It's important to remember that PDA doesn't occur in isolation. A preterm infant is likely to have problems related to immaturity of the lungs themselves. In addition to shortness of breath, PDA symptoms include increased work needed to breathe, which in turn burns more calories and may interfere with feeding, resulting in poor weight gain. If the ductus arteriosis remains open, the infant has a risk of developing heart failure, bleeding in the lungs, problems with lung development, or infection of the inner lining of the heart, called *infective endocarditis* (Neish, 2006).

About 3,000 infants are diagnosed with PDA each year in the United States. Although more common in premature infants, PDA does occur in some full-term infants. PDA is twice as common in girls as in boys (Neish, 2006). Infants with genetic disorders such as Down syndrome and those whose mothers were exposed to rubella, or German measles, during pregnancy are also at higher risk (Zipes, Libby, Bonow, & Braunwald, 2007).

The turbulent blood flow accompanying PDA causes a characteristic heart murmur that is heard on physical exam. PDA can be diagnosed definitively by a chest x-ray and a specialized form of ultrasound called *echocardiography* or by other imaging techniques.

If symptoms of PDA are not severe, a physician may decide to wait rather than intervene surgically (Zahaka & Patel, 2002). Should PDA persist beyond 28 days, it will most likely not close on its own. In neonates, medication may be given to constrict the muscle in the wall of the ductus arteriosus and promote closure. If the medications do not work, corrective surgery can be performed and the PDA tied off.

Retinopathy of Prematurity. Retinopathy of prematurity (ROP) is an abnormal growth of blood vessels in the eye. Most cases are mild and heal themselves with little or no vision loss.

When an infant is born, it passes from the uterus, a low-oxygen dark place, into a world of oxygen and light. The eye responds to these changes by growing extra blood vessels in the retina or back of the eye. This blood vessel growth begins around 6 weeks after birth, usually increases until 10 to 12 weeks after birth, and then begins to decline.

ROP occurs mainly in babies born before 32 weeks and can lead to vision loss. Every baby who is born at a gestational age less than 28 weeks will have some retinopathy. The more preterm the baby, the more sensitive the retina. If the blood vessels grow too much, they may cause the retina to separate from the back of the eye, resulting in severe problems with vision or even blindness.

Every infant born more than 8 weeks preterm will be examined by an ophthalmologist. These exams continue until the blood vessels decrease. If growth continues or causes problems, the condition may be treated with either a laser or freezing, called cryosurgery, to prevent separation of the retina from the back of the eye.

Anemia. Nearly every preterm infant becomes anemic during the first 2 months of life, which means they do not have enough red blood cells. Normally, a fetus stores iron during the later months of pregnancy and uses it to manufacture red blood cells. Infants born preterm may not have had enough time to store iron.

A neonate loses blood through frequent blood tests and through the normal process of red blood cell replacement. Babies with anemia tend to develop feeding problems and grow more slowly. In addition, anemia can worsen any existing heart or breathing problems.

Most infants who are sick or weigh less than 3 pounds at birth, will need a blood transfusion to keep the blood count normal and/or extra iron in their diet to aid their bodies in making new red blood cells. In addition, anemic infants may be given medication to increase red blood cell production.

Jaundice. Preterm infants are more likely than full-term infants to develop jaundice because their immature livers cannot effectively remove bilirubin from the blood. In addition, premature infants may be more sensitive to the ill effects of bilirubin excess. Bilirubin is a natural product that results from the breakdown of hemoglobin, a protein in red blood cells that carries oxygen.

Babies with jaundice have a yellowish color to their skin and eyes. Usually, jaundice is mild and not harmful, but if the bilirubin level gets too high, it can cause brain damage.

Blood tests will indicate when bilirubin levels are too high. When this occurs, the infant is treated with special lights in a process called phototherapy that helps the infant's body eliminate bilirubin. Occasionally, an infant will need a blood transfusion.

Immunological problems. Neonatal immunological problems can lead to many forms of infection. When an infant is born, it leaves the protective world of the mother's immune system and must begin to build its own immunity. Preterm infants have immature immune systems that are inefficient at fighting off bacteria, viruses, and organisms that cause infection. Serious infections commonly seen in premature infants include pneumonia, or lung infection; blood infection, or sepsis; and meningitis, an infection of the membranes surrounding the brain and spinal cord.

The early signs of infection are often subtle and may include increasing incidents of apnea, changes in breathing behavior, and poor feeding or poor digestion. Diagnosis is confirmed by laboratory tests, and the infection will usually be treated with antibiotics.

Feeding and digestive problems. Preterm infants may experience difficulty feeding and serious digestive problems. All infants lose weight during the first days of life as their bodies eliminate extra fluids and struggle with new demands. Once an infant begins to receive nutrition either intravenously or via nursing or bottle feeding, it will begin to gain weight slowly. Preterm or low birth weight babies may take several weeks just to regain their birth weight.

Preterm or small infants are not able to suck and swallow until they reach approximately 32 weeks of gestational age. Even then, some infants will be too weak or will tire quickly when trying to suck. In addition, all babies need to learn the difficult task of coordinating sucking, swallowing, and breathing. This takes time and practice with many feedings.

The way for preterm infants to overcome many of the problems associated with prematurity is to grow and mature, and this is accomplished through feeding, digestion, and nutrition. At first a preterm infant may be too weak or too immature or experiencing too much difficulty breathing to nurse or be bottle fed effectively.

The preterm infant will be given intravenous (IV) fluids immediately after delivery. The IV fluid contains a sugar solution for immediate baby energy.

Total parenteral nutrition (TPN) is a method of feeding that bypasses the gastrointestinal tract with infants who cannot feed by mouth. A necessity for very small or very fragile infants, TPN contains a mixture of fluids, electrolytes, calories, amino acids, vitamins, minerals, and fats. Blood and urine tests help alert the medical staff to needed dietary adjustments.

Usually, an IV line is placed into a vein in the infant's hand, foot, or scalp. An alternative is an umbilical vein in the navel area (Behrman, 2004). Because their veins are very small and thin and can break down quickly, if an infant requires long-term high concentrations of nutrients, an IV called a *peripherally inserted central catheter* (PICC) is inserted into larger veins located centrally in a baby's body. Sometimes it is necessary to place a central line in a neck or groin vein surgically.

TPN is not without risk, and the infant's levels of blood sugars, fats, and electrolytes must be monitored carefully. Problems can develop if the TPN or IV lines become dislodged or clogged. The use of IVs can also result in serious blood infections or blood clots. In addition, prolonged use of TPN may lead to liver problems (American Society for Parenteral and Enteral Nutrition, 2002). As an infant matures, TPN is gradually decreased and mouth feeding increased. Very small premature babies often need several weeks of TPN before they are ready for oral milk feedings.

An infant who is too small and weak to suck but able to digest milk may have a tube passed through the mouth or nose to allow milk to drip directly into the stomach or intestine by gravity. Very small babies may be fed small amounts continuously so their stomachs never overfill. A feeding tube called a nasojejunal tube can also be passed through the nose and stomach and into the intestine allowing feeding without filling the stomach.

A preterm or low birth weight infant's digestive system is immature and doesn't work very well initially. The amount of milk a baby is fed is usually increased very slowly.

Breast milk has the advantages of being easily digested and of protecting an infant against infection because of the mother's immune system. Unfortunately, breast-feeding requires stronger sucking than bottle feeding. Mother's milk, collected by a breast pump, may be fortified with extra protein and calories and fed to an infant by bottle or other means. In some cases, formulas for preterm infants or special formulas for infants with allergies or immature digestive systems may be used. As an infant grows stronger and bigger, breast-feeding becomes easier.

Necrotizing enterocolitis (NEC) is a serious and potentially dangerous intestinal problem found in some preterm infants. As the name suggests, the disorder is characterized by temporary or permanent *necrosis*, or death, of intestinal tissue. Usually occurring two to three weeks after birth, NEC can lead to feeding difficulties, abdominal swelling, and other complications. Although NEC affects the gastrointestinal tract, in severe cases it can damage multiple organ systems.

The most common gastrointestinal medical/surgical emergency occurring in neonates, NEC prevalence rates range from 0.3 to 2.4 cases per 1,000 live births in the United States. The disorder affects nearly 10 percent of infants who weigh less than 1,500 grams, with mortality rates of 50 percent or more depending on severity (Springer & Annibale, 2007).

The exact etiology of NEC is unknown, but outbreaks seem to follow an epidemic pattern within SCNs, suggesting an infectious agent. To date, a specific organism has not been isolated.

If NEC is suspected, x-rays of the baby's intestines are taken, feedings are stopped, and the baby is given antibiotics. If the diagnosis is confirmed, antibiotic treatment continues and the baby is not fed for as long as 10 days. Sometimes surgery is necessary to remove damaged sections of the intestine. Once an infant has begun to recover, it is fed intravenously until such time as it can either begin or return to oral liquid feedings.

TRANSITIONING TO HOME

Infants mature at different rates and hospitals have differing discharge criteria but in general, a preterm or low birth weight baby is released when several conditions are met:

- Can maintain its temperature in an open crib,
- Can take all feedings orally from the bottle or breast, and
- Has been free of apnea for a week.

Even then, a special needs infant may require special adaptive equipment to thrive.

For many parents, transitioning from the hospital to home is extremely stressful. Some parents will feel overwhelmed by their potential responsibility, and if the child has obvious problems, the parents and family will be in various stages of adjustment, ranging from denial to acceptance.

An infant may require more frequent feedings or have special nutritional needs. In addition, some babies may be especially susceptible to various infections. For example, as you might assume, infants with chronic lung disease may be very susceptible to upper respiratory infections. In addition, many children will have chronic otitis media.

My grandson, whom I have mentioned previously, had extreme acid reflux, which often made him cranky and irritable, and he slept for only short intervals. The acid reflux made feeding difficult, and he was only comfortable in certain positions. His arching of his back to ease the pain from reflux only exacerbated his tendency to go into an extension pattern from his cerebral palsy.

Premature infants may require special attention outside the home during their first year of life (Bromberger & Permanente, 2004), including

- Follow-up by a pediatrician to monitor weight gain and development,
- Childhood immunizations to protect against infection,
- Neurodevelopmental monitoring and checking for signs of developmental problems,
- Check-ups of vision and hearing for retinopathy and infant hearing loss, respectively, and
- Visits to and by physical and/or occupational therapists and SLPs.

In addition, specialists, such as the SLP, may make home visits to begin early intervention, or the child may go to an infant stimulation program.

Outcomes for Preterm and/or Low Birth Weight Infants

The increasing survival rates of children who are born very preterm is accompanied by greater risk of neurological disabilities and cognitive dysfunction. Although fewer than 1 percent of babies in this country are born at less than 28 weeks, these infants have the most complications. Overall prognosis remains poor. In general, outcomes improve with increasing gestational age, although for any given length of gestation, survival varies with birth weight (Tucker & McGuire, 2004). Other factors, such as ethnicity and gender also affect survival and the risk of neurological impairment.

Approximately 80 percent of infants born at 26 weeks and 90 percent of those at 27 weeks survive to 1 year. Unfortunately, about a quarter of these infants develop serious lasting disabilities, and up to half may have milder problems, such as learning and behavioral difficulties (American College of Obstetricians and Gynecologists, 2002). Interestingly, although preterm and low birth weight children are at risk for more cognitive difficulties, such as learning disabilities and intellectual disability, they are not at an increased risk for *specific language impairment* (SLI), especially when their test scores are adjusted for prematurity (Resnick et al., 1998; Rice, Spitz, & O'Brien, 1999; Tomblin, Smith, & Zhang, 1997). You'll recall from other courses or reading that SLI is characterized by late language emergence (LLE) related to working memory deficits.

At age 5 years, 49 percent of children born at 24–28 weeks of gestation, or extremely preterm, have some disability. In absolute numbers, however, more children born at 28–32 weeks, or very preterm, have disabilities although the overall percentage (36%) is lower (Larroque et al., 2008). Cerebral palsy is present in 9 percent of all children born very preterm, and 32 percent are intellectually disabled. In the very preterm group, 5 percent have severe disability, 9 percent moderate, and 25 percent mild disability. Special health care/ education resources are used by 42 percent of children born at 24–28 weeks and 31 percent of those born at 28–32 weeks, compared to only 16 percent of those born full term.

Although babies born at 28–32 weeks have survival rates of 95 percent and are less likely than infants born earlier to develop serious disabilities, they remain at increased risk for learning and behavioral problems. Late preterm infants, 33–36 weeks, are usually healthier than babies born earlier, and they are nearly as likely as full-term infants to survive. Although late preterm babies are unlikely to develop serious disabilities resulting from premature birth, they may still be at increased risk for subtle learning and behavioral problems (Raju, Higgins, Stark, & Leveno, 2006).

The outcome for preterm infants of multiple pregnancies, such as twins or triplets, can be better than for singleton births of the same length gestation. Because preterm multiple births are more likely to be the result of spontaneous preterm labor, the frequency of adverse factors, such as severe intrauterine growth restriction, placental abruption, and fetal or maternal infection, is lower than for preterm singles.

Communication Development

As mentioned, most preterm and low birth weight infants develop typically, but for those with extended stays in the NICU/SCN or with disabilities development may be more challenging. Early parental interaction may be disrupted, affecting early turn-taking, game-playing, and sound-making.

In part, early word acquisition is fostered by a child's ability to pair sounds with referents, something that begins within the first months of life as children attend to both sights and sounds simultaneously. Preterm children born at 32–36 weeks have a delay in their sensitivity to this pairing, which may account for later delays in word learning (Gogate, Maganti, & Perenyi, 2014).

A child who experiences language delay because of preterm birth or low birth weight may regain lost ground in this area, just as many do in other areas of development. Other disabilities or undiagnosed conditions may hinder this catch-up. Despite the potential for developmental delays and disorders, 8- to 10-year-old children born at 32 weeks or later or 1,500 grams or higher, while scoring significantly lower that TD children on standardized language tests, are, as a group, still within the normal range. In addition, no significant differences are found in language sample data (Smith, DeThorne, Logan, Channell, & Petrill, 2014). It is important to keep in mind, however, that these children are not extremely preterm or low birth weight.

Early Identifying Signs and Behaviors

Early identification of possible health or developmental problems is extremely important. Typically, the identification of a young child's developmental deficits occurs gradually over time as the child's delays become evident. This usually occurs when the infant or toddler fails to meet milestones of typical development. The family often reports an initial concern when their child is 7–8 months of age (Bailey et al., 2005). Unfortunately, in the typical scenario, the child is referred for EI services nearly seven months later.

Obviously, there is great variability. Infants with syndromes with well-known physical characteristics, such as Down syndrome, and some motor disorders are detected at birth. Other impairments may take much longer to be identified. Sadly, there are income disparities, and children from low-income families are identified significantly later than their middle-income peers (Mandell, Listerud, Levy, & Pino-Martin, 2002). For children without an established risk, the most common reason for referral for EI services is failure to acquire first words (ASHA, 2006). Given that first words occur around 12 months of age, parents and other health care providers may not become concerned until the child is 18 or even 24 months old. By that time, we are already two years behind the problem.

When identification begins shortly after birth and continues with regular visits to the pediatrician, EI may begin very early in a child's life. The first signs of a potential difficulty may occur shortly after delivery.

 Given the importance of the Apgar score, watch this video to explore what it is.

APGAR, AN INFANT'S FIRST EXAM

The Apgar is a score given to a newborn by a physician or nurse at one and five minutes after delivery. The total score of 0–10, based on a 0–2 score in each of five different categories, is a quick means of assessing a newborn's general status and adaptability to extrauterine life. If there are concerns, indicated by successive low scores or a drop in the second score, a third may also be given. A decreasing score at times two and three may indicate that an infant was

TABLE 2.7 **Apgar Scoring**

The child is rated in each category and given a score from 0 to 2. The scores for all five categories are totaled for an overall Apgar score of 0–10.

CATEGORY	SCORE = 0	SCORE = 1	SCORE = 2
Color	Blue, pale	Extremities blue while rest of body completely pink or other skin tone	Completely pink or other skin tone
Heart rate	Absent	Below 100	Over 100
Respiratory effort	Absent	Weak, irregular	Good, crying
Muscle tone	Limp	Some flexion of extremities	Active motion
Reflex irritability (catheter in nostrils)	None	Grimace	Cough/sneeze

initially fine but is experiencing increasing distress. The criteria for scoring are presented in Table 2.7. At-risk neonates will be examined further and their development and health monitored.

Although efforts have been made to correlate the Apgar score with future development, there are no long-term data. Low scores do not inevitably signal significant developmental problems in the future, but do suggest significant distress during labor and delivery that warrant close observation of the infant.

This said, children scoring below the 10th percentile on language development measures at 18 months seem to have had lower Apgar scores at birth (Marschik, Einspieler, Garzarolli, & Prechtl, 2007). Percentile is rank or order, so the 10th percentile represents 10 from the bottom in a theoretical group of 100 children.

Conclusion

A developmental epidemiological approach can inform prevention efforts with young children. *Developmental epidemiology* is a medical term for seeking to untangle the entwined trajectories of symptoms, environment, and individual development. More specifically, developmental epidemiology involves following defined groups of individuals, such as children with ID, through stages of life to determine early antecedents and developmental paths.

Evidence from research studies identifies specific antecedent risk factors as predictive of later developmental patterns. Through developmental epidemiology, professionals hope to be able to identify children at birth who are most at risk for a future developmental disability. Although we don't use the term *epidemiology* in the field of speech-language pathology, many SLP researchers are engaged in the search for antecedents that indicate the presence of ASD or other disorders in very young children. Early identification means the EI services can begin at a younger age.

Although infants and toddlers are largely dependent on adults to recognize and initiate treatment for their difficulties, these adults may not recognize early indicators of a disability. Failure in early identification may mean that a child does not receive treatment until her or his problems become obvious.

Within child-focused services, such as speech and language pathology, intervention programs need to consider strategies for reducing the effects of identified risk factors. This means that if you decide to work in an EI setting, you will also need to be actively involved in advocating for strong and widespread maternal health and education and neonatal screening programs as well as the availability of EI services.

 Click here to gauge your understanding of the concepts in this chapter.

3

A Model for Early Communication Intervention

Ideally, our knowledge of both development and evidence-based practice (EBP), plus the evolving child-parent interaction of individual clients, influences how we shape ECI services. In the next few pages, I'll try to provide a brief rationale and some reasoning for how this can be accomplished. This chapter frames the discussion in the rest of the text, so we'll discuss it all in more detail in subsequent chapters. First we'll discuss a model for ECI based on EBP and on legal requirements and regulations discussed in Chapter 1. Then we'll turn to the content and strategies we might employ and the role of the environment. Finally, after a discussion of the role of the SLP, we'll look at an example of an ECI program.

ECI is not one size fits all. Successful family-centered and caregiver-implemented intervention must be based on caregiver decision-making. We, as SLPs, can empower caregivers to make decisions about the outcomes and the activities and routines to be used for intervention. With our help, caregivers can decide when, where, how, and with whom intervention strategies will be used.

The Evolving Model of ECI Service Delivery

The goal of many but not all of the few existing ECI programs in the early 1970s was to develop an extensive receptive and expressive spoken vocabulary for use in communicating. Note that the emphasis is on spoken symbols or words and belatedly on the use of these symbols to communicate. This is where I began my professional life.

At the time, linguistics was still locked in a debate between *behaviorists*, who characterized language-learning as similar to other types of learning, and *structuralists*, who characterized language-learning as rule-learning that was not subject to behavioral principles of modeling, imitation, and reinforcement. Primarily because behavioral techniques had been used for at least two decades to teach self-help and other skills to individuals with intellectual disability (ID), early programs with nonsymbolic children adopted the same procedures to teach language.

Teaching was often accomplished in isolated teaching situations using very behavioral methods of stimulus-response. Unfortunately, many children, especially those with severe disabilities, did not automatically generalize from these very structured methods to everyday use. For example, vocabulary was often taught within a naming or answering function, in response to cues such as "What's this?" and responses such as "Good talking."

As mentioned, there is no one approach for all children and families. Behavioral models are still with us and work well with some children. For example, the Picture Exchange Communication System, or PECS, used primarily with children with autism spectrum disorder (ASD), initially begins with structured identification of pictures and builds to requesting using those pictures. Ideally, PECS' representations are used in more functional communication.

Unfortunately, responses learned in those early 1970s behavioral approaches for teaching communication did not naturally carry over to more functional communication forms, such as declaring and commenting. It became evident that while some progress was made, vocabulary items needed to be trained for more than a single communicative function or purpose and for more than response to a specific cue.

In the meantime, developmental data began to strongly suggest a social pragmatic theory of typical language acquisition that could be used in intervention with young children (Carpenter & Tomasello, 2000; Tomasello, 2001). According to such a model, language skills emerge out of a child's nonverbal understanding of the world. Such understanding develops during multiple shared social experiences in which a child's and a partner's attention are jointly focused on events or objects. These periods of joint attention were especially important as a framework within which a child experiences language.

More importantly, linguists began to recognize that words are acquired to fulfill the intentions previously expressed nonverbally, primarily through gestures. Children use single words to express a variety of early intentions. It was reasonable to assume, therefore, that intervention should focus on nonverbal strategies for communication as the initial step in training verbal communication.

It seemed, and still seems, logical that subsequent intervention should focus on mapping symbolic forms of communication onto these prelinguistic functions or intentions.

For children with developmental disabilities, communication in the form of gestures, such as reaching and pointing, and facial expressions, eye gaze, body movements, and vocalizations can signal intentions as varied as seeking notice, requesting, or rejecting.

If we target these intentions, it was reasoned, intervention would become *functional*, fulfilling the child's need for communication while at the same time building on communication uses already in place. In addition, the motivation for learning symbols would be embedded in the preexisting uses these symbols served. For example, if a child can request using gestures, the requesting intention is already in place, so words such as *cookie* and *juice* can be "grafted" onto this function.

FUNCTIONAL COMMUNICATION

The use of symbols or actions to express basic wants and needs and to obtain desired outcomes is called functional communication. In other words, the communication "works" or functions for a child to accomplish her or his goals, often through the mediation of a listener or communication partner, typically a parent. This approach has also been called *environmental* and *ecological* and has been shown in various permutations to be effective in communication training with young children (Fey et al., 2006; Hancock & Kaiser, 2002; Kaiser & Delaney, 2001; Kaiser, Hancock, & Neitfield, 2000; Smith, Warren, Yoder, & Feurer, 2004; Yoder & Warren, 2002).

Initial intervention may focus on requesting or rejecting objects or actions using vocalizations or gestures. Later intervention targets other intentional communication, such as commenting or requesting information, and the use of symbols to express existing intentions.

When, as sometimes happens, a child's nonsymbolic behaviors are socially unacceptable (such as screaming or hitting), socially stigmatizing (such as taking an adult to the water fountain and then just standing there), or difficult to interpret, the SLP often attempts to modify these behaviors into other, more conventional ones. Change is justified because use of such forms can limit both communication and the number of potential partners and may result in communicative breakdown (Brady & Halle, 2002). Note, however, that the behavior is targeted for change but the intention is retained.

It's important for SLPs to consult and work closely with a child's family to determine if a nonsymbolic form of communication is acceptable and effective. If so, it should be strengthened and encouraged. If not, such as hitting when desiring a toy or food, the SLP and family should examine acceptable modifications.

To be effective communicators, children need to learn to initiate communication and to respond to others in acceptable ways and to recognize and repair breakdowns. A child's communication is greatly affected by the ways in which caregivers interact with him or her. Children whose caregivers respond frequently to their communication attempts have better language than those whose family members are not as responsive (Rollins, 2003). As mentioned throughout this text, parent-child or caregiver-child interaction is also a focus of intervention efforts.

A transactional model of typical communication and language development, in which the parent and child are both contributing partners, is widely accepted and suggests a functional model for intervention. Attention to both parent and child factors is more effective than focusing solely on a child's behaviors in isolation. A child's nonsymbolic communication reveals the child's ability both to acquire language and to elicit parental language-facilitating responses. In ECI, if we target both child nonsymbolic communication behaviors and parental responses to these behaviors, then we should be able to facilitate a child's language development.

In contrast, direct language instruction may be of limited value for a nonsymbolic child who does not possess the cognitive and social skills needed. It is better with these children to enhance nonsymbolic communication and build the motivation for later language-learning through the uses of language for communication. Parents can be trained in the use of language-facilitating responses to these child communication behaviors. Data indicate that the frequency of nonsymbolic communication behavior in a child with developmental disability (DD) predicts later language development (Calandrella & Wilcox, 2000).

GENERALIZATION

In the ideal situation, intervention attempts to facilitate an individual's ability to respond across many situations. That's called *generalization*, or carryover. Generalization of both child and caregiver behaviors across contexts can be enhanced through (Kashinath, 2006)

- Sufficient exemplars,
- Common stimuli, and
- General case programming.

These three strategies are interrelated. Training *sufficient exemplars* means extending intervention to several different situations or involving different individuals. For example, the word or sign *juice* can be used to request at home with Mom and also to comment or seek confirmation ("Juice?") with the preschool teacher.

Common stimuli, such a toys, food, or everyday items, can occur in several contexts. Beginning with the assessment, parents are encouraged to recommend their child's favorite toys and everyday items. Our goal is for communication occurring in the home to be demonstrated in the evaluative setting. In intervention, the SLP and family target these items for the very reason that they occur frequently.

Finally, general case programming incorporates aspects of the other two. General case programming uses strategies, such as caregiver cuing and responding, and the selection and sequencing of teaching to build generalized responding across contexts. There are five steps in implementing general case teaching (Kashinath, 2006):

- Identify all possible contexts in which a child will be able to perform the skill being taught. For example, a request for assistance, such as signing "Help," can be used to open a juice carton, to put on boots, and to obtain an out-of-reach toy. Ideally, contexts for use of the behavior being taught would be relatively diverse, including snack time, dressing, and bathing, and also include a variety of play routines preferred by the child and family.
- Select teaching and test contexts that include the range of possible situations.
- Sequence teaching examples from easy to more difficult, and teach general use before more specific. For example, requesting "Cookie" when a cookie is before a child may be easier than requesting one shut away in a cabinet. Likewise, responding to "What do you want?" is easier for a child than initiating a request on her own, especially if the desired item is out of view.
- Teach within the identified contexts using a variety of strategies. Ideally, teaching occurs in the locations in which the behavior is routinely seen or would be expected to occur. Embedding intervention in daily activities or routines is part of an ecological systems perspective that views the activities and settings of family life as contexts within which learning opportunities happen naturally.
- Test or monitor in new or untrained contexts to make sure generalization occurs.

In all three generalization strategies—training sufficient exemplars, programming common stimuli, and general case programming—instructional opportunities are embedded in activities in which a child is expected to use the learned behavior subsequent to intervention. By embedding intervention in use environments, we can facilitate generalization.

These approaches presume that an SLP and caregiver will collaborate in identifying possible contexts within which the child has a need to perform the behaviors being taught. For example, if a child is being taught to comment about the environment, the SLP attempts with the help of the caregiver to identify situations in which this communication behavior might occur in the home, in the early intervention (EI) classroom or daycare setting, and on outings. Shared features across contexts, such as the way in which care providers cue and prompt the child, must be identified and included in the intervention plan. As much as possible, instruction is then embedded within these contexts.

To promote generalization, the SLP can embed intervention in daily routines by

- Selecting teaching routines with each parent-child/caregiver-child dyad that are simple and representative of the situation in which the teaching strategy is to be used, and

- Embedding intervention within multiple daily routines to facilitate parents' and caregivers' use of teaching strategies across different routines (Kashinath, 2006).

Incorporating these two components will help promote generalization of both the parent strategies and child learning.

Artificially created, one-to-one structured teaching situations within a center-based EI program are rare occurrences in the typical daily lives of families of children with disabilities. Even when such programs are optimally responsive and sensitive to a child's needs and abilities, they do not represent the typical life of the family. As much as possible, intervention ideally focuses on assisting caregivers to facilitate a child's communication within daily routines and activities rather than in more formal teaching situations that do not occur naturally (Mobayed, Collins, Strangis, Schuster, & Hemmeter, 2000; Woods, Kashinath, & Goldstein, 2004). Intervention that occurs throughout the day in natural settings also decreases parental stress and results in greater gains in child communication than intervention requiring designated time periods of one-on-one work with children (Koegel, 2000).

A note of clarification is in order here. My comments on naturally occurring teaching situations are not meant to totally dismiss the value of more formal training. Some children may benefit from more formal teaching situations, especially when new skills are being introduced, but it is crucial that the newly learned skill be placed within an environmental context in order for it to "work" for the child.

FAMILY-CENTERED INTERVENTION

Home-based intervention programs have been used successfully with children with varying disorders and with their parents. For example, preschool and early school-age children with Angelman's syndrome (Angelman, 1965), a rare genetic disorder found in 1 in 10,000 live births and characterized by severe intellectual disability, have been taught to use gestures through home-based intervention using parents as agents of change (Calculator, 2002). All training took place in the home at times parents cited as most productive and least disruptive of the family routine.

A family's daily routines and activities are unique, creating specific interactions that shape a child's development. In general, routines, such as feeding and bathing, are an important part of everyday family life and an ongoing natural learning environment.

When identifying routines to use for intervention, a family can select anything that the parent and child often do together (Weitzman, 2005). Such routines offer parents and caregivers a naturally occurring and supportive framework within which they can use specific teaching strategies that facilitate their child's development (McWilliam, 2000). Embedding intervention within daily routines is also consistent with current educational practices and legal requirements that services be provided in the least restrictive environment (LRE), mentioned in Chapter 1.

A routine can be of the frequent, daily type, such as diaper changing and feeding; game-playing; or a repetitive activity of a parent's choosing. In general, routines have four components (Weitzman, 2005):

- Purposeful or theme-based
- Predictable, with frequently repeated serial steps
- Shared and interactive
- Having clearly defined roles that are sometimes interchangeable

The repetitive nature of routines makes them an ideal way to foster early interactions and initial communication.

INDIVIDUALIZATION

Of course, the efficacy of your intervention will vary as a result of several factors. One important aspect of intervention is the contextual fit between a caregiver's current strategy, a child's communication goal, and an identified routine. Instead of teaching all caregivers the same teaching strategies, an SLP and caregiver select specific teaching strategies for each caregiver-child dyad and the specific needs of the child (Kashinath, 2006).

Children with different personalities and etiologies respond differently to intervention. For example, children with Down syndrome (DS) have communication and language skills that are delayed in comparison to their mental ages. On the other hand, many young children with other forms of ID tend to have communication and language ages similar to their mental ages. As a consequence, children with DS often encounter more obstacles in acquiring communication and language than do other children with similar severities of ID.

CONCLUSION

That was a lot of information! Hopefully, you are now getting some idea of why ECI can be a challenging but rewarding task for an SLP. Your professional fulfillment comes in crafting an intervention plan that fits each child and family and seeing that plan succeed. This is not the last time we'll refer to the information you've just read. It will be the basis for what follows in the rest of the text. Like any good intervention, we'll build one step at a time.

In the following sections, we'll discuss several issues that help define the overall ECI approach with nonsymbolic and minimally symbolic children. These include program content, intervention strategies, and the role of caregivers and professionals. At the end of the chapter, we'll look at an example of an EI program into which we might place our ECI model.

 The evolving model of EI and ECI contrasts with earlier models of intervention. Explore that contrast by watching this video.
https://www.youtube.com/watch?v=OpxGC6G0HMY

Content for Improving Communication

As with the overall approach just discussed, the content of early communication programs has also changed over the last several decades, reflecting the changing demographics of the population served and philosophical and practical changes. Initially, during the 1950s, programs for older nonspeaking individuals primarily consisted of language stimulation. Mature language was used in the belief that both children and adults who were nonspeaking just needed more examples of language. Under the influence of behaviorism, the emphasis changed to actually teaching language to be used in spoken communication. In this bottom-up approach, symbols were taught and then combined into longer utterances through imitation.

As educational mandates changed and deinstitutionalization occurred in large residential centers for those with severe and profound ID, more and more low-functioning individuals began being served. At about the same time, due to advances in prenatal and neonatal care, there was an increase in the number of infants and toddlers with handicapping conditions. Unfortunately, many of these individuals were unsuccessful in acquiring language through the behavioral methods in vogue at the time.

In the 1970s, SLPs began to target presymbolic skills in the hope that nonspeaking individuals could be taught the prerequisites needed to acquire language. For example, we might teach visual and auditory attending, physical imitation, object permanence, and symbolic play. This approach was complicated by the lack of research on exactly which prelinguistic skills were essential.

At this point, beginning in the late 1970s, several factors came together to change yet again the ways in which professionals viewed intervention with nonsymbolic children.

- Communication professionals began to focus on a child's current nonsymbolic communication, reasoning that intervention should build on the communication already in place.
- Legal requirements mandated that children receive intervention services from birth.
- Sociolinguists emphasized the importance of early communication for the later development of language and speech. Increasingly, professionals recognized the extensive communication system that exists for infants and mothers prior to development of symbolic communication.

■ Augmentative and alternative communication (AAC) techniques and equipment promised that increasing numbers of individuals would be able to acquire useful and meaningful communication as a complement to or supplement for spoken language. For many nonsymbolic individuals, AAC was used to establish an initial communication system.

These changes have brought us to the current state, reflected in this text, in which SLPs and other professionals work within a child and family's de facto communication system, expanding and extending a young child's communication attempts. Presymbolic communication provides an important foundation for development of symbolic communication or language (Brady, Marquis, Fleming, & McLean, 2004; Brady, Steeples, & Fleming, 2005; Calandrella & Wilcox, 2000; Iverson & Goldin-Meadow, 2005; Smith, Mirenda, & Zaidman-Zait, 2007; Watt, Wetherby, & Shumway, 2006).

Today, we still rely on teaching prelinguistic skills but not as an established curriculum. Instead, teaching these skills is a fallback position when a child seems to be experiencing difficulty communicating. Emphasis has shifted to early communication.

Let's look at how this process might work. For example, assume that as an SLP you are working with a child who vocalizes spontaneously, trying to get the child to incorporate these sounds into gestural communication already used by the child. Your goal is simultaneous gestural and vocal communication. Because the vocalizations occur randomly, you might decide to use imitation to increase the likelihood of the vocalizations' being produced when the child gestures. Notice that the goal is still functional communication, not imitation for its own sake. As the SLP, I would not elect to teach imitation to every child at this point unless it is warranted to move communication forward. That's the key. Prelinguistic skills are only taught as an assist for moving communication skills forward.

You might opt first to teach physical imitation, such as clapping hands, to establish the notion of using others as a model. Physical imitation is theoretically easier to teach than vocal imitation because the behaviors can be shaped through hand-over-hand physical prompts. Physical imitation is not a communication goal per se but a prerequisite behavior. Physical imitation is a means to the end of better communication. Once the child is imitating reliably, emphasis can shift to vocal imitation and we return to the original communication goal.

The focus of intervention, as discussed in the next several chapters, will be on improving a child's communication in the form and clarity of the message and in early child meanings. What we have termed presymbolic skills will be trained as needed to help advance the primary goal of improved communication.

Intervention Strategies

Very young children do not respond well to either formal or group instruction. For this reason, we will try to minimize the use of both in intervention. Instead, our emphasis will be on incidental teaching or intervention in the situational context in which communication occurs or has the potential to occur. While this model is somewhat disconcerting for SLPs who prefer to have more control, it is more ecologically sound, more natural, and easier once the SLP and parents determine techniques that work with the individual child in question. Let's look at an example.

Suppose that a child relies on vocalizations and gestures to request desired objects even though he can say a few single word approximations in imitation. Let's further assume that the words are *cookie, juice, ball,* and *car*. During the day, the parent, SLP, and other caregivers can manipulate the environment so that there are several times when the child is in a situation to request these objects naturally, such as meals and play times. In these situations, the child is prompted to imitate the word along with the gesture in order to complete the request. Verbalizations can be increased by parceling out food in small bits of cookie or sips of juice and awaiting requests for the ball or toy car before each is pushed back to the child. Vocalizations will not be accepted for any object for which the child has a word.

For the adults in this situation, the uncertainty is that we have no way of guaranteeing that the child will request these items. The adults have less control than they might have in a more formal instruction situation. This said, whenever a vocal or gestural request does occur, the adults will all respond in a similar fashion. The result is that the input for the child is consistent, although the adults must be ready at all times to prompt the required behavior. Once the adults have learned how to respond, however, this technique can be used with other words and other requests as the child's repertoire increases. In this way, the teaching is very flexible and can be adapted to any situation.

Specific strategies with promise fall into one of three general groups: responsive, directive, and blended (ASHA, 2008b). As we look briefly at each, you'll notice some overlap. We'll just mention these approaches here and expand on the methods used in Chapter 6.

RESPONSIVE INTERACTION STRATEGIES

Responsive interaction approaches typically include models of the target communication behavior without an obligation for the child to respond. They include

- Following a child's lead,
- Responding to a child's initiations, both verbal and nonverbal, with natural consequences,
- Extending a child's topic,
- Engaging in self-talk and parallel talk,
- Providing meaningful feedback, and
- Expanding the child's utterances with models slightly in advance of the child's current ability within typical and developmentally appropriate routines and activities.

I'll explain each of these strategies in subsequent chapters. For now, just know that responding with expansion to slightly more mature utterances is the most powerful because the adult response immediately connects the child's communication to more mature communication that serves the same purpose. For example, a child's single-word utterances can be expanded into two-word utterances. If a child says "Juice," the adult might expand into "Want juice" or "Spill juice" if it is appropriate to the situation.

DIRECTIVE INTERACTION STRATEGIES

Directive interaction strategies include several teaching strategies possibly best represented by behavioral principles. I'll explain these too in Chapter 6, but for now behavioral teaching strategies manipulate antecedents and consequences that surround the desired behavior. Another way to say this is that adults will alter cues and prompts in a systematic way to elicit the behavior and also manipulate what follows the behavior to give corrective feedback and to strengthen the desired response while weakening others. For example, the adult might hold a cookie in front of the child and ask, "What do you want?" If the child says "Cookie," the adult can give the child the cookie and verbally respond in a positive way. Notice that this method is adult manipulated and controlled.

BLENDED STRATEGIES

Blended approaches, which go by names as varied as naturalistic, contemporary behavioral, or hybrid intervention approaches, have evolved from the observation that more structured behavioral strategies frequently fail to generalize to more functional and interactive environments. Blended strategies are the approaches we've been discussing in this chapter. They include teaching in natural environments using strategies for modeling language and responding to children's communication that derive from typical mother-child interactions.

Role of a Child's Environment

Even though I might work with a child during home visits or in a childcare or EI center, my ability to affect that child's communication development is limited by the amount of time I can spend with the child relative to that of other caregivers and peers in the child's life.

These others are essential allies who, with training and monitoring, can become effective language facilitators.

A child's ability to function within the family is a strong predictor of both current overall functioning and future development. In order to function effectively, a child must interact with family members in a mutually rewarding manner. Together, the family, SLP, and other team members can make collaborative decisions regarding the design, content, and intervention methods for a child's ECI services and supports.

FAMILY-CENTERED SERVICES

The EI term *family-centered*, discussed in Chapter 1, refers to a set of beliefs, values, principles, and practices that support and strengthen a family's ability to enhance a child's development and learning (Boone & Crais, 2001; Dunst, 2001, 2004; Polmanteer & Turbiville, 2000). Families provide a lifelong context for a child's development. Individualization of services includes aligning services with each family's unique characteristics.

The family, rather than the individual child, is the primary recipient of ECI services, and the extent of a family's involvement is a family choice. Some may desire a family-focused in-home approach while others opt for either a more child-centered or center-based approach. Ideally, family-centered practices offer more active roles for families in the planning, implementing, interpreting, and decision-making of service delivery.

It is important to stress at this point that for cultural reasons, some families may opt for a program focused exclusively on the child. Their cultural beliefs may view all types of impairment as residing primarily in the affected person, or they may see family-centered intervention as suggesting that the parents are somehow deficient in their child-rearing. Other factors may include cultural notions of the role of children and the nature of disability.

Effective ECI practices are based on a model of child development that assumes the acquisition of communication occurs within a familial, social, and cultural framework. Within this context, intervention is based on (Roth & Baden, 2001; Sandall, Hemmeter, Smith, & McLean, 2005)

- Real everyday experiences,
- Caregiver-child interaction,
- Family concerns, and
- An individual child's age, development, cognitive level, learning style, strengths, and interests.

In this way, ECI promotes communication for young children through social interactions. This type of authentic learning has the potential to maximize children's acquisition of functional communication and promote generalization to natural, everyday contexts (Roper & Dunst, 2003).

Natural environments extend beyond a child's home and include settings where a child and family would typically be present (ASHA, 2008b). These include family centers, such as a local YMCA or community recreation programs; childcare centers; favorite family outings and parks; and family activities such as food shopping or attending a church, mosque, or temple. These family-identified community settings and activities are a potentially important source of learning (Dunst et al., 2001; Dunst, Hamby, Trivette, Raab, & Bruder, 2000).

What works with one family may not work for another. It's important, therefore, for an SLP to let the family identify what it considers to be frequent activities and routines.

While it may seem obvious, embedding intervention in daily routines is based on the assumption that the child is able to participate. This is essential because (Wilcox & Woods, 2011)

- Children must be able to participate to learn,
- Learning increases participation in daily activities, and
- Caregivers can mediate teaching and their child's learning as it occurs.

An emphasis on daily activities and routines naturally requires the use of flexible and adaptable strategies as individualized situations occur. Naturalistic intervention strategies can include (Hancock & Kaiser, 2006):

- Environmental arrangement to provide opportunities for communicating with familiar toys and everyday objects,
- Child initiation encouragement and following a child's attentional focus and interest,
- Promotion of requests by interspersing preferred and nonpreferred activities/ routines,
- Choice offerings and encouragement of choice-making,
- Use of natural reinforcers,
- Use of expectant waiting or time delays,
- Use of contingent imitation, and
- Structured predictability and turn-taking within the activity.

These strategies can be embedded in predictable activities and provide multiple opportunities for intervention while not interfering with that activity or routine. We'll discuss how to accomplish each of these in later chapters.

When intervention is begun early in life, several issues need to be considered. First, families are still coming to terms with their young child's disability and often seek a broad variety of interventions to help their child. These interventions may include seeking out highly publicized programs or attempting to use multiple types of speech-language therapy. Second, a family will be taking on a primary role in ECI in addition to their other, often overwhelming, parenting responsibilities. Fulfilling this primary interventionist role may require external supports.

Language use environments ideally extend beyond the immediate family. Let's discuss a rationale for a family-centered model and three groups of potential ECI partners: parents, childcare providers, and peers.

A RATIONALE FOR THE FAMILY SERVICE MODEL

Within the last few decades, the makeup of the American family has changed considerably. Today, SLPs serve children from traditional two-parent families, single-parent families, extended families, adopted and foster care families, and those with parents of the same gender, plus children living with other relatives such as grandparents. According to U.S. Census Bureau population estimates, there are approximately 75,000,000 children under the age of 18 in the United States (U.S. Census Bureau, 2013). Of these, 39 percent are considered to be children of color, including African Americans, Latinos, Native Americans, Asian Americans, and those of two or more races or identified as other than white non-Latino. Understanding these and other influences that shape children is a key factor in developing collaborative interventions.

Two theories, *family systems theory* and *ecological theory*, can help us understand why as SLPs we are interested in the entire family and not just the child with a communication impairment (Rogers-Adkinson & Stuart, 2007). Let's visit each briefly, and then we'll come back to working with families.

Family Systems Theory

The family systems theory, introduced by Bowen (1978), suggests that individuals, such as children, cannot be understood in isolation. Rather, we need to consider an individual as part of an emotional unit, known as the family.

Families are systems of interconnected and interdependent individuals in which each member has a role to play and rules to follow. Members respond to each other according to their role, which is determined by unspoken relationship agreements. Within this system, patterns develop as members' behavior is caused by and, in turn, causes other family members' behaviors. Maintaining patterns of behavior may lead to balance or unbalance in the family system.

Imagine what might happen when a child with disabilities appears in a family. The resultant change in roles may maintain the stability in the relationships or lead to a different equilibrium or even disequilibrium. The emerging pattern of interaction can lead to dysfunction.

Given this model, it's not difficult to assume that behaviors, even maladaptive ones, such as screaming in order to obtain something, can be maintained or modified through patterns of interaction within a family (Davis & Malone, 2001). The goal of communication intervention, therefore, is to evaluate and either strengthen or change those patterns of behavior that relate to communication development.

Ecological Theory

While there are some overlaps, the ecological theory goes beyond the family unit addressed in family systems theory. Initially introduced by Urie Bronfenbrenner (1979), the social ecological model describes four interdependent environmental systems—*macro, exo, meso,* and *micro*—that contain cultural, community, organizational, and interpersonal or individual influences within which children develop. The most important ecologies or environments for development are systems that contain direct relationships between a child and caregiving adults. Figure 3.1 presents a schematic diagram of the social ecological model. Note that each sphere operates fully within the next larger one.

Beginning with the largest sphere, the four systems are described as follows:

- *Macrosystems* are cultural contexts. Culture is the "way of life" of a group that is passed down from generation to generation. As such, culture includes codes of conduct, dress, language, rituals, spiritual beliefs, behavioral norms, and child-rearing practices.
- *Exosystems* indirectly affect a child's development. They include external networks, such as community structures and local educational systems, that influence the microsystems.
- *Mesosystems* are the organizational or institutional factors that structure the environment within which the interpersonal relations of the microsystem occur. Think of mesosystems as the norm or rule-forming component of a group or organization, such as a school or a church, temple, or mosque.
- *Microsystems* contain the factors within a child's intimate and immediate environment. Primary microsystems for children include the family, peer group, classroom, childcare, and neighborhood and include personal roles such as mother, brother, and teacher.

The child is at the center of the ecological model. As in family systems theory, a child is affected by and, in turn, affects the settings in which she or he spends time. Development occurs through a process of progressively more complex interactions between a child and

FIGURE 3.1 **Schematic of Social Ecological Model**

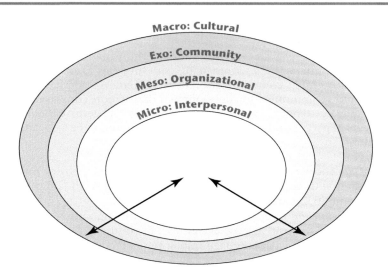

the persons, objects, and symbols in the child's immediate environment. The quality of a child's development is determined by what she or he experiences in these settings.

Effective interactions occur on a fairly regular basis at the microsystem level over extended periods of time. Interactions occur when individuals within a system, such as family members, coordinate their efforts.

From an ecological perspective, the child with a communication impairment is affected by and affects the interactions of others, especially within the family system. The family, therefore, has the potential for creating and/or modifying interactions and optimizing a child's development.

It's important for you, as a future SLP, to recognize the significance and interactions of all these systems. All of us—the child, caregivers, and you—function within these spheres.

WORKING WITH PARENTS

Young children learn best when participating in an activity while a caregiver interprets or facilitates (Hancock & Kaiser, 2006; Wetherby & Woods, 2006). An SLP can help parents understand how their young child learns to communicate and enable parents to make decisions about the best times to interact with their child throughout the day.

Parents are capable of learning and implementing multiple teaching strategies that result in positive outcomes for young children (Bibby, Eikeseth, Martin, Mudford, & Reeves, 2001; Kaiser et al., 2000). Parent-implemented intervention with young children has been linked to

- Increases in verbalizations,
- More spontaneous speech,
- Increased use of target utterances,
- Longer intervals of engagement,
- More responsiveness in target tasks, and
- Decreases in disruptive and noncompliant behaviors.

In general, inclusion of parents as language facilitators maximizes the chance that intervention is consistent and frequent and takes place in functional contexts (Goldstein, Walker, & Fey, 2005).

Parental Interaction Style

Studies have documented qualitative differences between the interactional styles of parents of typically developing (TD) children and those of children with disabilities (Pino, 2000). The communication style of many parents toward their children with disabilities tends to be more directive and less conversational than that of parents of TD children. In part, this style reflects the need to get through the day with a child who may be less responsive and need more direction.

There is broad consensus among professionals who work in ECI that more conversational parent-child interactions within daily activities can exert significant positive influence on a young child's communication development. A directive adult style is less conducive to a child's communication development than a more conversational style. The very child who may need more conversational exchanges isn't getting them.

Four aspects of parent-child interaction have been found to be associated with child language development:

- *Amount of parent-child interaction.* In general, parents spend less time interacting with their children with communication difficulties (Alston & St. James-Roberts, 2005; Hammer, Tomblin, Zhang, & Weiss, 2001).
- *Responsiveness to child communication.* Although the amount of maternal responsiveness is related to positive language growth in children, mothers are less responsive to their children with language impairments (Yoder, McCathren, Warren, & Watson, 2001).

- *Amount and quality of linguistic input.* In general, the richness of parental language used with a child has a positive effect on the child's language development (Hoff & Naigles, 2002; Rowe, 2008; Weizman & Snow, 2001). This richness is diminished when the child has slower language development.
- *Use of language-learning support strategies.* Parental support strategies include talking about things in the immediate environment, describing relationships, and expanding or recasting a child's utterances. Parents of children with language impairments use few and less mature language support strategies (Vigil, Hodges, & Klee, 2005).

Remember that communication is a two-way street. These are not bad parents.

Differences in joint attending and in a child's clarity of communication and responsiveness can contribute to differences in parents' behavior. Teaching parents to modify their interaction styles and linguistic input is an important aspect of ECI.

Collaboration

Parents or caregivers are in a unique position in ECI. They are both team members and the primary agents of change at the same time that they are *clients, patients, consumers,* or whatever term is preferred by the servicing agency. The SLP is concerned with changing adult behaviors concurrent with changing the child's.

As an SLP, you'll be challenged to use evidence-based intervention in consultative processes in which you'll collaborate with a child's significant communication partners (Woods, Wilcox, Friedman, & Murch, 2011). Your role will be to support caregivers in becoming competent and confident in their ability to help their child develop communication.

In ECI, an SLP assumes multiple roles relative to infants and toddlers and their families. These will be discussed at the end of the chapter. While some of these roles will seem familiar, others, such as collaborating with caregivers, will not. Embedding communication goals into a family's daily routines and helping caregivers learn to use communication intervention strategies require an SLP to be both a teacher and a learner.

Together the SLP and parent/caregiver support the child's development (Dunst & Trivette, 2009a). The nature of a truly individualized family-centered approach requires a bidirectional teaching and learning relationship (Woods et al., 2011).

The majority of home visits by professionals are predominantly child focused rather than interactional and involve caregivers as passive observers (Peterson, Luze, Eshbaugh, Jeon, & Kantz, 2007; Wilcox, Guimond, & Kim, 2010). There is a greater likelihood that caregivers will act as effective communication facilitators if they are involved in problem-solving and planning.

All too often professionals rather than family members act in the role of decision-makers. This is especially true with families with low SES or culturally diverse backgrounds. More than 20 percent of respondents in a nationwide survey of families with children enrolled in EI programs expressed a desire for more involvement in decision-making, especially in determining goals and services for their child (Bailey, Hebbeler, Scarborough, Spiker, & Mallik, 2004).

The greatest gains in intervention are through activities identified by caregivers (Dunst et al., 2000; Raab & Dunst, 2007). In addition, the generalization of intervention strategies is best when caregivers are encouraged to participate in decision-making by suggesting interactional opportunities for the child within a variety of activities and routines throughout the day (Kashinath, 2006; Wetherby & Woods, 2006).

In similar fashion, parents and caregivers can identify child interests that can become the vehicles for intervention, thus increasing the potential number of opportunities for intervention to occur. Placing intervention within a child's interests also increases the child's motivation to participate. In addition, interest-based child learning opportunities have a positive effect on child behavior (Raab & Dunst, 2007).

To be effective in collaborative consultation with families, you'll need skills in reflective listening, questioning, problem-solving, modelling, shaping, fading, providing meaningful feedback, and prompting, as well as providing more holistic approaches that promote communication in general (Hanft, Rush, & Sheldon, 2004). Consultation is triadic, involving the SLP, caregiver, and child. Each participant contributes, and the flow of information is bidirectional.

The manner in which you communicate with parents can make or break the collaborative model. Table 3.1 contains a few strategies that may lead to a successful collaborative effort.

An SLP keeps the avenues of communication open by actively encouraging and soliciting caregiver participation, input, and leadership (Buysse & Wesley, 2005; Campbell & Sawyer, 2007; Hanft et al., 2004). I tell my students that as SLPs, our goal is to put ourselves out of business by equipping and empowering parents to support their child's communication development in natural environments without us. Bidirectional communication is key to successful ECI.

TABLE 3.1   Strategies for Interacting Successfully with Caregivers

STRATEGY	DESCRIPTION	EXAMPLE
Engaging caregivers	Be open, welcoming, and friendly. Discuss familiar topics with caregivers, such as child-care and daily activities that are familiar. Try to see caregivers as whole individuals.	"You mentioned last week that feeding is difficult. How's that going now? What do you think would make that easier for you?"
Collaborative planning	Joint planning is an excellent opportunity for participation and decision-making by the caregiver. This includes collaborative planning for the next visit.	"I hear you saying that you're pleased with Jerome's progress. What seems like the next place to go with his language?"
Active listening	Sometimes it's just good practice to be quiet and let caregivers talk. Help the parent identify rough patches or bumps in the road that may pose a "problem." By just listening, you convey that you share a caregiver's concern. Once the caregiver has identified a concern, we have the makings of collaborative problem-solving within which alternatives can be explored together.	"As I listen to your concerns about preschool placement, I hear you saying that individualized services are your biggest concern? Am I correct? [Allow for parental confirmation] Okay, let's discuss the options."
Thoughtful questioning	Caregivers often respond well to open-ended questions that focus on specific activities or routines. Follow up with more probing questions. Reflective questioning encourages the caregiver to think about the action or strategy he or she performed and to integrate the information for future use.	"Did you notice how Kelly became more active when you talked to her? Why do you think she did that? Is that different from what was happening before? How?"
Suggesting	This strategy can help caregivers gain independence. Essential parts are: • Build on something the caregiver has shared about a method tried. • Provide an explanation for your recommendation. • Link the suggestion to a goal important to the caregiver. Leave room for the caregiver to participate in the problem-solving process.	"I've noticed when Kenny uses his computer he slumps in the chair. Have you noticed? Have you tried any other seating arrangement? Something that would free his hands. What do you think?" [Caregiver response] Yeah, I agree. Sitting straighter might make it easier for him to touch the computer screen and to see you when you talk to him. Should we try?"
Commenting	Comments and explanations help explain techniques being used to the caregiver. You might talk about what you observe and how it might be modified. This strategy conveys a sense of collaboration. Focus both on what you observe and on the training objective in ways that expand the program.	"Shawnee really likes that car. I wonder if we could get him to turn-take with it as he does with the ball. What do you think?"

Strategy	Description	Example
Making observations	In a conversational tone, the SLP points out something the caregiver may not have noticed or thought was important but may be important in the future.	"I noticed that you played with Monica one toy at a time. I think that's a great idea. As you know, she's easily distracted. We'll need to remember not to overwhelm her when we begin to offer her choices of toys."
Explaining	It's important for caregivers to understand why you are recommending certain targets and strategies.	"I think you would agree that the last thing you need is one more thing to do. Am I right? Well, for that reason, I'm going to recommend that we do our communication training within the things you're already doing. It will also help Sammy participate in those activities."
Sharing	Carefully explain how a strategy or technique worked with a child at a similar juncture in intervention. Avoid direct comparisons; no two children are alike.	"I think it's a great idea to have Jodi ask for small pieces of snack during snack time. How about if we brainstorm on other ways to have your daughter request at other times during the day."
Thinking aloud	This is an indirect way of giving the caregiver the choice of trying something or not and asking for his or her input; it is collaborative in nature as long as you are sincere in offering the choice. The best answer is the one the caregiver believes will work.	"What do you think would happen if you just held back a bit on placing all Ilana's toys in the tub as soon as she gets in? Do you think you might be able to get her to request them with a gesture or a sound?"
Soliciting	Caregivers' competence and confidence are increased when their ideas are accepted and expanded. Just remember that every caregiver has a limit and you must respect those limits.	"We're making great progress. I have some ideas, but where do you think we should go next?"
Linking to family priorities	Try not to overwhelm parents with suggestions. Linking each to a family priority will aid retention.	"Erik is really making lots of sounds when he plays. You've been doing a terrific job. But I know you want him to say words. What do you think of trying to add some meaning by adaption some of these into real words? For example, we could use 'baw' (/bɔ/) to stand for 'ball.' Then he'll have a word and a use for it. Can you think of any other possibilities?"
Adapting	It's important for you to understand the family's availability and the variables that affect routines within the home.	"I agree with you, Sean does make more sounds during bath time. Are you the one who typically bathes him? How long does he usually play in the water? Do you think there would be enough time for you to play a little turn-taking game with sounds with him?"
Offering feedback	Feedback is best when it is immediate, within context, and related to a strategy the caregiver is using. Remember that it is positive in tone even when you are correcting something. If done thoughtfully, feedback can help parents to modify their behavior. Be specific, and provide feedback that addresses the behavior and possible outcomes for the child and parent.	"When Lee said 'Doggie,' you repeated the word and then added something to it. I heard you say, 'Yes, doggie. Doggie's barking.' When you do that, you strengthen her talking at the same time that you give her additional information. It's a great way for her to learn. Can I show you something else you might try?"

continued

TABLE 3.1 **Strategies for Interacting Successfully with Caregivers** (*continued*)

STRATEGY	DESCRIPTION	EXAMPLE
Summarizing	You can use this technique to pull ideas together and to aid collaboration.	"I think we have a plan for moving forward. You had some great suggestions. I think I heard us say we wanted to introduce more vocal imitation and continue to encourage her use of gestures. Is that your understanding?"
Praising	All of us like praise and encouragement. They motivate us. Just remember to keep your accolades honest and sincere. Praise is not false flattery. It's positive feedback.	"I honestly think both you and your son are improving. You seem more confident, and I welcome your suggestions. Some have been really insightful."

Sources: Campbell and Sawyer, 2007; Dunst and Trivette, 2009a; Hanft et al., 2004; Wilcox and Woods, 2011; Woods and Lindeman, 2008; Woods et al., 2011; http://tactics.fsu.edu.

Parental Factors

It is imperative that parents be considered clients as well as communication and language facilitators or trainers. They will have successes with their child and failures. As an SLP, be mindful of and address parental feelings of inadequacy and frustration as well as feelings of success.

Parents of a special needs or medically fragile child are under a lot of pressure. Early intervention has been found to have both positive and negative effects on parental stress. In general, more intensive interventions with low-functioning children who make only limited progress can have the greatest potential of increasing parental feelings of anxiety, inadequacy, and stress. It's important to be sensitive to parents' emotions as intervention progresses.

Parent-SLP interaction likely will change across time and location. An SLP meeting parents in the NICU/SCN may find them in denial or in an overly optimistic state. For example, during the first few months of life, babies with Down syndrome are less likely to be identified as such by strangers. This can foster parental denial. Parents report that this honeymoon period lasts for the first six months or so and that their infant seemed "just like" other children at that age. With my grandson Dakota, this denial by my daughter lasted well into his second year of life. Parents in this state are not ready to discuss intervention.

Once parents accept that their child is different, they may become angry and blameful or begin to search for a magic cure. At this stage, parents may again not wish to discuss intervention.

Finally, nearly all parents will accept reality and be more open to SLP suggestions. As you can imagine, you'll need to be alert for subtle changes in parental attitudes that signal a shift in attitude and to alter your style accordingly.

Treatment effects vary as a function of pretreatment *maternal responsivity* and education level (Yoder & Warren, 2001b). Maternal responsivity is the ability of the mother to respond and motivate her child to communicate. In general, parent-child interactions without structure result in very few opportunities for parents to be responsive. Introducing greater structure through intervention helps increase opportunities for parental responses (Yoder & Warren, 2002).

Adult Learning Styles

Individual differences in the characteristics of both child and parent influence the nature of their interaction (Kelly & Barnard, 2000). It would seem most efficacious, therefore, to build on each dyad's interaction style and on the existing teaching strategies in each parent's repertoire. In other words, designing intervention that considers each parent's learning style, as well as the parent's teaching and interactional strategies, is a more efficient teaching approach than a generalized, one-size-fits-all type.

Unfortunately, we have little evidence on the best way to teach or promote implementation of intervention practices by caregivers (Fixsen, Naoom, Blasé, Friedman, & Wallace,

FIGURE 3.2 **Facilitating Adult Learning**

- Make certain that learning priorities, expectations, outcomes, and roles are clear, relevant, and established collaboratively.
- Build your relationship with the caregiver gradually and carefully because it's vital to success.
- Focus on the learner's knowledge and interests and on relevant observable outcomes.
- Teach specific strategies one at a time and provide a rationale, examples, and practice.
- Monitor progress of both the child and the adult.
- Apply easy-to-use measures of behavior.
- Demonstrate, practice, coach, and critique in multiple contexts in which the parent will use the strategies.
- Help parents, through self-reflection and individual goal-setting, to apply their knowledge and skills in novel situations.
- Solicit parent feedback by inviting questions and comments.
- Increase learning, opportunities for use, and decision-making through active caregiver participation and input.
- Foster deeper understanding and increase learning capacity and confidence through the use of repetition.
- Join in the parent-child interaction gently rather than pushing in.
- Build on and teach through the caregiver's strengths.
- Provide specific evaluative comments and meaningful feedback.

Sources: Roberts et al., 2010; Trivette & Dunst, 2007; Trivette, Dunst, Hamby, & O'Herin, 2009; Woods et al., 2011.

2005). Adult learning is a complex process, involving changes in behavior, knowledge, skills, and attitudes. This includes the acquisition and mastery of knowledge, the application of this learning to one's own experience, and the intentional use of the knowledge with novel problems (Knowles, Holton, & Swanson, 2005).

An SLP should consider adult learning styles when working with parents and other caregivers. Common adult learning guidelines are presented in Figure 3.2. Let's expand on some of these points.

As mentioned previously, intervention goals and methods should reflect the family's priorities. Parents may focus on issues other than communication and feeding. These topics need to be addressed thoroughly prior to or parallel with discussion of the communication concerns of the SLP. Through consultation, the intervention team, including the family, can jointly establish intervention parameters. It is also important for families to understand the consultative role of the SLP.

Within this role, an SLP can find ways to join caregiver-child activities rather than expecting the caregiver to join SLP-child interactions or to simply observe the SLP and child. Real parent-child interactions offer an SLP the chance to observe and to offer real-world suggestions for enhancing communication.

All of us learn best when what we are taught is close to what we already know. Caregivers know their childcare routines, and placing learning within these activities facilitates progress. It's easy for caregivers to make limited modifications or to incorporate new opportunities for interaction.

Much of the information about development and communication intervention is complicated and academic. An SLP who spouts too much academic information or uses professional jargon chances losing caregiver cooperation. Instead, an SLP can provide enough information to justify intervention but refrain from sounding too bookish or pedantic.

The SLP-caregiver relationship must be based on mutual trust and understanding. This will not occur on the first visit. As a parent gains confidence and begins to see improvement in a child's communication skills, he or she will begin to trust the SLP's advice and will be motivated to learn even more.

An SLP can foster the relationship by openly discussing expectations for intervention with the parent(s) and developing a relationship as co-interventionists (Roberts, Kaiser, & Wright, 2010). Parent expectations and priorities can be discussed and parent participation encouraged. It helps to view parents as experts on their own child. Their experiences within intervention need to be continually assessed and their opinions validated.

Finally, SLPs must be careful not to overwhelm caregivers with too many intervention tasks. SLPs will need to be mindful of the need to build confidence and not increase a parent's feelings of inadequacy or failure. It does no one any good to add to a parent's anxiety.

It's best to introduce intervention techniques slowly, no more than one or two at a time over the course of intervention. At each meeting, one or more techniques can be presented for talking to children, cuing their communication behavior, teaching, and responding to their behavior. If too many techniques are taught all at once, parents become overwhelmed and all too often do not follow through.

Families with a History of Maltreatment or Neglect

Working with children in families where they have experienced maltreatment or neglect can be uniquely challenging because these families may have complex histories, including different cultural perspectives and interactions with the social welfare system.

Trust is critical to collaboration with these families. A family that has encountered the child welfare system may feel uncomfortable with professionals visiting the home or asking about childcare. As an SLP, it's essential for you to specify your role with family members in order to build trust (Rogers-Adkinson & Stuart, 2007).

Effective communication requires that an SLP develop good interpersonal communication skills and tailor communication to family preferences and needs. This includes (Rogers-Adkinson & Stuart, 2007)

- Listening empathetically to the family members and other stakeholders,
- Brainstorming service options with family members and other stakeholders,
- Respecting cultural diversity, and
- Maintaining confidentiality as specified in the Family Education Rights and Privacy Act (FERPA), which requires professionals to treat client information as confidential and to disclose it only with the consent of parents or guardians.

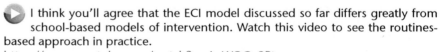 I think you'll agree that the ECI model discussed so far differs greatly from school-based models of intervention. Watch this video to see the routines-based approach in practice.
https://www.youtube.com/watch?v=sL_WOCu3Ptg

A Hybrid Approach to Family-Centered Intervention

The traditional model of speech-language pathology services evolved within the public school system and required children to be taken from their class a few times each week for a half hour of intervention services. It is now recognized that a more efficient and effective way to provide these services is a combination of some one-on-one intervention, using this older model, along with services in the child's classroom enlisting the aid of other language facilitators (Owens, 2014). Called a "push in" model of intervention, this approach posits that children benefit more from services provided in the context where language is likely to be used on a daily basis. Ideally, in this model, teachers and SLPs collaborate in identifying potential language targets. Intervention is ongoing through the efforts of teachers and parents who are trained by the SLP. Similar hybrid approaches exist in ECI.

Models for inclusion of parents in ECI range from individual to small group. For a number of reasons, initially legal but increasingly supported by evidence-based research, a hybrid model has evolved as the most efficacious means of providing ECI services. The components are similar to what we find in schools, but the emphasis is placed more heavily on parents and families in recognition of their important status in the lives of young children.

In this hybrid model, the SLP sees the child two or three times a week at home or in a childcare, EI, or preschool program. During these visits, the SLP works with the child and also instructs caregivers in the best methods of training the mutually agreed upon target behaviors. Parents and teachers are further trained within group or individual meetings where targets are selected, objectives modified, and training continued.

We'll discuss specific intervention techniques in the next several chapters. For now, let's explore a possible model for individual training sessions with the child and caregiver and group meetings with parents.

Assuming that the team, including the parents, has identified the initial targets for training, the SLP and parents can review these and modify them as needed. The SLP explains the model of intervention using multiple examples, demonstrates parent-child intervention, answers parents' questions, and explains the necessity to keep data in order to assess progress and aid planning. Finally, parents are helped to identify potential teaching situations in their daily interactions with their child.

INDIVIDUAL INTERVENTION SESSIONS

In individual intervention sessions, whether in the home or other LRE, the SLP and parent collaborate in finding the best techniques for both parent and child and in planning intervention that will occur until the next meeting. Intervention sessions with individual caregiver-child dyads may consist of the following format:

- Review with the parent any data kept on child responsiveness to the intervention.
- Observe the parent and child in an interaction, routine, or activity.
- Gently join as a participant in the routine or activity, but do not take charge.
- Critique the parent's behaviors, building on those that are working well.
- Directly and explicitly teach and demonstrate within a routine or activity what to do, why it is important, and how it can be done.
- Discuss with the parent child-based goals and teaching strategies to select for the intervening days.
- Model for the parent strategies for the new or revised goals, explaining what to do and encouraging the parent to ask questions.
- Have the parent practice while the SLP guides, observes, and provides feedback in the form of suggestions on what to continue doing and what to consider altering based on the parent's input, prompts, reflective questions, or encouragement.
- Collaboratively take turns interacting with the child and trying different strategies, while offering needed feedback.
- Determine how and when to implement the strategy.
- Agree on what data will be kept in the intervening days.
- Brainstorm new ways to create even more opportunities for communication.
- Model for the parent new ways to talk with or stimulate the child, and have the parent attempt these new methods
- Critique the parent's performance.

As you can see, there's plenty to accomplish in a short amount of time. Keep in mind that this is only one possible model. I have borrowed from the excellent article by Woods et al. (2011), which I would encourage you to read, and my own experience.

The process should be friendly and informal. Most importantly, the SLP focuses on increasing the caregiver's competence and confidence. We'll be discussing teaching techniques later in the intervention chapters.

GROUP INTERVENTION SESSIONS

Group sessions with parents will vary in format, sometimes including the child while at other times only parents or other family members. Parent participation can be increased if childcare is provided while parents and professionals meet.

Wilcox, Bacon, and Greer (2005) offer a wonderful online resource for structuring these meetings when the intervention target is single word production. Their site, listed in the bibliography, offers handouts, self-assessments, and other materials for parents. The following discussion borrows heavily from this fine resource, supplemented with input from other knowledgeable SLPs and my own experience.

If working with groups of parents and children, six to eight parent-child dyads may be optimal. Larger groups make it difficult for an SLP or other facilitator to attend easily to each individual parent-child dyad and for each parent to participate in discussions and demonstrations.

Although parents and children need not be homogeneous in their characteristics, it's best to focus on a narrow range of child functional ages or abilities. This will facilitate the use of materials and activities that will promote engagement if children have accompanied parents to the group meeting. There is the added advantage that parents can learn from each other. Figure 3.3 presents a possible format for successive parent meetings. If it is not feasible for parents to meet in groups, the material presented in the following section can also be covered in individual sessions.

In the first meeting, it's important to provide parents with a general overview of the training to follow. They need to understand their role, the format of intervention sessions whether in the home or a center, and the use of recordings for training purposes. After introducing himself or herself, the SLP should ask parents to introduce themselves, to briefly describe their child, and to share their hopes for the results of the intervention program. At this initial meeting, the SLP will want to stress the importance of parents in intervention and provide a brief parent-friendly overview of communication and language development.

Techniques should be explained and demonstrated before parents are asked to attempt each one. Recording parent behaviors may be useful for critiquing their performance. As an SLP, keep your presentation positive, and give praise liberally when warranted. Some general principles for talking with young children are presented in Figure 3.4.

In subsequent sessions, the SLP can help parents (Wilcox et al., 2005)

- Identify what their child is already doing to communicate,
- Identify the best time to teach for each parent-child dyad,

FIGURE 3.3 Play Group and Parent Class Training Agenda

Sensitivity: Tuning in to Opportunities for Language-Learning
   Session 1 Group meeting: *Overview and Introduction: Teaching Your Child*
   Session 2 Group meeting: *Creating Opportunities for Teaching*
   Session 3 Group meeting: *Using Daily Activities to Teach Language*
   Session 4 Individual meetings in your home
   Session 5 Group meeting: *Encouraging Communication*
   Session 6 Group meeting: *Encouraging Communication during Play*

Contingency: Responding to Children's Communications
   Session 7 Group meeting: *Talking to Young Children*
   Session 8 Individual meetings in your home
   Session 9 Group meeting: *Imitating, Interpretating, and Expanding*
   Session 10 Group meeting: *Responding to Your Child's Communications*
   Session 11 Group meeting: *Options for Responding*
   Session 12 Individual meetings in your home

Consistency: Self-Monitoring Skills and Encouraging More Complex Language
   Session 13 Group meeting: *Strategies to Further Enhance Children's Language*
   Session 14 Group meeting: *Identifying More Complex Communication and Language*
   Session 15 Individual meetings: *Reviewing Progress and Planning Future Goals*

Source: Based on the model presented in Wilcox et al., 2005.

FIGURE 3.4 **Guidelines for Talking with Young Children**

Be animated. Use exaggerated facial expressions, voice variations, and movement.

Be positive. The tone of your voice as well as the things you say have a tremendous impact because young children learn to interpret intonation very early.

Communicate at eye level. Being at the same level enables a young child to read the messages in your face and to learn the value of face-to-face communication and of paying attention to others. Face-to-face communication is more egalitarian and interactive.

Listen, take turns, and know when to stop. Knowing how to listen is just as important as being an enthusiastic and responsive conversational partner. Listening shows that you are interested in what a child is saying, even if it's not words. The best conversations with young children include a combination of quiet listening and simple talking; each of you taking a turn in a natural, easy manner. It's important to strike a balance.

Provide rich input. Varied activities, comprehensible language, educational play, and rewarding interactions provide challenging, fun, and interesting experiences. Stay on the edge of the curve so that your child is neither bored nor overwhelmed. Challenge a child to stretch her vocabulary by staying one step ahead. Talk about what's happening in your immediate surroundings to enhance the child's comprehension.

Pick the best time to communicate, and get the child's attention first. The best interactions with a child occur when the child's awake, alert, and quiet or making noises. Watch for a child's cues that he or she is open to communication, such as eye contact, indicating I'm ready to engage in play or a chat. When a child shows interest in something, slide into the activity and talk about it. Before beginning your own interaction, get the child's attention first. Sharing attention with another person is a precursor to sharing topics in conversation.

Always respond. Whenever possible, respond to *all* vocalizations and verbalizations. In general, good responses:

- Affirm that you're paying attention.
- Reinforce the child's efforts.
- Clarify the child's intentions.
- Provide evaluative feedback.
- Model longer or more adult-like phrases.

Noticing and responding to a child's communication attempts teaches a child that communication is important and reinforces the child for trying.

Speak in short two- to four-word phrases. Children on the cusp of talking understand one- or two-word expressions best. Longer utterances exceed their memory. Once children begin talking in single words, they can usually understand short two- or three-word phrases.

Speak slowly, pause between words, and keep your vocabulary small. Children's vocabularies begin to grow slowly. Use words that describe things that the child encounters most frequently, things that are part of her or his world.

Repeat words, but vary your language slightly. Repetition helps language-processing. One or two repetitions should do the trick, and comprehension improves when the words represent something present, visual, and interesting.

Focus on one topic, and follow the child's lead. It's confusing for a child to talk about more than one thing at a time until he or she is about 18 months old, so keep your conversations focused. Early communication is always most effective when focused on an object, action, or event that's happening in front of you. Let the child indicate an interest in something by looking, reaching, or picking something up, and then talk about it. If the child says a word, turn that word into a topic of conversation.

continued

Gesture and sign to aid comprehension. Gesturing is a natural accompaniment to and enhancement for spoken language. Natural gesturing holds a child's interest, enhances your message, and helps a child understand your words. The simpler the gesture is to do, the more likely a child will be able to copy it and use it to communicate. Be consistent; that also helps. Signs, such as those used in the Deaf community, can also be used like natural gestures. Children pick up sign language when they're exposed to it, just as they do natural gestures. A few other guidelines:

- Don't overwhelm the child with signs or gestures.
- Speak at the same time you gesture.
- Sign and gesture in context.
- Offer repeated exposure.
- Encourage imitation.
- Sign and gesture only important words.

Limit your questions. Besides requiring an answer that a child may not know, questions are more difficult to process than statements because of the grammar. In general, *what* and *where* type questions, such as *"What's that?"* and *"Where's doggie?"* are relatively easy for toddlers who are using single words.

Source: Information from Owens, 2004.

- ■ Reflect on how parents can encourage their child to communicate,
- ■ Describe their routine during activities and identify opportunities for their child to use targeted skills,
- ■ Describe how to create opportunities for communication and to encourage use of the targeted skills,
- ■ Role-play teaching following a model by the SLP, and
- ■ Design an intervention plan.

The SLP can use video or other digitally recorded examples of teaching and incorporate examples observed during home visits.

USING DAILY ROUTINES

The teaching techniques that parents use with their child do not need to be elaborate or formal. Simple is best. Daily activities provide the best time for language-learning because the child knows the routine, making participation easier, and has experienced the same actions and words repeatedly within each routine.

The SLP can help parents identify ordinary daily routines and play, such as pushing the child on a swing, changing a diaper, or bathing the child, that create opportunities for communication. Common problems encountered in routines include a parent (Weitzman, 2005)

- ■ Moving too quickly so the child doesn't have a chance to interact,
- ■ Being inconsistent with words and actions,
- ■ Stopping before the child is ready,
- ■ Having incorrect or inappropriate expectations for the child, and
- ■ Changing routines before the child is ready.

The child's turn may consist of an action, a sound, or a facial expression that the parent attempts to highlight within the routine. Once the child knows his or her part in the routine, the adult can wait expectantly for the child to take a turn. If the turn is not forthcoming, the adult may need to cue the child to respond.

Within routines, communication can be spurred in several ways (Owens, 2014; Wilcox et al., 2005):

- ■ Omitting or incorrectly performing a familiar or necessary step in an activity or routine

- Not supplying an item needed in a task
- Missing a turn
- Providing options for objects or activities
- Pausing and waiting for a response in a situation in which the child needs assistance

Other, more direct techniques, such as providing a model or requesting a behavior, can also be presented to parents. Once a child has experienced repeated success with his or her turn in a routine, the parent can plan a different turn or change the routine to encourage initiation by the child.

Consistency and timely responding are equally important. If the target behavior is not elicited or is incorrect, parents will need to learn responses for correcting the behavior. On the other hand, correct responses can be reinforced in order to strengthen these behaviors.

A parent might be taught to expand on the child's behaviors and to encourage the child to imitate in turn. A child's nonsymbolic behavior, such as pointing, can also be interpreted verbally by the parent ("Yes, you see the doggie"), adding meaning to the child's attempt. At a symbolic level, expanding a child's utterance into a longer utterance can stimulate the child's development, while replying can be reinforcing and can keep the child participating. All of these techniques will be discussed in detail in subsequent chapters.

Unlike you, parents are not students in communication sciences and disorders courses, so they should not be expected to write detailed lesson plans. Intervention plans are much simpler.

In preparing an intervention plan, the parent first identifies a routine as a good teaching milieu and then describes the steps in the routine. Next, parents determine what props may be needed to support language teaching opportunities. Finally, with help from the SLP, parents identify ways of creating opportunities for their child to use the targeted behavior. Finally, the parent and the SLP review the parent's response options. These form the basis of the plan.

The family and the SLP discuss the plan, followed by an SLP model of appropriate techniques, role-playing by the parents, and a critique by the SLP. This provides a great opportunity for brainstorming other techniques that might work. This may lead, in turn, to a revision of the plan by the parents and the SLP. In this way, intervention evolves as circumstances change.

Teachers, Classroom Aides, Childcare Providers, and Peers

Children who participate in daycare programs make gains in both receptive and expressive language skills. The best programs offer developmentally facilitative activities and have both high levels of staff training and optimal levels of social and linguistic responsiveness to children's communication attempts. In particular, adult responsiveness is believed to play a key role in accelerating language acquisition (Doherty, Lero, Goelman, Tougas, & LaGrange, 2000). Before I earned my doctorate, I worked in a program that included my spending part of each day in two preschool classrooms using an environmental model of intervention.

A DIRECTIVE CLASSROOM STYLE

Unfortunately, many childcare providers dominate conversational interactions, leaving few opportunities for children to contribute to the conversation (Girolametto, Hoaken, Weitzman, & van Lieshout, 2000). In both one-on-one and large group interactions, adult utterances include many commands and closed questions. A closed question elicits a yes/no answer or a single word reply.

This directive adult style affects the frequency of a child's conversational contributions. Within these interactions, children are minimally verbal, communicate infrequently with caregivers, and address few utterances to peers (Girolametto et al., 2000). By placing few cognitive demands on a child to communicate, such directive interaction inhibits children's language acquisition.

In group interactions, childcare providers' responsiveness is highly dependent on the context and less so on children's language abilities. For example, caregivers provide more responsive input in a play dough activity than in a shared reading experience with the same child (Girolametto & Weitzman, 2002). The play dough activity promotes adult-child interaction that is less directive than book reading. In turn, children with developmental disability (DD) interact more frequently in the play dough activity, although, in general, these children may interact infrequently both with childcare providers and with peers (Girolametto et al., 2000).

Although childcare providers use similar interactional strategies with both toddlers and preschoolers, they use more labeling ("Doggie") with toddlers and more topic extensions ("Then what happened?") with preschoolers. In general, the language used with children with DDs is often directive and not finely tuned to the child's language level.

AN INTERACTIVE CLASSROOM STYLE

An interaction style facilitates a child's participation in conversations with both caregivers and peers. Three major components of an adult interactive communication strategy are

- Child-oriented techniques designed to foster frequent episodes of joint or shared activity around the children's interests,
- Interaction-promoting techniques intended to encourage balanced turn-taking and peer interaction, and
- Language-modeling techniques.

In interactive language stimulation, childcare providers use naturalistic interaction strategies that are associated with accelerated language development in typically developing children. An interactive style

- Focuses on increasing children's initiation of interactions,
- Provides higher levels of responsive language,
- Limits use of directives,
- Extends turn-taking, and
- Promotes peer interactions.

Examples of published intervention programs that try to encourage a more interactive style include (Girolametto, Weitzman, & Greenberg, 2003)

- Developmental Language Intervention (Cole, Mills, Dale, & Jenkins, 1996)
- INclass Reactive Language (INREAL; Weiss, 1981)
- It Takes Two to Talk: The Hanen Program (Pepper & Weitzman, 2004)
- Learning Language and Loving It: The Hanen Program (Weitzman, 1992, 1994)
- Responsive Education and Prelinguistic Milieu Teaching (RPMT; Yoder & Warren, 2002)

Within each, language stimulation occurs in social interactions facilitated by the quality and quantity of adult speech.

Individual teacher or childcare worker training sessions would have a similar format to those involving individual parent-child dyads. Group training for teachers is best handled in an in-service format. Initially, these in-service meetings contain much information on the model and a rationale as well as intervention methods. The content of the initial teacher meetings will overlap with that of the group parent meetings previously discussed. Over time, however, as teachers become familiar with their role and as more and more children become involved, the need for group teacher meetings should lessen.

Initially, staff can be taught to observe, to wait, and to listen for a child's initiations; to talk face to face; and to follow a child's attentional or conversational lead or topic by imitating, interpreting, or commenting on the child's behavior or verbalization (Girolametto, Weitzman, & Greenberg, 2004). Interaction-promoting techniques may be as simple as pausing to allow the child time to take a turn. Turn-taking can also be increased through the use of adult questions that demonstrate an interest in the child or the focus of the child's attention.

Other interaction-promoting techniques include learning to chain comments and questions in order to facilitate a child's turn or continue a topic. This format is similar to *turnabout* techniques used by parents of typically developing preschoolers. For example, if a child says, "Go eat," the adult might respond, "Go eat! You must be hungry. Where should we go?"

The best questions are appropriate to the child's language level. It may be best to keep rhetorical questions with obvious answers ("Are you playing with the car?") to a minimum. Although they do encourage a question-answer exchange, they tend to violate one of the basic purposes of a question, which is to obtain unknown information. Finally, childcare providers can be taught to encourage participation by children in small group activities and to adapt their responses in order to draw a child into conversation.

Childcare providers who have received specialized training in crafting conversations are more likely to provide responsive social contexts for language-learning (Doherty et al., 2000). Specifically, daycare staff who are taught to be responsive to children's initiations, to engage children in interactions, to model simplified language, and to encourage peer interactions subsequently wait for children to initiate, engage them in turn-taking, use face-to-face interaction, and involve children more frequently than do caregivers who have not received training (Girolametto et al., 2003). In turn, children talk more, produce more combinations, and talk to peers more often. That's good!

CHILD PEERS

Children in childcare situations spend more time with peers and talk more often during these interactions than children without this experience. Participation by young children in peer groups can exert a positive influence on their development of both peer interaction and communication skills.

Among TD children, peer interaction skills emerge during toddlerhood. By age 3, children engage in social pretend play with peers and negotiate conflicts. This development requires underlying knowledge and skill in play, social cognition, and language (Abbeduto & Short-Meyerson, 2002). Within childcare centers, development of social competency can be influenced by responsive adults who model, coach, and reinforce peer interaction incidentally during daily activities.

Seeking social interaction with child peers is a critical developmental competency established early in life and increasing throughout the early childhood years. Successful peer interactions are an important context and mechanism for the acquisition of social, language, and cognitive competencies, making such interactions an important aspect of early childhood development. Consistently positive peer interactions have been found to be an important route for enhancing children's development, while peer interaction problems have been shown to be a primary predictor of future social difficulties (Brown, Odom, & Conroy, 2001).

In inclusive daycare or preschool, children with disabilities exhibit significantly less social behavior than their TD peers and, as a result, are often socially isolated (Odom et al., 2001). Difficulties with peer interactions cause these children to be at risk for social withdrawal and aggression (Paul-Brown & Caperton, 2001). Children experiencing difficulties in peer interactions may wander aimlessly, engage in solitary play, be uninvolved in social activities, lack friendships, and be aggressive in peer interactions. Those who have significant behavioral problems with peers, such as aggression or negative verbal interactions, are at high risk for peer relationship problems and later psychopathology.

To forestall the negative consequences, peer interaction intervention should be an integral part of early childhood programs. Positive peer interactions are especially important for children with communication impairments (Paul-Brown & Caperton, 2001).

It's unrealistic to expect childcare providers to engage in formal structured training throughout the day. One alternative is for childcare providers to facilitate peer interactions during play (Girolametto et al., 2004). As a result, young TD children and presumably children with **communication impairment (CI)** will initiate interactions with peers and engage in extended peer play sequences more frequently. Verbal support strategies to facilitate children's interactions with their peers may include both indirect referrals, such as alerting children to common interests or offering praise, and direct referrals, such as telling a child what to say to a peer, inviting children to play together, making specific suggestions, or prompting a child to talk with a peer.

Children with disabilities can make positive gains in interactive skills by being included with and learning from their TD peers (Kohler, Strain, & Goldstein, 2005). The extent of positive effects depends on the social repertoire of the individual child with disabilities. In general, those with some appropriate play and verbal skills make greater social gains than children who lack these skills.

Evidence-based practice (EBP) suggests that peer-mediated procedures represent the largest and best developed interventions for addressing the social interaction skills of young children, especially those with ASD (McConnell, 2002; Odom et al., 2003). Typically developing children model social overtures and buddy play behaviors that can generate positive responses from children with disabilities.

We have to remember that while TD peers can play a role in intervention, they are still very young children. Interactional strategies must be simple and direct.

PEER STRATEGIES

The most effective peer interaction interventions include the systematic use of a combination of strategies, including instructions to children, prompts of certain behaviors, modeling, rehearsals, reinforcement, feedback mechanisms, and discussions. Sadly, teachers in preschool programs use peer interaction intervention strategies infrequently. Instead, preschool teachers are more likely to employ general classroom interventions, such as environmental arrangements and group discussions. In addition, Individualized Education Programs (IEPs) only infrequently mention social goals and interventions.

Classroom-wide Strategies

At the very least, teachers can use (Brown et al., 2001)

- Classroom-wide developmentally appropriate practices in their inclusive classrooms, and
- Affective interventions that influence children's attitudes.

Classroom practices are a context for providing individualized early childhood services to both young children with disabilities and those without.

Teachers and early childhood environments can be supportive of young children's peer interactions both through arrangement of learning centers that encourage young children's engagement and through individualized intervention that promotes emerging peer-related social competence. Supportive conditions for enhancing young children's engagement and development include (Brown et al., 2001)

- Appropriate classroom materials,
- Well-planned learning centers,
- Responsive teachers, and
- Socially responsive peers.

Although these arrangements are a critical foundation, without further individualized intervention it may not be sufficient to improve peer interactions of children with DD.

A second classroom-wide strategy for supporting young children's social interactions is affective interventions that promote positive attitudes about peers with disabilities. Figure 3.5 presents some approaches for building antibias classrooms (Brown et al., 2001). Scientific research is still needed to identify the most effective of these antibias strategies.

FIGURE 3.5 **Approaches for Building Antibias Classrooms**

- Create inclusive classrooms.
- Monitor your own behavior; children learn by example.
- Answer children's questions about difference openly, honestly, and simply without being dismissive of their concerns.
- Treat difference as natural and expected.
- Encourage structured play activities, small group assignments, and heterogeneous ability groups.
- Promote awareness of disabilities through educational materials, posters, and books.
- Recognize the differing abilities of all children.
- Acknowledge that children recognize individual differences.
- Actively listen to children's comments around difference.
- Read positive and realistic books about children with disabilities.
- Guide children's discussions about disabilities.
- Avoid language that may support stereotypes and prejudices.
- Demystify disabilities; allow children without disabilities to explore adaptive equipment, and provide experiences that teach about specific disabilities.
- Invite students and individuals with disabilities to discuss their lives.
- Deal with children's misconceptions, stereotypes, and hurtful comments openly, without using guilt or shame.
- Celebrate similarities as well as noting differences.

Sources: Brown et al., 2001; Kupetz, 2008; Levitch & Gable, 2015.

Individualized Peer Strategies

Classroom-wide interventions can be augmented with individualized intervention strategies. SLPs and classroom teachers can use less intrusive and more natural peer interaction before moving on to more complex, demanding interventions (Brown et al., 2001). Less intrusive and more natural intervention requires the fewest changes in routines. Four suggested individualized interventions, arranged from least to most intrusive and structured, are (Brown et al., 2001)

- Incidental teaching of social behavior,
- Friendship activities,
- Social integration activities, and
- Explicit teaching of social skills.

Let's discuss each intervention strategy in more detail.

Incidental teaching of social behavior. Incidental teaching is a naturalistic, child-directed intervention strategy used during unstructured activities. Usually incidental teaching occurs when a child has shown an interest in something and an adult or peer mediates the situation. A meta-analysis of 56 intervention studies concluded that naturalistic interventions resulted in improved communication skills for young children in the early stages of communication development (McLean & Woods-Cripe, 1997).

During incidental teaching, adults can provide models of social behavior and encourage peers to model appropriate responses. Teachers and SLPs can also support peer interactions by systematically prompting social behavior. For example, when a child is standing to one side but looking at another child playing, the teacher can prompt the child to initiate an interaction by asking to join the play. Incidental teaching is an opportunity to expand teaching into functional and realistic social situations. If incidental teaching is not sufficient to improve children's social behavior, SLPs and teachers can try additional individualized interventions, such as friendship activities, social integration activities, and explicit social skills training.

Friendship activities. Friendship activities are naturalistic interventions for improving young children's peer interactions. In friendship activities, teachers and SLPs adapt early childhood songs, games, and activities to promote social interactions. Strategies include

- Encouraging peer interactions,
- Modeling peer social behavior with opportunities for children to observe positive peer interactions,
- Rehearsing social behavior related to peer interactions, and
- Acknowledging and praising children's peer interactions.

Teachers can encourage children to make friendly statements, to interact positively, to compliment, to smile, to give encouragement, and to share.

Although embedded in common classroom activities, friendship activities provide an opportunity for individualized intervention. In addition, TD peers receive teacher reinforcement for their social responsiveness to classmates with communication difficulties. Typically, friendship activities occur daily within groups of children for about 10 to 15 minutes.

Similar to incidental teaching, friendship activities provide additional opportunities for a child to acquire social skills or to elaborate or generalize previously learned social behaviors within common classroom activities. Although a slightly more intensive intervention strategy than incidental teaching, friendship activities need not replace incidental teaching, which can provide an important way to generalize children's social behavior to less structured, more child-directed social contexts.

Friendship activities have been found to generalize to nonintervention free play periods. For some children, however, incidental teaching and friendship activities are not sufficient to promote peer interactions. In this case, more structured and intensive social integration activities and explicit social skills training may be needed.

Social integration activities. Social integration activities, or environmental arrangement interventions, require teacher planning and some special education expertise. Social integration activities provide systematic teacher and peer support for young children with social interaction difficulties. Teachers arrange for children with limited peer interactions to be in brief, daily, direct contact with children who are socially responsive and competent. Within these supportive contexts, children can (Brown et al., 2001)

- Observe their peers in social interactions,
- Become part of those social interactions with their peers, and
- Benefit from repeated positive peer interactions.

The effectiveness of social integration activities is dependent upon careful teacher planning so that activities enhance the probability of positive social interactions.

Social integration activities have the following basic components (Brown et al., 2001):

- Selection of students
- Implementation of peer activities
- Introduction of play themes
- Partial withdrawal to become monitors and supporters

In selecting students, more typical peers than those with social interaction difficulties will lead to more successful interactions. Activities can be brief and within defined play areas within the classroom to provide multiple opportunities for positive play experiences and peer interaction. Sociodramatic play activities of familiar daily situations, such as going grocery shopping, can be supportive of peer interactions. High-quality functional play activities, such as eating lunch; constructive activities, such as using clay or painting; and games with rules can all be vehicles for interaction. The SLP, teacher, or aide can use prompts and scaffolds to encourage children to interact. Play may be preceded with suggestions about how to play, or in sociodramatic play, adults can assign roles. Adults can suggest play ideas, comment, or when needed, directly prompt play (Brown et al., 2001).

In general, children who participate in social integration groups have more frequent peer interactions, higher language scores, higher social competence ratings, and increased social "status" than those children who do not participate. For those children needing more structure and more teacher-directed intervention, more explicit training may be a next step.

Explicit teaching of social skills. Characterized by relatively intensive training of specific social strategies, explicit social skills training goes by various names, including *stay-play-talk* (English, Goldstein, Shafer, & Kaczmarek, 1997; Goldstein, English, Shafer, & Kaczmarek, 1997), the Cognitive-Social Learning Curriculum (Mize, 1995; Mize & Ladd, 1990), and others. These have been shown to be effective in teaching social interaction skills.

TD preschool children can be taught to maintain mutual or joint attention with a playmate, to comment on the ongoing play activities, and to acknowledge their partner's efforts to communicate through a method called *Stay with your friend, Play with your friend, and Talk with your friend*, or simply *stay-play-talk*. In buddy skills training, peers without disabilities are taught a sequential behavioral chain that includes moving closer to a child with peer interaction difficulties, saying the child's name(s), and maintaining proximity while talking and playing. Teachers act as "buddy coaches" to remind the TD children with the simple mnemonic "Stay, play, and talk with your friend."

During training sessions across daily activities, adults can use a combination of teaching methods including discussions, adult modeling, guided practice, and independent practice with adult feedback. After peer strategy training and practice sessions, training can be conducted with typical peers and children with social interaction problems within activities, such as free play, snack, and large group play.

Children with peer interaction problems are also taught a modified stay and play strategy. Training includes learning to

- Establish eye contact,
- Suggest play activities,
- Initiate conversations,
- Offer or ask for help, and
- Expand the content of the speech of the child with disabilities.

In typical training (Kohler, Greteman, Raschke, & Highnam, 2007).

- The teacher introduces and models a skill,
- The TD peers practice the skill with each other, and
- The peers practice the skill with the child with CI.

In addition, the teacher provides prompts and praise and makes ongoing reference with visual reminders that illustrate strategies, such as standing close to your buddy, saying your buddy's name, touching your buddy's arm, and exchanging toys.

During actual peer interactions, more direct adult strategies might include the following (Girolametto et al., 2004):

- Mentioning a rule governing peer interaction (*We share the toys*).
- Rephrasing or restating a child's utterance to another child (*Jeun-Li said she wanted to feed the baby*).
- Prompting children to talk with each other (*Ask Maria if you can use the crayons*).
- Inviting children to interact (*Nicole, please make dinner with Matt*).
- Telling children to help each other (*Mohammed, Tony needs some help*).

Indirect verbal strategies might include

- Providing positive verbal reinforcement for peer interaction (*That was nice to help Michelle wash dishes*).
- Alerting peers to situational information (*Kathy has play dough cookies for everyone*).

These strategies can facilitate communication between peers and invite peers to interact together. Among all the behaviors used by peers, comments and requests for action have the highest probability of generating a positive response from the children with ASD or other DDs.

In the Cognitive-Social Learning Curriculum, training is based on

- A child's awareness of appropriate social goals and strategies,
- Opportunities to respond to peers socially, and
- Discrimination of peers' reactions to social interactions and modification of responses.

The curriculum focuses on four critical social behaviors used by young children to initiate, maintain, and elaborate peer interactions:

- Engaging in prosocial behaviors that invite participation,
- Asking questions,
- Commenting on play, and
- Offering peer support.

Recognizing that many young children's peer interactions are script based and automatic, SLPs and teachers train child social and verbal behaviors.

For children with severe multiple impairments, idiosyncratic behaviors, or AAC use, SLPs may need to shape more conventional behaviors in order for these children to participate in peer interactions. At the same time, peers may need to be taught to interpret less sophisticated, unconventional, or AAC interactions.

Role of the SLP as a Member of the Team

Among young children, development across several areas is highly interdependent. Intervention in one area affects others. Infants and toddlers acquire new skills across domains simultaneously and synchronously rather than in isolation. This fact means that ECI should be part of a *comprehensive* approach for meeting family and child needs.

A comprehensive approach should include all the supports or resources a child needs and is eligible to receive. As a result, an SLP may be only one of several professionals working with a child and family. SLPs can play a key role with their specialized knowledge of typical and atypical early development of communication, language, speech, feeding/swallowing, hearing, cognition, emergent literacy, social/emotional behavior, and the use of assistive technology (ASHA, 2008b).

As you know, in a *transdisciplinary* model, all team members, including the family, work closely to plan the assessment and the subsequent intervention. Ideally, team members provide training to one another about key behaviors to observe and document and also consult with one another regarding interpretations and recommendations.

Typically, as mentioned in Chapter 1, one team member known as the primary service provider (PSP) and the family members are responsible for the day-to-day implementing of intervention. The team, in consultation with the family, selects the appropriate team member to serve as the PSP based on the needs of the child, relationships developed with the family, and the professional's special expertise. Coordination of services is achieved when the team's message is uniformly delivered by a PSP. Having said all this, it should be noted that according to ASHA (2008b), "It is not appropriate or suitable for SLPs to be asked to train others to perform professional level services unique to SLPs or for SLPs to perform services outside of their scope of practice." As the PSP, you walk a fine line.

Early intervention is a dynamic process, requiring continual assessment and monitoring of a child's development and intervention efficacy. These data are used to inform ongoing changes in service delivery. Coordination and integration of services are key components of effective EI implementation. Belief in and ability to practice family-centered care are central to effective collaborative relationships between parents and service coordinators. Even when an SLP is working independent of other professionals, such as in private practice or home-based services, referral and consultation with other professionals and additional caregivers are essential.

As part of the EI team, SLPs are uniquely qualified to help families enhance their child's communication development. According to ASHA (2008b), an SLP has the following primary functions in ECI:

- Prevention;
- Screening, evaluation, and assessment;
- Planning, implementing, and monitoring intervention;
- Consultation with and education of team members, including families and other professionals;
- Service coordination;
- Transition planning to ensure a seamless transition process for families moving from one program to another;
- Advocacy to raise awareness about the importance of EI; and
- Awareness and advancement of the knowledge base in early intervention through experimental and clinical research.

Aside from their obvious responsibilities in assessment and intervention, SLPs are expected to participate in consultation with and education of team members, including families and other professionals; service coordination; transition planning; advocacy; and awareness and advancement of the knowledge base in early intervention. Because much of this text is concerned with assessment and intervention, I'd like to take a few paragraphs to explore these other responsibilities.

Role changes require changes in thinking. Before we talk about the new role for the SLP, you might want to explore different ways of thinking in this video on changing the intervention mindset.
https://www.youtube.com/watch?v=jA6IOf9A298

CONSULTATION

In ECI, SLPs work in collaborative partnerships with families and caregivers and, in consultative relationships, share essential information and support with team members, including the family and other caregivers and other agencies and professionals (Buysse & Wesley, 2005). Consultation includes providing information that promotes the parents' and other caregivers' abilities to implement communication-enhancing strategies within everyday routines that create increased learning opportunities and participation for the child. The SLP is also responsibile for educating family members about the importance of early communication development and intervention and the role of the family in their child's communication development.

To accomplish this task, you'll need to convey information in a manner that is consistent with individual family members' preferred ways of learning. Coaching, video/digital feedback, modeling, parent workshops, and didactic training sessions are the most successful strategies (ASHA, 2008b). It is important that adult teaching strategies be appropriate to each family's cultural, linguistic, and educational background and learning style.

Use of a consultative style does not relieve an SLP of responsibility for intervention progress. This requires ongoing monitoring and input to ensure progress and appropriate implementation of chosen methods.

SERVICE COORDINATION

Service coordination is defined in Part C of IDEA (2004) as an ongoing, active process for assisting and enabling families to access services and ensuring their rights and procedural safeguards. The service coordinator, which in many instances is an SLP, is responsible for ensuring that every child and family receives

- A multidisciplinary evaluation and assessment,
- An IFSP,
- Provision of services in natural environments, and
- Service coordination.

Unfortunately, families report that service coordination is the least satisfactory aspect of their early intervention services (Dunst & Bruder, 2002). Families often report that multiple service providers do not communicate with each other and at times provide conflicting information.

One of the primary responsibilities of the service coordinator is acting as the single contact person for the family. Once a referral is made, a service coordinator is assigned so that she or he can be actively involved in every step of the IFSP process. As such, the service coordinator or PSP may be the first person within the early intervention system encountered by families and can influence their trust and expectations of the system as a whole. Without good coordination, intervention services are likely to be fragmented.

Models of service coordination vary by state. For example, in some states an individual person, such as the SLP, may perform the dual roles of service coordinator and primary service provider (PSP). In other states, these two roles may be performed by separate agencies or professionals. Early intervention models for each state can be found on the National Early Childhood Technical Assistance Center (NECTAC) website, which you can access by typing "nectac" into your online search engine.

TRANSITION PLANNING

A major goal of IDEA (2004) is to ensure a seamless transition process for families moving from one program to another and timely access to appropriate services. The transition process should be as smooth and positive as possible for the family. Although there are several types of transitions, such as NICU/SCN to home-based intervention and home-based to center-based programs, the most dramatic transition occurs when the child moves from early intervention to school-based services, typically at age 3 (ASHA, 2008b). It may be stressful for a family to transition from a home-based, one-on-one service delivery model to a school- or center-based classroom model. They may fear that they will lose the personal attention of ECI services.

Families and other team members should begin to consider the transition to preschool services at the time of the first IFSP and are required to provide a date for a transition plan on the original IFSP document. During initial meetings, the team attempts to

- Clarify the family's expectations,
- Establish priorities for future services, and
- Discuss possible options and settings for future placement.

During these meetings, the service coordinator ensures that the parents have an opportunity to ask questions and are presented with all possible options. The SLP may have various responsibilities related to helping the family explore the options and preparing the child and family for the transition.

ADVOCACY

Advocacy activities that raise awareness of the importance of EI and ECI are essential. Mechanisms include

- Working closely with other professionals;
- Writing research articles, textbooks, and other resource materials to provide accurate, timely information;
- Being involved in local, state, and national efforts to influence public policy; and
- Developing and distributing information on EI to families, health care professionals, and others involved in the care of young children. (ASHA, 2008b)

AWARENESS AND ADVANCEMENT OF THE KNOWLEDGE BASE

Here's where you come in right now. Higher education institutions have a responsibility for staying abreast of advances in the discipline, including implementation of EBP and provision of meaningful opportunities for students to gain knowledge and experience working collaboratively with other professionals. In fact, there is a positive relationship between the amount of interdisciplinary preparation and the degree to which SLPs seek out inter-disciplinary opportunities after they graduate (Crais et al., 2004; Mellon & Winton, 2003).

Practicing clinicians also have the responsibility to engage in ongoing professional development. In addition, SLPs who provide clinical services and those who conduct research have a responsibility to work collaboratively to enhance the knowledge base by

- Identifying risk factors and researching prognostic indicators more precisely;
- Clarifying the interaction between risk and resilience factors that affect early communication difficulties;
- Extending the use of EBP to the prevention and treatment of developmental communication difficulties;
- Developing and refining methods to increase the accuracy of detecting children in need of services;
- Carrying out scientifically sound studies to demonstrate and quantify the efficacy and effectiveness of current ECI approaches; and
- Creating, field testing, and evaluating new methods and procedures for enhancing ECI (ASHA, 2008b).

Through shared responsibility, EI providers, families, and higher education faculty can ensure a strong and positive impact for EI services.

An Example of Early Intervention: Parents Interacting with Infants (PIWI)

As promised, we're going to look at an ECI program as an example of this intervention model. The Parents Interacting with Infants (PIWI) model, an innovative approach at the University of Illinois, offers a strong example of transforming beliefs about families and their children into a set of guidelines and strategies. The PIWI model gives us some assumptions from which we can begin. These are presented in Figure 3.6. Because a healthy

---

FIGURE 3.6 **Assumptions of Parents Interacting with Infants (PIWI)**

- Parent-child interaction is a critical context for early learning and development.
- Parents' perceptions of themselves as competent parents come from early interactions with their children.
- The characteristics of the parent-child interaction are influenced by characteristics or behaviors of the child, the parent (e.g., depression), and the environment.
- Characteristics of the parent-child interaction contribute to the mutual nature of a developmentally supportive interaction.
- Characteristics of the parent-child interaction affect the relationship between parent and child and the benefits of EI.
- Developmentally supportive interactions are responsive to intervention that increases the parent's ability to interpret and respond to the infant's emotional, social, cognitive, and communicative cues.
- The ability to interpret and respond to the child's cues is dependent on knowledge and understanding of the child's perspective, dispositions, and temperament.
- Interactions between the SLP and parents provide a frame for parents to view their interactions with their child.
- Mutuality and partnership between the SLP and parent influence a parent's sense of confidence and competence as a parent.
- Responsive, supportive interactions among team members enhance competence, growth, and fulfillment.

Source: Information from McCollum et al., 2001.

parent-child relationship is at the heart of optimal early development, that relationship offers an effective focus and context for EI.

It's through strengthening of the parent-child relationship that we can enhance developmental opportunities for the child. This is accomplished through planned and guided observation of a child by the parents and through professional observation of the parent-child interaction. When the focus becomes the parent-child dyad, it changes the role of the SLP to that of interactional facilitator who attempts to promote parent-child interaction while supporting both members of the dyad.

Based on these assumptions, child goals might include (McCollum, Gooler, Appl, & Yates, 2001):

- Develop, maintain, practice, and master interactional skills;
- Explore and master the physical and social environment;
- Gain confidence in one's ability to influence events in the environment; and
- Through experience with interpersonal relationships, develop a healthy perception of self.

For parents and caregivers, the goals might include (McCollum et al., 2001):

- Gain knowledge of their child's development;
- Understand their role in this developmental process;
- Observe, develop, and practice interactional skills with their child;
- Within natural play and caregiving routines, address their child's IFSP goals;
- Develop a perception of self as parent;
- Become invested in and proud of their child's development and learning; and
- Experience joy in their mutual interaction.

One of the first things you probably noticed is how different these goals are from those found in traditional speech-language pathology with older children, which, given the caseloads found in many schools, is often reduced to some level of performance in learning to apply some morphological ending or language structure. This is not to belittle the very important need of many children for such intervention in order to be successful both academically and socially. But when our focus is very young children and their families, intervention is very different.

Accomplishment of these goals should be guided by your intervention philosophy. A service-providing philosophy is a simple statement of beliefs from which service provision flows. The best intervention is based on a vision and on principles that bring EI services into sharper focus. It's much more than just grabbing your little ECI language kit and marching off to save all the children of the world . . . or at least those on your caseload. Again, let's look at the PIWI model for some guidance.

If one of our basic assumptions is that parent-child relationships are critical for early development, then our overall model is one in which professionals collaborate with parents in providing developmentally appropriate and supportive environments for their child. This is accomplished by

- Expanding on a family's knowledge and understanding of their child,
- Building on natural interaction styles, and
- Acting on parent preferences.

Intervention is based on a belief, supported by scientific research, that a child's development is enhanced when parents recognize and enhance their own important developmental roles.

You might recall from your language acquisition text that early development is embedded within significant relationships and daily routines of the family and occurs through interactions with others in which the child is an active participant and learner. If you believe this, then intervention should focus on the parent-child interaction and on the parent's and child's strengths and be based on developmentally and culturally appropriate parent-child activities and interactions. Individual goals identified by parents can be blended into these interactions with adaptations to enhance a child's ability to engage.

Of course, there should also be a philosophy related to SLPs and facilitators. In general, an SLP's primary role should be to support and enhance parent-child relationships through collaboration. This is accomplished through supportive relationships with both parents and children and through providing meaningful and pleasurable opportunities for interaction. In addition, the SLP and other professionals function as resources for one another and for families.

From these beliefs flows a final one on the atmosphere that best reflects the family-centered, developmental approach to EI. This should be a commitment to the importance of the parent-infant relationship in the provision of personnel, time, and resources needed. In addition, staff should be committed to self-education and growth and to the fostering of team and individual development.

Conclusion

If you're thinking that you've heard some of this before, you're correct. Much of what was said in this chapter fits into the overall model of EI in Chapter 1, as it should. Remember that the provision of EI services must follow the legal requirements of family inclusion and intervention in the least restricted environment. ECI must fit within EI. In many cases, the justification for family inclusion and intervention in the LRE is stronger for ECI than for EI overall. If we want communication to generalize to the child's typical use environment, then it naturally flows that we should include those environments and the persons in them into our intervention.

A meta-analysis of parent-implemented language intervention studies with young children concluded that (Roberts & Kaiser, 2011)

- Intervention should focus on socially communicative interactions between parents and children,
- Parents should be taught to increase their use of specific linguistic forms through models and expansions,
- Parents should be trained at home and across everyday routines,
- Parent-implemented interventions may be effective for children with a range of intellectual and language skills, and
- Training parents about once per week may be sufficient to improve child language outcomes.

Both the content and the manner of parental interaction are important, as is general parental responsiveness.

 Click here to gauge your understanding of the concepts in this chapter.

4

Assessment of Early Communication Intervention: What to Assess

LEARNING OUTCOMES

When you have completed this chapter, you should be able to:

- Describe the role of parents and caregivers in early communication assessment.
- List the behaviors of interest in an informal assessment of communication.
- Explain the difficulty is assessing young children for autism spectrum disorder (ASD).

Terms with which you should be familiar:

Arena assessment
Attention-following
Communication breakdown
Contingent caregiver response
EI assessment
EI evaluation
Functional equivalence
Hyper-reactivity
Hypo-reactivity
Intentional communication

Item-based constructions
Joint attention
Lexical density
Pivot schemes
Proto-declaratives
Recognitory gestures
Reinforcing combinations
Representational gestures
Supplemental combinations
Word combinations

Y ou're about to discover that assessment of young children is not like any other type of communication evaluation in speech-language pathology. If you are a speech-language pathologist (SLP) student or professional who prefers a more "cookbook" procedure and the use of standardized tests, you may find early childhood assessment a challenge. And yet, if you like tasks that sometimes test your professional skills and problem-solving abilities, early communication assessment can be incredibly rewarding.

I recall once being escorted into a child's bedroom by his mother. It was like any other small child's room: crib, brightly painted walls, child furniture. The child, however, was very different than the room suggested. He was approximately 12 months of age, lying in a puddle of drool, seemingly oblivious to us standing right next to the bed. My task was to figure out how, with the parents' help, we could enable him to engage his world actively. No standardized test was going to work here.

Instead, the mother and I began by examining how he responded to the sights and sounds in his world and by identifying his attempts to influence these events. We noted his behavior in response to sound and light toys and to his mother's speaking to him. When he showed interest in a noisy object, I stopped the noise to see if he would indicate in some way that he wanted the noise and lights to continue. He showed only fleeting interest. After several attempts, he reached for the object when I stopped it. I activated it again. Repeated trials indicated that we might have a place to begin.

This example may be more severe than many you're likely to encounter, but hopefully, this example helps you appreciate that when it comes to EI assessment, "We're not in Kansas anymore, Toto!" You cannot pull your favorite standardized test out of your tote bag of materials and be done with it. By the same token, for those of you who are creative, are curious about the world, and think you might like the challenge, early communication assessment and intervention may be the right fit for you.

I wouldn't be honest if I didn't admit to a certain amount of frustration that is also part of early childhood communication assessment. Sometimes I get it wrong. Yep, we all do. On some occasions, I miss something. I make recommendations that are sometimes inappropriate or even unworkable. That's part of problem-solving too.

Early childhood communication assessment is not an exact science. It's a combination of science and art. The science comes in our attempts to systematically collect and objectively analyze what we experience. The art occurs in creating opportunities for communication to occur and in designing intervention strategies.

Federal legislation and state regulations have increased the importance of early intervention (EI) and focused especially on the diagnostic process. The goals of an assessment are to

- Collect developmental data,
- Identify the priorities, concerns, and resources of the family,
- Determine eligibility for EI services,
- Synthesize a plan for intervention,
- Enlist the caregivers' collaboration in intervention, and
- Monitor progress.

As we've mentioned, the movement toward more family-centered services necessitates a modification in more traditional roles for SLPs and other professionals. This is in recognition that family members are the primary decision-makers for themselves and that this necessitates their active participation in their child's assessment.

Current recommended practices within EI focus on comparing a child's skills across and within different developmental domains to provide a clearer picture of the child's overall development and to identify the child's relative strengths and challenges (Crais & Roberts, 2004). In addition to being required by law, this type of developmental "profiling" is thought to provide the best overall portrait of the child. At each step in assessment and intervention, a child's profile of skills should be used to help families and professionals make the most informed decisions.

A child's linguistic skills are built on a foundation of prelinguistic skills that not only serve as an indicator of the child's current skill level but are a strong predictor of the child's potential for language competence later. For very young children, especially those who are not talking, it is important to identify the key components of prelinguistic communication, such as vocalizations, symbolic play, gesture use, initiating and responding to joint attention, parental interactions, and familial history of language and/or learning impairments (Hadley & Holt, 2006; Mundy et al., 2007).

For many children, early language difficulties are already evident well before the second birthday (Määttä, Laakso, Tolvanen, Ahonen, & Aro, 2012). Delayed early expressive language and a minor delay of overall language performance plus symbolic difficulties are early signs of potential language disorders.

Our charges—the infants and toddlers we serve—are small and often sick or with multiple handicaps, and their caregivers may be confused and overwhelmed by their child's needs. We tailor our assessment to these realities.

An assessment is the child's and family's introduction to the EI process. The manner in which we, as professionals, interact with the family and the child can mean all the difference between a satisfying and fruitful experience that can lead to future collaboration if needed and a situation that leaves a family confused, frustrated, and possibly hostile.

If we hope to have the family as allies in our quest, we need to ensure that we structure our assessment to do just that. The assessment process is a vehicle for acquainting parents and caregivers with their role in the child's future intervention and for helping them become allies and partners with professionals in the EI process. In addition, the assessment experience can affect the family's views on both the child's abilities and their skills in meeting their child's needs. There's a lot riding on every assessment.

Typically, the assessment process for communication is a two-step affair, but the lines between them are blurry. First, the transdisciplinary team is interested in a more global or overall assessment. This may be followed by assessment of skills in different areas, such as communication. This two-step process is not carved in stone, and communication assessment may occur either as a portion of an overall evaluation or as its own separate assessment. In either case, the SLP is interested in the input from others on the transdisciplinary team.

Evaluation versus Assessment

In part, professional involvement is influenced by the way in which the SLP and other team members define assessment. Part H of the IDEA specifies that an EI evaluation must be conducted to determine a child's eligibility for services. This requires identifying a child's level of developmental functioning in a manner that is comprehensive, nondiscriminatory, and conducted by qualified personnel. Traditionally, evaluations are structured and formal and rely on the use of standardized instruments.

In contrast, *assessment* is the ongoing process of identifying a child's unique needs; the family's priorities, concerns, and resources; and the nature and extent of the EI services needed by both. As such, assessment activities are usually less formal and rely on the use of multiple tools and methods with the close cooperation of families and professionals. Typically, assessments focus not on what is *wrong* with a child but on identifying what levels of support are needed for the child and family to be successful.

Assessing early communication involves a dynamic model that threads its way between normative testing and more flexible nonstandardized approaches. The strength of normative testing is its strong external validity vis-à-vis the age at which certain behaviors can be expected. In contrast, nonstandardized approaches do not compare a child's existing system of communication with others. Instead, nonstandard approaches attempt to describe individualistic interactional behavior that by its nature defies standardization. These descriptions lead to hypotheses about patterns of interactional behavior in varying contexts and about how the child responds to different and changing stimuli.

Let's begin to sort this all out by first discussing a model for EI assessment, the role of caregivers, and then what to assess. In the following chapter, we'll discuss how to assess and some special considerations.

I had to make some tactical decisions when I designed this chapter. I've decided to leave assessment for augmentative and alternative communication (AAC) for later in the text. This is somewhat arbitrary but seems to make pedagogical sense. Keep in mind that as an alert clinician, you'll most likely already be making some tentative decisions about AAC even in the early stages of the assessment mentioned here.

Transdisciplinary Model of Assessment

Many young children need to be assessed by more than one professional and may have disorders in several developmental areas. In most cases, the SLP will be a central figure in these evaluations and in subsequent intervention decisions. The question then becomes how to coordinate the interaction between these various professionals and parents in order to have the true team assessment required by law rather than a fragmented one. As you know from Chapter 1, a transdisciplinary model of assessment has evolved over the past several years as a way of integrating input and providing a holistic assessment of the child and family.

In short, a transdisciplinary team approach is one in which there is a conscious effort to pool expertise and freely exchange insights and ideas. This is best accomplished if parents and professionals observe the entire evaluation and simultaneously assess the child, a method dubbed arena assessment. Instead of the child's being separately assessed by each discipline, a common sample of the child's behavior is collected and recorded as all observe the process. In a transdisciplinary approach, professionals who are accustomed to viewing a child through individual disciplinary lenses learn to see a child holistically as an integrated being. In the process, professionals draw their inferences from a common core of data.

To SLPs more familiar with standardized testing, the rather open-ended data collection methods common to this model can be a little disconcerting at first and may, on the surface, seem to yield very little. I remember a group of graduate students bemoaning our lack of test scores and, by implication, our lack of information, at the same time that I was thrilled by how much we knew about the young child's cognitive and communicative ability.

PLAY-BASED ASSESSMENT

Early communication data are frequently collected through both free and structured play with the child and via caregiver interviews and questionnaires. In other words, the assessment with the child is play based rather than test based, and the methods of collecting data are varied.

There are some assessment tools available to an SLP that can aid in a play-based assessment. For example, the *Transdisciplinary Play-Based Assessment* (Linder, 1993) offers a model for assessment with results that highly correlate with more structured measures such as the *Bayley Scales of Infant Development, Second Edition* (Bayley, 1993) (Kelly-Vance, Needelman, Troia, & Ryalls, 1999). Other assessment tools that have a play component or can be easily adapted to a play mode are listed in Figure 4.1 (ASHA, 2008b).

In addition, the *MacArthur-Bates Communicative Development Inventories* (Fenson et al., 2006) contain a list of play behaviors that parents can check off. We'll have more to say about these assessment tools later.

In structured play, the partner attempts through manipulation of the context to elicit specific behaviors from the child while using a play mode. For example, while playing, an adult, either a professional or a parent, may roll a ball under or behind another object to see if the child will search for it or may play an imitation "game" to see if the child will follow suit. Throughout, the process of interaction takes precedence over the product or result. A failure by the child to comply or a partial reply by the child is still good information.

It is all too easy to assume that the word *play* implies an open-ended free-for-all in which data are collected haphazardly. Nothing could be further from the truth.

FIGURE 4.1 **Assessment Tools That Have a Play Component or Can Be Easily Adapted to a Play Mode**

Assessment, Evaluation, and Programming System (Bricker, 2002)

Carpenter Play Scale (R. L. Carpenter, 1987)

Casby Scale (Casby, 2003)

Communication and Symbolic Behavior Scales Developmental Profile: First Normed Edition (Wetherby & Prizant, 2002)

Infant-Preschool Play Assessment Scale (I-PAS) (Flagler, 1996)

MacArthur-Bates Communicative Development Inventories (Fenson et al., 2006), which contain a list of play behaviors that parents can check off

McCune Play Scale (McCune, 1995)

Rossetti Infant-Toddler Language Scale (Rossetti, 1990)

Symbolic Play Test (Lowe & Costello, 1988).

Source: ASHA, 2008b.

CONCLUSION

When we bring together all of the new concepts introduced above and in previous chapters, we have a *transdisciplinary play-based arena assessment*. The list of advantages for this type of assessment over other more structured, discipline-specific methods includes

■ Naturalistic,
■ Ecologically sound,
■ Context based, and
■ Child centered.

I had the good fortune to participate in an excellent transdisciplinary play-based arena-style assessment conducted by the fine faculty and students at the University of Pretoria in South Africa. While an SLP played with the child, faculty and students from several disciplines observed through one-way glass. At the same time, another professional interviewed the mother in the same room as the child, and a third recorded the entire event. At some point during the assessment, the mother joined her child on the floor to engage in play. In the observation room, there was a lively discussion throughout the evaluation and much note-taking on both the child's and the mother's behaviors. Suggestions were passed from the observation room to the professionals in the other room when specific information was desired.

Following this phase of an evaluation, team members, including parents, meet to formulate a report integrating observations and proposing a transdisciplinary intervention plan, called an Individualized Family Service Plan, discussed in Chapter 1. As you'll recall, parents are an integral part of the team rather than simply receivers of the team's recommendations. Let's investigate the parents' role more thoroughly.

Role of Parents and Caregivers

As I'm fond of saying ad nauseum, thanks to my training with Dr. Jim MacDonald, now retired from Ohio State University, "We can't teach only one person to communicate." Communication by its nature requires at least two people. In practice, this means that we must teach a child ways to signal needs and desires while at the same time teaching caregivers—usually parents—to encourage and respond to these attempts by the child. This is another way of saying that our approach will be environmental or ecological. This was summed up on a sign that used to hang in my office that read, "Communication training without the environment is like toilet training without the potty."

I give parents credit for helping their child attain her or his current level of communicative skill, but I also recognize that what the parents are doing may not be enough to move their child forward from this point. If so, as an SLP, I hope to be similar to the person who enters a room and finds the one puzzle piece that those engaged in the puzzle-making have been unable to locate.

Public Law 99-457, Education of All Handicapped Children Act Amendments (1986), and the Individuals with Disabilities Education Improvement Act (IDEIA) (2004) highlighted the need for greater family participation in early intervention. In order for families to be empowered, they must be full participants and real decision-makers in the EI process (Dunst, 2002). If assessment and intervention recommendations are to be "owned" by a family, these proposals must match the family's notions of appropriateness and importance.

The changing demographics of an increasingly diverse United States require that SLPs respect each family's unique sociocultural characteristics (Barrera & Corso, 2002). Our task is to help family members identify those early intervention practices that mesh with the family's cultural perceptions of its role. In doing so, we can attempt to avoid cultural bias and activities that are misunderstood, inappropriate, and unsupported by families.

When parents are asked about specific assessment practices, they indicate receiving fewer chances to participate than they would have liked (Crais & Belardi, 1999). Unfortunately, despite legal requirements to do otherwise, some service providers continue to offer only limited roles for parents in the evaluative decision-making processes (McWilliam, Snyder, Harbin, Porter, & Munn, 2000). Although caregiver decision-making and participation are uneven within and across EI programs, parents routinely report having relatively little input in their child's assessment. You can change that.

A RATIONALE FOR PARENTAL INVOLVEMENT IN ASSESSMENT

The assessment process is an introduction for the family to the early communication intervention (ECI) process. Assessment may be the first or one of the initial contacts between you as an SLP and the family. Your behavior at that time determines whether or not a family becomes vested in their child's communication development program. In essence, the family's experience during the assessment determines if parents will become your allies, and their cooperation and partnership are vitally important.

Traditionally, parents have served as informants and describers of their child's behaviors during assessments. When surveyed, parents and professionals differ widely in their perceptions of family participation both in the assessment process and in assessment decisions (McWilliam et al., 2000). In general, parents state that they want more control over decisions made during their child's assessment (Crais, Roy, & Free, 2006). A lack of parental participation in an early communication assessment may be the result of (Bruder, 2000)

- A belief by SLPs that testing can only be administered in a standard manner,
- The hesitancy of SLPs to give up the role of primary decision-maker, and
- The notion that parents lack the knowledge and expertise to adequately participate in the child's assessment.

Research, however, has documented that parents can be both reliable informants and valuable team members and can be very accurate in reporting current and emerging behaviors of their child (Crais, Douglas, & Campbell, 2004). For example, one study found that mothers could very accurately describe the communication behaviors of their young children with fragile X syndrome (Brady, Skinner, Roberts, & Hennon, 2006).

There are numerous reasons that families are critical to the assessment process. Family members

- Have unique knowledge of their child's special needs;
- Know the variety of people, settings, and conditions of their child's interactions;
- Can suggest alternative ways to elicit behaviors; and
- Are a wealth of knowledge on their child's developmental history.

Through the combined efforts of family members and professionals, a larger sample of behaviors may be available for analysis. For example, when parents, teachers, and SLPs are asked to suggest vocabulary training for children, each contributes words unique to his or her interactions with the child, resulting in a more well-rounded vocabulary.

Families can also gain from their participation in the assessment process. They may gain increased understanding of their child's abilities and needs or may increase their ability to handle stressful care provision issues. Participation may also foster increased awareness of development and of their child's strengths and weaknesses.

The active participation of the child's caregivers enhances the validity of an assessment. By using families as co-assessors, you can efficiently gain more, and more varied, information than you could alone. In fact, the input of caregivers can both enhance and shorten an assessment.

Given that care providers are most often the primary agents of change in ECI, their participation in assessment can benefit both intervention planning and implementation. Without consensus between caregivers and professionals on assessment procedures and outcomes, however, parents are less likely to follow the recommendations made by SLPs.

INVOLVING FAMILIES IN AN ASSESSMENT

Although numerous family-centered principles have been identified, the implementation of these principles in actual practice has been difficult to gauge (McWilliam et al., 2000). Wide agreement exists between caregivers and professionals on family-centered practices, but a gap exists between what families and professionals view as actual implementation and how each might like it to occur ideally (Crais et al., 2006). This may be especially true if parents feel that they are not invited to meetings, not asked to review reports and make suggestions, and not requested to make written observational notes. Figure 4.2 presents family-centered practices that can provide an expanded role for families in the assessment process.

To help families with this new role, a portion of the assessment should include evaluation of the caregivers' strengths and weaknesses and consideration of the roles they will play in intervention. More on how this can be accomplished will be discussed in this chapter and the next.

FIGURE 4.2 **Family-Centered Practices That Expanded the Role for Families in Assessment**

- Inviting parents to a meeting with the whole team before the assessment
- Inviting caregivers to participate in preassessment planning
- Asking parents about previous assessments, including how they felt about the results and the most/least successful activities or techniques used in the assessment
- Identifying the family's most important concerns
- Asking the family to observe or write down observations of the child before the assessment
- Asking the family what the child does well
- Offering the option for the family to write down observations during the assessment
- Asking parents to identify strategies to use in assessing their child
- Making and accepting positive comments about the child
- Having caregivers complete an assessment tool and comment on its use and findings
- Asking whether the behaviors observed were typical of the child
- Summarizing and explaining all assessment results
- Asking if the family agrees with the assessment results
- Collaboratively identifying next steps for the family and professional
- Having parents preview the written report and suggest changes

TABLE 4.1 **Assessment Settings**

	HOME-BASED	CENTER-BASED
Benefits	More comfortable for family More natural family setting Fragile or young child's health better protected Family routines can be preserved Sibling interactions may be present Greater likelihood of gaining meaningful insights	Greater access to entire professional staff and selected experts on an ad hoc basis Opportunity for parents to interact with other families Ready availability of services All members present for immediate team conference
Drawbacks	Wide range of possible responses, including possibly disinterested parent Home setting can be extremely distracting Inability of all team members to attend Travel time for professional staff who do attend	May be extremely difficult for family with a medically fragile child Family may need to obtain childcare and/or transportation Travel time for family Extra time taken from family schedule or work

Parental accuracy in describing a child's behavior can be increased through a checklist format, such as circling the words a child produces, rather than a free-form report or diary, such as writing down the words. In fact, parents using a checklist of their child's vocabulary may be as accurate as formal testing in identifying the words a child understands and produces.

In order to accommodate families, EI centers may need to modify the ways in which assessment and intervention occur. For example, to enable families to participate fully in an assessment, centers may need to provide childcare services, meals, and private areas for changing the child or for just being alone for short periods. In some cases, it may be best to assess a child in the home environment. There are advantages to assessment in either a center or in the home. There are also drawbacks to each. These are presented in Table 4.1.

FAMILY CONCERNS, PRIORITIES, AND RESOURCES

IDEA 2004 requires that programs provide an opportunity for a family to identify their concerns, priorities, and resources related to enhancement of their child's development. Some key objectives that guide the gathering of information may include (ASHA 2008b; Bailey, 2004):

- Identify the family's concerns
- Identify what they hope to accomplish through the assessment
- Determine how the family perceives the child's strengths and needs
- Determine the family's values, structure, and routines as they affect the child
- Identify the family's priorities
- Determine how service providers might assist the family with these priorities
- Identify the family's resources relative to the priorities
- Identify the family's preferred role in service delivery and decision-making
- Establish through this process a supportive and collaborative relationship that informs intervention

Each of these outcomes should be addressed in an assessment and throughout the intervention process. Let's discuss each briefly.

Families' concerns vary with each family and are influenced by characteristics of the family, culture, community, and experiences (Winton, Brotherson, & Summers, 2008). Because the family knows their child and their family circumstances best, it is important for professionals to honor the family's perspectives. Some families may have very specific concerns to be addressed, while others may be less sure of what they want from the service system. Families may be less likely to talk about certain concerns, such as marital issues or difficulties, especially in the early phases of service delivery.

It is important to gather information about how the family perceives their child's strengths and needs relative to their own beliefs, values, and everyday experiences. This requires having the family identify the ways that the child functions within the daily environment.

Although professionals may not always agree with family members, identifying their priorities for the child and the family is important for future planning and intervention. Priorities reflect values, and it would not be uncommon for professionals and families to have differing priorities. It isn't necessary that everyone agree as long as they understand and honor each other's viewpoint.

Professionals can consider the range of resources that might be available to a family. These include formal supports, such as social services, and informal supports, including family members, neighbors and friends, and community and religious organizations. Existing and potential resources and supports are important for intervention planning.

Not all families desire to take the same roles within service delivery and decision-making. Some families may prefer very active roles, while others prefer to have professionals take the lead. The specific roles are less important than the way those roles are identified and used. Families can be offered choices, and professionals can individualize services and supports to match the family's preferences, which may vary with different components of ECI service delivery or over time (Bailey, 2004). A family's priorities will be influenced by their perceptions and experiences with the EI systems, their beliefs about their child, and other sociocultural factors (Applequist & Bailey, 2000; Chen & McCollum, 2001).

Finally, professionals need to take their lead from the family as to the type of relationship preferred. Relationship-building is one of the more important elements of ECI and family-centered services. At the very least, SLPs can be friendly and positive, responsive, oriented to all family members, and sensitive. Although building good relationships with families is important, participatory practices that build competence and confidence are key in parental empowerment and full partnership (Dempsey & Dunst, 2004).

Before we begin to discuss assessment of a child with communication impairment, it might be good to remind ourselves of a typically developing (TD) child, such as this 2-year-old using two-word utterances.

Informal Communication Assessment

Initially, you may have assumed that there is little to assess in nonverbal children because they may not be talking yet. Actually, the opposite is true. The difficulty comes in trying to winnow down all the possible behaviors and to note only the most important ones. At the present time, researchers are attempting to identify the most significant early communication developments that affect early language. One of the values of evidence-based practice is that we are beginning to recognize which child behaviors seem to have the greatest impact on later communication intervention.

Although some efficacy studies exist, there is little research that definitively concludes that teaching any one behavior results in more rapid development of speech and language. For this reason, I will target those behaviors mentioned most frequently in the professional literature and found to be important in my own clinical experience. Other professionals, including your professor, may have had similar or quite different experiences and will, hopefully, share these with you.

In the following sections, we'll explore the information that we hope to gain from an evaluation of both the child and caregivers. In each section, I'll provide a rationale for the choices I have made. We'll discuss

- The communication behaviors of the child, including the caregiver-child interaction, and
- The nonsymbolic and symbolic child behaviors of interest.

To begin this discussion, it may be helpful to look at children with ASD. Multiple factors seem to contribute to the development of language skills in young children with ASD and may give us a place to begin. Of importance are (Bono, Daley, & Sigman, 2004; Charman, Baron-Cohen, et al., 2003; Stone & Yoder, 2001; Woods & Wetherby, 2003)

- Functional and symbolic use of objects,
- The number and type of gestures,
- Ability to initiate joint attention,
- Presence of verbal imitation skills,
- Number of words produced, and
- Number of words comprehended.

Several studies of young children with ASD also report an association between attention, imitation skills, and language (Bono & Sigman, 2004; Dawson et al., 2004; Siller & Sigman, 2002; Stone & Yoder, 2001). This appears to be true regardless of a young child's cognitive status or the severity of autism characteristics (Smith, Mirenda, & Zaidman-Zait, 2007). In fact, attention, imitation skills, and the use of gestures appear to be more important than intelligence as predictors of later language development among children with ASD.

Two additional prerequisites for the development of language would seem to be the motivation to convey a message, called communicative intent, and the ability to think at a symbolic level. Many young children with ASD have difficulties with both (Prizant, Wetherby, & Rydell, 2000).

DESCRIPTION OF COMMUNICATION

All humans communicate. I begin with that assumption. It may be unintentional, such as crying, or intentional, such as a gesture, but from the time we're born, we are enveloped in a world of communication and treated by others as natural communicators. Both unintentional and unconventional at first, an infant's communication behaviors become increasingly intentional and conventional during the first year of life.

Younger TD children at certain stages of development and many of those with developmental disabilities can be said to be either *nonsymbolic* or *presymbolic*, using few or no conventional symbols in the form of words, signs, or picture symbols (Wetherby, Prizant, & Schuler, 2000). Instead, nonsymbolic children interact using gestures, vocalizations, echolalia, and for some, problem or challenging behavior. Sadly, without symbols, many attempts to communicate will be misunderstood or unsuccessful.

Terminology

I would be doing you a disservice if I didn't acknowledge that there is a professional debate going on as to the use of the terms *nonsymbolic* and *presymbolic* to describe our clients not using symbols. I prefer *nonsymbolic* in recognition that some individuals, especially those with severe communication deficits, may never attain truly symbolic communication. In this way they are technically not presymbolic. I will use *presymbolic* when referring to behaviors of TD children prior to symbol acquisition.

One additional term should also be mentioned. Some professionals prefer *prelinguistic*. Of course, the use of language involves much more than the use of symbols. Remember, language involves symbols and rules for combining and using those symbols. Linguistic communication occurs when a child develops a generative system for creating word or symbol combinations. That will develop later. It may seem like splitting hairs, but a progression for children with communication impairment might be as follows:

- ■ Nonsymbolic
- ■ Prelinguistic/symbolic
- ■ Linguistic

While that may seem logical, no professional I know uses this terminology to distinguish differing levels of attainment. Be warned, you are stepping into a minefield where different terms may be used to refer to the same thing. For simplicity, I'll stick to *nonsymbolic* and *symbolic* in reference to our clients.

Much nonsymbolic communication between children with developmental disabilities (DDs) and caregivers is termed *idiosyncratic*, meaning individualistic in an eccentric sort of way. The child's attempts to communicate, possibly through screaming to signal a desire for something or making a consistent sound to indicate dislike, have evolved over time and are unique to the child and caregiver. That's idiosyncratic.

Often occurring within established routines, idiosyncratic communication may be incomprehensible to others outside the immediate context. In other words, the child does not have behaviors that can be used in communication within a larger circle of potential partners. In short, no one else understands the child's communicative behaviors. The child simply does not use the conventional means of communication used by everyone else. Our challenge is to unravel these behaviors, to identify their meaning and intent, and then to use what we can while moving the child to more conventional ways of communicating that will be comprehensible to a wider group of potential communication partners.

Conventional Communication

Often college students wonder why we don't just leave the child's system in place and teach others to accept the child's behaviors. At some points in intervention, we will do just that. But the rationale for going to a more conventional system is simply that other people—teachers, aides, other family members—usually will not make the effort to learn another system of communication for each individual child. They're not evil people, just distracted by other concerns or too busy. Imagine being a teacher in a class of 10 children and trying to interpret 10 different communication systems.

Think about the majority culture's response to the Deaf Community. Why doesn't everyone who is hearing just learn to sign so they can communicate with people with deafness? We just don't. Now imagine trying to convince everyone to learn the communication method of individual children.

While it might be possible for a babysitter to learn the child's method of communication, it isn't feasible or desirable for the preschool teacher to learn different modes of communication for each child. And how will the children communicate with each other? From an intervention perspective, if a child is already expressing his or her own meanings and intentions in an idiosyncratic way, then we have a base from which to build new, more widely used ways to express those already present communication functions. It's important to realize that we are not teaching new replacement behaviors, but rather modifying old ones.

Let me personalize this. I was speaking to the mother of a young woman with ASD. The mother had home-schooled her nonsymbolic daughter, and as a family, they had developed their own communication system. Her daughter was now at the age where her parents wished to have her reside in a community residence with other adults with developmental disabilities. Unfortunately, no one else understood the elaborate communication system used within the family. This was a real dilemma because the level of independence desired by the family required that their daughter be able to communicate with others. Although a seemingly simple solution might be to change her daughter's communication prior to placement, this will not be an easy task given almost 20 years of using her own method. While this is an extreme case, it highlights the need to think long term. To only think of the immediate future is to undervalue the lives of those with communication impairments.

Of most importance for future communication development is intentionality, or goal-directed communication behavior. Intentionality signals that the child is aware that people are a means for attaining a desired end. With intent, the performance of communicative signals becomes purposeful and goal oriented. It is within the context of intentional presymbolic communication that the TD infant, in a desire to be better understood, modifies his or her communication behavior to become more conventional. The result is greater communication success.

With this background in mind, during an assessment an SLP attempts to describe as well as possible the present communication system of the child and caregiver. Of importance are the

- Forms and means of communication, and
- Communication success.

Of course, successful communication depends on more than just the child. Success requires a responsive partner. We'll discuss caregivers in more detail in the following sections. For now, let's briefly discuss forms and means and success.

Forms and means of communication. Communication forms are both intentional and unintentional behaviors performed by a child in the presence of a caregiver. The means may be physical, vocal, or both. Physical, or nonvocal, signals may include eye contact, facial expression, communication distance, body movements or contact, gestures, and even aggression to self or others. Vocal signals can range from soft sounds to screaming and crying.

A positive relationship exists between the early use of various means of communication and later language skills in children with communication delays and those with ASD (McCathren, Yoder, & Warren, 2000; Zwaigenbaum, Bryson, Rogers, Brian, & Szatmari, 2005). Gesture use among "late talkers" can help predict which children will attain more typical development. It is important, therefore, that all forms of communication be identified in an assessment.

Although we'll discuss children's use of language later, it's worth noting here that the form and means of communication may be related to the function or use of communication. Both early language form and function follow orderly developmental progressions in TD children (Nathani, Ertmer, & Stark, 2006; Oller, 2000). During the prelinguistic and early linguistic period, some forms of vocalization are more tightly linked than others to specific language functions (Iyer & Ertmer, 2014). Other forms and functions vary freely. Individual child variation exists. This said, it may be helpful during an assessment to note whether specific phonological forms are used with specific communication functions. If so, this information may help to inform how an SLP proceeds in expanding a child's communication abilities.

Functional Equivalence. Before we move on, we should spend some time describing functional equivalence and its relevance for communication assessment. If two behaviors have the same effect on the environment, they are considered to be *functionally equivalent* (Carr, 1988). For example, a child may either tap a potential listener on the back or scream to get attention. These behaviors are functionally equivalent if they produce the same outcome. Similarly, a child may seek to escape from an activity either by screaming or by kicking her legs. Again, the behaviors are functionally equivalent if they both achieve the same end. In both cases, attention-seeking and escaping, we can assume that each behavior has been reinforced in the past by producing the child's desired outcome.

Functionally equivalent behaviors are in competition with one another, and depending on situational conditions, one will prevail and be expressed. The specific behavior expressed will be the most efficient one for that situation. The relative efficiency of a behavior, called *response efficiency*, can determine use of that behavior by a child. Response efficiency refers to the relationship between effort and outcome (Halle & Drasgow, 2003).

In general, a child will attempt to use the most efficient way to obtain a desired outcome. Several factors are important in determining efficiency (Halle, Brady, & Drasgow, 2004):

■ Response effort
■ Immediacy of outcome
■ Consistency of outcome
■ Quality
■ History of punishment/ignoring

Effort is the amount of energy required to produce the response. For example, speech may require great effort for a child with cerebral palsy (CP) compared to indicating a picture using a laser pointer attached to a headband.

Immediacy is the quickness with which a child obtains the desired outcome. If tantruming produces the desired end more quickly than pointing, then tantruming becomes the child's communication behavior of choice.

Consistency refers to the frequency with which the desired outcome is obtained. If throwing food on the floor gets the desired response while saying "No" requires two or three attempts before food is removed, then throwing food is more efficient.

Quality refers to the strength of the caregiver's response. If caregivers respond with a large amount of juice to quiet a child who is yelling but only with a small amount when a child signs "Juice," then screaming is more efficient.

Finally, history relates to consequences that reduce the likelihood of the child's response. Child communication behaviors that have been punished or ignored in the past are less efficient and less likely to be used. If, for example, the child's sign "No" was ignored but a tantrum was reinforced by ending a nondesired activity, the sign's efficiency is decreased.

It should be obvious from this discussion that the frequency of all five factors is highly dependent on the behavior of the partners with whom a child interacts.

If you're following this discussion, then it should have dawned on you that when we teach a child a new way of achieving the same desired end, the old behavior and the new are functionally equivalent and in competition with one another. In this situation, response efficiency becomes very important, and each SLP becomes a detective, trying to figure out the variables that affect each behavior. During an assessment, an SLP will attempt to look behind the child's behaviors, even disruptive ones that may be used to communicate. Relax for now; we'll talk about how to intervene in a few chapters from now.

Let's just take a moment to recognize how some forms of challenging behaviors may arise. For some children, unacceptable forms of behavior, such as hitting or biting, can become more efficient than other, socially accepted behaviors. Depending on the degree of unacceptability, these behaviors can affect both the child and the family. Families may feel helpless to control their child's behaviors and are judged poorly by others because of these behaviors. The family's social life may be restricted because of or in anticipation of the child's challenging behavior (Fox, Dunlap, & Buschbacher, 2000). In addition, these behaviors can negatively affect relationships within the family.

Challenging behaviors can also negatively affect assessment and intervention services. It is difficult for a child to attend to interactions while acting out.

When differing behaviors all produce the same outcome, such as obtaining an object, then these responses are said to form a *response class*. All members of a response class are functionally equivalent. A defining feature of a response class is that anything that affects the probability of one member will affect the probability of all members. In other words, functionally equivalent responses are in competition with each other.

We now recognize that some challenging behavior, even self-injurious behavior, may be an attempt to communicate (Durand & Merges, 2001). Given a child's limited behavioral resources, the behavior may enable nonsymbolic children to influence people in the environment in desired ways.

The research literature contains numerous examples of challenging behaviors that have signaled messages such as the following (Bopp, Brown, & Mirenda, 2004):

■ "I want X" (Robinson & Owens, 1995; Sigafoos & Mirenda, 2002)
■ "I want social interaction/attention" (Light, Parsons, & Drager, 2002)

- ■ "I don't want X" (Sigafoos, O'Reilly, Drasgow, & Reichle, 2002).
- ■ "Hello" or notice me (Robinson & Owens, 1995)

While some behaviors serve a single function, others serve multiple functions.

Let's look at an example of how this might occur. Suppose during group snack, Carlos looks at the teacher, vocalizes, and points to a box of cookies but is ignored. He makes a second attempt with the same outcome. Finally, he begins to scream and struggle to reach the cookies. The teacher responds by saying "Carlos, stop screaming. Here's your cookie." Having achieved his desired outcome, Carlos is more likely to scream in the future to achieve his end.

If his first two socially appropriate attempts had been honored by the teacher, Carlos may not have resorted to screaming. By ignoring the first two attempts, his teacher has made these forms less likely in the future. In contrast, the teacher's immediate responding to his third, inappropriate behavior (screaming) made it more likely to occur again in a similar situation. Although unintentional, the teacher's behavior has taught Carlos that screaming is an effective communication strategy. In similar fashion, the parent who decides that prompting a word is too much trouble and just accepts a vocalization has made the same error.

Although a child has begun to communicate, the method or form of that communication may be inappropriate, unacceptable, or below the level desired, such as a vocalization when capable of producing a word. Sometimes unknowingly, communicative partners reinforce a nonconventional or socially unacceptable communicative form, resulting in that behavior's being functionally equivalent or having the same function as an acceptable form of communication.

In defense of parents and teachers who are interacting with the child, we need to recognize that no one starts out trying to teach challenging behaviors to children. Parents and teachers are busy, and sometimes it takes a scream or a self-injurious behavior to obtain their attention. Unwittingly, the adults may be teaching unacceptable means of communication. When my grandson began hitting himself as his mom, my daughter, left the house, we had to think quickly how to honor his request that she remain without reinforcing the hitting.

It's important to note that not all challenging behavior is taught. I worked with a child who hit his head when he experienced painful headaches. It was most likely his attempt to make the pain less.

Communication success. Stated simply, communication success occurs when a communicator's goal is attained. For example, a child requests an object through gesturing and subsequently receives it. Nothing succeeds like success for strengthening a behavior. Success, therefore, is a factor in functional equivalence. If tantruming gets you what you want, you're more likely to tantrum the next time. Success doesn't occur automatically. Sometimes a child's message is not understood. On other occasions, a caregiver may decide not to comply. The communication is still successful as long as the caregiver acknowledges that the message was understood, as in "No, honey, you can't have a cookie until after dinner." Communication failure, on the other hand, may encourage a child to modify or change the behavior.

Initially, infant communication meets with little success, owing to the TD child's lack of skill. With little success to bolster these behaviors, a child often abandons early attempts. With maturation and increasing success, the typical 7- to 11-month-old infant who encounters communication difficulties abandons her or his attempts less often and increases the use of augmentations, simplifications, and substitutions. Augmentation is adding more behaviors, such as a vocalization; simplification may include dropping a behavior. In substitution, a child may abandon one gesture or vocalization and try another. In other words, the infant's behavior becomes more flexible to meet the needs of the situation and to accomplish a desired goal. If, after age 1, a child continues to abandon interaction all together or to simply repeat the behavior over and over, it may signal a potential communication problem (Hanson & Olswang, 2005).

The success of a child's communication depends as much on the communication partners and the environment as on the child. Efficiency improves with the advent of intentional or goal-oriented behavior, demonstrating that the child understands that objects and persons can be used to achieve an end. Intentionality, the use of purposeful communication signals to influence others, is evident when a child exhibits behaviors that indicate deliberate pursuit of an objective. In general, when compared to unintentional behaviors, intentional nonsymbolic communication, such as gesturing, is less ambiguous, more efficient, and more successful.

Our task as SLPs is to describe communicative or potential communicative behaviors as best we can and to attempt to determine how they are used by the child and/or interpreted by caregivers as communication. And as mentioned, there are no one-size-fits-all tests that do this for us. This is where your real clinical skill comes into play. I'll offer as much guidance as I can when we discuss how to accomplish this.

Caregiver-Child Interactions

Parents' and other caregivers' behaviors are also evaluated within the context of interacting with the child. It is within this interaction that most of the work of intervention will occur, so the quality of that interaction will be an important factor in a child's learning to communicate more effectively.

Part of any evaluation is determining the sensitivity, responsiveness, and interpretation of intent by caregivers in response to the child's attempts to communicate. Responsiveness includes

- Contingency, or the relatedness of the response to the behavior of the child;
- Consistency of the adult response; and
- Timeliness, or the quickness with which the adult responds.

All of these factors add to the quality of the caregiver-child interaction.

Sensitivity includes noticing the sometimes subtle behavior of the child as he or she displays interest or attempts to interact with an object or a person or to communicate in some way. Parents who are either distracted or more intent on completing some task may miss chances to interact with their child.

Caregivers can develop and improve their sensitivity (Siegel & Wetherby, 2000; Snell & Loncke, 2002). In turn, a child can learn the impact of certain behaviors through the responsiveness of others, primarily caregivers. This requires caregivers to be more than just sensitive. Consistent caregiver responses provide consequences that encourage or discourage behaviors.

Caregivers often interpret a child's behavior as meaningful and purposeful even when it is not meant to be by the child. Over time, certain behaviors, even challenging or aggressive ones, can take on this interpretation based on the caregivers' responses to the behavior. As mentioned, in part, a caregiver's response can determine functional equivalence.

Just as important may be behaviors of a child that are missed. A child may signal a desire with eye contact. If a caregiver misses this behavior, it may become lessened. In frustration, a child may scream. If the care provider responds at this point, the screaming behavior may be strengthened.

A **contingent caregiver response** is one based on the perceived intent of the child. In this way, the response is related to the child's behavior. For example, as a child struggles to reach a desired toy, a contingent adult response might be to say, "You want train? Mommy help," as she hands the toy to the child. Such a response provides labels for the object and the child's behavior, while handing the toy to the child strengthens the reaching behavior as a signal of desire.

Over time, as a child's behavior, such as pointing, is responded to in a consistent manner, the behavior becomes a signal of the child's intent. In this way, even random or idiosyncratic behaviors can take on meaning.

Social responsiveness in caregivers is demonstrated in several ways. A few are presented in Figure 4.3 (Siegel & Wetherby, 2000). It's important to remember that all forms of communication occur within a cultural context. Caregiver responsivity may vary widely by culture and country of origin. We cannot assume that the behaviors of the majority culture in the United States or any country are the norm for everyone. SLPs need to be

FIGURE 4.3 **Social Responsiveness of Caregivers**

- Individualized structuring of situations to support or guide a child's performance
- Following a child's lead, such as commenting on an object to which a child has pointed
- Establishing joint or shared attention with a child
- Waiting for or prompting communicative responses or initiations from a child
- Outwardly interpreting a child's intent, such as saying "Oh, you want to pet the doggie"
- Complying with a child's interpreted intent, such as giving a requested object
- Seeking clarification of a child's failed communication attempts by looking confused or asking "What?"
- Shaping increasingly clear and more conventional behaviors, such as a recognizable gesture, from a child before responding

Source: Information from Siegel & Wetherby, 2000.

mindful that Western patterns of interaction and parenting may conflict with those of other cultures.

Caregiver interviews and environmental observations may suggest preferred materials, partners, settings, and activities that promote a child's interest and communication. Similarly, data can suggest environmental shortcomings in need of improvement.

PRESYMBOLIC BEHAVIORS

During the presymbolic period, a TD child learns to initiate communication for a variety of purposes and to attend jointly with a partner. Communication becomes purposeful and increasingly symbolic. Let's look at what we know and try to determine what we might wish to assess.

For TD toddlers, early communication predicts later language performance in the preschool years (Chiat & Roy, 2008; Watt, Wetherby, & Shumway, 2006). Especially important factors are

- Early receptive language skill,
- Use of a range of conventional gestures,
- Communication for joint attention, and
- A child's inventory of consonants.

Aspects of early language acquisition among TD children have their roots in these children's presymbolic interactions. Our knowledge of the presymbolic-linguistic relationships enables early identification and monitoring of children at risk and informs intervention.

Of most importance in predicting later language skills in TD children and children with DDs are the following presymbolic behaviors:

- Joint attention and attention-following of gazing and pointing
- Variety and complexity in symbolic play (Lyytinen, Poikkeus, Laakso, Eklund, & Lyytinen, 2001)
- Intentional communication and the use of gestures and vocalizations (McCathren et al., 2000). The use of gestures correlates with later receptive language abilities (Watt et al., 2006). Gestures may, in fact, serve as a bridge from understanding language to actively producing language. The extent of early pointing predicts the level and rate of vocabulary growth two years later (Brady, Marquis, Fleming, & McLean, 2004; Calandrella & Wilcox, 2000).
- Complexity of presymbolic vocalizations, including variety of consonants and syllable structures

FIGURE 4.4 **Signs of Possible Early Communication Delay**

- Six-month or greater delays in comprehension as well as production
- Limited response to own name and to language
- Few spontaneous vocalizations
- Limited variety of consonants in babbling
- Few spontaneous imitations
- A lack of object or symbolic play
- Limited communicative gestures or vocalizations
- Low rate of nonverbal communication
- Requesting as the sole communicative intent
- Difficulty gaining access to peer interactions
- A preference for adults over peers
- A family history of language delays or reading problems

Sources: Ellis & Thal, 2009; Paul, 2007; Paul & Roth, 2011a.

■ Rate of intentional verbal, gestural, and vocal behavior, which predicts spontaneous word productions within two years (Calandrella & Wilcox, 2000)
■ Receptive language, or the number of words and phrases understood by a child. Numerous studies have demonstrated that receptive language is a significant predictor of later expressive language skills (Lyytinen et al., 2001).

Children delayed only in the use of words are more likely to catch up on their own compared to those delayed on several of the other factors mentioned. For those with delays in several areas, problems in communication and language usually persist. Among late talking toddlers or those with specific communication deficits, several factors may signal chronic delay. Signs of delay are listed in Figure 4.4.

In addition, there are other presymbolic behaviors that, while not important per se for development, may be important for intervention. Chief among these are

■ Functional use of objects as a way of learning concepts, such a *spoon-ness*, and
■ Motor imitation.

While neither behavior is sufficient for communication growth, each provides a method for enhancing teaching and learning. As you might expect, imitation is a valuable teaching tool.

It should be obvious that there is some overlap between the assessment of a child's current method of communication and the presymbolic skills mentioned above. For example, while some children may already be communicating with gestures, others may have to be taught.

Some presymbolic behaviors are more important than others. For example, presymbolic communication behaviors such as pointing may mark important presymbolic development. When a child points to a novel or interesting item, it often results in adults' responding by labeling items or providing additional verbal input. Such input can lead to increased verbal understanding. In other words, children who comment on the environment with a point have greater opportunities for input, which in turn increases verbal understanding or receptive language.

Let's look in greater detail at some of the areas mentioned. Of importance will be the manner of assessment and the specific behaviors to note. We'll take them in the more developmental order of attention and joint attention, motor imitation, functional use, intentional communication, vocalizations, and symbolic play. Then we'll turn our attention to symbolic behaviors. During an assessment, we're not as interested in developmental age as in describing a child's abilities in these areas.

Attention, Joint Attention, and Attention-Following

The ability to consider a partner's attentional focus and to draw a partner's attention toward objects and events of mutual interest is the basis for development of social-conversational skills, social relationships, and language. Typically developing prelinguistic infants learn to

- Orient to a social partner,
- Coordinate and shift attention between objects and people, and
- Share and interpret emotion or affect.

These behaviors usually precede intentional communication.

It is a tenet of education that the ability to focus and sustain attention is vital for learning. For example, it is assumed that the unusual characteristics of attention in children with ASD influence development, especially in socialization and communication.

Researchers have divided attending behavior into the broad categories of orienting, sustaining, and shifting focus. Orienting is the initial physical adjustment toward a stimulus, usually reflected in gaze-shifting or head-turning. Sustaining attention is the ability to maintain attention by ongoing regard of the stimulus. Shifting attention is disengaging from one stimulus and then reorienting to a new one.

Triadic gaze (TG), or shifting gaze back and forth between an adult and an object or event of interest, is one signal of coordinated joint attention. Appearing at about 9 months in TD children, TG is believed by some developmental experts to signal a transition from preintentional to intentional communication (Beuker, Rommelse, Donders, & Buitelaar, 2013; Mundy & Newell, 2007). TG may, therefore, reflect a child's growing ability to integrate his or her behavior with that of others (Mundy & Acra, 2006).

Patten and Watson (2011) offer an excellent review of research and subsequent intervention for attentional deficits among children with ASD. In short, we can summarize our knowledge as follows:

- Orienting impairments have been observed in infants who are later diagnosed with ASD as early as 8–10 months of age and persist through childhood and adulthood (Renner, Klinger, & Klinger, 2006; Werner, Dawson, Osterling, & Dinno, 2000).
- Sustained attention in children with ASD is characterized by remaining fixated or overfocused on a particular stimulus while ignoring other stimuli to a greater extent than TD children and peers with other disabilities (Landry & Bryson, 2004; Liss, Saulnier, Fein, & Kinsbourne, 2006; Zwaigenbaum et al., 2005). While this exaggerated or overselective attention exists, visual fixation does not assure processing and may, in fact, indicate difficulty with stimulus encoding.
- Difficulties in shifting attention are related to a relative inability to disengage from a stimulus that a child has already focused on in order to attend to a new stimulus (Landry & Bryson, 2004; Leekam, Lopez, & Moore, 2000).

Joint attention. The ability to coordinate attention between people and objects for social purposes is called joint attention. The behavior emerges in early infancy and develops through the first 18 months of life. Attention-following refers to a child's ability to change the direction of head and eyes in response to adult focus. Early gestures of showing or pointing to an object are ways to draw another's attention or respond to a partner's gaze or point (Tomasello, 1988).

In joint attention, TD infants coordinate their attention between a social partner and an object or event. Joint attention behaviors thus allow children to share, follow, and direct focus of communicative partners, as in following a partner's line of regard, usually a pointing gesture.

Within attentional episodes, infants learn to use behaviors such as eye gaze, affect or emotion, and later gestures to respond to, initiate, and maintain shared reference. In this way, children are able to establish referential understanding and learn the meanings of words by accessing different types of social information from communicative partners (Hollich, Hirsh-Pasek, & Golinkoff, 2000; Tomasello, 2001, 2003).

Although children with ASD orient less frequently than TD children to all types of stimuli, they do so even less with social stimuli, such as voices and faces (Dawson et al., 2004; Kuhl, Coffey-Corina, Padden, & Dawson, 2005; Osterling, Dawson, & Munson, 2002; Paul, Chawarska, Fowler, Cicchetti, & Volkmar, 2007). Differences between social and nonsocial stimuli exist. Children with ASD shift attention more between two objects than between two people or between an object and a person (Swettenham et al., 1998). In similar fashion, children with ASD demonstrate decreased duration of attention to objects when the objects are held by a person (Osterling et al., 2002). Auditory attention to the human voice is also reported to be less for children with ASD than for TD children (Paul et al., 2007; Zangl & Mills, 2007).

The ability to share attention requires orienting toward a stimulus and sustaining and shifting focus. In addition, among children developing typically, rates of responding to others' attempts to establish joint attention at 6 to 18 months of age predict both receptive and expressive vocabulary at 30 months (Morales et al., 2000). Children, such as those with ASD, who seem unable to follow a speaker's referential focus may make inaccurate symbol-referent pairings or fail to match symbols with their appropriate referents.

Typically developing infants communicate to indicate a shared interest in an object or activity. Initiation of joint attending is associated with better early receptive and expressive abilities. Gestural and/or vocal initiative behaviors, called proto-declaratives, indicate a desire to share attention with a partner. That desire is the root of human communication. Failure to develop proto-declaratives has been associated with severe communication disorders (Lord & Risi, 2000).

The importance of joint attending cannot be overstressed. For example, young children with ASD seem to have a unique impairment in the development of joint attention (Leekam et al., 2000). They initiate joint attention less than children with other developmental disabilities. In turn, core deficits in joint attention skills limit the ability of young children with ASD to learn new words.

Difficulties with joint attention affect other developmental areas, especially for children with ASD (Prizant, Wetherby, Rubin, & Laurent, 2003).

- *Limitations in coordinating attention and affect* result in difficulties in orienting and attending to a social partner, shifting gaze, sharing emotional states, following and drawing another person's attention, and participating in reciprocal interactions.
- *Limitations in sharing intent* result in difficulties in directing signals to others, gaining another's attention, communicating intentionally, and repairing communicative breakdowns.
- *A restricted range of communicative functions or intentions* results in less communication for social purposes.
- *Difficulties inferring another's perspective or emotional state* results in problems monitoring the appropriateness of verbal and nonverbal behaviors, selecting appropriate topics, providing sufficient background information, and appropriately reading and responding to others' expressions of emotion.

The child's emerging ability to direct joint attention contributes uniquely to later expressive language (Watt et al., 2006). For example, being able to initiate joint attention at 14–17 months predicts expressive language outcome four months later (Mundy & Gomes, 1998). Initiating joint attention requires a child, through gestures and eye contact, to direct another's attention for the purpose of sharing (Mundy & Newell, 2007).

Motor Imitation

Imitation is one of the initial ways by which children learn. In addition, motor imitation contributes to language development. Imitation is used by presymbolic TD children to coordinate attention between social partners and objects within interactions.

Some forms of imitation are present in very young infants and continue to develop during the first two years of life. Imitation appears to be a strategy used by infants to acquire and master both new linguistic and new motor behaviors, although the exact nature of this relationship is unknown (Masur & Eichorst, 2002). TD infants with more early spontaneous verbal imitation skills have larger vocabularies, and those with early verbal imitation have better expressive vocabulary skills later.

Among children with ASD, improvement of motor imitation skills appears to be correlated with more advanced language abilities. This seems to be especially true for imitation of oral and facial movements.

Although motor imitation will be important in intervention, no one specific action, such as clapping hands, will turn a nonsymbolic child into a talker. Instead, it is the underlying concept of using others as both models and teachers that is important. In intervention, we can build on general motor imitation and train oral and vocal imitation.

A word on sensory and motor processing and ASD. Young children with ASD demonstrate more sensory impairments than young children with other DDs (Wiggins, Robins, Bakeman, & Adamson, 2009). These sensory differences seem to be significantly related to stereotyped interests and behaviors. More specifically, young children with ASD have more tactile and taste/smell sensitivities and difficulties with filtering auditory stimuli. Problems with adjustment to auditory sensation might be noted in the more frequent hands over ears behavior seen in infants later diagnosed as having ASD (Loh et al., 2007).

Because of neurophysiological factors, children with ASD have difficulty modulating arousal and regulating emotion (Anzalone & Williamson, 2000; DeGangi, 2000). It is possible that heightened states of arousal and emotion and a limited ability to learn and interact may result from a low threshold for physiological stimuli and from emotional reactivity, termed hyper-reactivity. In heightened states of arousal, a child may exhibit *flight, fright, and fight* reactions. The child might attempt to escape from overly stimulating environments. In contrast, under-arousal—a high threshold for physiological and emotional reactivity, or hypo-reactivity—results in passivity, lethargy, and an inability to process social and environmental experiences. Some children may experience shifting states, either cyclically or unpredictably, that result in complex patterns of behavior that can affect socio-emotional development.

Motor impairments are also common in children with ASD. Compared to TD peers, children with ASD have significant deficits in both gross and fine motor movement and in praxis, or conceptualizing, motor planning, and problem-solving (Dawson & Watling, 2000). These motor impairments, in turn, are associated with social, communicative, and repetitive behaviors characteristic of ASD. In fact, dyspraxia may mark neurologic deficits that underlie ASD. This could explain why imitation skills, especially oral-facial, are difficult for these children. There is also evidence that tics; dyskinesia, or impaired, uncoordinated, or jerky movement; and akathisia, or involuntary motor movements, are all associated with repetitive stereotypic ASD behaviors such as body-rocking, repetitive self-injurious behavior, and compulsive behavior (Bodfish, Symons, Parker, & Lewis, 2000; Dziuk et al., 2007).

Preschool children with autism are significantly more impaired in overall imitation abilities, oral-facial imitation, and imitations of actions on objects than TD children or those with fragile X syndrome or other developmental disorders (Rogers, Hepburn, Stackhouse, & Wehner, 2003). For children with ASD, imitation skills are strongly correlated with autistic symptoms and development of joint attention. Deficits in imitation skills are mainly evident when the imitation task is presented in a spontaneous context, suggesting a need for consistency on the part of the child (Ingersoll, 2008).

Functional Use

Unlike adults, children generally only talk about things they know. In contrast, adults—especially politicians—seem to have opinions on all sorts of things that they know absolutely nothing about. Using a toy truck or a spoon for its intended purpose means that a child is beginning to form a concept of—beginning to "know"—that object by its use, and we can build upon that knowledge in intervention. Ask a young child "What's an apple?" and you're likely to hear "Something you eat." That's object use or function!

For young children, it generally follows that conceptual knowledge leads to receptive understanding followed by expressive language. That's not a hard-and-fast rule, just a general guideline. And of course, a child's somewhat superficial concept of spoon is a long way from your much fuller understanding.

Children with communication problems may have unformed or incomplete object and action concepts. For example, some children with ASD or other DDs use items in a purposeless or indiscriminate manner, indicating a lack of differentiation of objects. In these cases, all toys may be used to bang on a table, with little differentiation based on each object's unique purpose.

Don't misunderstand me; I'm not interested in forcing every child to play in the same purpose-driven manner. But I am concerned about a child's knowledge or conceptual base that is part of early symbol meanings.

Intentional Communication

Presymbolic communicative behaviors include facial expressions, body or limb movements, gestures, vocalizations, and sometimes even challenging behaviors, such as aggression, that children use to communicate. In general, TD children progress from preintentional to intentional presymbolic communication before they attain intentional symbolic communication.

Although preintentional behaviors often have a communication effect on an interactive partner, they lack deliberate communication intent from the child. These preintentional acts result in communication only because interactive partners attribute meaning to them. In contrast, intentional communication behaviors are produced by a child with the intent of conveying information to an interactive partner. A child's attention to an interactive partner is the primary characteristic differentiating preintentional from intentional nonverbal communication.

Intentional communication is any child gesture and/or vocalization that is either conventional or symbolic in form and produced in combination with a behavior that demonstrates coordinated attention to both an object or event and a person simultaneously. The ability to communicate for a variety of purposes is an important milestone of presymbolic communicative development and necessary for the development of higher level communication skills (Brady et al., 2004).

The frequency and type of intentional communication are important factors in identifying children with communication impairment and are predictive of language outcomes among these young children. Higher rates of nonsymbolic intentional communication are associated with better language development (e.g., Calendrella & Wilcox, 2000). A slower rate of intentional communication may indicate a communication deficit. Similarly, a limited variety of interactive gestures at 9 to 12 months may signal later diagnosis of ASD or other DD (Colgan et al., 2006).

Presymbolic gestures. Many professionals in early child language recognize two categories of gestures: deictic and representational. *Deictic* gestures establish reference by calling attention to or indicating an object or event. These gestures can only be interpreted by their context and can be used with a variety of objects and events. In turn, deictic gestures can be divided into contact and distal gestures. Considered "early" gestures, *contact gestures* require contact between a child and object/caregiver, such as giving a toy or taking an adult's hand. In contrast, *distal gestures* require no contact with the caregiver/object and include pointing and reaching. Distal gestures typically appear later (10–12 months of age), but not always. Deictic gestures account for nearly 88 percent of the gesture repertoire in young infants and toddlers.

Between 8 and 9 months, TD infants begin to use eye gaze to direct others' attention. Later a child gains more efficient means, such as gestures and words. The emergence of joint attention abilities in the 9-month-old is a crucial indicator of communicative competence. Early in development, infants also use vocalizations paired with gestures to communicate. Between 8 and 12 months, gestures and gestural-vocal combinations predominate. Approximately half of deictic gestures between 8 and 11 months are accompanied by vocalizations. Even as children enter into the one-word stage, gestures with or without vocalizations continue to play an important role.

Although gestural communication can be extremely effective, conventional gestures somewhat limit a child to the "here and now," to making reference only to physically and temporally present topics by pointing to, looking at, and/or touching referents. Because these conventional gestures are made only in the presence of a referent, or the thing to which they refer, they do not qualify as symbolic.

Representational gestures. The second type of gestures, *representational* or symbolic gestures, both establish reference and indicate semantic content. They often appear after the emergence of a few deictic gestures (Crais et al., 2004). Representational gestures can be object-related gestures that signify some feature of the referent, such as a cupped hand to mouth to represent *drinking,* or can also be culturally defined, such as waving *bye,* that represent some action or concept rather than a specific object.

Typically, representational gestures emerge within familiar games and routines that parents and other caregivers use to engage children. Games such as "Itsy Bitsy Spider" and routines such as exaggerated blowing and hand-waving to signal "hot food" contain many interactive opportunities for the child to observe and produce representational gestures.

Compared to deictic gestures, representational gestures are more dependent on modeling by caregivers. Their use, therefore, may be more reflective of parents' cultural beliefs and practices than are deictic gestures.

Representational gestures can be used to refer to objects and events outside the immediate context. As such, these symbolic gestures can be used either in the absence of or as an accompaniment to speech to express concepts that are also expressed verbally. For example, a child might pretend to eat as a signal for hungry or imitate throwing with an empty hand as a signal for *ball.* Like words, symbolic gestures undergo a process of *decontextualization,* meaning they gradually rely less and less on the immediate context. Symbolic gestures seem to incorporate functional elements of word meaning, as in miming throwing a ball, rather than perceptual elements, such as making rounded hand shapes, thus demonstrating the importance of understanding functional use, mentioned previously.

Gestural intent. Another important aspect in the development of gesture use is the communicative function or intent of the gesture. The median age for emergence of common communicative functions is presented in Table 4.2. These data represent groups of children, and an individual child may not follow the same order.

For our purposes, intentional communication is defined as the use of

- ◼ Coordinated attention to an adult and an object combined with either unconventional gestures or vocalizations, or
- ◼ Conventional gestures or symbols directed toward an adult.

TABLE 4.2 **Gestural Development**

AGE OF APPEARANCE	GESTURE	VARIABILITY
6–7 months	Protesting Showing off	
7–13 months	Requesting objects Requesting actions Requesting assistance	Different types of requests appear, including reaching toward a desired object, placing an object in an adult's hand for assistance, and pulling on an adult's hand to obtain something.
8–10 months	Showing objects	
9–10 months	Pointing to actions Pointing to objects	
10–13 months	Giving	
There is wide variability across children and intentions.		

Sources: Crais, Day Douglas, & Cox Campbell, 2004; Owens, 2016.

Intentionality is recognition by the child that his or her behavior is having an effect on a listener and is characterized by persistence and by monitoring of a communication partner's behavior. Of interest are the

■ Level of development of the intent to communicate,
■ Type of behavior displayed by a child,
■ Range of intentions, and
■ Caregiver's response.

Development begins with unintentional behavior that nonetheless expresses a child's needs, desires, or interests, such as crying, reaching for an object, or sharing a toy with an adult. The infant communicates with the adult without really intending to do so.

Frequent intentional communication indirectly or directly contributes to the language development of children and predicts later language levels in children with disabilities. This may occur for several reasons (Yoder & Warren, 2001b).

■ Gestures and vocalizations serve the same intentions as early words. Later, words fill the intentions already expressed nonverbally.
■ Presymbolic and linguistic communication may rely on the same cognitive developments, such as means-ends or the understanding that a desired object can be acquired via indirect means, such as a person. Children with mental retardation who receive direct training on means-end relations acquire more language in subsequent intervention than children who receive only language intervention.
■ Children who produce relatively complex and frequent vocalizations, often while gesturing, may have more advanced neurological development for speech planning and functioning.
■ Intentional communication may elicit maternal responses that in turn facilitate later language development.

As children's behavior becomes more intentional, they tend to communicate to

■ Regulate the behavior of others by requesting or protesting;
■ Engage others in interaction through social routines, greeting, or showing off; and
■ Establish joint attention by directing another's attention to an object, event, or topic and then possibly commenting or requesting information.

Although all three processes occur in children with DDs, behavior regulation is often the most prevalent, social interaction less so, and joint attention even less. Examples of the three types of gestures are presented in Table 4.3.

Gesture-language link. Gestures, speech, and language are related both neurologically and developmentally (Bates & Dick, 2002). This may be the result of neural overlap in the control for speech and gestures and of the spreading of neural activation from one brain region to another. Although I will attempt to explain the linkage and how this can be used in intervention, interested readers should consult the excellent review provided by Capone and McGregor (2004) for more details.

Early in development there is a synchrony in an infant's hand and mouth activity. For example, in the Babkin reflex, a newborn will open its mouth when pressure is applied to a palm. Later, repetitive hand movements, such as banging objects, and reduplicated babbling emerge at about the same time. After the first year, gestures expand an infant's communication beyond single words.

Gestures mark the emergence of intentional communication and are used to obtain and maintain attention and to communicate, which in turn creates opportunities for learning language. The first intentional behavior to emerge is showing off to attract attention to oneself. Young infants will repeat behaviors that were previously successful in gaining attention from caregivers. Showing off is very individualistic and will vary across children. This is followed by the use of objects to obtain caregiver attention and by other deictic gestures, such as giving, pointing, and requesting.

TABLE 4.3 Types of Gestures

Gesture Category	Gesture	Development
Behavior regulation	Protest	Pushing away is gradually accompanied or replaced by shaking head "no."
	Request actions	Reaching to pick something up or miming an action, such as petting a dog, is modified by pointing, taking adult's hand, or giving an object.
	Request objects	Reaching for object, pulling adult's hand toward object, or pointing to obtain object is gradually modified to request reaching while opening and closing hand.
Interaction	Representation	A gesture represents, or stands for, an event, such as waving "bye," clapping when excited, or using an object for its intended purpose. This often begins in imitation and is modified into a more communicative gesture, such as clapping for excitement or accomplishment
	Seek attention	Showing off is very individualistic and begins early. Other examples of attention-seeking include banging an object, making a noise, or taking adult's hand.
	Social games	Occurs through participation and later by initiation.
Joint attention	Signaling notice	Comment or draw attention by showing or giving an object. Gradually the child learns to follow the pointing of others and then to direct others by pointing.

Sources: Crais, Day Douglas, & Cox Campbell, 2004; Owens, 2016.

Within deictic gestures, gradual distancing from contact with the object to more distal forms occurs and underlies symbolic development. Within showing, children move from showing objects in their hands to showing objects that are not being manipulated by either partner. Shortly after this occurs, infants give objects to a partner and referentially point. Spontaneous distal pointing toward an object or event outside the child's immediate proximity is later related to comprehension of an object's name.

In general, infants attend to and use gestures that adults in their environment produce (Goodwyn, Acredolo, & Brown, 2000; McGregor & Capone, 2001; Namy, Acredolo, & Goodwyn, 2000). When parents use gesture-word pairs in daily caregiver-child interactions, their infants begin to use symbols earlier (McGregor & Capone, 2001). In addition, infants who are explicitly taught to use gestures demonstrate greater use of them (Goodwyn et al., 2000). Both findings are important for intervention.

Commenting and requesting are the two most frequent communication intentions expressed by TD presymbolic children through gestures. Commenting, which involves the expression of shared interest toward both the referent and the social partner, may be used to initiate joint attending. Both requesting and commenting are positively related to comprehension and production of language in TD children and are long-term predictors of language development (Blake, 2000).

In presymbolic requesting, a child uses gestures and/or nonword vocalizations, while attending to an adult, to ask the adult to get an object or to perform an action. Requesting is defined as behavior that works through the mediation of an adult listener to enable a child to gain or maintain access to objects, activities, or interactions, revealing that a child understands that communication is effective in getting his or her needs met (Sigafoos & Mirenda, 2002). In addition, requests may elicit language-facilitating verbal responses from the child's caregivers. Among young children with various intellectual disabilities, the frequency of requesting is positively associated with their later language.

Presymbolic commenting also consists of gestures and/or nonword vocalizations coordinated with attention to an adult. The purpose, however, is to share an interest or positive affect about an event or object. This motivation to share is very important for later language development and may be the primary reason why children learn to talk. The frequency of presymbolic comments also predicts later linguistic skill in children with a variety of etiologies.

Gestures are also a source for and an expression of semantic knowledge and can provide a glimpse into a child's evolving semantic representations (Capone, 2007). In other words, for many children, semantic relations are represented mentally earlier than speech alone would indicate. Thus, assessment of gestures is one possible way of determining a child's semantic knowledge when oral language is limited and possibly unreliable.

Gestures and communication impairment. For children experiencing difficulty acquiring language, the level of presymbolic development can be predictive of later language development (Capone & McGregor, 2004). In addition, recognition of a child's level of presymbolic gestural development can be important for subsequent intervention. For example, children with developmental delays but the ability to point show greater growth in language than children who don't point (Brady et al., 2004). Thus, the level of expressive gesture use can provide an index of presymbolic communication development.

Many young children with developmental disabilities rely on presymbolic gestures with or without vocalizations as their primary means of communication. For example, they may push away undesired objects. Even given their importance, the acquisition of communicative gestures alone may not be a sufficient basis for the acquisition of symbolic communication. For a variety of reasons, not all individuals who communicate through gestures are able to transition to using symbols, such as words or signs. The difficulty seems to lie in learning the one-to-one correspondence between an arbitrary symbol and its referent.

Although several well-respected assessment instruments, including the *Communicative and Symbolic Behavior Scales* (CSBS) (Wetherby & Prizant, 1993) and the *Rossetti Infant Toddler Language Scale* (Rossetti, 1990), include intentionality items, some standardized assessment tools are inappropriate or of only limited value for children and families with individualized presymbolic means of communication. Some older, more traditional assessment tools focus solely on the child and do not include family members as participants in the assessment other than as providers of interview and questionnaire responses.

When normative measures focus on developmental milestones, they provide little information relevant to intervention. In addition, assessment tools based on the behavior of TD children may not accurately describe the individualistic nature of communication that doesn't easily fit into preestablished categories of behavior.

Gestures and Children with ASD. The gestural development of children with ASD often is impaired. For example, a child's use of gestures may not be accompanied by eye contact. Although challenging behavior found in some children with ASD can take many forms, it often is for the same purposes—protesting, requesting, or seeking attention—found in the gestures of TD children.

Lack of or less use of gestures in infancy indicates a decreased desire to communicate. When we examine the gesture use of infants with ASD, for example, some interesting patterns emerge. At 9–12 months, infants with ASD are less likely to use joint attention gestures than infants with developmental disabilities (DD) or those developing typically (TD). Joint attention gestures involve directing another person's attention to an event, object, or person solely to share interest. This is usually accomplished by pointing or by holding up an interesting item. Nine- to 12-month-old infants with ASD are also less likely to use behavior regulation gestures than their TD peers. Used to control another person's behavior, behavior regulation gestures include reaching to request an object, pushing an object away, or shaking the head to indicate protest (*No!*).

At 15–18 months, infants with ASD are less likely than infants with DD to use both joint attention and social interaction gestures. Infants use social interaction gestures to direct another person's attention to themselves. An infant can accomplish this in a number of ways, such as waving her arms, covering her face to indicate wanting to repeat *peeka-boo*, or giving kisses. Not surprisingly, 15- to 18-month-old infants with ASD are less likely than TD infants to use all three types of gestures (Watson, Crais, Baranek, Dykstra, & Wilson, 2013).

As noted previously, there are three general purposes of gestures: behavior regulation, interaction, and joint attention. Although total gesture use by 9- to 12-month-old children with ASD is similar to that of TD children, use at 15–18 months is approximately 40 percent that of TD children (Neitzel et al., 2003). The distribution by function also differs, with the largest discrepancy seen in joint attention and behavior regulation gestures. Fewer children with ASD use these types of gestures, and those that do, use them less frequently.

Gestures and Children with DD. Although TD children express both requests and comments at an early stage of presymbolic development, children with DDs often show a more restricted range. Further, the range of communication functions and the level of gestural development seem to be related. For example, children with communication difficulties who communicate with contact gestures and vocalizations rarely initiate joint attention or comments. In contrast, children who use distal gestures frequently express comments as well as requests. The emergence of commenting is extremely important for the subsequent development of communication and language.

Among at-risk infants, the emergence of deictic gestures appears to follow the same developmental sequence as found in TD children (McGregor & Capone, 2001), although somewhat delayed. Despite immature gesture ability, older children with persistent language impairments use gestures to compensate for deficits in their expressive language (Evans, Alibali, & McNeil, 2001).

For children with Down syndrome (DS), gesture production is a relative strength compared to their receptive and expressive language abilities. Toddlers with DS produce both conventional (e.g., bye-bye) and deictic gestures (e.g., pointing), enact play schemes, and use expressive and symbolic gestures (Chan & Iacono, 2001). In addition, children with DS benefit from intervention that makes use of this manual modality. For example, 7-year-olds with DS respond to a teacher more often if the teacher uses gestures than if he or she uses speech solely (Wang, Bernas, & Eberhard, 2001).

Children with neuromuscular deficits such as CP may gesture in very limited ways. Often their movements are extremely subtle and can be easily missed. Failure of caregivers to respond to their children's gestures may cause a decrease in these children's attempts to initiate communication.

It's important in an assessment to describe a child's gesture use in terms of the types of gestures used. Red flags include decreased gesture use at 9–12 months and lack of or decreased use of social interaction gestures at 15–18 months (Watson et al., 2013).

Gestures and intervention. When documenting gesture use in children, professionals need to consider several important aspects of gesture development, from both an assessment and an intervention planning perspective. These are (Crais, Watson, & Baranek, 2009)

- Frequency of gesture use,
- Communicative function,
- The pairing of eye gaze and vocalization with gestures,
- Transition from contact to distal gestures,
- Transition from gestures to verbalization, and
- Communication repair.

Let's discuss some of these for a moment.

Frequency of Gesture Use. The frequency of intentional communication is an important factor in identifying children with communication deficits. The amount of gesture use by infants and toddlers is related to later verbal development. With a responsive adult,

TD 12-month-olds communicate intentionally about once a minute, 18-month-olds approximately twice per minute, and 24-month-olds about five times per minute. A slow rate or a lack of intentional communication may signal deficits. Further, to express their intentions, 12-month-olds use primarily gestures and/or vocalizations, 18-month-olds use a combination of gestures, vocalizations, and words or word approximations, and 24-month-olds use primarily words or word combinations. In general, children with DD gesture less than TD children (Watson, Baranek, & Crais, 2005).

Communicative Function. The communicative function expressed by children's gestures can also be used to help in decision-making. In general, a limited *variety* of intentional communicative acts in infants and toddlers at about 24 months of age has been shown to be related to later diagnosis of ASD and other developmental disabilities. A limited variety of communicative gestures as early as 12 months of age may indicate risk for communicative disorders (Colgan et al., 2006).

Transitions. The transition from contact to distal gestures may be related to the symbol acquisition process. The lack of or delay in distal gestures can signal a concurrent lack or delay of language.

The transition from the use of gestures to a predominant use of words is another stage that should be noted. Before the use of words to name, children produce "recognitory" actions associated with objects such as bringing a cup to the lips, demonstrating functionality (Bates & Dick, 2002). These gestures serve as gestural labels or gestural names similar to early verbal naming.

Communication repair. As noted, young children with significant disability often have limited or restricted communication repertoires. Often the form of these behaviors is unconventional, ambiguous, and idiosyncratic, making them difficult for partners to understand. As a result, the potential for communication breakdowns is great. **Communication breakdown** refers to situations in which children attempt to communicate but their communication does not result in their intended outcome (Halle et al., 2004). For example, breakdown may include child requests that are not followed by the objects or events requested, joint attention attempts by a child that are not followed by a comment or appropriate response by a partner, and child protests that are not followed by escaping or avoiding an undesired item or event. Poor intelligibility and a lack of specificity can lead to frequent breakdowns (Brady & Halle, 2002).

For nonsymbolic children, their ability to repair breakdowns successfully determines the level of control they can exercise over their environment. Because they cannot communicate clearly or readily with language, young children with disabilities often use informal gestures, facial expressions, body movements, and nonsymbolic vocalizations to communicate (e.g., Keen, Sigafoos, & Woodyatt, 2001). The intent behind these communication attempts may not be easily discerned by a child's communication partners, leaving these same partners to guess at how to respond. One study of TD children found that even among 5- to 7-year-olds, as many as 40 percent of their initiations are followed by a communication breakdown (Steeples, 2002).

When a child's communication attempt is difficult to understand, communication partners frequently respond by requesting clarification, often in the form of a question, such as "What?" or "Do you want ____?" When a partner does not respond within a reasonable amount of time, possibly because he or she is focused elsewhere, a child does not receive a clear signal that a repair is needed. In another example, the partner may not wish to acknowledge the child's communication, such as requesting candy just before dinner, and may shift the topic to one deemed more desirable. In these cases, children may abandon their original communication.

Of importance for assessment of intentional communication is the possible persistence of the child. Persistence indicates a child's intention to communicate. Similarly, a tantrum may signal frustration that a communication partner did not acknowledge that intent. I remember an instructional video in which the speaker was making this very point about persistence while unaware of the child in the background insistently continuing to signal *more* again and again.

Oral Motor Abilities

Coordinated oral motor patterns are used in the production of speech sounds. Disorganized or dysfunctional patterns are related to several established risk categories, such as cerebral palsy and Down syndrome, and can lead to deficits in speech and language (Nobrega, Borion, Henrot, & Saliba, 2004).

Poor oral and manual motor planning correlates with lower expressive language in children with ASD. This correlation is not found when general gross motor planning is compared to language use. Similarly, basic oral motor functions, such as control of oral secretions, do not differentiate. Instead, voluntary nonverbal oral skills, such as imitating lip puckering, often differentiate verbal from nonverbal children. Finally, motor imitation ability, more than other abilities such as play level or joint attention, predicts speech at age 4 (Stone & Yoder, 2001).

For these reasons, an SLP is interested in both the structure and function of a child's oral motor system. At the very least, an SLP should observe the child, ask parents about the child's feeding and swallowing skills and sound productions, and then compare what is observed or reported with what might be expected developmentally (ASHA, 2008b). Feeding and swallowing will be discussed in detail in Chapter 10.

Some infants and toddlers may need more in-depth assessment. Although there are no standardized tests of the full range of oral motor skills, common informal assessment tools include the following:

- *Carolina Curriculum for Infants and Toddlers With Special Needs* (Johnson-Martin, Attermeier, & Hacker, 2004)
- *Oral Motor Assessment* (Sleight & Niman, 1984)
- *Preschool Oral Motor Examination* (Sheppard, 1987)
- *Pre-Speech Assessment Scale* (Morris, 1982)

An informal summary of oral motor development is presented in Table 4.4.

It's important to remember that many oral motor assessments involve imitation, a cognitive skill. When a young child cannot imitate oral movements, the SLP must consider cognitive as well as oral motor skills.

Vocalizations

Production of early sounds and words, especially the diversity of sounds and syllable types, has been found to be particularly important for later expressive language. Although babbling is the random production of both individual speech sounds and consonant-vowel (CV) syllables, the sounds that predominate are also the most frequent sounds found in children's first words. Among TD children, new words are added when the child develops a phonological template or format for those words from his or her existing repertoire of sounds and syllable structures. The child's phonological repertoire is a factor in determining the words that he or she chooses to say. Children tend to avoid words they cannot pronounce.

By 16 months of age, TD children are using a greater proportion of consonants than vowels, and babbling contains more than one syllable. The inability to use more than one consonant by 24 months of age is related to delayed language.

Semantics and phonology have a reciprocal relationship, with each affecting the other. For example, children with small vocabularies also have restricted use of both sounds and syllables.

Vocalizations and communication impairment. Children identified as language delayed have significantly lower scores on all phonetic measures than do children developing typically. In general, the more delayed a 2-year-old child is in phonological development, the more at risk the child is for continuing delays at age 3 (Perry Carson, Klee, Carson, & Hime, 2003).

While babbling sounds are important, an SLP is more interested in the speech sounds and syllable structures a child can produce at will. It is these structures that a child will use to form her or his first words. In typical development, the sounds /p, b, w, m, h,

TABLE 4.4 Oral Motor Development

AGE (Mo)	FEEDING POSITION	FOOD TYPES	SUCKING	SWALLOWING	COORDINATING SUCK, SWALLOW, & BREATHING	JAW MOVEMENT	LIP MOVEMENT	TONGUE MOVEMENT
1–2	Supine; head slightly raised	Liquids	Whole jaw suck	Suck-swallow pattern with slight tongue protrusion	Two or more sucks, then pause for breathe or swallow	Undifferentiated	Undifferentiated	Undifferentiated
3	Semi-sitting	Semi-solids	Sucking with increased tongue movement	Primitive suck-swallow pattern; some food pushed out of mouth, more volitional swallow	Up to 20+ sucks with no obvious pause for swallow; breathing pauses infrequent	Sucking pattern, no independent chewing pattern	Sucking pattern, no independent chewing pattern	Sucking pattern, no independent chewing pattern
4–5	Sitting supported	Pureed foods & soft cereals; liquids	Sucking strength increases			Reflexive phasic bite-release pattern with soft solids; chewing primarily up-down		Strong tongue protrusion
6	Sitting unsupported in high chair or infant seat	Pureed foods; liquids	Sucking from cup with some loss; spoon accepted	Swallows liquid from cup; food not pushed out by tongue	Long sequences of suck-swallow-breath; suck from cup with loss of liquid	Wide jaw extension; up-down chew more variable with some diagonal movement	Lips may be open during swallow, draw in slightly for chewing; "kisses" pouts; "kisses"	Extension-retraction during drinking from cup, up-down pattern during chewing

7	Pureed foods; liquids			Extension-retraction of tongue while chewing			Lateralization with gross rolling or horizontal movement when food placed to side
8	Pureed, ground, or junior canned foods; mashed table foods	Solid foods from spoon				Upper lip assists food removal from spoon; closure with semi-liquid chew and swallow	
9	No external support needed		Extension-retraction of tongue lessens but continues	Long sequences of continuous sucking from cup; some difficulty coordinating swallowing and breathing continues	Phasic bite present for firmer solid foods only; variations in amount and speed of vertical chew; some diagonal chew	Active in chewing; upper comes down and forward; both draw inward when chewing	Lateral movements for food placed to side; begins to transfer food from middle to side
10		Liquid from cup				Move inward when spoon removed	
12		Chopped easily chewable table foods and meats		No extension-retraction of tongue with swallow, chews food of uneven consistency	Up-down and backward-forward during sucking; sustained controlled bite of soft solid	May be open during swallow of liquids; uses teeth and gums to remove food from lower lip	Extension-retraction rare during sucking; intermittent tip elevation during swallow; can transfer food from center to sides during chewing

continued

TABLE 4.4 **Oral Motor Development** (*continued*)

Age (Mo)	Feeding Position	Food Types	Sucking	Swallowing	Coordinating Suck, Swallow, & Breathing	Jaw Movement	Lip Movement	Tongue Movement
15					Well coordinated suck-swallow; food transferred side-to-side while chewing	No phasic bite; smooth rotary chew diagonally	Lip and cheek assist during chewing	
18	Sit at table in child seat	Coarsely chopped table foods, including some meats and raw vegetables		No loss of food or saliva while swallowing solid foods; seals lips		Sustained controlled bite of hard solid foods with related head or limb movement	Upper lip seals on edge of cup; chew with lips closed intermittently	
21					Swallows solid foods with combination of textures		Easy lip closure during liquid swallowing; lip movement and closure during chewing	Tip elevation during swallowing, no protrusion; can transfer food from side to side
24			Drink from cup without biting edge	No loss of liquid during swallow	Tongue depression and elevation independent of jaw	Controlled sustained bite; mouth opening consistent with food thickness; circular rotary chew	Easy lip closure with no loss of liquid during swallow	Sweeping movement to clean lips; tip elevation consistent during swallow; transfers food rapidly

Sources: Information taken from Carruth & Skinner, 2002; Carruth, Ziegler, Gordon et al., 2004; Gisel, 1991; Owens, 2016; Wilson & Green, 2009; and Wilson, Green & Weismer, 2012.

g, k/ predominate in VC (*Up*), CV (*Hi, bye*), CVCV-reduplicated (*Mama, baba*), and CVCV (*Cookie, baby*) structured words, although many other permutations are possible.

During assessment of a nonsymbolic child, an SLP is not concerned with the typicality of the sounds and syllables. In other words, /m/ and CVCV are nice to have but not essential. After all, there are few hard-and-fast standards. These sounds and structures mentioned for TD children are simply the easiest to produce, given the abilities of most 1-year-olds. In intervention, the SLP is not going to attempt to mirror typical development, but rather to build the child's initial lexicon or personal vocabulary from the phonological structures present to reflect the unique things the child wants to and is able to talk about. It is important, therefore, to accurately describe a child's individualistic sound and syllable repertoire and the child's ability to turn-take with sounds and to make sounds when requested to imitate an adult.

One measure of vocal development is the number of nonword vocalizations with a consonant-vowel syllable that occur in combination with a gesture or attention to the message recipient. These measures of vocal communication are also associated with later language in children with a variety of handicapping conditions. Of importance are a child's oral motor skills for speech.

In intervention, an SLP will attempt to form an initial lexicon based on the concepts the child understands, such as *push truck* or *roll ball*, the words that the child "comprehends" or can match to an object or action referent, and the sounds and syllables the child can reproduce. If, for example, a child has an interest in or enjoys playing with a ball, can roll or throw the ball—even if in an unconventional manner—can find the ball among other objects when asked, and can say /bɔ/, then *ball* may be an appropriate word to attempt to have the child say. One of the challenges in ECI will be to keep track of all these variables in order to accurately program a child's burgeoning repertoire of words. It will be important to keep an updated list of the child's sound and syllable repertoire in order to facilitate selection of new words at the same time as training new sounds.

Those children who are unable to produce developmentally appropriate consonant and vowel sounds and words and are limited to one or two vocalization types may be exhibiting childhood apraxia of speech (ASHA, 2008b; Shriberg et al., 2003). In some cases of severe phonological delay or disorder, a child may become a candidate for AAC.

Another of my grandsons had childhood apraxia of speech and was severely limited in his speech production. Most words were reduced to CV syllables and were produced in imitation. Through the early use of signs accompanying speech intervention, he now, at age 6, is very intelligible.

Sound-Making and ASD. The frequency of speech sound vocalizations by 18- to 24-month-old children with ASD correlates significantly with developmental levels and predicts expressive language outcome at age 3 (Plumb & Wetherby, 2013). Many young children with ASD exhibit different patterns of vocalization from those of TD children and children with developmental disabilities (DD). In general, children with ASD use a significantly lower proportion of speech sound vocalizations and a significantly higher proportion of atypical vocalizations than children with DD. Atypical vocalizations might include atypical phonation, such as a loud nondistress yell, a grunt, a high-pitched squeal, or a growl (Sheinkopf, Mundy, Oller, & Steffens, 2000). In addition, children with ASD use a significantly higher proportion of distress vocalizations than either the TD children or those with DD. Distress vocalizations, associated with a negative emotional state, include crying/whining and loud, long, intense screaming.

Level of Play

Although no specific play skills are prerequisites for acquisition of language, the two areas of development are parallel in many ways. For example, first words appear along with single play schemes, such as a child feeding a doll with a spoon. When children begin to combine words, they also combine play schemes, such as self-feeding with a spoon and then drinking from a cup. It's not surprising, therefore, that the level of symbolic play at 14 months predicts later language skills at both 24 and 42 months (Lyytinen et al., 2001). In addition, higher levels of play are associated with better comprehension. Assessing a child's play provides a nonlinguistic benchmark against which the child's linguistic performance can be compared (Paul, 2007). Possible levels of play are presented in Table 4.5.

TABLE 4.5 **Levels of Play**

TYPE OF PLAY	ACTIONS	EXPLANATION	AGE (MONTHS)
Exploratory: Infant examines environment through a combination of sensory modes.	Mouthing, banging, shaking, and poking	Initially actions are indiscriminate and objects are treated randomly. Gradually, single objects are differentiated and play preserves the physical or conventional characteristics of the objects, such as rolling a ball.	2–10 months
Relational: Infant uses objects in combination but without regard for the attributes or functions of the objects.	Pushing, stacking, nesting, and piling	Takes objects apart and recombines, such as removing pieces from a puzzle. Gradually, combinations reflect the environment, such as putting objects into box.	10–18 months
Functional: Child is influenced by social or cultural properties of objects.	Pretending actions, such as feeding doll	Focus gradually moves from self to dolls or puppets, to objects, and then to another person.	12–18 months
Symbolic: Child uses object attributes that are not present or substitutes objects.	Using slipper as cell phone or putting doll to bed on a block	Object substitution, such as a cup for a car, becomes agent play in which a child moves a doll or object as if it were capable of action.	18–30 months
Role: Adopts role	Pretending to be another person, such as Mommy	Evolves gradually as child becomes aware of self and of individual differences	30–36 months

Sources: Baranek, Barnett, Adams, Wolcott, Watson, & Crais, 2005; Knox, 1997; Libby, Powell, Messer, & Jordan, 1998; Lifter, Sulzer-Azaroff, Anderson, & Cowdery, 1993; Owens, 2016.

Hearing

The impact of hearing loss on a child's speech and language development can be great. Therefore, children suspected of communication difficulties should undergo comprehensive audiological assessment and ongoing monitoring (ASHA, 2008b). Although many children with severe hearing loss are identified through newborn hearing screening, those with mild or unilateral losses may go undetected. In addition, some children may experience late onset or progressive hearing losses. As in other areas of development, early identification and intervention can result in improved developmental outcomes (Moeller, 2000).

Motor and Cognitive Skills

Cognition, motor control, and communication abilities are interrelated, and children who have or are at risk for motor or cognitive disabilities are likely to have speech and language deficits (Abbeduto & Boudreau, 2004). For example, some children with cerebral palsy have difficulty vocalizing or using spoken language even when linguistic abilities are not affected. Therefore, a child's cognitive and motor abilities should be a consideration when assessing and intervening with these and other children who have or are at risk of having communication impairments.

As SLPs, we are interested in cognition and motor abilities as they relate to communication. In other words, SLPs should not use a child's overall cognitive or motor level of functioning to make decisions about the need for speech and language services. There are several reasons for this. First, a young child often receives very different scores from different tests. Second, many tests of cognition have a verbal component that confounds results for nonsymbolic children.

In addition, we must be cautious in our use of test results because some states make children ineligible for SLP services unless language abilities lag well behind cognitive abilities, sometimes by as much as two years. Such cost-cutting measures are wrongheaded and can actually increase costs in the long run. We know that children without a language-cognitive discrepancy can benefit from communication intervention that may forestall future problems (Carr & Felice, 2000).

The SLP is interested in cognitive and motor skills as they relate to communication. Cognitive areas of interest may include areas such as sensorimotor learning, levels of play, means-ends, and object permanence. Oral motor abilities including sound-making, but sucking, chewing, and swallowing are also important. If an SLP is considering a child for AAC, then other motor abilities, such as hand movement, must be assessed. This assessment will be covered in Chapter 7.

Feeding and Swallowing

Feeding and swallowing are needed for nutrition, health, and development. They are also precursors to the development of early oral communication (Kent & Vorperian, 2007). In addition, early feeding difficulty may be an indicator of neurological deficits that can result in communication difficulties and delays (Hawdon, Beauregard, Slattery, & Kennedy, 2000; Selley et al., 2001). The incidence of feeding and swallowing difficulties in children with disabilities is higher than in TD children (Eicher, 2002).

Information about a child's past and current feeding can be helpful in determining risk (ASHA, 2008b). More specifically, the SLP is interested in

- Type, amount, and frequency of meals,
- Variety and consistency of foods eaten, and
- Evidence of difficulties sucking, chewing, or swallowing, or
- Presence of gagging or drooling.

Both observation of the child's feeding and swallowing and more formal assessment are important. Chapter 10 gives a more detailed discussion of pediatric feeding and swallowing difficulties and assessment.

SYMBOLIC BEHAVIORS

Once a child is using symbols, whether as words, signs, or some form of AAC, the focus of an early communication assessment changes somewhat. In addition to some of the previously mentioned areas of concern, we now focus on symbols and the ways in which a child uses them to communicate. As an SLP, you're interested in the number of words the child understands and expresses but also in the breadth of use in questions, declarations, and the like. Let's discuss the areas of a communication assessment that are particularly relevant for a young child using symbols: gestures and play, receptive language or comprehension, and the form and pragmatic functions of expressive language.

Gestures

From infancy, gestures supplement and predict spoken language skills (Capone & McGregor, 2004). Even after words emerge, gestures are still used to communicate. I bet you've used your share of gesturing today, and you have excellent spoken language skills. Within just a few months, children combine gestures with words to express relations that will later be expressed by two words (Goldin-Meadow & Butcher, 2003; Iverson &

Goldin-Meadow, 2005; Özçalişkan & Goldin-Meadow, 2005). For example, a child may express "Want cookie" by using a requesting gesture and saying the word "Cookie."

TD toddler communication consists of a combination of gestures in isolation, speech, and gesture-speech combinations (Iverson & Golding-Meadow, 2005). In general, TD toddlers use gestures in isolation more often than do older children.

Types of gestures. At around 12 months, new gesture types begin to develop. Recognitory gestures are play schemes in which an object is used for its intended function. These are discussed in the section on play. In general, TD infants with more object gestures in their repertoire tend to have larger vocabularies and more early spoken words. Usually, these gestures are performed as actions associated with objects. Only rarely, do these gestures represent perceptual qualities, such as two fingers on the head to represent a rabbit.

In contrast, *representational* or *symbolic gestures*, which usually emerge prior to having attained 25 single words expressively, do not manipulate the referent, as in recognitory gestures, but instead symbolize a referent. For example, a child may run with his or her arms extended to symbolize an airplane. A TD child usually acquires three to five representational gestures that refer to multiple referents, are produced spontaneously, and are not part of a rehearsed routine. Development of empty-handed, representational gestures seems to parallel symbolic speech development.

In later toddlerhood, representational gestures decrease as words take their place, but deictic gestures, mentioned earlier, and words, such as a point and the word "this" or "that," increase. Pointing is increasingly integrated with spoken language as a complement to speech during the second and third years of life.

Bootstrapping. Early gestures and spoken vocabulary are generally mutually exclusive, so gestures will be gradually replaced by words. TD children's development never goes in reverse order, replacing a word with a gesture. It's believed by many child development specialists that gestures facilitate communication until articulatory and phonological systems develop further. Increasingly, gestures are used by TD children to supplement, clarify, or provide a context for spoken language performance (McNeil, Alibali, & Evans, 2000).

Gestures are used as a bootstrap for spoken language. Gestures often function as words that are not yet part of the child's spoken repertoire and can in this way expand a child's lexicon or personal dictionary. For example, the child may see a butterfly and extend an index finger, making it flit about as the butterfly moves. This representational gesture evolves into semantic relations expressed in supplemental gesture-speech combinations, such as *bug fly*. Similarly, a child might say *mommy* + point to car, which precedes those same relations heard in speech combinations later, such as *mommy car* (Özçalişkan & Goldin-Meadow, 2005).

Single gestures and gesture-word combinations used by TD toddlers at 16 months of age are significantly correlated with total vocal production at 20 months. Gesture-word combinations also facilitate comprehension in young children (McNeil et al., 2000). Of particular importance is the relationship between combinations of deictic or representational gestures with other gestures or words. As you might expect, multi-element combinations of more than two items increase with age.

Gesture-word combinations. Two-symbol combinations initially may be expressed by both gestures and words. These gesture-speech combinations serve different purposes.

- Reinforcing combinations convey matching information, such as pointing to juice and to glass to indicate wanting juice poured into the glass as the child says "Juice glass." Reinforcing combinations consist of deictic gestures, such as pointing or showing an object, in combination with a spoken word.
- Supplemental combinations convey different cross-modality information, such as the representational gesture of holding a cup up and saying "Juice" to convey "Want juice" or "More juice." Supplemental combinations consist of
  - Pointing or showing an object plus a spoken action, adjective, or *different* noun, such as pointing to a dog while saying "bite," or
  - An action gesture or head-nodding plus a noun, such as gesturing "throw" while saying "ball."

Two-gesture combinations are rare at 16 months of age as speech supplants gesturing.

The two-symbol formation found in supplemental combinations is associated with advances in expressive language. For example, TD toddlers who produce supplemental information in their gestures will produce more spoken words than those who only produced reinforcing combinations. This said, the use of supplemental combinations may be rare for some children (Duchesne, Sutton, & Trudeau, 2005). As a child moves toward complete understanding of an utterance, the relationship between what is conveyed in gesture and in speech changes systematically.

Comprehension and Receptive Language

Children usually understand many words before they start to speak. Among TD infants, comprehension at 13 months of age predicts both receptive vocabulary and expressive grammatical complexity, as measured by mean length of utterance, at 28 months. Comprehension throughout the second year of life continues to play an important role in both receptive and expressive language acquisition (Watt et al., 2006).

Among children with atypical language development, comprehension skills at 12–24 months of age are a significant predictor of later comprehension and production ability (Lyytinen et al., 2001; Wetherby, Allen, Cleary, Kublin, & Goldstein, 2002; Wetherby, Goldstein, Cleary, Allen, & Kublin, 2003). Interestingly, comprehension predicts language production in both speech and AAC (Chapman, Seung, Schwartz, & Bird, 2000). Comprehension skills, especially comprehension vocabulary size, can also identify which children are most likely to develop language more typically (Paul, 2000). Children with language production difficulties but normal comprehension are more likely to catch up in their language production than are children with poorer comprehension (Thal, Tobias, & Morrison, 1991).

Synchrony of cross-sensory (auditory-visual) perception plays an important role in learning to map words onto referents. TD full-term preverbal infants as young as 2 months are highly sensitive to naming that occurs simultaneously with the movement of objects (Gogate, Prince, & Matatyaho, 2009). In contrast, preterm infants are delayed in developing this synchrony (Gogate, Maganti, & Perenyi, 2014). This may be related to the word-learning delays found in older preterm infants.

A young child with ASD may fail to look up or orient to his or her own name and to respond to speech directed to him or her (Zwaigenbaum et al., 2005). This and other failures in comprehension are barriers to language development and are associated with later language deficits.

During assessment, both a child's nonlinguistic comprehension strategies, such as responding to routines and watching what others do, and linguistic comprehension skills can be examined. The ratio of words produced to those comprehended may be a crude measure of possible future word production. Although a small receptive vocabulary is cause for concern, a receptive vocabulary several times bigger than the expressive one may indicate poor oral muscular development, speech planning problems, or poor recall.

Play

Although recognitory gestures, found in play, do not necessarily display intentional communication, they do demonstrate early defining of objects based on their use and symbolic representation. In this way, recognitory gestures are an extension of functional play, mentioned in the presymbolic assessment section.

In general, toddlers who can imitate incongruent actions, such as drinking from a toy shoe, or who can link play schemes onto featureless objects, such as pretending a block is a car, have larger expressive vocabularies. In these symbolic actions, a toddler is able to abstract a gestural scheme from its referent just as an arbitrary word can represent that referent.

Context seems to be very important in helping TD toddlers link language and play schemes (Bates & Dick, 2002). The infant relies on these contextual cues for early comprehension. In contrast, both word comprehension and production of a single play scheme or word with no contextual support requires more mature cognitive processing and symbolic representation.

Play schemes can also serve a complementary function with speech. By 20 months of age, TD toddlers begin to replace object-in-hand play schemes with empty-handed gestures that depict the function of objects. For example, a child may pretend to talk on the phone by bringing her empty hand to her ear. The gradual distancing from contact with the object, mentioned previously with deictic gestures, occurs with play schemes, indicating the creation of abstract symbols within play.

Expressive Language

A third to a half of children with an ASD either fail to develop any functional speech or experience delayed development of functional speech and language (Wetherby et al., 2000). Nonverbal communication is frequently unconventional, such as screaming and hitting; is idiosyncratic or extremely individualistic; is difficult to understand; and leads to increased communication breakdowns (Halle et al., 2004; Keen, 2003).

Among children beginning to use symbols, there is a progression as words move from imitations of the speech of others to functional communication. For speech to qualify as communicative, it should be produced for the purpose of conveying a message to a partner. For communicative speech to be functional, it also should be frequent, flexible, and purposeful. In other words, *perseverative speech*—saying the same word repeatedly—and echolalia are not functional in most cases.

Single symbols or symbol combinations reflect the intentions previously expressed through gestures. A child who only imitates symbols has a severely limited use of his or her expressive vocabulary. Possible early intentions of speech are presented in Table 4.6.

A child's acquisition of new words is influenced by many. The traditional benchmark of an expressive vocabulary of 50 words and the production of two-word combinations by 24 months should be used carefully because 10 to 15 percent of all children fail to meet this mark although approximately half of these children appear to have typical, if low, development by age 3 or 4. We need to be especially careful when comparing a child exposed to two or more languages to the normative data, which almost exclusively represent the development of monolingual, English-speaking children.

Considerations for bilingual children. Monolingual children with poor vocabulary development at age 2 are at risk of morphological and syntactic difficulties (Lee, 2011; Rescorla, 2002). This relationship of early vocabulary size and later grammatical development is also true for bilingual children (Conboy & Thal, 2006; Marchman, Martínez-Sussmann, & Dale, 2004; Parra, Hoff, & Core, 2011). Interestingly, the relationship of early vocabulary and later morphological and syntactic learning seems to be language specific, not cross-languages (Marchman et al., 2004; Parra et al., 2011). In other words, it may occur in a child's first language but not in the second, or the reverse.

Bilingual children often have lower scores than monolingual peers when assessed in only one of their languages (Bedore, Peña, García, & Cortez, 2005; Bialystok & Feng, 2011; Hoff et al., 2012; Junker & Stockman, 2002; Thordardottir, Rothenberg, Rivard, & Naves, 2006; Vagh, Pan, & Mancilla-Martínez, 2009). Using a single-language vocabulary measure, for example, increases the likelihood of overidentifying bilingual children as having language impairment (LI) (Bedore et al., 2005). Nor do we have sufficient norms for bilingual children, given such variables as language dominance and age at which the child is exposed to the two languages.

Two possible measures of vocabulary in bilingual children are total vocabulary and conceptual vocabulary. *Total vocabulary* is the total number of the words a child knows regardless of language. In contrast, *conceptual vocabulary* measures concepts, not words, so the same concept represented in both languages is counted only once. Using these measures, *cat* in English and *gato* (cat) in Spanish would count as two for total vocabulary but only one for conceptual vocabulary.

Total vocabulary across bilingual and monolingual 2-year-olds is similar. In contrast, the conceptual vocabulary of bilinguals is significantly smaller and grows at a slower rate than total vocabulary scores. Total vocabulary measures, therefore, are a fairer and more accurate way to assess the vocabulary growth of young bilingual children (Core, Hoff, Rumiche, & Seño, 2013).

TABLE 4.6 **Early Intentions**

Broad Pragmatic Categories	Primitive Speech Acts (PSAs)	Early Verbal Intentions	Examples
(Wells, 1985)	(Dore, 1975)	(Wells,1985; Owens, 1978)	
Control	Requesting action	Wanting demands	*Cookie* (Reach)
		Direct request/ commanding	*Help* (Hand object or struggle)
	Protesting	Protesting	*No* (Push away or uncooperative)
	Requesting Answer	Content questioning	*Wassat?* (Point)
Representational	Labeling	Naming/labeling	*Doggie* (Point)
		Statement/declaring	*Eat* (Commenting on dog barking)
	Answering	Answering	*Horsie* (in response to question)
		Reply	*Eat* (in response to "The doggie's hungry)
Expressive		Exclaiming	Squeal when picked up
		Verbal accompaniment to action	*Uh-oh* (With spill)
		Expressing state or attitude	*Tired*
Social	Greetings	Greeting/farewell	*Hi*
			Bye-bye
Tutorial	Repeating/practicing	Repeating/practicing	*Cookie, cookie, cookie*
Procedural	Calling	Calling	*Mommy*

Measures of expressive language. Through several means of assessment, an SLP can attempt to collect data on the child's

- Phonotactic abilities, or production of sounds, sound combinations, and syllable structures,
- Ability to imitate words,
- Expressive vocabulary,
- Communication breakdowns,
- Multiword combinations,
- Word combination patterns, and
- Pragmatic functions or intentions.

Let's discuss a few of these in detail. The particulars of how to measure some of these areas will be discussed in Chapter 5.

Many measures of early language result in a list of words that the child seems to understand and that the child produces. While this is important, to stop here is to severely restrict the description of what the child knows and can express through symbols. For example, from the earliest stages of vocabulary growth, children produce words for a variety of purposes.

One measure of a child's ability to use many different nonimitative words is lexical density, which reflects both talkativeness and productive vocabulary size (Yoder & Stone, 2006a). Lexical density is the number of different signs and/or words a child uses in a communication sample. This value reflects the diversity of meanings that a child uses for frequent communication purposes. In Chapter 5, we'll discuss how to calculate lexical density.

Communication breakdown is also of concern in assessment. When a speaker is faced with a breakdown in communication, he or she resorts to repair strategies, such as repeating or modifying the initial communication act. Thus, communication repairs can be viewed as an early indicator of intent to communicate, as the primary way in which a child influences people in their environment, and an important clinical measure (Meadan, Halle, Watkins, & Chadsey, 2006). For that reason, the SLP will want to note when breakdown occurs and to observe the child's repair strategies.

Although early symbol combinations initially may reflect imitation or be word specific in nature, productive multisymbol expression quickly falls into patterns that reflect underlying meaning and symbol combination strategies. In a sense, these early symbol combinations are an early grammar upon which later syntactic grammar will be based.

Multiword combination patterns. Most children begin to combine words at about 18 months, when their vocabularies reach between 50 and 100 words. Vocabulary size may be a better marker than age of when word combining should begin. Children with productive vocabularies of more than 100 words who are not combining words are at risk for communication delays (ASHA, 2008b).

A natural concern is the way in which we describe these combinations. This is not just a philosophical discussion, because we will be using our characterization of a child's multiword combinations to plan the direction of intervention, including new combinations and longer ones.

The more traditional way of describing early word combinations is with the early semantic rules, such as *agent + action* and *negative + X*, first described in detail by Roger Brown and others in the early 1970s.

The semantic approach is appealing because most practicing SLPs know these categories, which are relatively easy to teach to young children. We should keep in mind, however, that these are analytical and theoretical categories for discussing early language and may not actually be relevant or even meaningful to young children, especially those with language impairment.

The second and newer approach comes from constructionist linguistic theory. According to Michael Tomasello, a psychologist, and other constructionists, young children use at least three different methods of combining words (Tomasello, 2003). These are called *word combinations*, *pivot schemes*, and *item-based constructions*.

Let's discuss both descriptive methods and ways in which they might be employed. It might be helpful to conceptualize the semantic approach as the "what," or the content for teaching early language, and the constructionist approach as the "how," or the method for teaching multisymbol utterances.

Semantic approach. The older semantic or semantic-syntactic concept consists of two sets of rules based on the ways in which they expand. We don't have space here to discuss the origin of these rules or the cognitive base from which they supposedly evolve, but most older language development texts will entertain this discussion. The two-word semantic rules are presented in Figure 4.5.

The initial group, from *demonstrative + nominative through experiencer + state* on Figure 4.5 are theoretically expanded from single words which already represent the semantic function. In other words, a child can already express negation with words such as "No" and expands into two-word utterances by adding another word. The semantic function remains unchanged. For example, "No" might be expanded to "No juice" but the meaning is still *negation*. The second group, consisting of the final three, is different in that *agent*, *action*, and *object* each represent distinct semantic categories. Unlike the first group, two-word utterances are created by combining categories rather than adding another word. While this distinction may seem like splitting hairs, it does appear to have some reality for children. In general, combinations of the first type are easier for children and tend to develop first. Of course, there is much individual difference across children.

FIGURE 4.5 Early Semantic Rules

Nomination: Naming a person or object using a single word or in the form *Demonstrative + Nominative*.

Examples: *Choo-choo, Kittie, That horsie, This book*

Location: Marking a spatial relationship with a single word or in the form *X + Locative* in which *X* may be any word.

Examples: *Kittie bed, Throw me, Come here*   Adult: Where kittie?

Child: *Bed*

Negation: Marking nonexistence, rejection, and/or denial with a single word or in the form *Negative + X* in which *X* may be any word.

Examples: *No, Allgone, No ride, No ni-night, Allgone juice*

Modification: Modifying noun-like words or concepts with single words or in the form *Modifier + Modified*.

Possession: Marking that an object belongs to or is frequently associated with an individual.

Examples: *Mine, My kittie, Mommy sock, Baby ball*

Attribution: Using descriptors for properties not inherently part of an object.

Examples: *Big, Hot, Yukky peas, Little doggie*

Recurrence: Marking reappearance or expected reappearance of an object or event.

Examples: *More, 'Nuther, Again, More juice, 'Nuther cracker*

Notice: Attempting to gain attention or signal some event in single words or in the form *Introducer + X*.

Examples: *Hi, Bye-bye, Hey Mommy, Hi man*

State: Mark feeling with single word or in form *Experiencer + State*.

Examples: *Tired, I tired, Doggie sleepy*

Action: Marking an activity with a single word or in the forms *Agent + Action* or *Action + Object*.

Agent: Marking that an animate entity initiated an activity.

Examples: *Mommy (throwing), Daddy eat, Doggie bite*

Object: Marking that an animate or inanimate object was the recipient of action.

Examples: *(Throw) Ball, Eat cookie, Ride bike*

Three-word combinations recombine the two-word rules. Thus *Agent + Action* could be combined with *X + Locative* to form *Agent + Action + Locative* as in *Mommy throw (ball) me*.

The advantage of using the semantic method is that the categories are easy for adults to conceptualize and teach. Recordkeeping is facilitated when many words fit nicely into categories that can be combined into even longer utterances. For example, *agent + action* (Mommy eat) and *action + object* (Eat cookie) can be combined into *agent + action + object* (Mommy eat cookie). Grammar, especially word order, has a semantic base, and later in development *agent + action + object* will morph into *subject + verb + object*, the form of the basic English sentence. The semantic word order "rules" may vary based on the language the child is learning, but the semantic relationships seem to underpin syntax nonetheless.

The use of the semantic categories corresponds to increases in mean length of utterance (MLU), which enables an SLP to track a child's progress. Growth in MLU is as follows:

- At 18 months: 1.0–1.6 morphemes
- At 21 months: 1.1–2.1 morphemes
- At 24 months: 1.5–2.2 morphemes

There is much to like in this more traditional theoretical approach, even though it may represent how adults conceptualize their world more than how children do.

Constructionist approach. Without going into great detail, and at the risk of misstating the theoretical position, let's just say that constructionists hypothesize that children do not learn rules per se but learn individual constructions, such as "Mommy eat," which eventually lead to rule generalization. In other words, children do not learn semantic rules, only individual constructions or combinations involving specific words. SLPs learned long ago that with young children it's difficult to teach a language rule per se. In intervention, SLPs teach individual examples and combinations, which is similar to the explanation of learning put forth by constructionists.

As mentioned previously, constructionists hypothesize that early word combinations may be of three types: word combinations, pivot schemes, and item-based constructions. These are presented in Table 4.7. Word combinations consist of nearly equivalent words that divide an experience into multiple units. The two words are not used in combination with other words. For example, a child has learned to label Daddy and a car and upon spying Daddy in the car says, "Daddy car." Initially, two-word combinations may be expressed as successive single-word utterances, as in "Daddy. Car." In a second example, one symbol might be spoken and the other conveyed by gesture. Either way, these forms serve as a transition to word combinations.

If you're following, you might have automatically thought, *Hmm, "Daddy car" represents the semantic rule x + location*, and you'd be correct. Hang on, the semantic and constructionist schemes are not necessarily mutually exclusive unless you're a linguist.

Pivot schemas have a more systematic pattern. Often one word or phrase, such as *want* or *more*, structures the utterance by determining the intent of the utterance as a whole, such as making a demand or requesting. This might be accompanied by an intonational pattern, such as an insistent sound to the utterance that also signals the intent. Other words, such as *juice*, or phrases, such as *go-bye*, simply fill in the blank or slot, so to speak, as in *More juice* or *Want go-bye*. In this way, one word is used with a wide variety of others as in *More juice, More cookie,* and *More apple,* even *More go-bye* and *More up.* Most likely, the categories reflect "things I want" or "things that disappear" depending on the word order and the specific words used, rather than reflecting semantic or syntactic categories. In fact, pivot schemes, unlike the semantic categories, do not appear to have any internal word order grammar, and thus "No juice" and "Juice no" would seem to have the same meaning.

Any EI-experienced SLP can confirm that use of a "carrier phrase" methodology, such as *Want X* or *More X*, is an excellent way to get lots of "mileage" from a few words. In fact, a major consideration in intervention is the choice between high usage–low specificity words, such as *more* and *want*, and low usage–high specificity words such as *cookie* and

TABLE 4.7 **Constructionist Multiword Utterance Patterns**

PATTERN	EXPLANATION	EXAMPLES
Word combinations	Equivalent words that encode an experience, sometimes as two successive one-word utterances.	Water hot Wave bye Drink cup
Pivot scheme	One word or phrase structures the utterance by determining intent.	Throw ball, Throw block, Throw airplane
	Several words may fill the "slot," as in "Want + 'things I want.'"	More juice, More cookie, More bottle
		Want blanket, Want up, Want out
Item-based constructions	Seem to follow word order rules. May contain morphological markers.	Baby eat, Hug baby, Baby's bed Daddy driving, Drive car, Drive to gran'ma's

juice. Use of pivot schemes is a productive strategy for producing many two-word utterances from a limited set of constructions.

Interestingly, and this is important for intervention, novel words used in pivot schemes by TD children do not seem to be used creatively to make other constructions. For example, a child might say "More cookie" but not use "cookie" to produce "Eat cookie." This will occur later. We can only conclude that at this point in development, each pivot schema is its own *grammatical island* and does not represent a grammatical rule. It tells us that in intervention, we must be certain to expand on these constructions and use words in many different ways.

In contrast, item-based constructions do seem to be following word order rules, but again with specific words. A child's word-specific, word-ordered constructions seem to be dependent upon how a child has heard a particular word being used. For example, some verbs may be used by adults in complex forms of several different types (e.g., *Eat__, Eat on__, Eat with __ , Eat all your __* and *__ eat*). Unlike pivot schemes, the item-based constructions of TD children contain morphological markers (*-ing, -s, -ed*), prepositions (*in, on, to*), and word order to indicate syntactic classes of words that are treated in certain ways. For example, only verbs receive a past *–ed* marker. These syntactic structures are not generalized but are learned and applied word by word after hearing similar words used in the same way by adults.

Although constructionists make a distinction between pivot schemes and item-based constructions, the two categories suggest a hierarchy for intervention in which words can be taught within pivot schemes and later broadened to item-based constructions. Although this is seemingly heresy to the linguist, it seems like a practical application for intervention. We'll discuss this approach later when we get to intervention. For now, you may want to try to interpret a child's two-word constructions based on semantic rules, constructions, or both.

Grammar

When children add verbs to their lexicons, they also typically begin to produce sentences. Approximately 70 percent of children between 24 and 26 months produce simple subject-verb (e.g., *Mommy eat*) and subject-verb-object (e.g., *Boy throw ball*) sentences (Klee, Gavin, & Letts, 2002). Limited use of verbs and of simple sentence forms by 30 months may indicate a risk for language impairment (Hadley, 2006). By age 3, a child should have a diverse verb vocabulary, be producing a broad array of simple sentences frequently, and exhibit some use of tense markers.

The first tense markers typically emerge within sentences between 24 and 26 months of age. Children with LI often use no or limited tense markers even at 36 months (Leonard, Camarata, Brown, & Camarata, 2004). The absence of tense morphemes or limited production of tense morphemes at 36 months is indicative of risk for language impairment (Hadley, 2006). Typical early markers include progressive *-ing*, third person singular *-s*, past tense *-ed*, and forms of *be* and *do* (Hadley & Short, 2005; Klee et al., 2002; Rispoli & Hadley, 2005).

▶ Although we will touch only lightly on specific assessment tools, you might want to explore how an assessment of a nonverbal child might look. Watch this video to see the Communication and Symbolic Behavior Scales being administered.

https://www.youtube.com/watch?v=JrO5aA9JjiA

Formal Assessment of Infants, Toddlers, and Preschoolers

Formal normative tests of language development are inappropriate for measuring language comprehension and production in children below age 3, especially those with ASD (Mirenda, Smith, Fawcett, & Johnston, 2003). Standardized tests, for example, adhere to

TABLE 4.8 **Communication Tests for Young Children**

Assessment Tool	Author(s)	Publisher or Journal
Ages and Stages Questionnaires (ASQ): A Parent-Completed Child-Monitoring System, Second Edition (2003)	Bricker, D. D., Squires, J., Mounts, L., Potter, L. Nickel, R., Trombley, E. & Farrell, J.	Baltimore, MD: Paul H. Brookes
Assessment, Evaluation, and Programming System: AEPS Measurement for Birth to Three Years (Volume 1), Second Edition (2002)	Bricker, D. D. (Ed.)	Baltimore, MD: Paul H. Brookes
The Bayley Scales of Infant Development, Second Edition (BSID-2) (1993)	Bayley, N.	San Antonio, TX: The Psychological Corporation
Carolina Curriculum for Infants and Toddlers with Special Needs, Third Edition (2004)	Johnson-Martin, N. M., Attermeier, S. M., & Hacker, B. J.	Baltimore, MD: Paul H. Brookes
Communication and Symbolic Behavior Scales (1993)	Wetherby, A., & Prizant, B.	Chicago: Riverside
Infant-Toddler Language Scale (1990)	Rossetti, L.	East Moline, IL: LinguiSystem
Language Development Survey (1989)	Rescoria, L.	*Journal of Speech and Hearing Disorders, 54,* 587–599
MacArthur-Bates Communication Development Inventories (2007)	Fenson, L., Marchman, V. A., Thal, D. J., Dale, P. S., Reznick, S., Bates, E.	Baltimore, MD: Paul H. Brookes
Maternal Behavior Rating Scale (MBRS) (1986)	Mahoney, G. A., & Finger, I.	*Topics in Early Childhood Special Education, 6,* 44
A Manual for the Dynamic Assessment of Nonsymbolic Communication (2002)	Snell, M. E., & Loncke, F. T.	Unpublished manuscript, University of Virginia at Charlottesville. This informative paper is available by typing "people.virginia.edu" into your online search engine and "snell" in the search box.
Observation of Communicative Interaction (OCI) (1987)	Klein, M., & Briggs, M.	*Journal of Childhood Communication Disorder, 4,* 91
Preschool Language Scale, Third Edition (PLS-3) (1992)	Zimmerman, I. L., Steiner V. G., & Pond, R. E.	San Antonio, TX: The Psychological Corporation
Receptive-Expressive Emergent Language Test, Third Edition (REEL-3) (2003)	Bzoch, K. R., League, R., & Brown, V. L.	Austin, TX: PRO-ED
Sequenced Inventory of Communication Development–Revised (SICD-R) (1984)	Hedrick, D. L., Prather, E. M., & Tobin, A. R.	Los Angeles: Western Psychological Services
Speech and Language Assessment Scale (1993)	Hadley, P. A., & Rice, M. L.	*Seminars in Speech and Language, 14,* 278–288
Transdisciplinary Play-Based Assessment: A Functional Approach to Working with Young Children (TPBA) (1990)	Linder, T.	Baltimore, MD: Paul H. Brookes

Longer explanations are available in Appendix B.

inflexible performance criteria that are often difficult for young children. They're static. For example, regardless of their language and cognition abilities, children with limited hand and arm control are unable to complete 70 percent of the items on the cognitive scale of the Bayley–III (DeVeney, Hoffman, & Cress, 2012).

In contrast, alternative parent-completed vocabulary checklists, such as those in the *MacArthur-Bates Communicative Development Inventories, Second Edition (MCDI-2*; Fenson et al., 2006), have proven to be both valid and cost effective for assessing vocabulary size and development (Dale, Price, Bishop, & Plomin, 2003). Measures of vocabulary are also useful for examining individual differences in children independent of developmental level.

By its very nature, nonsymbolic communication lacks convention. Each child-caregiver dyad is in the ongoing process of negotiating the individualistic interactional behaviors that "work" for them. There are no rules here. These nonsymbolic interactions are not confined by what appears in normative testing. By definition, nonsymbolic interactions are often idiosyncratic and multimodal (both vocal and gestural).

In general, formal early childhood assessment protocols fall into two broad categories, age-related and task-related. Age-related tools attempt to describe a child's behavior based on the development of typical children. Questions are often grouped within certain age brackets. While the results may be helpful for establishing an age equivalence, often required by governmental agencies such as school systems or used to establish eligibility for services, these same results help little in establishing ECI goals. In contrast, task-related tools attempt to determine a child's performance of certain behaviors that are considered important for the development of symbolic communication. We identified some of these in the previous section. These measures yield a performance level relative to step-like intervention goals.

Not all measures, even those supposedly assessing the same behaviors, will yield the same results, especially for young children. For example, one study of toddlers with severe expressive impairments found that although receptive language scores were better than expected, given the children's cognitive or overall developmental scores, receptive language scores were less advanced on the *MacArthur Communication Developmental Inventory* (Fenson et al., 2006) than on the *Battelle Developmental Inventory* (Newborg, Stock, Wnek, Guidubaldi, & Svinicki, 2005), suggesting that the tests measured different aspects of receptive language (Ross & Cress, 2006).

Evaluations are more ecologically sound when caregiver input is included (O'Neill, 2007). Thus, both the Institute of Medicine (2001) and the American Academy of Pediatrics (2012) have recommended that parental/caregiver experiences be incorporated into clinical decision-making. For example, a parent report measure of language ability, such as the *MacArthur-Bates Communicative Development Inventories*, Level III (CDI–III), can reliably discriminate children with LI from those developing language typically (Skarakis-Doyle, Campbell, & Dempsey, 2009).

With these cautionary thoughts in mind, you might want to look at some commercially available assessment tools and tests as well as some that have appeared in professional journals. The list of tests presented in Table 4.8 are explained in more detail in Appendix B.

Early Identification of Children with ASD

It is extremely important to diagnose ASD in infants because ECI with these children can be particularly effective. Early identification of children with ASD allows for early intervention in comprehensive, intensive programs addressing communicative, educational, developmental, and behavioral needs.

The importance of earlier identification can be seen in the progress made by children who subsequently receive ECI (Harris & Handleman, 2000; Simpson, 2005). In general, early identification and intensive intervention services before age 3 are associated with better communicative, academic, and behavioral outcomes at school age.

Although ASD is sometimes diagnosed before 3 years of age, such early diagnosis is still rare (Brian et al., 2008; Chakrabarti & Fombonne, 2005). The mean age for diagnosis in the United States is between 3 and 5 years, and many children are not diagnosed until school age (Mandell, Novak, & Zubritsky, 2005). The delay between initial evaluation and definitive diagnosis of ASD may be 13 months in some cases (Wiggins, Baio, & Rice, 2006). Closing the gap in time between initial parent concern, initial evaluation, and age of diagnosis would greatly reduce the age of entry into intervention.

One reason for the delayed diagnosis is that the criteria used for conventional diagnosis are often based on older children. In addition, some symptoms, such as repetitive movements, occur frequently in TD infants as well, making definitive diagnosis more difficult. Further, some characteristics of ASD vary widely across individual infants and may be unusual but not necessarily problematic. Tremendous variability exists in the nature, timing, and stability of early signs in ASD (e.g., Bryson et al., 2007). Finally, it is difficult to distinguish autism from other childhood disorders, such as intellectual disability, at a young age (Bailey, Hatton, Skinner, & Mesibov, 2001).

With still limited but increasing frequency, children with ASD are being identified under 3 years of age based primarily on deficits in communication, social reciprocity, and repetitive behaviors. Because there is currently no recognized biological marker for ASD, screening and diagnosis must be based on behavioral features (Johnson & Myers, 2007).

Diagnosis before age 2 is still rare. The barriers to early identification of infants and young toddlers include

- Little knowledge of early development of children with ASD,
- Need to identify both typical and atypical behaviors, and
- Still emerging knowledge on the markers that identify infants and toddlers with ASD.

Luckily, some of the best minds in the fields of speech-language pathology, cognitive and behavioral sciences, neurology, and education are attempting to identify markers and describe early development of these children.

The American Academy of Pediatrics (AAP) recently recommended that all children be evaluated with a standardized broadband screening tool at 9-, 18-, 24- and 30-month visits, and an ASD-specific screening tool at the 18- and 24-month visits. Unfortunately, we still lack reliable tools with which to do so (Johnson, Myers, & The Council on Children with Disabilities, 2007).

The primary methods used in early identification of infants and toddlers with ASD have been (Matson, Wilkins, & Gonzalez, 2008).

- Evidence-based assessment scales using established criteria for differential diagnosis, and
- Cognitive/developmental descriptive studies that attempt to identify behavior patterns of infants who later evidence ASD.

The diagnostic team will need to draw information from a variety of sources in order to identify early behavioral markers that are most predictive of an ASD diagnosis. The problem is complicated by our lack of knowledge of which early behaviors have diagnostic significance and by the variable ages at which some behaviors emerge.

Research into early behavioral markers is hampered because it is extremely costly to follow a large group of infants and toddlers to see if early diagnoses are fruitful. In a longitudinal study of younger siblings of children with ASD, several factors have emerged for 18-month-old children (Brian et al., 2008). Surprisingly, behavioral items, such as difficulty transitioning from one activity to another, seem to be more important than speech and language for early identification, because many children with ASD are nonverbal. Early behavioral markers include (Brian et al., 2008)

- Lack of response to name (e.g., Wetherby et al., 2004; Zwaigenbaum et al., 2005),
- Poor eye contact (e.g., Dawson, Osterling, Meltzoff, & Kuhl, 2000; Stone, Conrood, & Ousley, 1999),
- Lack of social smiling (e.g., Charman, Swettenham, Cox, Baird, & Drew, 1998),
- Lack of shared enjoyment/social interest (e.g. Charman et al., 1998),
- Atypical motor behavior (Loh et al., 2007; Watt, Wetherby, Barber, & Morgan, in press), and
- Atypical sensory responses to the environment (Bryson et al., 2007).

Information on these and other behaviors can be gathered by the diagnostic team as outlined in Chapter 5.

Eligibility for Services

Before we finish this chapter, we should discuss the issue of eligibility for services. School districts are responsible for providing EI services for children either within their district or from agencies under contract with the district. Of course, parents are always free to seek help from SLPs in private practice or working in preschool or EI programs. With tight budgets, school districts try to monitor closely those children who will receive government-mandated services.

As professionals, we need to be wary of some common "eligibility" criteria that may be used to deny access to services. These criteria are used despite the lack of scientific evidence for their appropriateness.

One of the most insidious and widely used, called *cognitive referencing*, is based on the discrepancy between cognitive and communication functioning in children with intellectual disability (ID). In short, those who support cognitive referencing believe that children with ID should not receive SLP services if their language skills are commensurate with their cognitive level. In other words, if the child has a mental age of 2 years and a language age of 2 years, no services are needed regardless of the child's chronological age. The result of cognitive referencing can be intermittent services as a child falls behind, necessitating intervention, catches up because of intervention, and then is no longer eligible, which begins the slide to once more being behind. While this criterion may save money, it hardly benefits children to the full extent possible. If anything, young children respond best to consistent intervention.

In short, cognitive referencing is not an appropriate criterion for eligibility decisions. In fact, language intervention benefits children with ID/DD even when no language-cognition discrepancy exists. The American Speech-Language-Hearing Association has urged its members to advocate for the use of other eligibility criteria and to work actively to overturn cognitive referencing policies (ASHA, 1996, 1999, 2000, 2004a). This is where your role as an advocate is very important.

Conclusion

The short list of assessment areas of concern for an SLP includes:

- Forms and means of child's communication
- Child's communication success
- Contingency, or the relatedness of adult responses to the behavior of the child, consistency, and timeliness
- Functional use of objects
- Motor imitation
- Joint attention and attention-following of gazing and pointing
- Intentional communication and the use of gestures and vocalizations
- Oral motor abilities and feeding and swallowing

- Hearing
- Level of play
- Cognitive and motor abilities
- Comprehension and receptive language
- Expressive language

Most of these areas have multiple levels and measures.

Now we know the *what*; it's time for the *how*, the organization of the assessment. We'll need to explore ways in which we can elicit data on the communication behaviors of the child, the caregiver-child interaction, and nonsymbolic and symbolic behaviors mentioned in this chapter. That's a lot to accomplish, and we may have a very small window of opportunity with a child who is ill or has multiple impairment, or one with ASD.

✓ Click here to gauge your understanding of the concepts in this chapter.

5

Early Communication Assessment Process

LEARNING OUTCOMES

When you have completed this chapter, you should be able to:

- List the steps in an early communication assessment.
- Explain the importance of preassessment planning and preliminary data collecting.
- Describe what to look for in an interactional observation.
- Explain how to conduct a play-based interactional assessment.
- Explain how assessment procedures may differ for children with specific disorders.

Terms with which you should be familiar:

Communication temptations	Scaffolding
Dynamic assessment	Zone of proximal development
Mediated assistance	

We have most of the pieces for an assessment of a nonsymbolic or minimally symbolic child. What is needed is to organize our assessment in a logical manner to give us the information that we need to describe how an individual child communicates with those in her or his environment. In other words, we need to plan our assessment to get the best and most information possible. Planning is essential to this entire process.

In some settings, a speech-language pathologist (SLP) begins involvement in the neonatal intensive care unit (NICU) or special care nursery (SCN) by promoting specialized feeding and swallowing techniques and educating parents about early communication development. Other SLPs may become involved when the infant visits the follow-up clinic or is referred for evaluation. Some children will be identified through comprehensive "child-find" systems. In each situation, an SLP must evaluate a child's performance in as detailed a manner as possible for the level of assessment required. While not all levels of assessment and analysis would apply to every child, a similar assessment plan might be appropriate.

SLPs are responsible for selection and development of age-appropriate screening and assessment procedures (ASHA, 2008b). Let's look at a possible model for a thorough communication assessment. Assessment for a child's potential AAC use will be discussed separately in Chapter 6.

You can offer communication opportunities, and you can simplify a task to ensure success, but ultimately it is up to the child. Your task is to figure out how you can fit into a young child's pattern of behavior.

Whether the measures used in an assessment are yours or someone else's, they should be valid, meaning they should measure what they claim to measure. For example, measurement of communication skills, such as gestures, should not be confused with performance of the fine motor skills needed for a pointing response. In a situation in which a child exhibits motor deficits, you as the SLP will need to identify alternative ways in which the child indicates responses other than by pointing with an extended finger, hand, and arm (Crais, 2011).

A word of caution: Just like you and me, children have their bad days. When, as a toddler, my grandson Dakota's acid reflux was particularly bad, it was all but impossible to get him to do anything but whine and cry. So . . .

- Stay flexible,
- Be creative,
- Trust the caregivers, and
- Rely on your team.

Stowing your glasses out of reach, tying up your hair, and not wearing dangling earrings can also be good proactive strategies for the tantruming child.

For the braver souls among us, let's proceed. We'll discuss communication screening and a full communication assessment, including the various steps that might logically lead the assessment team to recommendations.

Communication Screening

In the United States, as mentioned previously, children in the established risk category are eligible for services under IDEA 2004 Part C. Although children in the at-risk category are also eligible, states have varying criteria for eligibility. Availability of services for these children also varies by locale. It is the responsibility of SLPs to integrate knowledge of at-risk factors with the results of screening tests and, if needed, with more thorough results from communication assessment (ASHA, 2008b).

Screening is a process for determining whether a child is likely to show deficits in communication and/or feeding and swallowing development. More specifically, screening helps SLPs identify young children at risk so that evaluation can be used to establish eligibility and to determine the appropriate in-depth assessment. This responsibility requires SLPs to possess knowledge of typical development and individualistic variation in interactive styles, especially among children from culturally and linguistically diverse backgrounds (ASHA, 2008b).

The first contact most families have with an SLP or an early intervention (EI) team may be through this eligibility determination process. Handled thoughtfully, these contacts can provide the first opportunity to develop a relationship with a family. Often, these early meetings are information-sharing events. Because many young children are not speaking when parents become concerned, much of the SLP's assessment may focus on presymbolic behaviors.

Screening is the first step in possible receipt of services, so it is extremely important that the measures used be valid, reliable, sensitive, specific, and representative, whether they are standardized or criterion-referenced in nature (ASHA, 2008b).

- *Validity* is the extent to which a test measures accurately what it purports to measure when compared to other measures and to evidence and theory.
- *Reliability* is a measure's consistency under similar conditions—its stability over time for the same child and/or for different judges.
- *Sensitivity* refers to a measure's ability to identify children who actually have difficulties.
- *Specificity*, in contrast, is a measure's capacity for accurately identify children who do *not* have a problem.
- *Representativeness* of the results is achieved through a large and diverse norming sample in which the child being evaluated is represented by similar children.

These criteria, difficult to obtain in early communication assessment, are typically discussed in the examiner's manual that accompanies the test. Given our population of infants and toddlers, few validated measures are available. This requires that SLPs be creative and flexible.

Screening formats include both direct assessment of the child and parental report using a standardized instrument. Either format may be used alone or in combination, providing the measures used have adequate psychometric or data-collecting properties (ASHA, 2008b). Of course, the validity of the screening process increases with a combination of measures. Several screening tools, along with comments, are presented in Table 5.1.

As a new SLP, you might be reluctant to use the parental report format. You can relax. Parent-completed screening measures are appropriate and useful. In addition, we cannot stress enough that most parents have been shown to be reliable and accurate reporters of their children's communication and general development when using structured reporting formats (Stott, Merricks, Bolton, & Goodyer, 2002).

Results of the screening should be shared with the family who, in turn, should be encouraged to ask questions. If a child passes the screening, the SLP should make sure the family understands that (ASHA, 2008b)

- Screening is only a general estimate of the child's performance at a point in time,
- Continued monitoring of the child's progress over time is important, and
- The family should return for further screening or a full evaluation if their concerns persist or new concerns arise.

When a child fails a screening, an evaluation is typically conducted to determine if he or she meets eligibility criteria for services under IDEA and state guidelines.

To increase validity of the screening, the SLP can ask the family if the results reflect the child's typical performance or if there are other factors affecting the situation, such as the child's health. If parents or caregivers believe that the screening was not an accurate reflection of their child's abilities, further evaluation may be needed. SLPs and families should work together to identify the next steps in the evaluation process.

FAMILIES WITH CULTURALLY OR LINGUISTICALLY DIVERSE BACKGROUNDS

As in any assessment of language performance, you have to consider whether a child who appears to have a problem is demonstrating a language *difference* or a *disorder* (ASHA, 2008b). This is especially important if a child comes from a background that is culturally or linguistically different from the normative sample used in the screening tool.

TABLE 5.1 **Screening Tests for Infants and Toddlers**

TEST	COMMENTS
Battelle Developmental Inventory, Second Edition (Newborg, 2005)	Direct assessment of child. Spanish version available. High concurrent validity, interrater reliability, and internal consistency (Johnson, Cook, & Kullman, 1992; McLean, McCormick, Bruder, & Burdg, 1987). Moderately high sensitivity and specificity (Glascoe, 1993).
Birth to Three Assessment and Intervention System, Second Edition (Ammer & Bangs, 2000)	Direct assessment of child.
Capute Scales: Cognitive Adaptive Test and Clinical Linguistic and Auditory Milestone Scale (Accardo & Capute, 2005)	Direct assessment of child. Spanish and Russian versions available.
Communication and Symbolic Behavior Scales Infant and Toddler Checklist (Wetherby & Prizant, 2002)	Parental report. High sensitivity and high specificity reported in manual.
Denver Developmental Screening Test II (Frankenburg & Dobbs, 1990)	Direct assessment and some parental report. Spanish version available. High sensitivity; low specificity (Glascoe, Byrne, Ashford, Johnson, Chang, & Strickland, 1992)
Early Language Milestones Scale, Second Edition (Coplan, 1993)	Direct assessment of child. High sensitivity and high specificity with high-risk children. High sensitivity and moderately high sensitivity with low-risk children. (Coplan, Gleason, Ryan, Burke, & Williams, 1982)
Early Screening Profiles (Harrison et al., 1990)	Direct assessment of child and parental report.
Language Development Survey (Rescorla, 1989)	Parental report. Moderate to high sensitivity and specificity, increasing with age (Klee et al., 1998). High validity with the *MacArthur-Bates Communicative Development Inventories* (Rescorla, Ratner, Jusczyk, & Jusczyk, 2005).
MacArthur-Bates Communicative Development Inventories, Second Edition (Fenson et al., 2006)	Parental report. Spanish version available. Words and Gestures and Words and Sentences forms correlate from low to high with behavioral assessments for children with profound hearing loss (Thal, DesJardin, & Eisenberg, 2007)
Pre-Screening Development Questionnaire (PDQ-II) (Frankenburg & Bresnick, 1998)	Parental report. Spanish version available. PDQ-I has French version.
Screening Kit for Language Development (Bliss & Allen, 1983)	Direct assessment of child. Normed for standard English and African American English.

In these cases, an SLP can pay particular attention to the properties of commonly used tools to determine their applicability. In many cases, a standardized measure is not available in the native language and a parent report measure may be more appropriate. Although translations of parent report measures are less problematic than translations of actual tests, these translations also may not account for linguistic, dialectal, or cultural differences and must be used with care.

The location and format for screenings are important and will affect a child's performance. This is especially true when the SLP has a sociocultural background different from that of the child and family. In this situation, when possible, it may be better to frame screening activities within the events and activities of the local community (Lynch & Hanson, 2004).

Some EI programs use cultural guides or cultural-linguistic mediators to facilitate communication between professionals and families (Barrera, 2000; Lynch & Hanson, 2004; Moore & Pérez-Méndez, 2006). Although a mediator is knowledgeable about the family's culture and/or linguistic community, the SLP is still responsible for familiarizing families with available services and supports (ASHA, 2004c).

Let's move to our main topic, a thorough early communication intervention (ECI) assessment. Remember that an assessment is a structured, step-by-step process in which each step informs the next.

Steps in Early Communication Assessment

By its very nature, a typical ECI assessment encompasses more in-depth observations and information-gathering than do eligibility evaluations or screenings. Our overall assessment goals, as stated in the previous chapter, are

- To describe the child's communication abilities,
- To relate those abilities to partners in familiar environments/contexts,
- To describe the communication behaviors of the child's partners,
- To identify the child's responses to various facilitative prompts, and
- To discover promising intervention techniques.

In practical terms, this means that we need to collect assessment information on a child's communicative skills, the partners' skills, and the facilitative characteristics of varying communication contexts (Snell, 2002).

Ideally, as we know, the assessment is completed within a transdisciplinary context that assesses a child across all developmental domains. As with any type of communication assessment, planning and organization are important and help answer the question "What do we want to know, and how can we best obtain that information?"

MULTIPLE MEASURES

Traditionally, assessment involves the use of standardized tests. Designed to provide information under a "standard" set of conditions, these measures do not allow examination of a child's behaviors within daily interactional contexts. This characteristic limits the generalization of results to natural environments, especially for very young children (Neisworth & Bagnato, 2004). In addition, standardized measures often limit the role of family members and do not focus on spontaneous communication (ASHA, 2008b).

For these reasons and others, many professionals recommend against standardized testing as the sole source of information and suggest instead a blend of standardized testing and nonstandardized assessment (Boone & Crais, 2001; Neisworth & Bagnato, 2004; Paul, 2007; Wetherby & Woods, 2006). This is especially true of our very youngest clients.

Children with nonsymbolic communication are best assessed using multiple non-traditional approaches that individualize assessment to suit the child in terms of tasks, materials, procedures, and assessors. In general, such flexible, individualized assessment includes (Snell, 2002)

- Familiar contexts, objects, and individuals;
- Active involvement of the child;
- Variety of information sources, those familiar with the child;
- Information collected over time;
- Manipulation of the environment to increased child and caregiver communication; and
- Going beyond current performance and probing child's learning potential.

Several approaches for assessing early communication exist, including interviews, naturalistic observation, ecologic-functional assessment, elicitation tasks, and dynamic assessment. We'll get to each of these shortly.

Assessment tools and procedures should be age appropriate, culturally sensitive, and individualized for the child and family. Because our goal is to obtain the best description

FIGURE 5.1 **Schematic of the Assessment Process. Each step logically flows from the previous one as we refine and sharpen our description of the child.**

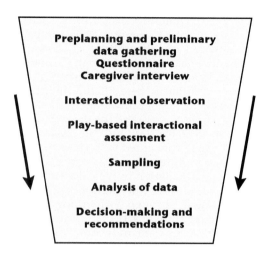

Preplanning and preliminary
data gathering
Questionnaire
Caregiver interview

Interactional observation

Play-based interactional
assessment

Sampling

Analysis of data

Decision-making and
recommendations

possible of a child's functional communication abilities, we are interested in the observations of both professionals and caregivers. These can be obtained in a variety of ways. At the very least, the assessment process should include the following steps:

- Preplanning and preliminary data gathering
  - Questionnaire
  - Caregiver interview
- Interactional observation
- Play-based interactional assessment
- Sampling
- Analysis of data
- Decision-making and recommendations

Like any good detective, the assessment team discovers more and more as they advance. As mentioned, each step informs the next as the team hones its description of the child's and caregiver's behaviors and their interactional style. Figure 5.1 illustrates the process graphically. We'll discuss each step in order later.

TRANSDISCIPLINARY TEAMS

Traditional assessments are often conducted exclusively by professionals who share their findings and make recommendations rather than building consensus with family members. In the process, caregivers may be reduced to mere observers, reinforcing notions of parental incompetence and leading to parental feelings of disenfranchisement.

In contrast, as you know, the transdisciplinary teams in EI work collaboratively, pooling members' knowledge and skills across discipline boundaries and including the family's concerns and expertise. The transdisciplinary model seems well suited to EI because it emphasizes functional goals and family-centered intervention in a variety of natural settings.

One way to build a consensus and a collaborative relationship is to share assessment information in an ongoing way throughout the assessment. Before each task, professionals can explain its purpose to parents, and as each is completed, families and professionals can share their impressions and discuss their findings. Collaboratively, the team can begin to generate ideas to enhance assessment and to plan intervention.

ECOLOGICAL VALIDITY

An assessment is ecologically authentic to the extent that it provides information about the behavior of a child in her or his typical and natural settings and indicates what a child knows and can do (Neisworth & Bagnato, 2004). Family members and childcare providers are the primary sources of information within these natural environments.

A child may inhabit a variety of differing environments, such as the home, childcare setting, babysitter's apartment, and a center-based intervention program, to name a few. When a child has multiple caregivers, the SLP can discuss daily activities and routines with each. The interactions that reach across these settings and different partners are a necessary part of an early communication assessment. By recognizing different caregivers' expectations and interactions, an SLP can enhance intervention in these differing milieus. Family members may have impressions or observations that differ significantly from those of professional team members.

Communication is a dynamic process, and the three elements, the child, the partner and their shared environment, are in constant flux (Siegel & Wetherby, 2000; Snell & Loncke, 2002). In an assessment, we're concerned with the entire communication dynamic and as interested in the behaviors of the caregiver as we are in those of the child.

Information on a child's participation in typical activities and routines is obtained primarily from the caregivers. Ideally, this information is supplemented with direct observations in the natural environment. Through both informal observation and discussion, an SLP gathers information about a child's participation and the ways in which communication affects that participation. A key element is contextual factors that may enhance or constrain participation (Wilcox & Woods, 2011).

The SLP and caregiver can collaboratively identify situations in which (Wilcox & Woods, 2011)

- Communication breakdowns cause participation difficulties, and
- Children's communication skills can be facilitated to enable or enhance participation.

It's important here to not focus solely on the negative. Equally important are those activities and routines that are going well. These events promote the acquisition of new skills and can help in generalization of these skills to different activities and routines. For example, given my grandson's severe acid reflux, mealtime and for a few hours after were not periods when interactions were optimal. Other activities, such as riding in the car, at other times were more positive.

Let's start at the beginning of the assessment process and explore each step. As we proceed, we'll discuss ways to mesh flexible nonstandardized approaches with more formal, structured methods. This is a joint exploration by all team members. Ideally, there are several opportunities for both the child and caregivers to interact in a variety of ways across several situations in which potential communicative behaviors occur both spontaneously and in response to elicitation.

The Importance of Preassessment Planning and Preliminary Data Collecting

Preassessment planning, the process by which families and professionals set the parameters of an upcoming assessment, is a critical factor in determining how an assessment will be conducted and perceived. Although collaborative planning prior to formal assessment is still not widely used, it's favored by many families and professionals (Crais, Roy, & Free, 2006).

In the initial preassessment meeting, professionals should discuss with a family the issues of confidentiality and the rights of participants during the assessment process. Parents should understand that the assessment will be recorded for further study and comparison and be encouraged to sign the necessary waivers.

The goals of preassessment planning are to (Boone & Crais, 2001)

- Identify the family's assessment expectations, wants, and/or needs;
- Explore the family's priorities and preferences;

- Identify strength areas and activities of the child; and
- Determine the roles family members wish to play in the assessment.

In an initial contact with the family, professionals begin to gather information about parent concerns and questions and to identify what parents wish to gain from the assessment. Other information might include

- Best time(s) and location(s) for the upcoming assessment,
- Preferences for the evaluative approaches to be used in the assessment,
- The child's favorite activities and toys, and
- Other people that parents might wish to include in the assessment.

Ideally, the initial meeting will be followed by both a questionnaire and an interview or interviews with family members.

Not all families will readily embrace an active role in assessment planning and implementation. Some will be more hesitant and expect professionals to take the lead. When professionals actively listen to family members' concerns and show genuine appreciation for the family members' knowledge of the child, parents often become more willing to be involved. Active listening is attending to a parent, making good eye contact, providing verbal and nonverbal feedback and validation (*um-hm, yes, I understand*), and not interrupting to provide advice.

During the preassessment planning phase, professionals and families will also want to explore when and where it would be best to share information following the assessment. Time should be spent discussing sharing of results both within the team and with others who might benefit from this knowledge. Parents are often reassured to find that they are the ones to determine where results will be sent.

All of these considerations help families become full participants in the transdisciplinary team. Additional ideas for family involvement are contained in the excellent reviews in Barrera and Corso (2002), Boone and Crais (2001), and Crais et al. (2006).

QUESTIONNAIRE

A portion of the preliminary data collecting includes gathering information on the child's birth, medical and developmental histories, and current behaviors. This information can be collected efficiently through questionnaires and follow-up interviews with caregivers.

At the initial preassessment meeting, parents can be alerted to the questionnaire and its purpose. Professionals can impress upon parents the importance of this initial data collection as a first step that will influence everything that follows. Because parents observe large samples of their child's behaviors in naturalistic settings, their input can enhance both the validity and reliability of assessments (Fenson et al., 2006).

For a variety of reasons, some parents do not read. As the SLP, you can offer parents a choice by saying, "Would it be helpful if we went through the questionnaire together?" You can then read the questions to the parents. Some parents, especially refugees, may come from cultures in which reading is not common even in the native language. Offering to complete the questionnaire with the parent removes any awkwardness or embarrassment on the part of the family.

The strength of parental reports is that parents are highly motivated observers of their infant's behavior. One weakness is that most parents have a very limited comparison sample with which to rate their child's behavior as typical or atypical. For this reason, it's best if questionnaires focus on describing behaviors rather than on making comparisons of the child's behavior with that of typically developing (TD) children. Giving parents the ages at which certain behaviors are typically attained may bias their responses and cause some unneeded angst. Ideally, both questionnaires and interviews would consist of a combination of open-ended questions that allow caregivers to elaborate and specific questions that ask for descriptions of behavior.

The validity of parental responses describing behaviors can be increased by using a preprinted format containing frequently occurring behaviors rather than an open-ended recall or speculative format. For example, regardless of socioeconomic status, parents can be very effective reporters on the words their child understands and expresses if they have a list of possible words from which to choose. The SLP can explain that the list contains possible words, not expected ones. Tasks that ask parents to list words from their memory are less reliable (Furey, 2011). One caution is that the use of standard questions may not provide individualized information about a specific child's participation in daily activities and routines.

For Spanish-speaking families, the parent report format of both the *Inventarios del Desarrollo de Habilidades Comunicativas Palabras y Enunciados* (INV–II; Jackson-Maldonado, Bates, & Thal, 1992; Jackson-Maldonado et al., 2003) and the Spanish version of the *MacArthur-Bates Communicative Development Inventories* (CDI) *Words and Sentences* form have high sensitivity and high specificity in identifying children with expressive language delays (Guiberson, Rodríguez, & Dale, 2011). The results of these parent inventories correlate well with results on the Spanish version of the *Preschool Language Scale, Fourth Edition* (SPLS–4; Zimmerman, Steiner, & Pond, 2002).

A sample questionnaire/interview is presented in Appendix C. You'll note that the questions presented in this appendix assume some level of communication and may alert parents to previously overlooked behaviors. The questionnaire is roughly divided into five areas:

■ Family priorities and preferences
■ The child
■ The child's current communication
■ The partner's communication behaviors and strategies
■ The communication environment

By focusing on communication within everyday routines and contexts, the questionnaire reinforces the notion that communication is part of each family's day and that intervention can occur in the context of everyday events. Hopefully, you can see how such questions early in the process can subtly introduce the notion of intervention within daily routines.

Some questions may be uncomfortable for caregivers if the SLP has not explained the purpose of the questionnaire and its relevance for intervention. Parents may also worry that professionals are judging their parenting or caregiving skills. This can be especially true for parents with linguistic and cultural backgrounds that differ from that of the SLP. These concerns may be addressed in preplanning meetings or via phone or written correspondence.

Once the questionnaire is returned, professionals can study the results to determine what information needs clarification or further exploration. In this way, the questionnaire can provide a framework for the caregiver interview to follow.

CAREGIVER INTERVIEW

An interview based on the questionnaire can further focus an assessment on a child's interests and abilities and on caregivers' priorities. In addition, the interview process provides the SLP with an opportunity to explain the concept of activity- and routine-based intervention and the importance of families in participation-based outcomes (Wilcox & Woods, 2011). The SLP can also attempt to ascertain from family members what seems to work and what doesn't in terms of their child's participation in interactions (Campbell, Milbourne, & Wilcox, 2008; McWilliam, 2000).

Although conversational in tone, interviews are not freewheeling unorganized chats. Organization provided by the questions helps professionals gain the caregiver's perspective across all areas of communication and inform the subsequent steps in the assessment process.

In the following section, we will focus on parents, although separate interviews with different caregivers, such as teachers, are also extremely important. Information may be corroborated by different informants, increasing the accuracy of the assessment. Even differing answers can be useful because they may highlight the different ways caregivers interact with the child. For example, a parent may state that a child initiates interaction frequently while a childcare provider reports no such initiations. Such disparate information may provide insight into different communication environments.

Format of a Caregiver Interview

The SLP should begin by thanking the family for completing the questionnaire. This is also an opportunity to restate the purpose of the assessment process. Parents can be reminded of the confidential nature of all information disclosed and of the different steps in the assessment process and a rationale for each. It also helps to stress the contribution all team members, including the family, can make. Professionals can discuss the options available and help family members decide on their roles within these events.

As with the other initial steps in assessment, the interview can help build rapport between caregivers and the rest of the transdisciplinary team. This is essential. To do this, the interviewer(s) can communicate in a positive manner, express genuine interest, and

- Stress the importance of parents in the process,
- Reflect on parental expertise on the development of their child, and
- Emphasize that there is still much to be learned about the child's and family's communication.

It's best if the interview is recorded digitally for future reference. An example of how you might begin an interview is presented in Figure 5.2.

Some parents may be uncomfortable with the interview format despite your best efforts to put them at ease. In these cases, there are alternative information-gathering strategies that may be more appropriate, including (Wilcox & Woods, 2011)

- Moving from an interview format to a conversation, and
- Engaging in problem-based discussion.

The somewhat more relaxed format of a conversation may facilitate the collection of information. I encourage you to read the excellent review on this process in Wilcox and Woods (2011).

When questionnaires, interviews, and even focused conversations yield only superficial or minimal information, problem-based discussions in the form of *What do you do when . . .* may be helpful in identifying priorities and intervention contexts (Dunst & Trivette, 2009a; Hanft, Rush, & Sheldon, 2004). The SLP may begin by directly asking what routines or activities are difficult. After learning about a difficult situation, the SLP can ask the parent to discuss strategies he or she has used to address the problem. In the process, caregivers can identify effective strategies and supports that may be helpful in intervention. It is also helpful to have caregivers identify activities in which the family would like to participate.

The interview is a two-way street, and parents should be encouraged to ask as well as answer questions, especially as they relate to the assessment process to come. The interviewer can explain why specific questions are being asked or why more information is needed for answers previously given on the questionnaire. Parents can be encouraged to elaborate on their responses and to provide examples. In turn, these responses may open new avenues of inquiry. In this situation, it's fine to stray from the order of the questionnaire and to let parents take the lead from time to time.

Interview Information Desired

In interviews, parents are asked how their child communicates basic needs, such as rejecting or wanting something. Information is also gathered on the communicative forms and functions or uses that the child routinely exhibits in specific contexts. You'll also want to explore any challenging behavior, especially how caregivers responded to it and possible functions it may serve for the child.

Using open-ended questions, such as those in Figure 5.3, an SLP can help family members describe the issues most vital to them. For example, a question such as "What

FIGURE 5.2 **Example of How to Frame an Interview with Parents**

Mr. and Mrs. Smith, I'm Bob Owens, a speech-language pathologist on the early intervention team. [Shake hands] We met during the preplanning meeting. Please have a seat and make yourselves comfortable.

Can I get you anything? Coffee? Water?

[No, we're fine, thank you.]

Okay. How are you feeling?

[A little nervous. We don't know what to expect.]

I understand. Well, it's perfectly natural to feel anxious. Don't worry. Remember, you've never done this before. Even for me, every child is different, so every communication evaluation is too.

Before we begin, I want to thank you on behalf of the EI team for your help and coopera-tion. You know your child better than anyone else, and your input is invaluable. You're the experts when it comes to Billy. Thank you so much.

Tell me a little bit about what you would like to happen today. What questions would you like answered with today's evaluation?

[We really want to know why he isn't talking yet. We thought we were doing everything we should but . . .]

Thank you. That's one of the primary questions we have in common. We'll try to answer that question as well as describe how Billy does communicate and how we can help him. There's a lot of variation in children's development, and sometimes despite our best efforts, some chil-dren take their time. I can't promise a definitive answer, but we'll keep your question foremost in our thoughts as we proceed.

You'll recall filling out our questionnaire about your son Billy's communication. I apologize for the length, but we're trying to piece together a portrait of how your son communicates. Our purpose is to describe Billy's communication as best we can, and you've gotten us off to a good start.

I do have a few areas I'd like to explore further with you based on your responses to the questionnaire. This will help to clarify my own thinking. As with all aspects of this evaluation, your remarks are confidential and will not be shared with anyone except team members. If you feel that something is especially sensitive, please let me know.

The interview is just one more step in the assessment process that began in the planning meeting and will continue with an observation and play assessment. At each step, we'll stop to make sure that you understand what we'll be doing and why. Please feel free to ask questions as we proceed, including during this interview.

This entire process should be a two-way street in which information flows both to and from you and Billy. Only in that way can you be fully participating members of the team. So please ask if you are unsure or need more information.

You and Billy are a communication unit. What we hope to do is to describe how commu-nication occurs within that context. We want to explore Billy's interests and the activities and events in his and your daily lives.

Before we begin, do you have any other questions about Billy or about the assessment process that I can answer for you?

---

do you hope to obtain from an assessment?" can highlight family concerns, which may or may not differ from those of professionals.

During interviews, an SLP can ask about successful and unsuccessful ways to moti-vate communication in the child. Later, the SLP can observe strategies to further iden-tify those that seem to work and those that do not. For example, parents are occasionally under the misguided notion that making sounds is impolite or disruptive and should be inhibited. These unfortunate assumptions may have a profound impact on intervention.

Interestingly, the interview process may indirectly benefit the child and family by altering parental perceptions of and interactions with the child. For example, one fam-ily I interviewed had been punishing their child for screaming until it was noted in the

FIGURE 5.3 Open-ended Questions for Caregivers

Family Concerns

What are your concerns about your child, and in what areas would you like more information?

What kinds of information would be most helpful?

What are your expectations for this assessment?

What do you hope to gain from this assessment?

Family Preferences

What other locations, contexts, and people should we include in our information gathering?

Are there other people you would like to assist with your child during the assessment?

How would you like to participate in your child's assessment?

Source: Information from Crais, 1994.

interview that this behavior was quite possibly one of the child's only nonverbal means of communicating.

If the child was assessed previously, team members will also want to know

- The types of activities used,
- Which activities provided the most useful information, and
- What that information was.

If the child received some type of intervention, families or teachers should also be asked what methods worked in changing the child's behavior and what did not.

In addition, the team will want to establish an approximate communication age for the child, if only to have a gauge against which to note improvement. When comparing a child's communication to developmental language milestones, it is important to remember the wide variation among TD children. The "established" ages are means.

Appendix E offers a possible format arranged by developmental age. In using this format or similar commercially available ones, the interviewer should not disclose the age at which these developmental milestones typically occur in order not to bias the parent's answers. The SLP can begin inquiring at the age he or she believes the child to be functioning, given parental responses so far. There is no need to continue to ask questions at higher levels of development once they begin to produce a string of negative responses.

Appendix E also presents some commonly recognized criteria for concern. These are guidelines for SLPs and should not be shared with parents at this point in the assessment.

Remember that a child born preterm whose age is below 36 months should be evaluated based on his or her age corrected for prematurity. In other words, a 16-month-old child born three months premature should be compared to other 13-month-olds.

Parents with culturally or linguistically diverse backgrounds may view development, and specifically their child's development, in ways that differ from the majority culture. Possible additional interview questions for these parents are presented in Figure 5.4. The SLP may want to ask additional related questions relevant to the family's specific ethnic group. This will require some research or consultation with ethnic community members.

THE EVOLVING ASSESSMENT PLAN

The assessment plan should evolve collaboratively. Keeping the family involved at each step ensures that they will be familiar with each task and understand the rationale for each.

FIGURE 5.4 **Possible Additional Interview Questions for Parents from Culturally or Linguistically Diverse Backgrounds**

- What things are important for your child's language learning?
- How do you and the other children in the family help in your child's language development?
- What activities or experiences seem to improve or encourage your child's use of language?
- With young children, speech-language therapy is often accomplished through play. Do you think that it is important for children to play? How is play viewed in your culture?
- Who plays with your child the most at home? How much time do you spend playing with your child during the day?
- As a parent, do you think you would enjoy participating in your child's speech-language intervention if it is needed?
- Is there anything that you think the team should know about you or your family that would help us serve you and your child better?

Source: Information from Kummerer, Lopez-Reyna, & Tejero Hughes, 2007.

Usually, the questionnaire and subsequent interview provide an extensive description of the child's communication behaviors, the partner strategies, and communication contexts. Because each person who interacts with the child forms a unique communicative context, information supplied by different caregivers should be summarized separately. It is important to note where different informants confirm as well as contradict each other.

At this point, team members can review all information and begin to form hypotheses about the child, caregivers, and contexts. These hypotheses may be confirmed through observation and later tested in the upcoming play-based assessment. Jointly, team members will decide which situations are most likely to elicit the best examples of the child's and caregivers' communication. It's important that parents understand the rationale for suggesting one context over another. Within these contexts, the team will want to be alert for subtle behaviors of both the child and caregivers.

Interactional Observation

The purpose of the observation is to confirm and possibly extend information gathered in the questionnaire and interview, ideally in a variety of contexts. Team members will want to attend to (Snell & Loncke, 2002)

- The child's communication behavior. *What forms does the child use? What function or purpose do these forms serve for the child?*
- The parent or other caregiver's responsive behaviors. *How do they respond?*
- Environmental facilitators and determinants. *In what context or under what conditions do certain forms and functions occur?*

While we might tend to focus on the first two, it's also important to remember the influence of context in determining behavior.

It's best to record all observations using either analog or digital technology in order to increase the reliability of analysis, especially of subtle child behaviors. Because the environment can be such an important factor, the team may want to view live interactions supplemented by recorded interactions from a variety of settings. Recordings can be used in analysis and later during intervention for demonstration, discussion, and comparison purposes.

One goal is to identify situations in which a child communicates most. Children may respond differently to different social partners and situations. Of course, because of their familiarity with the child, parents and teachers are excellent resources for this information (Bornstein, Painter, & Park, 2002). Familiar adults can also describe situations in which they have more or less difficulty understanding the child, and explain how they respond in each situation and how the child responds in turn.

Parents and teachers can suggest contexts and materials likely to produce optimal child performance (Brady, 2003). In general, reliability is increased if the evaluation occurs in several contexts that are natural and familiar to both the caregiver and the child. It might be advisable, for example, to record the child in daycare or a preschool classroom and at home as well as in a more clinical setting.

Remember that familiar activities provide scripts that make it easier for a child to participate (Owens, 2014). The more structuring or manipulating of the natural context that occurs, the less likely the child's behavior is to mirror naturally occurring communication.

With a 2-year-old who was demonstrating behaviors characteristic of autism spectrum disorder (ASD), our team asked if the family had digital recordings of him as a younger infant that we could view. Although his mother had attributed his behavior to a temporary moderate hearing loss that had occurred shortly after his first birthday, some members of our team suspected that behavioral signs of ASD may have appeared at an earlier date.

THE OBSERVATION PROCESS

So far in the assessment, the interaction between team members and the child has been minimal. This will be true of the observation as well. It's difficult at first for those of us who like to be actively involved to sit back and observe. I have to remind myself that we are interested in typical patterns of communication between the child and his or her routine partners. That doesn't include me—not yet anyway. Besides, observation, if done well, is not a passive process, and we'll have plenty to do recording information, conferring with team members, including the parents, and forming hypotheses.

Prior to the interaction, the adult partner needs some gentle guidance and a reminder that we want a representative or typical sample of the child's behavior. Parents sometimes attempt to have their child perform. This is not typical behavior. Other parents may attempt to do everything for their child or to anticipate the child's needs, especially while the "cameras are rolling." If this is typical caregiver behavior, it's very important information, but if it's not, it biases the data. A partner who is asked to wait and give the child an opportunity to initiate and then goes right back to being too "helpful" may be alerting us to a caregiver behavior that will need some tweaking during intervention.

Parents also need to know that recording and observation can be halted if the child becomes noncompliant or overly upset. It's important that parents understand that their concerns are honored throughout the assessment and intervention process. In extreme cases, the team may need to exit and rely solely on recorded information and observation. Ideally, the team can observe from a different space or behind one-way glass.

Although the tone of the observation is informal, it's sometimes helpful during the interaction to ask partners to do certain things in order for the team to assess the child's responses. For example, a parent may be asked to delay a response to the child, pretend not to understand, or ignore the child's behavior. At other times, it may be interesting to tempt the child by having an interesting toy or tasty treat just out of reach.

Throughout the session, team members record their observations of the child, caregiver, and environment. Team members are encouraged to make free-ranging comments as well as noting specific behaviors using a checkoff form similar to that in Appendix F and available on the text website. These on-the-spot observations will be refined as the team reviews the recordings of the session.

JUDGING COMMUNICATION SUCCESS AND INTENTIONALITY

During observations, the forms and functions of the child's behavior, as well as communication success, are noted and compared with the descriptions from the interview. The SLP documents the frequency of communication opportunities and the responsiveness of the child's communication partners.

Intentionality is particularly difficult to determine, and lack of intentionality is often judged by what is missing. For intent to be present, three observable things should occur:

- The child performs a signal or form,
- The signal is directed toward another person, and
- The signal appears to indicate some communication function.

That last one can be particularly difficult to judge.

As you'll recall, the key element in determining intentionality is coordinated attention that first focuses on an object, action, or event and then shifts to the partner and back. This coordinated attention requirement can be very subtle because it involves an indication of a desire to engage rather than direct engagement. Given the sometimes limited movement of children with more severe developmental disabilities, coordinated attention may be especially difficult to determine.

Changes in either the rate or magnitude of a behavior may be better criteria for judging intentionality in children with neuromuscular deficits. For example, a young boy with severe cerebral palsy (CP) in a low communication context may immediately stiffen his body, arch his back, extend his arms, and vocalize when a cup of juice is placed near him but out of reach. Although he doesn't turn and gaze purposefully at a caregiver, the change in the magnitude of the child's behavior may signal an attempt to gain attention or to express intent.

CAREGIVER-CHILD INTERACTIONS

Throughout this text, I stress the importance of caregiver interactions with young children. It's primarily through observation that professionals begin to form their hypotheses about the quality of the parent-child interaction and its potential as a vehicle for change. Some parents fail to notice their child's intentional behavior. Others assert that intentional behavior exists when the evidence is weak or nonexistent.

Caregiver behaviors can be significant barriers to a child's development of useful communication. Caregivers who anticipate and fulfill a child's requests, fail to pause so a child can express himself or herself, dominate the interactions, provide few opportunities for choice-making, and/or speak at a level of complexity too high or too low for a child may be limiting their child's communication. In addition, a caregiver's lack of understanding of his or her child's communication can also pose a challenge for intervention.

For many parents, an assessment will be the first time that their parenting behavior has been objectively critiqued. It's important, if we wish to keep parents as contributing members of the intervention team, that we be very careful with our analysis and feedback. Forming constructive comments is not easy, especially if the interaction is poor. I would couch my comments in *Did you notice . . .* statements or *Is there another way . . .* questions. We can empower parents with questions such as *How do you think . . .?*

Parameters of Caregiver Behavior

Parental interactive style is important for a child's language development. In general, a directive parent style provides less input and less interaction than a more conversational style. Possible categories and descriptions for use in an assessment are presented in Table 5.2. I've taken some liberties and modified descriptions, but the framework is essentially that of both Haebig, McDuffie, & Ellis Weismer (2013) and Fitzgerald, Hadley, and Rispoli (2013).

Although research has repeatedly demonstrated that an interactive style provides more language input to young children, a directive style may in some ways be beneficial for toddlers and preschoolers with ASD. For these children, parent directives that follow the child's focus of attention may predict better comprehension and production a year later (Haebig et al., 2013). Directives of this sort relate to the child's focus and convey an expectation that the child will change his or her ongoing activity in some way, such as "Push the truck." This input provides information on an action to accompany the object.

TABLE 5.2 **Describing Caregiver Interactive Styles**

STYLE	DESCRIPTION AND FORM	EXAMPLES
Conversational		
Initiative	Parent initiates conversation.	*Can I play with the babies too?*
Question	Parent continues conversation using questions.	*What should I do now?* *What did the teddy do?*
Comment	Parent describes child's action or focus of attention.	*Is Goldilocks sleeping in Baby Bear's bed?* Child playing with teddy. Adult: *You have the teddy.*
Reply	Parent replies to the child's communication attempt. May take the form of an imitation, expansion, or reply.	Child hands shoe to adult. Adult: *Oh, you want Mommy to put on your shoe.* (Reply) Child: *Shoe on.* Adult: *Yes, shoe on.* (Imitation) Child: *Shoe on.* Adult: *Your shoe is on.* (Expansion)
Description of own behavior	Parent describes his or her own action with a toy to which the child is attending.	*I'll color this one.* *Mommy is dressing the baby.*
Mapping	Parent describes what the child is doing.	*Jenna is reading her book to Teddy. "Goodnight, Moon. Good night, Teddy."*
Directive	Parent attempts to direct child either explicitly or indirectly.	*Get teddy.* *Don't touch that. Yuck.* *Can mommy see that?* *Should we play with the ball?* *Maybe we should put the book away.* *What would the doggie say?* *Did Jon* [Child's name] *drink all his milk?* *Baby needs her shoes.*

Sources: Haebig, McDuffie, & Ellis Weismer, 2013; Fitzgerald, Hadley, & Rispoli, 2013.

That said, parent comments on the child's focus of attention manifest in better language acquisition by the child in subsequent years. These data would suggest that some types of directives may serve an interactive function.

There are very few objective evaluative tools for assessing interactional quality. For the most part, professionals are left with descriptive tools and their own expertise. At the least, the assessment team should comment on the following parameters of the caregiver's behavior:

- Caregiver positioning relative to the child
- Caregiver affect

- Caregiver visual interaction
- Caregiver play style (animate, engaging, enthusiastic)
- Caregiver use of touch and distance
- Caregiver initiation of communication
- Caregiver attempts to elicit the child's behavior
- Caregiver vocalization and verbalization
  - Tone
  - Content (appropriateness)
- Caregiver responsiveness
  - Contingency
  - Consistency

With an infant, the team will also want to consider:

- Caregiver holding style
- Caregiver sensitivity to
  - Infant level of wakefulness
  - Infant mood and affect

Overall, the team is interested in the caregiver's ability to encourage interaction and communication by initiating and prompting the child and by responding contingently.

Contingent responding is based on the intention and meaning of the child's utterance. For example, if a child points at a dog, the adult might comment, "Yes, Mommy sees doggie. He's a big dog."

Occasionally, a child seems to be nonresponsive or noncooperative with a caregiver. This may result from the assessment situation, the child's state, the parent-child history of interacting, or all of these. For example, we may assume incorrectly that playing with a child is a natural behavior for parents. While this is true for many parents, it is not so for all. In situations where playing with a child is extraordinary, we should expect that both participants would seem awkward and ill at ease when asked to play "naturally."

Sometimes, a nonresponsive or noncooperative child signals something other than the current situation. For example, I noticed one male toddler's differing responses to males and females. While cooperative and smiling with women, the same child was quiet and withdrawn around men, especially his father. Upon gently mentioning this, we learned that the father had punished the boy for crying while the child was teething and experiencing severe acid reflux. In response, the child refused to interact with his father or reacted in a very apprehensive manner. This behavior was extended to all adult males.

Parental Responsiveness Factors

Sometimes the caregiver's responses in the questionnaire and interview do not match what the team observes. There are a number of reasons for this. First, no matter how much we try to have a natural interaction, the recording device has a telling effect on the participants. Look at your family's digital recording of the last big event, holiday, or trip, and you'll see how atypical behaviors often are when people know they are being recorded.

Second, the caregiver is keenly aware that professionals are watching and making judgments. I have observed parents who are very ill at ease as they fidget, giggle, and make silly remarks aside. Parents who are uncomfortable with their child's disability may also be embarrassed by their child's behavior, especially if the child is uncooperative during the assessment. Children too are affected by an audience and may be very reluctant to interact naturally on demand.

Finally, parents may consciously or unconsciously under- or overestimate their child's behavior on the questionnaire or in the interview for a variety of reasons. For example, a parent may attribute intent to a random behavior in the hope that the child is actually doing more than behavior would indicate. In contrast, a child's routine behavior may be overlooked and its communication potential missed.

FORMING HYPOTHESES

Ideally, the team, including the parents, will view the recorded session immediately after it terminates. These meetings can be lively and the recording may be stopped and replayed several times as each member has his or her say.

The team can share and discuss the analyzed data from all sources so far. The focus of the discussion should be on the communication system of the child and caregiver and on the behaviors of both partners. Because parents are a necessary part of the assessment team, professional comments should focus on ways to improve the interaction and not on criticizing it.

As the recorded interaction is viewed, caregivers can be encouraged to add their own comments, especially as they relate to ways of improving communication. One of the first questions for the caregiver after the observation ends is the extent to which the behavior of both partners was typical of daily interactions.

Working collaboratively, the team begins to formulate hypotheses. Issues to be addressed in the team's hypotheses are presented in Figure 5.5.

It's quite natural for team members to disagree. In these situations, the recorded events can be replayed and discussed. There may be some tension between disagreeing team members at this point. That's fine as long as everyone stays open to the process. Answers may be obtained as the assessment progresses.

FIGURE 5.5 Issues to Be Addressed in the Team's Hypotheses

- What is the form of the child's communication? Is it primarily vocal, verbal, or gestural, or signaled through gaze, facial expression, other, or a combination? Does it vary with the partner and the context? What are potential forms? Can other forms be taught or prompted easily?
- What intentions does the child express? Does the child request, comment, protest, or express other intentions? Are some intentions expressed solely in one form (form-specific)? What intentions are missing? Does there seem to be a need to express other intentions? Does the child resort to problem behavior when communication breaks down? What are potential intentions?
- Do the child and partner establish joint attending? Who typically initiates? How?
- Is the interaction balanced (equal number of turns, equal time)? Does one partner dominate? Is this related to the situation, or does it seem to be a pattern? How long are interactional exchanges? How many turns does each partner typically take on a topic? In an exchange? Who typically initiates interaction? How might a balance be reached?
- How are interactions initiated? What keeps the interaction going? Who keeps the interaction going? Why does it stop? Is the communication part of a routine, such as game-playing, feeding, changing, toy or object play, or the like?
- How did the partner encourage or prompt the child to communicate? Was this behavior appropriate? If not, how might it be changed? How did the child respond?
- Does the partner notice the child's attempts to communicate? Is the child's attempt acknowledged and encouraged or discouraged?
- Was the partner responsive? Contingent? Consistent? Are both the child and partner attentive to each other? How does the partner get the child's attention? Does the partner allow time for the child to initiate and respond? Does the partner acknowledge the child's communication attempts? How? Is the partner in a good position (facing child, same level, proximal) to communicate with the child? Does the partner facilitate or inhibit interaction? How? Is this behavior situational? Do the partners persist when the interaction fails or the message is not understood? How? How does the partner respond to the child's problem behaviors, if any?
- What effective and ineffective interactional strategies did the partner use? What potential interactional strategies could the partner use?
- Did the environment (location, materials, activity, and people) support or discourage communication? In what ways? If the environment is not maximally supportive, how might this be changed? What are potential changes in the environment that will challenge the child's communication?

Play-Based Interactional Assessment

After reviewing either the live or recorded interaction samples and formulating and refining their communication hypotheses, the team members plan the play assessment by

- Noting routines and activities familiar to the child that can be used in the assessment,
- Targeting communication forms and functions to be elicited from the child,
- Determining the best way to elicit these forms and functions by enriching and improving interactions and by introducing temptations and other communication variations,
- Deciding how the team will attempt to "stretch" the child's behaviors to assess the child's ability to learn,
- Targeting caregiver behaviors to be assessed, and
- Identifying needed materials.

The entire play-based assessment can be recorded for later review. The team will want information on behaviors not observed so far in the assessment.

An individualized play-based assessment consists of three steps:

- Building rapport through interacting with the child in preferred routines, following his or her lead, and being responsive to communication attempts
- Assessing through unstructured play while intentionally programming opportunities for a variety of early intentional behaviors
- Assessing directly in structured play mode the early presymbolic skills not evident so far in the evaluation

These steps optimize the assessment by providing opportunities to communicate in context with both familiar and unfamiliar partners. Although the structured portion is more directive in nature, it is still within a play mode.

It's best if caregivers or those who most frequently interact with the child participate in the assessment with the child. The SLP or other professional can coach the caregiver, giving suggestions or modeling what to do. In this way caregivers experience firsthand the methods that may be used later in intervention. If caregivers are hesitant or resistant, the SLP can interact with the child while the parent holds the child on his or her lap or sits next to the child.

A communication assessment of a young child includes both (Lichtert, 2003)

- Routines with a variety of highly motivating stimuli, such as food items or toys that make noise or move; and
- Play or seeming play activities, such as stacking blocks or putting a doll to bed, that are guided by an adult.

In addition, the situation (Halle & Meadan, 2007)

- Includes highly motivating stimuli that are individually determined,
- Focuses on the individual child and caregiver, and
- Presents repeated trials to the child.

Caregivers can be especially helpful in identifying activities in which the child participates and toys that the child enjoys on a regular basis.

Initially, the child is invited to sit down on the floor or in a chair to play because it's easier to assess a stationary "target." If the child insists on clinging to a parent, that's fine, and Mom or Dad can be invited to join the play. The child who seems unable to focus or sit is giving us good information. The SLP can ask parents how they settle their child and what activities are likely to entice the child into an interaction.

Guidelines for building rapport are presented in Figure 5.6. This first step in play-based assessment is essential if our goal is for the child to demonstrate his or her best performance. Developing a positive relationship with the child within an established routine

FIGURE 5.6 **Guidelines for Building Rapport Prior to Assessment**

Spend time in the child's natural, everyday environment. Get to know the child and family routines.

Become a positive reinforcer yourself by delivering preferred items and activities to the child noncontingently to the child's performance. If the child views you positively, he or she will attend to your presence and approach you.

Engage in positive, unstructured, and fun interactions with the child. This can be accomplished by

- Playing with the child using the most preferred objects and activities that were identified by caregivers;
- Following the child's lead during play, allowing the child's interests to determine the flow of activities; and
- Being responsive to the child's communication attempts by acknowledging them and attempting to discover and comply with their purpose.

Build routines similar to those to be used in the structured protocol of assessment.

- Create opportunities for communication through play with the child's preferred items.
- Program opportunities for communication to occur.

Source: Information from Halle & Meadan, 2007.

will motivate him or her to approach, stay, and play. Rapport-building need not be a separate event and can occur during the unstructured play portion as a natural part of inviting a child to play.

Activities will differ with each child and should be appropriate for the age and interests of individual children. I have worked with some children for whom I never could have guessed their play interests. Parents are a great source for this type of information.

DYNAMIC ASSESSMENT

Static assessments, such as norm-referenced tests, are designed to document a child's habitual level of functioning relative to a peer group. While this information is useful for qualifying a child for services, static assessments are not designed to examine the learning process or potential or facilitative adult strategies (Tzuriel, 2000).

Dynamic assessment, on the other hand, is designed to describe a child's optimal level of functioning and can help identify a child's potential and the amount of external support needed (Feuerstein, Feuerstein, & Falik, 2010). Teaching and adult assistance are an integral part. Dynamic assessment flows from Vygotsky's (1978) notion of the zone of proximal development, which recognizes that we all learn best things that differ only slightly from (are *proximal*, or close to) what we already know. Thus, adults offer assistance at a level just above a child's current functioning.

All assessment of the child's communication skills should attempt to accomplish two things:

- Determine the child's current level of communication, and
- Assess the child's ability to learn behaviors slightly advanced from the current level.

Once the child's existing communication system has been tentatively described, it's time to explore how modifiable it is. This task can be accomplished using a dynamic *test-teach-test* paradigm to examine the "teachability" of a behavior (Snell & Loncke, 2002). Young children with severe disabilities who look similar on static assessment actually may be very different when dynamic assessment techniques are used.

Within this test-teach-test dynamic assessment model, the child is

- ■ Tested for baseline performance to establish a level of performance, then
- ■ Taught the new or modified skill, and finally
- ■ Retested to determine if learning has occurred.

After observing how the child responds without assistance (test), the SLP provides limited assistance over several trials while looking for changes in the child's behavior (teach), and then withdraws the assistance and returns to the original situation to see if learning has occurred (test). While teaching, the SLP introduces a graduated amount of assistance over one or a series of trials.

Dynamic assessment rests on the concept that a child learns best when adults provide mediated assistance, or guidance in which the amount and type of assistance are individualized to suit the learner and task and are slightly different from what the child can do at present. Assistance might include (Olswang, Feuerstein, Pinder, & Dowden, 2013)

- ■ Varying the rate of presentation
- ■ Repeating cues
- ■ Supplementing with nonverbal cues such as pointing or gesturing
- ■ Using more and varied verbal cues such as *Touch the X, Show me X,* or *Where's X?*
- ■ Decreasing the communication distance from the child
- ■ Modeling or having someone model the desired response for a child
- ■ Physically guiding a child such as hand-over-hand manipulation of a toy
- ■ Manipulating the environment such as placing objects closer to a child
- ■ Allowing more time for a response
- ■ Helping a child complete the task

The SLP and team members can systematically explore how various mediation methods influence the child's communicative behavior to identify methods that work the best (Gutiérrez-Clellen, 2000).

Of particular importance are scaffolding strategies that appear to be most effective in eliciting a behavior. Scaffolding is the use of both verbal and nonverbal prompts to "frame" a behavior. For example, a parent may be able to prompt requesting by saying "What want?" or simply waiting.

Teaching would occur within an activity likely to elicit the behavior, such as a cookie in plain view to elicit requesting. The adult prompt or scaffolding would either immediately precede or follow the child's signal. It's important that the SLP or caregiver prompt the new signal in a manner appropriate for each child and that the adult wait for some response, reinforcing any approximation of the new signal.

Scaffolding can be specified so that a minimum of additional aid is given to prompt the child's success. In constructing a hierarchy of prompts, the team will decide the order of the prompts and the amount of time that will occur before the next prompt is given (Snell, 2002).

Let's assume we are trying to assess a child's ability to physically imitate. In the context of play, I might first ask the child to copy my movement, as in "Now Tzi-ki do." If the child failed to respond, I might give a verbal prompt along with my original hand model, as in "Tzi-ki clap hands." If there is still no response, I could present my model, give the verbal prompt, and place the child's hands in position. Finally, if all else fails I might present my model, give the verbal prompt, and physically assist the child to clap. When the child is successful, I would reinforce him and return to the original "test" condition "Now Tzi-ki do."

Even small changes in a child's behavior are significant. The SLP can target behaviors just beyond the child's observed performance level. For example, if the child gestures but in limited ways, the SLP may attempt to introduce other gestures or add a vocalization.

Determination of success is made on the basis of the child's performance. In dynamic assessment, the child is retested on either the same or a similar task to assess learning. In this way, the SLP can assess

- ■ A child's independent abilities,
- ■ The modifiability or reaction of the child to varying types of assistance, and
- ■ Possible intervention methods.

Ideally, when the play-based portion of the assessment is complete, the team will have a new description of the child's communication behavior and potential. In addition, the team has identified the ways in which that communication is malleable. Through observation, caregivers can also learn how to modify their own behavior to promote communication.

DESCRIBING COMMUNICATION

The avenue for enhancing communication and social interaction for young children is their existing system of meaningful interaction with others (Snell, 2002). Intervention is built on a child's existing nonsymbolic skills. In order to foster the growth of all communication skills, SLPs need to thoroughly understand a child's current communication system, including characteristics of the child's communication partners and environments.

Information gained from interviews with parents and care providers and from observations of their interactions with a child can be useful in (Chan & Iacono, 2001; Siegel & Wetherby, 2000)

- Establishing goals for the assessment;
- Designing the assessment to suit the team's goals;
- Describing a child's individualistic communication, such as the form of communication and the intentions expressed;
- Identifying those activities, people, and settings associated with a child's communication;
- Exploring ways to obtain the best, most representative, and contextually rich communication samples of a child and familiar partners; and
- Suggesting ways to individualize the assessment in order to optimize child and caregiver performance.

This information can be used in planning an authentic assessment, one that relies on real-life tasks within natural contexts as much as possible.

During assessment, the environment can be arranged to stimulate certain behaviors. For example, if parents report that their child frequently waves when certain people arrive, the SLP can simulate this event as much as possible to prompt the behavior. In addition, the SLP can attempt to stimulate functions that occur infrequently or are reported not to occur. If, for example, a child reportedly does not engage in joint attending, the SLP can place a visually intriguing object before the child or attempt to draw the child's attention.

Eliciting Communication Behaviors from the Child

Two possible techniques for eliciting communication behaviors from the child are communication temptations and context manipulation. Communication temptations are minor challenges to the expected occurrence of events in familiar situations. For example, the SLP might eat and comment on a delicious cookie but offer none to the child. This may stimulate the child to vocalize or reach out in order to obtain some. Once the behavior is emitted, the SLP attempts to shape the response into a more mature communication form. Several communication temptations are presented in Figure 5.7 (Wetherby & Prizant, 1989).

Context manipulation consists of environmental arrangements that may include but are not limited to (Owens, 2014; Wetherby & Prizant, 1989)

- Pausing in the middle of a favorite activity, such as listening to music;
- Pausing before completing an act, such as holding the spoon just in front of the child's face;
- Violating a routine, such as missing a child at snack time;
- Violating an object function, such as wearing gloves on your feet;
- Offering choices either visually or verbally;
- Not having enough items to complete a task, such as no plastic knives for cutting fruit for fruit salad or missing puzzle pieces;

FIGURE 5.7 **Communicative Temptations**

Await a response after . . .

Eating a desirable food item and not offering any.

Activating a wind-up or remotely operated toy, letting it deactivate, and handing it to the child.

Setting up a play routine and then abruptly changing the routine, such as rolling a ball then rolling something else.

Looking through a picture book and modeling naming the pictures.

Opening a bottle of bubbles, blowing bubbles, then closing the bottle tightly and handing it to the child.

Initiating a pleasurable social activity with the child, then stopping and waiting.

Blow up a balloon, letting it deflate, then handing the deflated balloon to the child.

Offering a food item or toy that the child dislikes.

Letting the child see you place a desired food item or toy in a clear plastic container that the child cannot open, then handing the container to the child.

Handing the child a cold, wet, or sticky substance.

Using an object in an unusual manner.

Imitating the child's sound-making.

See Wetherby & Prizant (1989) for a more in-depth description.

- Giving small portions of a favorite food or drink;
- Withholding needed assistance, such as help getting coats and boots on; and
- Sabotaging activities so children must ask for assistance, such as putting a small hole in a child's cup.

Within both temptations and contextual manipulation, the SLP waits for a short time for the child to initiate communication. If this does not occur, the SLP prompts a response. Because the potential exists for temptations and contextual manipulation to frustrate young children, it's important not to heap too many of these upon a child. The purpose is to explore more effective ways to communicate for both the child and caregivers. Different modifications of the child's and caregivers' behaviors are tried and then added or withdrawn based on their responses.

Intentional Communication

There is no one accepted standard for distinguishing preintentional from intentional communication. Instead, identification of a child's intent to communicate depends on several characteristics. Two critical aspects are the actual behavior of the child and the specific intention that child attempts to convey.

As you'll recall from your language acquisition course, the development of intent passes through several stages. In assessing early communication, however, placing a child in a stage of development is not as important as thoroughly describing his or her behavior. Stages in development of intent and adult mediation strategies are presented in Table 5.3.

Even professionals can be inconsistent in accurately and reliably judging the communicative intent of young children (Carter & Iacono, 2002). Decisions on intentionality should consider

- The actual behavior,
- The context, and
- The consistency of behavior over time.

TABLE 5.3 **Stages of Intentional Communication**

The physical component of gesturing is easy to teach through imitation. The intentional aspect of gesturing or its purpose is not as easy to teach and requires some flexibility and creativity. If a child does not demonstrate any intentional communication, assess to see if the child has a notion of means-ends or of using a creative means to reach a desired end, such a obtaining a toy by pulling an attached string.

LEVEL OF ASSESSMENT	EXPECTED RESPONSE	TEST FORMAT	POSSIBLE MEDIATED TEACHING FORMAT
Pre-intentional			
Means-ends*	Child will obtain object through desired means, such as pulling string.	Place an interesting or desired object just out of reach but with attached cord or handle within child's reach. An alternative is to place a busy box or kiddy gym before the child and await a response. You might cue with "Get X," "Find X," or "Where's X?"	If child does not respond or if response is inadequate, place the attached cord or handle in the child's hand and recue. If the response is still inadequate, provide an imitative prompt and recue. Should the child still not respond, you may need a more enticing object or a physical prompt, such as a hand-over-hand demonstration.
Intentional			
Requesting	Child will obtain object by reaching for it and establishing momentary eye contact with the adult.	Place an interesting or desired object within easy reach of the child. Talk about it when the child picks it up. Move the object just out of reach and await a response.	If child reaches even slightly, respond accordingly. If the child does not reach, ask "What do you want?" If the child's response is still unacceptable, ask "What do you want? and give an imitative prompt. If the response is still unacceptable, ask, give an imitative prompt, and provide a physical assist.
Protesting	Child will reject object by turning away or shaking head side to side plus momentary eye contact with the adult.	Place an interesting or desired object just out of reach. When the child makes a gestural or vocal request, hand an undesirable object instead and await a response.	If child reaches even slightly, respond accordingly. If the child does not protest, ask "Is that what you want?" If the response is still unacceptable or nonexistent, cue again and give an imitative prompt. If the response is still unacceptable, give an imitative prompt and a physical assist. Be sure to talk as you do this so the child understands that this is a method of rejection.
Signaling notice or pointing	Child will point to novel or interesting object before him or her.	Place a novel or interesting object in front of the child. Cue with name and "What do you see?"	Respond to any pointing approximation by talking about the object. If the child reaches with a grasping gesture, give the child the object but prompt a point with another object. You might give a verbal prompt such as "Point to X." If this is unsuccessful, provide an imitative prompt and finally a physical assist.

*Possible objects for means-ends include the following:

Any object attached to a string	Any out-of-reach object sitting on a napkin
Balloon on a string	Busy box or jack-in-the-box
Pull toys	Rubber ball on elastic cord
Toy fishing pole	Toys operated by remote switch

Consistency signifies the habitual nature and conventionality of a behavior and can be verified by asking caregivers. Standard indicators of intent may include:

- Eye gaze alternating between an object, event, or focus of attention and a listener, as in checking to ensure that the listener is attending
- Pause indicating a child is expecting a response
- Body orientation of a child, indicating the communication is being directed toward a partner
- Persistence in signaling a listener until the goal is reached
- Change in the quality of the signal if the intended effect is not achieved
- Ritualized signal or conventional form (e.g., pointing, shaking head, nodding)

Alternating gaze is particularly important because it signals that a child is considering the effect his or her behavior is having on the caregiver.

The range of intentions that a child is able to communicate is extremely important. While there is no magic number of possible intentions that predicts later success, the team is interested in the breadth of these intentions. Common early presymbolic intentions include but are not limited to the following:

- *Drawing attention to an object or event* by pointing or looking at the object or event, touching, picking up, or showing the object, and possibly vocalizing
- *Drawing attention to oneself* by "showing off" and possibly vocalizing
- *Giving an object* by pushing or handing it and possibly vocalizing insistently
- *Initiating play* by looking at the partner or toy, commencing play, and possibly vocalizing
- *Protesting* by expressing displeasure through refusal, tantruming, turning away, or shaking head side to side, and possibly vocalizing
- *Providing information* by pointing or touching and possibly vocalizing following an adult question or spontaneously
- *Requesting an object or action* by reaching or looking and possibly vocalizing insistently
- *Requesting assistance* by reaching, looking at, or handing an object and possibly vocalizing insistently
- *Requesting information* by looking, pointing, or touching and possibly vocalizing with rising intonation

Some children, especially those with a history of frustration with verbal communication, may have developed a somewhat elaborate sound and gesture system. For example, a child may tap her mouth repeatedly while making sounds to indicate a request to eat. It is critical that an SLP thoroughly describe the behaviors that signal a child's intentions and that these be corroborated by the child's family.

During the assessment, the SLP will want to create opportunities for different intentions, such as requesting, to occur. Figure 5.8 presents a possible dynamic assessment format for requesting.

Within the play framework, the SLP tries through a structured format to prompt other communication forms and functions from the child. Although planned in advance, the actual prompts used are determined by trial and error. The SLP introduces and withdraws prompts as needed by the child to be successful. Methods of eliciting and prompting other intentions were presented in Table 5.4.

Communication Breakdowns

Through structured probes within naturalistic interactions, an SLP can purposefully attempt to elicit not only communication success but also breakdowns (Halle, Phillips, & Carey, 1999; Meadan, Halle, & Drasgow, 2003). Intentional breakdowns by an adult provide an opportunity to examine behaviors that share the same function or are functionally equivalent. For example, an SLP might follow an interactive routine, based on previously collected data, to introduce situations in which breakdowns are likely to occur. Repeated breakdowns can lead to multiple repair strategies.

FIGURE 5.8 **Example of Dynamic Assessment for Requesting**

Some children are easily overwhelmed by stimulation, so it may not be good to offer a smorgasbord of objects. It may be better to remove toys or foods from a bag or box one at a time or to have one or two just out of reach.

The SLP can proceed as follows (Halle & Meadan, 2007):

- Remove a preferred object or toy, or pick it up and talk about it. For example, I might say, "(Child's name), I have ____ (ball, baby, car). It's fun to play with."
- Wait for a few seconds to see if the child responds. If the child does not respond, I might say, "No play?" and play with the toy alone.
- After some quick coaching of the parent, I could also say, "Mom, I have ____. It's fun to play with." Mom would then respond in the way we want the child to respond. In other words, she would model a request for the child.
- Cue the child again.
- If still no response, cue the parent again to respond.
- Cue the child again.
- If the child . . .
  - Requests in the desired manner, give the item to the child.
  - Requests the item in something less than the desired manner, model a response and cue again.
  - Does not respond within 15 seconds, remove the item and offer a new one.
  - Actively rejects the item, remove it from sight.
- After allowing the child to play for 30 seconds, offer a new item.

Some children will not respond to a model, and it may be necessary to use a physical prompt, such as moving the child's arm to form a gestural request. When this is done, the SLP can reinforce the child and return to the original cue, "(Child's name), I have ____ (ball, baby, car). It would be fun to play with." From here we can move to choice-making, or the child's selecting one of two objects to play with.

Of interest are the type and origin of breakdown, the repair efforts of the child, and the outcome. To repair, a child must recognize that a communication breakdown has occurred, use a repair, and recognize when successful communication is restored. The most common repair strategy for individuals with severe disabilities is repetition of the previous message. The SLP can signal that a breakdown has occurred in several ways. These might include (Snell, 2002)

- Looking confused by furrowing your brow;
- Asking "What?" or "Huh?";
- Not complying with a request or following a point;
- Acting confused as if misunderstanding; or
- Ignoring the child's attempt to communicate.

The SLP should pause to provide an opportunity for the child to repair, noting the type of repair and the success. Caregiver responsive behaviors may be better documented through naturalistic observation (Halle, Brady, & Drasgow, 2004).

SYMBOLIC ASSESSMENT

Although our discussion is dichotomized into presymbolic and symbolic assessment, in reality one flows into the other, and assessment begins at the level at which the SLP believes the child is functioning. Many of the areas assessed when children begin to use symbols are similar to or continuations of the areas of interest for nonsymbolic children. There is continuity over time. For example, the intentions expressed in gestures are later fulfilled by symbols.

TABLE 5.4   **Eliciting Communicative Intentions**

Intention	Task	Expected Child Behavior	SLP Response
Request for assistance	SLP presents two wind-up toys and offers one to child. Play with your wind-up toy.	Requests help to wind up the toy by holding the toy up, handing it back, or vocalizing, verbalizing, and/or gesturing accompanied by eye contact with SLP.	Takes wind-up toy, acknowledges that it is not working, winds it for child, and returns it.
Request for object	SLP presents markers and paper and offers paper to child but leaves markers out of child's reach as SLP begins to draw. Some children may respond best to food items.	Requests a marker by vocalizing, verbalizing, and/or gesturing toward the markers accompanied by eye contact with the SLP.	Acknowledges child's request and offers child a marker.
Comment	SLP places an unexpected object among others, such as a toy worm in a box of markers or a block among snacks, and awaits response. Similar task might involve using an object in an unacceptable way.	Draws attention to object by vocalizing, verbalizing, and/or handing object to SLP accompanied by eye contact. Establishes joint attending.	Acknowledges child's comment and replaces or removes unexpected object.
Clarification request	SLP presents two bottles of bubbles, giving child one permanently sealed with glue.	Requests assistance by holding bottle up, handing it back, or vocalizing, verbalizing, and/or gesturing accompanied by eye with SLP.	Responds with "Yes, bubbles are fun!" and awaits a response. (Similar response might be to ignore child's behavior.)
Directing attention	SLP activates remote-operated toy but ignores it. (Similar task would be any interesting, unusual, or unexpected event.)	Draws attention to object by vocalizing, verbalizing, and/or gesturing accompanied by eye contact.	Acknowledges child's comment and talks about toy.
Answering questions	SLP establishes routine of pulling objects from bag and asking "What's this?" (Similar task involves asking about actions—i.e., "What happened?") If child responds in gestural mode only, SLP asks *where*, *whose*, and *which* questions that can be answered with a point.	Responds with vocalization or verbalization accompanied by eye contact.	Acknowledges child's answer, comments, and plays briefly with toy and child.
Asking questions	SLP encourages child to participate in previous activity by asking SLP to identify toys. Alternative is to include objects not known by child and encourage child to seek answer by asking Mommy.	Asks vocal or verbal question such as "What?" or "What's that?"	Answers question, comments, and plays briefly with toy and child.
Protesting	SLP presents child's favorite treat and asks "What want?" or "What do you want?" Hands child a nonpreferred item instead.	Responds by vocalizing, verbalizing, and/or gesturing toward the treat. When nonpreferred item is handed instead, child may show displeasure by shaking head side to side, vocalizing, verbalizing, and/or gesturing toward desired treat.	Hands wrong item, then acknowledges child's protest by handing originally requested treat.

TABLE 5.4 **Eliciting Communicative Intentions** (*continued*)

INTENTION	TASK	EXPECTED CHILD BEHAVIOR	SLP RESPONSE
Responding to clarification request	In any of the above tasks, SLP can ask for clarification by saying "What do you need?" or "What?"	Responds with repetition of original response, possibly accompanied by increased loudness or heightened gesturing.	Acknowledges error and comments.
Greeting	SLP waves and says "Hello" and "Bye" to puppet as it enters and exits play. For child that does not relate to a puppet, have parent initiate greeting.	Waves accompanied by vocalizing or verbalizing.	Acknowledges greeting and responds appropriately.

Source: Information in part from Halle & Meadan, 2007.

Receptive Language

At the lowest level, the team is interested in a child's ability to associate a spoken word or symbol with the thing to which it refers, called the *referent*. Judgments of receptive language made on the basis of performance on a test may or may not reflect a child's actual competence and will vary with the level of contextual support provided. In part, this reflects confusion over exactly what comprehension means.

Within a play format using familiar objects, an SLP can informally assess a child's receptive language. This is complemented by parental report, checklists, and observation. Other formats for assessing receptive language in young children can be adapted for a play format. With many children, it won't be possible to test all words in a child's lexicon or personal dictionary, so we will sample a few and assess the child's ability to learn using the test-teach-test format as we have throughout the assessment. It's important to keep a list of words a child comprehends so these can be used to build the child's production and to test comprehension of longer utterances later in the assessment.

A child's incorrect or inconsistent responses or lack of responses do not conclusively indicate comprehension problems. Ensure that the child is attending and that responses are cued by auditory stimuli and not inadvertent nonverbal cues. Although nonverbal prompts will be included in the teaching phase, you must be careful when testing not to look at or gesture toward an object or person and thus accidentally give away the correct response.

All items should be tested several times, especially when responding is inconsistent. Because very young children comprehend best in the context of familiar routines and cannot apply labels to unseen entities, it's important to test both within routines in which these entities are expected and outside these contexts.

Prior to the assessment, the SLP can assemble an individualized vocabulary from questionnaires, interviews, and observation. Caregivers can be encouraged to bring familiar, easily recognizable toys and objects from home to use in the assessment. Familiar objects may include toys, clothing, eating utensils, and household items.

The SLP may want to assess a child's comprehension of (Miller & Paul, 1995)

- Person and object names,
- Actions and words that signify action, such as *up*, and
- Functional words such as *more* and *no*.

A possible format for dynamic assessment of receptive language is presented in Table F.1 in Appendix F.

By the end of the second year of life, children are beginning to have a syntactic understanding of three- and four-word relations, to answer questions beyond the simple *what* and *where* variety, and to follow one-step commands. A possible format for dynamic assessment of more advanced receptive language is presented in Table F.2 in Appendix F.

Expressive Language

In contrast to receptive language, expressive language is more easily observed. Expressive language assessment can be divided into analysis of

- Speech intelligibility,
- Phonotactic characteristics,
- Structure of gesture and speech combinations,
- Intentions expressed, and
- Vocabulary.

Several measures of speech can be applied to a speech sample. A possible format for dynamic assessment of single-symbol expressive language is presented in Table F.3 in Appendix F.

The key is collecting and eliciting sufficient quantity and variety to be able to make definitive statements. Luckily, the team is not limited to the more structured portions of the assessment and can garner data from observation and sampling as well.

Speech intelligibility. Some children, even in imitation, may be difficult to understand. There are several ways to quantify speech intelligibility using a recorded speech sample. These include percent of intelligible words and percent of correct consonants (PCC).

The percent of intelligible words is the easiest to calculate. Using at least a 100-word sample, one team member unfamiliar with the situation, writes down what he or she believes the child has said. Because context can influence such decisions, the team member should listen to but not view the interaction. Calculation is accomplished by simply dividing the number of intelligible words by the total words in the sample and multiplying this result by 100.

$$\frac{\text{Number of intelligible words}}{\text{Total number of words}} \times 100 = \text{Percent of intelligible words}$$

Although a rough estimate, the percentage does give some idea of how an unfamiliar partner may interpret the child's speech and a rough estimate of communication success.

Similarly, PCC is calculated by dividing the number of correct consonants by the total number of consonants and multiplying the result by 100.

$$\frac{\text{Number of correct consonants}}{\text{Total number of consonants}} \times 100 = \text{Percent of correct consonants}$$

If similar sounds, such as several stops, are affected, the SLP might wish to analyze further for phonological processes. Intervention could focus on consonant production along with building the child's vocabulary. These will be discussed in subsequent chapters.

Phonotactic characteristics. Phonological data can be gathered through a variety of methods, including recordings from home, caregiver report, observation, informal testing, and sampling. In some cases, sound and syllable combinations act as words for children within their own "self-designed" lexicon.

The SLP is interested in the repertoire of sounds and syllables that can be used by the team in selecting vocabulary targets and in building target words. At a minimum, the sample should consist of 50 consecutive vocalizations that include

- Voiced vocalic elements, or
- Voiced syllabic consonants.

The utterances are transcribed using phonemic transcription. Child cries, coughs, screams, and incidents of glottal fry are not transcribed. Any vocalization that cannot be transcribed confidently after several repeated replayings or that occurs simultaneously with other sounds rendering it inaudible or indistinct should also be eliminated.

Two possible measures are mean babbling level (MBL) and syllable structure level (SSL) (Morris, 2010). MBL is restricted to babbling while SSL, an extension of MBL, focuses on productive words.

TABLE 5.5 **Calculating Mean Babbling Levels (MBLs)**

LEVEL	DESCRIPTION
1	Consists of a vowel, voiced syllabic consonant, or CV syllable in which consonant is a glottal stop, a glide, or /h/
2	CV, VC, or CVC syllables with "true" consonants of a single type (manner or place)
3	Syllables with "true" consonants of two or more types (manner or place)

Source: Information from Olswang, Stoel-Gammon, Coggins, & Carpenter, 1987. See original for specifics.

MBL is an appropriate measure for children with fewer than 10 different words. MBL is calculated by analyzing the phonetic and syllabic properties of 50 child vocalizations recorded during a 30-minute parent-child play session. Utterance boundaries consist of one second of silence, by a nonspeech production, such as a scream, or by parental speech. In order to be included, a vocalization should be nonmeaningful, speech-like, and include one vocalic element (Morris, 2010).

Each vocalization is coded according to the values presented in Table 5.5. Average MBL is calculated by totaling the score for all utterances and dividing the overall sum by the number of babbled utterances. Average MBL values are also presented in Table 5.5. For a more in-depth discussion, see Morris (2010). The babbling of TD 9- to 12-month-olds mostly contains vowels with a few true consonants, as demonstrated by MBLs below 1.50. By 23 months, most vocalizations contain a true consonant, with some vocalizations containing two different consonants.

As with any measure, it is important to go behind the calculated value. While MBL may tell us something about the level of babbling, it does not describe the variety of phonemes produced.

The mean syllable structure level (SSL) can be calculated from the sample containing word production (Olswang, Stoel-Gammon, Coggins, & Carpenter, 1987; Paul & Jennings, 1992). Please refer to the references cited for a detailed description. Briefly, syllable structure levels are as follows:

Level 1: Word contains a vowel, a single voiced consonant (/g/), or a consonant-vowel (CV) syllable in which the consonant is /h, w, j, l, ɹ/.
Level 2: Word is composed of a VC, CVC with a single consonant (/kaɪk/), or a CV that does not fit the characteristics for Level 1.
Level 3: Word includes two or more different consonant types (/dɔgi/).

More important than placing the child's production at a level is an SLP's description of a child's sound system. SLL values for TD children are presented in Table 5.6.

Phonetic transcription of young children's speech is difficult. Note that MBL and SSL values are assigned based on phonetic characteristics, such as manner and place, and not on specific phonemes.

TABLE 5.6 **Mean SSL Values for TD Children**

MEAN AGE IN MONTHS	SSL	STANDARD DEVIATION	−1 SD
24	2.18	.21	1.97
28	2.34	.17	2.17
36	2.39	.1	2.29

Sources: Paul & Jennings, 1992; Pharr, Ratner, & Rescorla, 2000. Values for other ages are available in these references.

Structure of combinations. The term *combinations* implies that the child is using some two-symbol utterances, such as words, words and gestures, or signs or other augmentative and alternative communication (AAC) symbols, to express a variety of meanings. At this point in development, the TD child may no longer be limited to talking only about referents present in the context. A possible format for dynamic assessing of multisymbol expressive language is presented in Table F.4 in Appendix F. A possible recordkeeping form is presented in Figure 5.9. You may wish to return to the discussion of multiword utterances

FIGURE 5.9 Language Sample Analysis Form

Utterances	SEMANTIC/CONTENT — Nom	Loc	Neg	Pos	Att	Rec	Not	Sta	Act	Agt	Obj	Oth	INTENT/USE — Ans	Que	Rep	Dec	Pra	Nam	Sug	Oth	FORM — Ges	Sin	Voc	Ver	TYPE — Init	Resp
1. *More Juice*						2													2					2	2	
2. *Mommy push*									2	2									2					2	2	
3. *Mommy throw me*	3								3	3			3											3		3
4. *Eat cookie*									2		2					2					1			1	1	
5.																										
6.																										
7.																										
8.																										
9.																										
10.																										
11.																										
12.																										
13.																										
14.																										
15.																										
16.																										
17.																										
18.																										
19.																										
.																										
.																										
.																										
.																										
47.																										
48.																										
49.																										
50.																										
TOTAL SYMBOLS	8																									
TOTAL UTTERANCES	3																									
MLU (Divide symbols by utterances)	2.7																									

Nom Loc Neg Pos Att Rec Not Sta Act Agt Obj Oth | Ans Que Rep Dec Pra Nam Sug Oth | Ges Sin Voc Ver | Init Resp

Key:

Semantic Content
Nom = Nomination Loc = Location Neg = Negation Pos = Possession Att = Attribution Rec = Recurrence
Not = Notice Sta = State Act = Action Agt = Agent Obj = Object Oth = Other

Intent/Use
Ans = Answer Que = Question Rep = Reply Dec = Declaration Pra = Practice Nam = Name
Sug = Sugestion/Command/Demand/Request

Form
Ges = Gesture Sin = Sign Voc = Vocalization Ver = Verbalization

Type
Init = Initiate Resp = Respond

in Chapter 4 prior to use of an analysis similar to that in Figure 5.9. The use of Figure 5.9 will be discussed in depth in the sampling section later in the chapter.

Intentions. TD children express a great variety of communicative intentions in their early speech. The most frequent communicative intentions are requesting information, such as "Wassat?" and acknowledging what another has said, such as "Yeah" and "Uh-huh."

The team will want to describe the breadth of intentions expressed by a child. If we use the presymbolic categories mentioned previously, we might modify them for early speech as follows:

- *Drawing attention to an object or event* by pointing or looking at the object or event, touching, picking up, or showing the object, and verbalizing "Look" or the object name
- *Drawing attention to oneself* by "showing off" and verbalizing "Look" or calling a person's name
- *Giving an object* by pushing or handing it and verbalizing insistently "Look" or "Take" or using a person's name or "You"
- *Initiating play* by looking at the partner or toy, commencing play, and possibly verbalizing "Play" or naming the toy or a person's name
- *Protesting* by expressing displeasure through refusal, tantruming, turning away, or shaking head side to side, and verbalizing "No" or naming an alternative
- *Providing information* by pointing or touching and verbalizing a name or action either following an adult question or spontaneously
- *Requesting an object or action* by reaching or looking and verbalizing the object or action name or "More" insistently
- *Requesting assistance* by reaching, looking at, or handing an object and verbalizing insistently
- *Requesting information* by looking, pointing, or touching and verbalizing with rising intonation, as in "That?" "Wassat?" or "Where?"

Most children will use a combination of symbolic and nonsymbolic communication to express their intentions.

Vocabulary. Through a variety of methods, including parental report, you can compile a list of the words that a child comprehends and produces. These words will be the grist for early multiword utterances that can be taught in intervention. Data from TD children suggests the following growth in expressive vocabulary with age (Owens, 2016):

- At 18 months, 20–50 words
- At 20 months 150 words
- At 24 months, 300 words

Remember that there is wide variation across children, even those developing typically.

Normative data suggest that in a 20-minute conversational sample you might expect the following (Klee, 1992):

Age in Months	Total Number of Words
21	240
24	286
27	332
30	378
33	424
36	470

Unfortunately, you may not have a 20-minute sample, but rather bits and pieces. In this case, you may need to modify the procedure. Even without normative data, lexical density in shorter periods of time might be used to demonstrate changes in a child's speech over time.

One measure of vocabulary is *lexical density*, typically derived from a timed conversational language sample. Lexical density is the number of different nonimitative words used within that time period.

We have normative values for the number of different words in a 50-utterance sample. As you might expect, the number of different words spoken by TD children varies with age. In a 50-utterance sample we would expect the following (Klee, 1992):

Age in Months	Number of Different Words
21	36
24	41
27	46
30	51
33	56
36	61

If we divide the number of different words by the total number of words from the same sample, we can calculate type:token ratio (TTR), a measure of lexical density.

$$\frac{\text{Number of different words (NDW)}}{\text{Total number of words (TNW)}}$$

Because the total number of words will always be greater than or equal to the number of different words, TTR values will be one or less.

TTR can vary greatly for an individual child and is affected by the context and the conversational partner. For example, if the child and adult talk repeatedly about the same object or event, the same words may occur frequently, lowering the TTR score. It is best to collect a sample in more than one context. Although there are no normative values for TTR with children below age 3, TTR scores can be used for comparison over time.

Counting different words is time consuming. A website such as "Using English," designed to help older students with variation in their writing, can be helpful. Type "usingenglish" into your search engine and then click on "Resources" at the top, followed by "text statistics." Copy your entire sample without utterance numbering and drop it in the box. The calculation for TTR is done for you.

PRESYMBOLIC BEHAVIORS

Those presymbolic skills that may help a child acquire the means to communicate purposefully and meaningfully are not ends in themselves but are building blocks for symbolic verbal communication. That said, no child should be assumed to be incapable of meaningful and purposeful communication because he or she has not attained one of these presymbolic skills.

Joint Attention and Attention-Following

Joint or shared attention behaviors should be assessed for both (1) responding to another person's directing attention, such as a point, and (2) initiating attention of another person to an object or event by shifting gaze, labeling, using gestures, or a combination of these.

Caregivers can provide valuable information about the objects and actions that attract their child's attention. In general, novel, brightly colored, and noisemaking objects or toys will usually attract a child's attention. After the child notices the object or action, the SLP can attempt to share it and to keep the child's attention. A possible format for dynamic assessment of joint attention is presented in Table F.5 in Appendix F. Note the graduated guidance in which the SLP provides fewer prompts as the child is able to respond to less input.

At this level of assessment, responding to the SLP's directive behavior is most important and can be used in intervention. Without the ability to follow someone else's initiation, a child will have difficulty focusing attention during intervention. In contrast, a child's initiating of attention blends naturally into initiating gestural communication and may be at too high a level at this point in development.

Motor Imitation

As mentioned in the previous chapter, motor imitation is an important developmental milestone as well as one of the primary modes of teaching with young nonsymbolic children. Being proficient in imitation is related to observing and noting the behavior of others, a basic component of social skills and peer play.

The team may be interested in a child's ability to imitate single (clap once) and multiple acts that are both similar (clap-clap) and dissimilar (clap-touch). By imitating two behaviors, the child demonstrates limited working memory, which will be important in stringing syllables and, more importantly, words together.

A possible format for dynamic assessment of motor imitation is presented in Table F.6 in Appendix F, reflecting graduated guidance by an adult. Note that there are several levels of prompting. A physical assist or prompt can range from a mere touch to fully performing the act with the child by manipulating his or her body.

As an SLP, be flexible is your assessment. If I rub my stomach and ask the child to "Rub tummy," I may get a response in which the child rubs his or her own stomach or one in which the child rubs mine. Either one is acceptable.

Children with cerebral palsy or other motor programming and control difficulties may be unable to respond to traditional infant imitation tasks, such as clapping hands. Of importance is not the specific behavior but the notion of imitating others. For this reason, the team should pick behaviors that the child has performed spontaneously and attempt to have the child imitate someone doing that behavior. The SLP can monitor the child's behavior for attempts to comply.

You may evaluate a child who is able to vocalize or use AAC but is seemingly unable or unwilling to imitate physically in the precise way requested. We do this child a great disservice if we concentrate intervention at the motor imitation level when we could be working with the communication we have. It is better advised to work on the motor behaviors needed to activate an AAC device while concentrating on communication behaviors.

Oral Motor Skills

Speaking is constrained as much by the physical mechanisms of speech production as by the ability to connect symbols to the things to which they refer. The team can note all volitional oral movement by the child and attempt to elicit oral motor imitation. For some children, oral imitation devoid of sound production will be difficult, and the two can be paired during the assessment. Oral motor imitation might also be facilitated with the use of objects, such as a lollipop to assess tongue control. If the team suspects oral motor abnormalities, the SLP might wish to assess the child further using a tool such as the *Kaufman Speech Praxis Test for Children* (Kaufman, 2007).

The presence of abnormal oral-motor imitation skills may be associated with below-average general fine motor deficits (Newmeyer et al., 2007). If a child is having difficulty with oral motor imitation, the SLP may wish to assess fine motor imitation in general, such as opening and closing the hand or touching the thumb and forefinger.

A possible format for dynamic assessment of oral motor imitation is presented in Table F.7 in Appendix F. This format does not take the place of a thorough oral motor skills assessment, including noting muscle tone and strength; range, speed, and coordination of motion; and dissociation, or the ability to move structures such as tongue and lips independently.

Children with oral motor problems will most likely also have difficulty with eating and swallowing. In Chapter 10, we'll discuss oral movement and feeding and swallowing in detail. Let's continue with presymbolic behaviors and save that discussion for later.

Sound-Making

The team will want to collect a list of the sounds the child makes and see if the child can produce these sounds volitionally in imitation, both alone and in connected syllables. These sounds will become the building blocks for words.

By this point in the assessment, the team should know if the child has the notion of using others as behavioral models. Because we already know from dynamic assessment whether the child can imitate single and two-step physical behaviors, inability to do this orally may indicate an oral motor control problem. A possible format for dynamic assessment of sound production is presented in Table F.8 in Appendix F.

This is not an evaluation of articulation. At this point, approximations are fine. We can shape them into phonemes later. A nice sharp /g/ may be difficult, but "revving up your motor" in a guttural growling /g-g-g/ works just fine for now.

If a child is having difficulty with sound imitation, the SLP may want to introduce oral imitation with objects or actions as a bridge to production of specific phonemes. Here's a short list of possibilities:

■ /h/ by blowing a whistle or musical instrument such as a harmonica
■ /m/ by wiping the child's mouth with washcloth
■ /a/ while chanting, having lips patted as in "war whoop," or bouncing
■ /b/ and /p/ by making raspberries
■ /h/ and /b/ while simulating greetings ("hi") and departures ("bye")
■ /m/ after small treat, such as mini M&Ms, while rubbing tummy

Vocalizations can also be added to physical movement that the child already imitates.

Functional Use

Functional use of objects requires that a child demonstrate evidence of object discrimination. In other words, the child should use actual or miniature objects in the manner in which they were intended or for their socially designed function. We must allow children a certain amount of latitude with functional use, given that most objects have more than one function. A possible format for dynamic assessment of functional use is presented in Table F.9 in Appendix F.

How a child interacts with objects is important. A child is beginning to move into the realm of intentional conversation when he or she

■ Gazes at a preferred item and then shifts gaze to an adult,
■ Explores objects and picks the relevant one in context,
■ Expectantly pushes an object toward an adult, or
■ Pulls or pushes an adult in a way that says "Do this with me."

Level of Play

Spontaneous, natural play is basic to child development. One of the primary contexts in which a child learns, play is also one of the best places for a child to demonstrate that learning. Of interest to the team are the type, level, and complexity of play skills. The diversity of object play has been shown to be a predictor of word frequency among nonverbal and low verbal children with ASD (Yoder, 2006).

There are various ways to assess a child's play. The choice of method depends on the individual child and family and on the outcome desired. Informal approaches include observation of the child during both solitary and partnered play and description of the child's behavior. Several checklists of play are available.

One measure of play is a child's level of engagement. This could roughly be categorized as unengaged, neutral, and engaged. While these categories do not correspond to developmental levels, they may provide a useful way of analyzing a child's behavior. A possible format for assessing levels of play is presented in Table F.10 in Appendix F.

The unengaged child would be inattentive or display negative behaviors such as pulling away, physically resisting, shaking head side to side (*No!*), or crying and whining. Some children will be too interested in other objects, such as a blanket, to break from these and join an adult in play.

Neutral engagement is characterized by looking at the adult or toy, possibly even smiling or vocalizing, but not interacting in the play sequence. The child might participate in routine play but not follow the routine. For example, in *Peek-a-boo* with a cover over the child's head, the child may pull the covering off as soon as it is applied rather than

TABLE 5.7 **Dynamic Assessment of Presymbolic Play**

Level of Assessment	Expected Response	Test Format	Possible Mediated Teaching Format
Familiar routines	Child begins game and anticipates outcome.	Using just intonation, both with and without words, say the initial line for familiar games in succession, such as "So Big," "I'm Gonna Get You," "This Little Piggy," and "Pat-a-cake."	Practice familiar routines with the child, take a short break, then begin again using both speech and intonation. If child does not comply by joining game, try again with body movement, such as crouching along with "I'm gonna get you." If child still does not comply, use a physical prompt, such as placing the child in position along with your verbal cue. When the child is successful with two routines, return to the test mode.
Functional play	Child plays with objects in a meaningful way.	Call child's name, say "Look," and name object(s). Cue child with "Let's play" or "What do you do with this?"	Respond to any child behavior that approximates appropriate play and demonstrates appropriate use of the object. If the child does not respond or responds in an unacceptable or indiscriminate manner, model an action with the object and try to engage the child in play or an interaction. If the child's response is still unacceptable, try to get the child to imitate by performing the action and then prompting the child to do it, as in "Cory, brush hair." After teaching a few actions with the objects, return to each one to see if the child will now demonstrate functional use.

waiting for "Where's Suzy?" In *Pat-a-cake*, the child may stick his or her hands between the adult's or touch the adult's hands randomly.

In contrast, the engaged child, will raise arms appropriately when playing *So Big* or bring hands to the adults for *Pat-a-cake*. In addition, the child may follow the sequence of events in *Pat-a-cake*, imitating the mother's motions. Fully engaged children also initiate games, such as lifting the arms to begin *So Big*, and participate in social routines, such as waving bye-bye.

As an SLP, remember that play skills and styles vary depending on the characteristics of the partners, the toys available, and the type of play (Cherney, Kelly-Vance, Glover, Ruane, & Ryalls, 2003). There are also cultural differences in the themes and communication functions found in the social pretend play of preschoolers and in the play of caregivers with their infants and toddlers.

As mentioned previously, parental play reflects a parents' beliefs and values about the role of play. Assessment expectations should be adjusted based on these parental assumptions. A possible format for dynamic assessment of play is presented in Table 5.7.

Symbolic play. Children developing typically display symbolic play at about the same time that they begin to speak. Sometimes play reveals what language does not. I was involved in an assessment in which a child did not speak or respond to the speech of others. When she and I began to play, she engaged in role play and imaginative play, clearly well beyond the level of her language. Something was holding back her language development. The team suggested a thorough audiological examination, which revealed a severe hearing problem.

Westby's scale for assessing development of children's play (Westby, 1998, 2000) integrates cognitive and communicative skills to describe seven stages of symbolic play corresponding to language development. A possible format for dynamic assessment of symbolic play is presented in Table F.11 in Appendix F. This will require creativity and flexibility by the SLP because each child has favorite toys and play scenarios.

Sampling

Spontaneous language samples may be useful as a qualitative method for assessing language problems, developing a sound inventory and a babbling analysis, categorizing sound errors and/or patterns, and making judgments about intelligibility. A sample is more than just a list of words a child produces. Instead, language samples can be used to determine language level and to describe to the best extent possible the form, content, and use of language. Figure 5.9 (page 172) is an example of a language sample analysis form that can be used when examining the form, content, and use of early utterances. Although the form in Figure 5.9 uses only 50 utterances, an SLP is not limited to that sample size and may desire a larger sample.

Using the form in Figure 5.9 or a similar one, the SLP can analyze each utterance for its semantic function, intention, and form. The format in Figure 5.9 is merely suggestive and can be as easy or difficult to use as an SLP desires. For example, if the child uses spoken words to request "More juice," the semantic function is *Recurrence*, the intention is *Request for an object*, and the form is *Verbal*. This utterance could be scored by placing the number 2 in each block as demonstrated in Figure 5.9, signifying a two-symbol utterance.

Not all utterances may be so easy to rate. While *Recurrence* can be either one symbol ("More," "Nuther") or two ("More cookie"), other forms expand by combining semantic categories. For example, the utterance "Mommy push" is a combination of the *Agent* and *Action* categories. In *Agent + Action*, *Action + Object*, and the rarer *Agent + Object*, the SLP might place a 2 in both affected categories, as in the second utterance in Figure 5.9. Longer utterances pose a similar problem. For example, "Mommy throw me" in response to "What do you want?", meaning "Mommy throws the ball to me," is *Agent + Action + Location*, and all three categories would receive a value of 3. These examples are merely suggestions.

There is no one agreed-upon method for rating early utterances. In fact, as you know from Chapter 4, many linguists question the very notion of semantic categories in early speech. A similar rating form could be used employing the constructionist categories of *word combinations, pivot schemes,* and *item-based constructions*.

Each utterance also has at least one means or form. Each form could be scored with the number of symbols sent via that mode. In the fourth utterance in Figure 5.9, the child signs "Eat" and says "Cookie." Under form, the child might receive a 1 for *Sign* and a 1 for *Verbalization*. By scoring the utterance in this way, the SLP is able to know how the child builds longer utterances.

One caution: It may not be readily apparent why certain utterances in Figure 5.9 are scored as they are, especially for intent. Figure 5.9 is meant as an example and not as a definitive model. I have rated utterances that, based on the child's production and on the contextual situation, do not fit in the suggested categories in this figure. In these cases, I add a new category of my own. And remember that an utterance such as "Eat cookie" could just as likely be a question, an answer, or a request, depending on context. All you can do as an SLP is try to your best ability to determine the parameters of an utterance.

After each utterance is rated, the number of utterances in each category and the number of symbols can be totaled within each column, as in Figure 5.9. By dividing the number of symbols by the number of utterances, the SLP can compute the MLU for each category. These data can then be compared to other child data from other segments of the assessment to determine nonexistent categories, low-frequency categories, and utterance length by category and form. This information can be very useful in planning how to expand a child's output.

Analysis of Data

After completing the assessment, the team tries to reach consensus on a description of the child's and caregiver's communication system, focusing on possible communication goals and objectives, including improvements in the environment and in the partners' interaction patterns.

At the very least, assessment outcomes should include comments on

- Communication forms that are already present, their meaning and effectiveness;
- Communication forms that the child and the partners have shown evidence of learning;
- The child's lexicon, or personal dictionary;
- The partner's responses to the child's communication forms; and
- The environment's ability to support communication.

Analysis of the data from dynamic assessment can show which strategies seem to facilitate communication and which do not.

Decision-Making and Recommendations

The team members review the results and discuss different intervention options. Although discussing sensitive assessment information with families can be one of the more difficult tasks associated with providing intervention services to young children, the importance of this step as a means of continuing to build consensus between families and professionals cannot be dismissed. Families who express dissatisfaction with their assessment experiences often report specific unhappiness with the way this information was shared. Mindful of this possible source of conflict, the team can try to share information in a way that is useful to families, that promotes their competence, and that facilitates consensus building.

It may be helpful for professionals to explore the degree of comfort family members have about sharing their own findings. Prior to the postassessment meeting, the family may need help in preparing their remarks. This may be aided if parents are provided with forms to help organize their thoughts around the major assessment questions to be answered.

Families who were more actively involved in all aspects of assessment are more likely to contribute to intervention planning and decision-making. In addition to specific questions about a child's communication, families can be given a list of general questions to consider before this discussion begins, such as

- What were your impressions?
- What area would you prefer to discuss first?
- What assessment activities went well?
- What assessment activities did not go as well?

The team might begin their meeting by asking families to respond to these questions aloud.

In a recent assessment of a child's communication, it was revealed that the mother had been to see several professionals before we met. As we began our discussion, we asked "What would you like to discuss first?" The mother burst into tears and responded that she was overwhelmed because no other professional had ever asked her opinion before.

Following this collaborative decision-making effort, team members write a report reflecting consensual goals and objectives and recommendations on intervention techniques that were successful or have the potential for success. The plan should reflect present communication priorities and target functional communication goals within the everyday environment of the child and family.

Outcomes

After obtaining information from caregivers regarding children's participation in activities and routines and assessing a child's communication skills, the team begins to develop desired communication outcomes. Family-centered EI outcomes are based on the caregivers' priorities and concerns and are attainable within a young child's daily activities and routines (Bernheimer & Weismer, 2007; Jung, 2007).

Of necessity, ECI focuses on enhancing or enabling children's participation in these activities and routines. If a child is already participating well, an SLP can help the caregiver embed opportunities for learning new skills within these activities. More specifically, the SLP focuses on communication to improve or enable participation, and learning opportunities in which a child can practice and learn new communication skills that are high priority for caregivers.

The team can attempt to answer the following questions (Wilcox & Woods, 2011):

- What are important daily activities and routines of the family that include the child?
- How can increased communication enhance or enable a child's participation?
- What skills does the child need to successfully participate?
- Might participation be enhanced through the use of augmentative or alternative communication or other forms of assistive technology?
- What activities and routines have the potential to provide a context for embedding communication learning?

As the caregiver and EI team consider these questions, they can generate tentative hypotheses or conclusions and then develop relevant outcomes.

Outcome statements can be framed within a participation-based perspective by specifying the activity and routine as well as the targeted skill. For example, *Georgeanna will participate in snack time by selecting what she wants to eat through pointing*. Note that the skill to be acquired or strengthened is placed within an interactive context. The measuring of achievement should be based on the child's participation and individualized for a given caregiver and child.

Specific Disorders

Some children, because of the nature of their disorder or because of their special circumstances, will require a different means of testing or additional analysis. Let's discuss these briefly prior to wrapping up this chapter.

CHILDREN WITH DEAFNESS AND BLINDNESS

Multiple and consistent observations in a natural setting are important for recognizing the meaningful verbal and nonverbal acts of a young child with deafness and blindness and for understanding changes over time. It is important to understand the events associated with the child's behavior, to recognize sometimes subtle or nonstandard communication signals, and to respond meaningfully to these behaviors. Team members should be alert to changes in mood, attention span, startle reactions, activity level, and responsiveness. Some possible observational rating scales include:

- *Child Behavior Checklist* (Achenbach & Rescorla, 2000)
- *Behavior Assessment System for Children* (BASC) (American Guidance Service, Inc., 1992)
- *Vineland Adaptive Behavior Scales* (American Guidance Service, Inc., 1984)
- *Bayley Scales of Infant Development*, 2nd Edition (The Psychological Corporation, 1993)

In general, when compared to TD infants, those with deaf-blindness may exhibit extremes in behavior from hyper-responding to passivity and near motionless behavior.

For a child with limited expressive communication, the SLP will want to observe the child's use of nonsymbolic systems, such as gestures, facial expressions, and body movements that may indicate needs. A systematic functional analysis can be accomplished in context to determine the purposes of these nonsymbolic behaviors. Functions of early expression can be the basis for training more sophisticated interactions, such as requesting and commenting (Stremel, 2000).

It's important that behavioral assessment and intervention be individualized. A child who has deaf-blindness may engage in unwanted and socially inappropriate behavior for a number of reasons, including communication deficits, developmental delays, and difficulties in interpreting environmental information. These behaviors limit a child's ability to interact and to influence others. The consistency, frequency, and intensity of negative behaviors need to be recorded. As an SLP, you'll want to try to identify the communicative function or use of challenging behavior so you can help the child develop a more socially appropriate method of communicating.

INTERNATIONAL ADOPTEES AND CHILDREN FROM FAMILIES SPEAKING A LANGUAGE OTHER THAN ENGLISH

International adoptees pose a special challenge for SLPs. Although bilingual children should be assessed in both languages, it's important to note that many children are from multilingual regions of the world in which the community language may not be the national one. In other words, a child from Thailand may not have been exposed to Thai.

SLPs and adoptive parents are advised to make inquiries through the adoption agency or international adoption support groups to determine the likely birth language. In many cases, assessment tools in a child's first language may not be available.

Although it may be easy for some to dismiss the importance of the first language for very young children, this position is shortsighted (Glennen, 2002). The prosodic, syntactic, and phonological differences between the birth and adopted languages must be compared before predictions can be made regarding language acquisition.

As you may recall from your language development course, at early stages of language development, children use prosodic and phonological patterns to help them segment speech into phrases and words. Beginning at birth, the process develops throughout the first year of life, so that by 10 months of age, the infant can recognize language patterns in the native language. These patterns are used by infants to fathom speakers' meaning. The adopted infant or toddler must learn to pay attention to these patterns in the new language. Only then can a young child focus on learning what the patterns mean. Because language acquisition is a developmental process, children will require adequate time and exposure to a second language.

I'm reminded of a dear friend who was asked to evaluate a child adopted from Russia who was reportedly not talking by age 2. According to the adoptive parents, their child produced only unintelligible babbling. My friend, who spent much of her life in Russia, recognized the child's Russian words immediately. The child was exhibiting a slower pace in learning English for reasons very different from those found in children with language disorders.

Many families living in the United States possess limited or no English skills. In these cases, a child and family's English proficiency should be considered before any evaluation is attempted. Of more importance than whether or not the parent can speak English is how often the parent talks to the child in either language.

Important assessment issues include the choice of evaluative measures, determination of whether an English-speaking SLP or bilingual SLP is better, and consideration of using an interpreter along with an English-only SLP. When possible, the evaluation team should consider the use of a standardized test in the family's language. Be aware that some instruments in other languages are simply literal translations of English tests that may not have been validated in those languages. In these cases, it is generally preferable to use nonstandardized measures. If language impairment exists, a child would exhibit a language delay in the primary language as well as in English.

CHILDREN WITH CHALLENGING BEHAVIORS

Young children are at risk of developing challenging behaviors, such as screaming, hitting, or self-abusive behaviors, because of delays in communication, language, and social development. These problem behaviors may remain if they "work" for the child by attracting attention or helping the child obtain a desired outcome (Horner, Carr, Strain, Todd, & Reed, 2000). Most SLPs are not behavioral specialists, but if the challenging behavior seems related to communication, the SLP and other team members can attempt to discover this relationship.

Although a TD child might be encouraged to express these intentions through speech, some children, such as those with ASD or CP, may have fewer conventional forms of communication and much more difficulty retrieving them within appropriate contexts. These children may develop the use of unconventional, sometimes challenging, behaviors as a means of communication. The two most common communicative functions of challenging behaviors are

- To request something, such as attention, an object, food or drink, assistance, or participation in an activity; and
- To avoid or escape something, such as discomfort, activity transition, or demands upon the child.

For example, my grandson Dakota, who has severe cerebral palsy and had no usable speech at the time, began hitting himself at around age 2 when his mother left the house or when he was in pain. In Chapter 4 we discussed *functional equivalence*. Dakota's hitting himself was the functional equivalent of protesting, which could have been signaled by shaking his head instead.

The goal of assessment is to understand the function or purpose of these challenging behaviors and when they are most and least likely to occur. Successful intervention depends on understanding the function(s) of the challenging behavior. A comprehensive functional assessment results in a clear description of the challenging behavior, the context(s) in which it occurs, the antecedents and consequences maintaining the behavior, and the communicative function of the behavior.

As we have discussed throughout this chapter, a thorough functional assessment, especially with challenging behaviors, includes multiple sources of information (Buschbacher & Fox, 2003):

- Interviews with parents, school staff, and significant others in the child's life;
- Direct observation;
- Review of relevant archival records; and
- Data analysis.

From these data, the SLP and team members form a hypothesis about the challenging behavior. At the very least, an interview should include information about when the behavior is most and least likely to occur, ongoing events in those contexts, and possible communicative function(s) of the behavior. Families and school staff are in the unique position of being able to provide this information. Variables that affect the behavior may be as seemingly unimportant as allergies or the amount of sleep.

It's important to observe the child within the contexts where the challenging behavior is likely to occur in order both to confirm information described in the interviews and to provide a baseline or quantifiable measure of how often the behavior occurs. During observation, the SLP or other team member attempts to describe the antecedent or preceding events, the challenging behavior itself, and the consequences as carefully as possible. In addition, the observer should describe contextual events that may increase the likelihood of the challenging behavior. Systematic observation may need to occur over time and to enlist the help of all relevant team members. If particular events within a context are determined to be related to the occurrence of the behavior, these events will need to be included in the planned intervention.

This type of functional assessment results in the development of a hypothesis, or several hypotheses, representing the team's best estimate of the function of the behavior and the relationship(s) between that behavior and the environment (Harrower, Fox, Dunlap, & Kincaid, 2000). The hypothesis should be methodically assessed to determine its accuracy.

These hypotheses are strengthened through direct observation in the child's natural environment. In general, observations involve watching a child in situations that appear to be associated with the occurrence and nonoccurrence of the problem behavior.

Finally, functional analysis has two parts: a careful manipulation of the antecedent and consequent events to measure their effect on the behavior, and a re-creation of situations that include some of the environmental conditions that may be related to the problem behavior. In each condition, a specific antecedent or consequent event is manipulated to gauge its impact on the frequency of the behavior over time. Functional analysis requires careful monitoring, especially in situations in which a behavior is dangerous to the child or to others.

Let's assume that Alejandro becomes self-abusive both in the classroom and at home. Through discussion with his parents and teachers, we find a pattern that suggests that these behaviors occur when he transitions from one activity to another, such as going from play to snack or from bath to bedtime. In both contexts, the adults precede the transition by saying "Okay, it's time to. . . ." When he becomes self-abusive, the teacher or parent sometimes lets him stay in the activity longer. The team might hypothesize that Alejandro's challenging behavior is a request to remain in the activity longer. The occasional granting of that request has strengthened the challenging behavior.

A hypothesis can be tested by manipulating the preceding and following events, such as transitioning him with no announcement, giving him another warning prior to announcing a transition, or allowing him to request more time in the current activity, and observing the effect on his behavior. The team might also remove all opportunity to continue an activity when he exhibits challenging behavior. Through careful observation and documentation, the team looks for subtle changes in his behavior that indicate that the adult behavior is having some effect. The next step is intervention based on these data, but that will have to wait for a chapter or two.

CHILDREN WITH MOTOR SPEECH DISORDERS

Some children exhibit motor speech disorders in addition to or separate from language impairment. My grandson Zavier, later diagnosed with childhood apraxia of speech (CAS), had excellent comprehension of language and the cognitive skills to engage in symbolic and imaginative play but had extremely limited speech. In contrast, his brother Dakota had both speech and language disorders, primarily caused by his cerebral palsy and associate intellectual disability. In general, motor speech problems such as these are disorders in the control and function of the oral muscular system caused by neuromuscular dysfunction and/or anatomical anomalies. In an evaluation, the SLP is particularly interested in

- Any gap between comprehension and poorer speech production,
- Structure and function of the oral mechanism, and
- A phonetic inventory.

These will be discussed more in Chapter 10.

> Although children with ASD have unique communication behaviors, an SLP is interested in many of the same communication behaviors. That's not to say children with ASD will all be the same. If you're interested in this population, you might want to watch this video on assessing the communication needs of a child with ASD. https://www.youtube.com/watch?v=Imd0QBtDy_w

CHILDREN WITH ASD

It is important that you not feel as if you must totally reinvent the manner in which you assess communication in children for ASD. Although these children present a unique behavior profile, we are still interested in many of the same behaviors, such as the manner in which they communicate and their ability to establish joint attention and display intentional communication. An SLP will want to pay particular attention to the items presented in Figure 5.10.

It is recommended that an individualized communication assessment protocol for a child with ASD consist of at least three steps (Halle & Meadan, 2007):

- Assess the child's preferences through both indirect procedures, such as care provider and client interviews, and direct procedures, such as observation while systematically exposing the child to differing stimuli (Hagopian, Long, & Rush, 2004). The goal is to describe the communication topographies of requesting, rejecting, and repairing, and to identify preferred and nonpreferred foods, objects, and activities.
- Build rapport through interacting with the child in preferred routines, following his or her lead, and being responsive to communication attempts.

FIGURE 5.10 **Possible Assessment Questions for Caregivers of Infants and Toddlers with ASD**

Does the child . . .

- Feel like other children when held?
- Look at you when called, talking, or playing?
- Avoid or ignore adults and other children?
- Spend relatively more time looking at objects than at people?
- Engage in reciprocal back-and-forth play, such as passing toys or rolling objects?
- Play simple games, such as Peek-a-boo or I'm Gonna Get You?
- Interact with objects or play with toys in the same exact way each time?
- Have limited or absent pretend play?
- Imitate other people's actions?
- Imitate other people's sound-making?
- Smile in response to a smile from others?
- Gesture?
    - Point?
    - Nod "yes" and "no"?
    - Hold objects for you to see?
    - Show things to people?
    - Lead an adult by the hand?
    - Make requests?
- Combine gestures and sounds?
- Give inconsistent responses to speech, such as response to name and/or commands?
- Use rote, memorized, repetitive, or echolalic speech?
- Memorize strings of words?
- Have any odd speech behaviors?
- Have repetitive, stereotypic, or odd motor behavior, especially in the hands or fingers?
- Have preoccupation with a narrow range of interests?
- Strongly attach to a specific object?
- Overly attend to parts of objects, such as the wheels on a toy car?
- Have a strong preference for performing activities in a specific way or sequence?

Sources: Filipek et al., 1999; Zwaigenbaum et al., 2005.

- ■ Assess through a structured protocol by intentionally programming opportunities for requesting, rejecting, and making repairs, the primary early intentional behaviors of children with ASD.

These steps optimize the assessment by providing opportunities to communicate in context with both familiar and unfamiliar partners. By varying the conditions in these contexts, the SLP can examine how the child's communication attempts differ in response to differing conditions. Of interest is a description of the child's intentional behaviors, their frequency, and their consistency across situations and partners.

Given the influence that the quality of a relationship can have on the interactions of children with disabilities, rapport building is extremely important (McLaughlin & Carr, 2005; Ogletree, Pierce, Harn, & Fischer, 2002). Frequently, children with ASD, especially young children, will not communicate optimally in unfamiliar settings or with unfamiliar partners. This would seem to argue for parents' being integrated into the assessment process. Others who will interact with the child should plan to spend several hours getting acquainted prior to the assessment.

It's extremely important that the SLP or adult interacting with the child be flexible and modify procedures according to the unique characteristics of the individual child. A sample protocol is presented in Figure 5.11.

Multiple opportunities for the child to communicate can be embedded into the many ongoing routines that occur regularly on a daily basis. If this is not possible, new routines

FIGURE 5.11 **Flexible Assessment Protocol**

1. Establish a play routine and develop a positive relationship with the child that will motivate him or her to stay and play.
2. Encourage child to sit with you. (A stationary target is preferable to a moving one.)
3. Remove a preferred object/activity and show but keep out of reach.
4. Cue child with "Let's play with . . ." or "Look, I have a . . ." and wait 5 seconds for a response.
5. If the child . . .

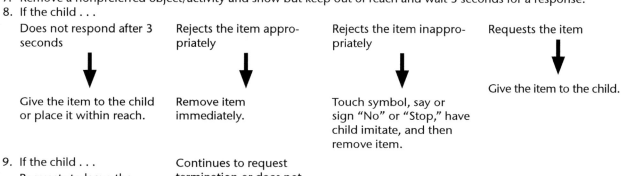

Does not respond	Rejects the item by indicating "No" or by pushing the item away	Requests the item with a reach	Does not respond after 15 seconds
↓		↓	↓
Model by playing the activity or with the object and wait 10 seconds for a response.	↓ Remove the item.	Give the item to the child.	Offer a new item or activity.

6. After playing with one item for 20 to 30 seconds, offer a new item.
7. Remove a nonpreferred object/activity and show but keep out of reach and wait 3 seconds for a response.
8. If the child . . .

Does not respond after 3 seconds	Rejects the item appropriately	Rejects the item inappropriately	Requests the item
↓	↓	↓	↓
Give the item to the child or place it within reach.	Remove item immediately.	Touch symbol, say or sign "No" or "Stop," have child imitate, and then remove item.	Give the item to the child.

9. If the child . . .

Requests to leave the session	Continues to request termination or does not want to return to the table
↓	↓
Attempt to redirect with a preferred item or activity to maintain child in session.	Honor by giving a 2-minute break and then start a new trial.

10. On about one-third of the request trials, look at the child and say "What?" to indicate a communication breakdown.
11. If the child does not produce a repair after 3 seconds, begin a new trial with a new object.
12. Repeat steps 10–11 once or twice during a session of 30 trials, on reject trials.

Examples of probes within everyday routines:

- Toothpaste in a "funky" dispenser but out of reach at tooth-brushing time
- Clothing child dislikes handed to child while dressing
- Favorite breakfast food on shelf child cannot reach in the morning
- Favorite tub toy just out of reach during bath time
- Dead batteries in favorite toy at playtime
- Missing favorite CD when listening to music
- Small quantity of easily consumed favorite treat at snack time

Source: Information from Halle & Meadan, 2007.

can be easily established. The reliability of assessment data is important for purposes of comparison, so the team will want to describe the child's behaviors carefully, as well as the preceding and following behaviors of others that may affect the child's behavior.

Although several more formal assessment tools are available at present, most are still under development or revision, and few have undergone the necessary reliability and validity trials. This is not a criticism but instead reflects the dynamic nature of early assessment of children with ASD that makes a one-size-fits-all assessment tool difficult to develop. Many are still works in progress. Several are presented in Table 5.8.

TABLE 5.8   Tools for Screening for ASD in Young Children

The Checklist for Autism in Toddlers (CHAT) (Baird et al., 2000; Baron-Cohen et al., 1992, 1996)	Consists of nine items reported by parents and five items observed by a health professional at the 18-month developmental checkup. CHAT identifies approximately one-third of children diagnosed as having ASD at age 7.
The Modified Checklist for Autism in Toddlers (M-CHAT) (Kleinman et al., in press; Robins & Dumont-Mathieu, 2006; Robins et al., 2001)	Consists of 23 parental report items. M-CHAT sensitivity is only slightly better than the CHAT.
The Early Screening of Autistic Traits Questionnaire (ESAT) (Dietz et al., 2006)	A 14-item screening instrument designed for use at 14–15 months of age. While the ESAT detects children with ASD, it does so at well below the expected prevalence rates.
The Infant-Toddler Checklist (ITC) (Wetherby & Prizant, 2002; Wetherby et al., 2004)	A component of the *Communication and Symbolic Behavior Scales Developmental Profile* (CSBS DP) (Wetherby & Prizant, 2002). The ITC includes 24 questions about developmental milestones of social communication and is a standardized tool that has standard scores at monthly intervals from 6 to 24 months based on a normative sample of nearly 2,200 children (Wetherby & Prizant, 2002). Results from follow-up studies suggest that the ITC has higher sensitivity and specificity than the other tools for catching 9- to 24-month-olds at risk for ASD.
The Autism Diagnostic Observation Schedule (ADOS) (Lord et al., 2000)	A semi-structured direct observational measure developed to identify early behavioral markers of ASD in infancy. Standardized activities are used to observe and systematically rate the occurrence or nonoccurrence of behaviors informative of the earliest emergence of ASD. Designed to take 15–20 minutes to complete, but administration times can vary depending on an infant's ability to engage with the examiner, as well as the infant's temperament, state, and developmental levels.
The Autism Observation Scale for Infants (AOSI) (Bryson et al., 2008)	A semi-structured assessment of communication, social interaction, and play/repetitive behaviors. Scores cover five domains: communication; social; play; autism-related behaviors; and nonspecific behaviors such as activity level, tantrums/negative behavior, and anxiety. Stability of an autism diagnosis is high when the ADOS is used with 2-year-olds.
The Mullen Scales of Early Learning–AGS Edition (Mullen, 1995)	A measure of cognitive and language development consisting of five scales, four of which (visual reception, receptive language, expressive language, and fine motor) assess different domains of cognitive ability, while the fifth scale measures gross motor development of infants and toddlers. An early learning composite (ELC) is calculated based on the first four scales for children aged 0–69 months.
First Year Inventory (FYI) (Reznick, Baranek, Reavis, Watson, & Crais, 2007)	Assesses behaviors in 12-month-old infants, including social orienting and receptive communication, social-affective engagement, imitation, expressive communication, sensory processing, regulatory patterns, reactivity, and repetitive behavior.

A few autism-specific screening tools have been used with a general population sample. No instrument or individual item shows satisfying power in discriminating ASD from non-ASD (Oosterling et al., 2009).

Conclusion

The sheer volume of information in this chapter should alert you to the challenge in thoroughly describing the speech and language of very young children or those with severely handicapping conditions. In practice, it is a problem-solving task and not a one-size-fits-all test administration.

For all your effort, you will still find that some children give you very little to go on. Some children will be locked into a body or a mind or a behavioral pattern that seems to mitigate against development of intentional and meaningful communication. We may wish that it were otherwise, but in the end we have to be realists. That shouldn't stop us from rolling up our sleeves and finding a way for this child to communicate better.

If you have tried your best through a variety of methods to assess a child's communication, then no matter how limited the results may be, you at least have a place, albeit tentative, to begin intervention. Should you find later that you were wrong, you can always revise your plans and projections. That's called flexibility, a characteristic of the best SLPs.

It's now time for you as an SLP and for the team, including the parents, to begin the longer task of intervention. Just as in the assessment, there will be frustrations as well as enlightening *ah-ha* moments. As an SLP, you'll learn to take the good along with the not-so-good and to remember that each improvement in a child's communication is one step further in helping the child become an independent, functioning member of society.

Even though we are moving to another phase, remember that assessment in the form of periodic probes and recordkeeping is an essential part of intervention. In addition, the mediation strategies used in our dynamic assessment can inform the teaching techniques used in intervention.

 Click here to gauge your understanding of the concepts in this chapter.

6

Presymbolic Early Communication Intervention

LEARNING OUTCOMES

When you have completed this chapter, you should be able to:

- Give examples of different intervention approaches within the spectrum of early communication intervention (ECI).
- Provide a rationale for each of the evidence-based strategies for eliciting speech-like vocalizations.
- Describe different strategies for enhancing communication.
- Provide a rationale for language stimulation.
- Explain strategies for teaching presymbolic skills.

Terms with which you should be familiar:

Behavior chain interruption	Fading
Enhanced natural gestures	Incidental teaching
Environmental sabotage	Mand-model
Expectant delays	Positive behavior support

The effectiveness of parent/caregiver-implemented intervention for children with a variety of developmental disabilities is well documented (Kaiser, Hancock, & Neitfield, 2000; Law, Garrett, & Nye, 2004; T. Smith, Buch, & Gamby, 2000; Woods, Kashinath, & Goldstein, 2004). Parents can learn specific intervention techniques, such as modeling, prompting, and reinforcing, to teach specific language forms and functions and also techniques to promote communication (Kaiser et al., 2000; Mahoney & Perales, 2005; Yoder & Warren, 2002). It is within such a model that we'll examine presymbolic intervention. In the following sections we'll discuss the spectrum of intervention, including evidence-based practice (EBP); enhancing presymbolic communication; and principles and techniques.

Spectrum of Early Communication Intervention

In Chapter 3 we discussed an overall philosophy for the delivery of intervention services. Within that spectrum are a variety of service delivery models. The selection of a specific service delivery model or a possible hybrid will vary based on the particular needs of the individual child and family. ECI service delivery generally varies by location, type of service delivery, and overall approach.

LOCATION OF INTERVENTION

It is generally believed and supported by empirical evidence that intervention is most effective when family involvement is maximized and when it occurs within the family's daily routines and activities.

As we know, federal legislation requires that early intervention (EI) services and supports be provided in the least restrictive environment, including those home and community settings in which children with and without disabilities participate. According to the Individuals with Disabilities Education Improvement Act (2004), EI services are to be provided in the natural environment unless satisfactory outcomes cannot be achieved in this setting. In fact, traditional clinical or medical models of service delivery may not be reimbursable unless they are delivered in consultation and collaboration with the family and can be justified as the best environment for intervention.

Although a family's home is the primary natural environment for a child, the number of children in single parent homes or with two parents working outside the home has necessitated expansion of EI services to a variety of early care and education settings (Stowe & Turnbull, 2001). Some children receive services in more than one setting. In general, the location of out-of-home services is usually determined by geographical location, child and family needs and resources, and family and other team members' preferences (Bruder, 2001).

Both home and community settings have value and afford many opportunities for adults to enhance a child's individualized intervention. Over time, the nature of EI services and supports will likely change as family and child needs change (Hanft & Feinberg, 1997).

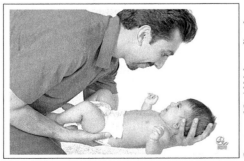

Courtesy of Omid Mohamadi and Mehdi Amiri.

TYPES OF ECI SERVICE DELIVERY

Service delivery models in speech-language pathology range from the traditional, one-on-one, direct clinical model to more indirect collaborative approaches. Although evidence-based research on ECI service delivery models is still in its infancy, there is a growing professional consensus toward service delivery options that are (Sandall, Hemmeter, Smith, & McLean, 2005)

- Individualized;
- Aligned with family priorities;
- Matched to the child's communication, speech, language, emergent literacy, feeding and swallowing, and social and emotional needs; and
- Consistently monitored.

ASHA (2008b) has outlined a model that is evidence based, family centered, individualized, culturally responsive, linguistically appropriate, developmentally supportive, and team based. In many locations, despite this professional recommendation, ECI intervention consists of more traditional models, which might include weekly home visits or half-day classroom programs with little child or family individualization (ASHA, 2008b; Hebbler, Zercher, Mallik, Spiker, & Levin, 2003; U.S. Department of Education, 2003).

In this text, we primarily discuss a consultative-collaborative model with service delivery in natural environments and a focus on functional communication within a child's and family's natural daily activities and routines (Paul-Brown & Caperton, 2001). This is an integrated model that includes the child, family, caregivers, and the speech-language pathologist (SLP) in collaborative roles in which team members work collectively to determine the most suitable location or locations for services and select the most appropriate intervention goals and strategies (McWilliam, 2005). This is not to negate the value of face-to-face SLP-child intervention, which can also occur within such a model.

INTERVENTION APPROACHES

As noted in Chapter 3, ECI approaches vary from those that *support* language acquisition and use to those that *enable* a child to expand her or his linguistic repertoires by acquisition of new words, morphemes, and grammatical structures (ASHA 2008b). In general, supportive strategies respond to a child's communication attempts by engaging the child in conversation around activities and materials of high interest to the child within the context of everyday activities and routines. While important to the success of enabling strategies, supportive strategies alone have not been found to have a significant impact on language development (J. Smith, Warren, Yoder, & Feurer, 2004).

More explicit enabling strategies use

- Direct cues and prompts within the context of an ongoing activity,
- Modeling, and
- Expansion of a child's utterances.

Designed to increase the frequency and complexity of a child's communication, enabling strategies fall along a continuum from *responsive* to *directive*. Responsive interactional strategies attempt to encourage a child's engagement and to provide opportunities for child-initiated and child-directed behavior and for reciprocal and balanced turn-taking between communication partners. In general, responsive interactional strategies facilitate learning with a child who already exhibits emerging word or grammatical structure knowledge.

In contrast, directive interactional strategies consist of adult-led interactions that attempt to elicit specific communication behaviors from a child while supporting the child to gain a desired response. Directive strategies are most useful for teaching new or complex behaviors that have not as yet emerged in a child's repertoire.

In reality, programs often use varying amounts of each enabling approach in an attempt to be more naturalistic. Of course, the ultimate test of which strategy is most appropriate is the effect it has on the individual child and family (Smith et al., 2002; Yoder

& Stone, 2006a, 2006b). Let's discuss each intervention approach in more detail before we get into the specifics.

Responsive Techniques

Responsive nonsymbolic interaction strategies model a target communication behavior without requiring a response and may include (ASHA, 2008b; Bricker & Cripe, 1992; Hancock & Kaiser, 2006; Warren & Yoder, 1998; Wilcox & Shannon, 1996, 1998)

- Self-talk and parallel talk,
- Following a child's lead,
- Contingent imitation,
- Responding to a child's nonverbal initiations with natural consequences,
- Providing meaningful feedback to a child,
- Expanding a child's behavior with models slightly in advance of the child's, and
- Extending.

Responsive techniques are used within typical, developmentally appropriate, functional, and meaningful routines and experiences dispersed throughout the day in the home and classroom.

In self-talk, an adult describes his or her own actions while engaging in play with a child, such as "Push car. Mommy push car." In contrast, parallel talk provides self-talk for the child as the adult talks about the child's action.

Following a child's lead means allowing the child to establish an interest or attempt to communicate and then responding in an appropriate way, such as naming an object or action that is the focus of attention, commenting on the child's behavior, and if welcome, joining in. For example, if the child reaches for a toy car, the adult might say "Car" or "Maurice has a car" or join in with "Push car to Daddy."

Adults can also be encouraged to use contingent imitation of a child's behavior. Data from typically developing (TD) children suggest that when this occurs there is a substantial likelihood that, in turn, the child will repeat the adult's imitation (Carpenter, Tomasello, & Striano, 2005).

Natural consequences flow from the situation. For example, a gestural request for a cookie might be followed by handing one to the child when possible or replying, "Yes, you want cookie. Eat banana, then cookie."

So far, all of our feedback has been meaningful because it provided a label, described the child's behavior, acquiesced to a request, or replied in another way. A nonmeaningful consequence would be either an off-topic comment or a stock phrase, such as "Good talking." Personally, I consider "Good talking" or similar phrases to break the link of conversational exchanges.

Expansions, which primarily occur following verbal behaviors, may also be motor, gestural, or vocal. For example, a gestural request in the form of a reach might be followed by an adult gesture-verbal response such as "Want juice." In contrast, extensions are replies that build on an action or utterance by providing additional information. For example, if the child reaches, the adult might respond with both expansion and extension, as in "Want cookie. [Expansion] Sierra likes cookies and milk. [Extension]."

Language models should be simplified and at a level slightly above the child's production, including expansions or slightly more mature versions of a child's previous utterance. Providing language input that slightly leads a child's language is called teaching within a child's *zone of proximal development*, something we discussed in dynamic assessment in Chapter 5. In short, we learn best if what we are learning is close to what we already know.

In order to use daily routines and everyday activities as a context for embedded instruction, an SLP can

- Identify the sources of learning opportunities that regularly occur in family and community life;
- Select, in collaboration with the parents and caregivers, desired levels of participation and desired communication by the child in these daily activities;

- Identify and plan motivational aspects of these routines and the child's interests within each; and
- Identify facilitative techniques that can be used to maximize the learning opportunity.

Evidence-based practice demonstrates that (Dunst, Hamby, Trivette, Raab, & Bruder, 2000; Raab, 2005; Raab & Dunst, 2004)

- A child's interest-based involvement in learning is associated with more positive and less negative child behavior, and
- Parent-identified child interests are associated with the largest child benefits.

These data support a family's input in identifying their child's preferred activities and materials to be used in intervention.

Responsive intervention strategies have been credited with modest gains in cognitive, communication, and socioemotional functioning in children with ASD and other developmental disabilities (Mahoney & Perales, 2005). In part, children's improvements are related to increases in parental responsiveness. Similarly, children who have not yet demonstrated productive, intentional nonverbal communication make significant gains in intentional nonverbal and symbolic communication when parents are trained to respond to their children's communication behavior and to prompt and cue more complex behaviors.

Directive Techniques

Directive interaction approaches include several adult-directed didactic teaching strategies, such as variations of a *prompt* or *prompt-cue technique*. We discussed these adult-mediated techniques in Chapter 5, under dynamic assessment. In short, these techniques come in the form of assistance or help that is provided to the child to facilitate an adult-desired response.

Prompts should be as natural as possible and occur throughout the day in the child's natural environments. A flexible technique, prompts may be planned and embedded in both typical routines and play or may be specific to a situation, such as a prompt for a treat at snack time. Prompts are individualized based on the child's needs and the scope of instruction.

In general, these directive techniques encourage a child to respond when his or her response is not spontaneous. To forestall the child's dependence, the SLP can

- Implement the procedures systematically through adults in the child's everyday environment,
- Provide only as much prompting as is necessary to elicit the behavior from the child,
- Fade prompting as the child becomes more independent,
- Plan for increased initiations by the child, and
- Design generalization opportunities in collaboration with the family and others who interact regularly with the child.

While cautiously optimistic about the results, we must acknowledge that prompt-cue strategies frequently fail to generalize to more functional interactive environments. For this reason, many SLPs prefer a blended or hybrid social interactive approach based on mother-child interactions involving TD children and similar to what you learned in your language acquisition course.

Blended Techniques

Blended responsive and directive interaction strategies or hybrid approaches heavily emphasize arranging the environment to promote communication in natural environments. Based on my experience as a clinician, hybrid or functional approaches, emphasized throughout this text, are my method of choice. Depending on the child and family, these more naturalistic language techniques may be used as the primary intervention, as an adjunct to more directive teaching, or as a generalization strategy (ASHA, 2008b).

During intervention, communication environments can be adapted in ways that support a child's early communication, such as encouraging more individuals to converse with the child, adding interesting materials and making them available to the child, and creating comfortable physical conditions. Although we must not neglect a child's safety, the environment should pose challenges that create a need and desire for communication. A variety of techniques might include, but are not limited to, the following:

- *Environmental sabotage.* Environmental sabotage involves manipulating the environment in such a way that a child's access to a desired object or activity is prohibited, thus creating an opportunity for communication. The partner can take actions to challenge a child, such as standing in the child's way, or remove elements, such as treats before snack time is complete. Care must be taken not to frustrate children when implementing this procedure.
- *Setting up communication opportunities.* Our goal is to encourage expression, play, engagement, and independence. Opportunities can range from creating situations to encourage requests for food, objects, or help to situations to encourage negotiation, refusal, or protesting.
- *Providing choices.* Choice-making is one of the earliest and most critical aspects of communication. Provide continuous opportunities for choice-making throughout the day, from snacks to objects or activities. Preferred and nonpreferred activities can be interspersed to encourage choice-making.
- *Waiting and listening.* Adults can encourage a child to initiate interaction by waiting expectantly, using a slow pace that allows lots of time for initiation, and listening to allow time to complete a message. This method works well in situations in which a child needs assistance that is withheld while the adult waits. For example, the adult might not supply all the items needed for a particular task, such as no plastic knives for cutting fruit or missing puzzle pieces.
- *Changing a routine.* Omitting or incorrectly performing a familiar or necessary step in an activity or routine is likely to get a response. Once a child has learned a routine or a predictable turn-taking activity, he or she anticipates what will come next, so changes elicit responses from the child.
- *Missing a child's turn.* At snack time, this one is sure to get a response. It also works well in games or sharing activities.
- *Violating an object function.* If a child knows an object's "purpose," he may become agitated enough by your wearing gloves on your feet to communicate this to you.
- *Time delay or waiting.* Use these at critical moments during natural routines to encourage spontaneous communication.
- *Interrupting behavior chains.* Mentioned previously, behavior chain interruption involves removing a needed object or ceasing the activity and awaiting or prompting a response to continue.

If the child produces some form of communication, the adult can accept it and respond in a manner that encourages more communication or attempt to modify that communicative behavior into more conventional communication.

Naturalistic approaches. There is a large body of evidence-based support for using naturalistic teaching methods across the day in different settings with a range of intervention agents. Teaching parents, teachers, siblings, and peers to implement naturalistic intervention seems to be an efficient strategy for promoting both learning and the use of new communication skills in everyday social contexts.

Examples of more naturalistic approaches include (ASHA, 2008b)

- Focused stimulation,
- Vertical structuring,
- Prelinguistic milieu teaching (PMT),

- ■ Responsive education/prelinguistic milieu training (RE/PMT), and
- ■ Enhanced milieu teaching.

Let's explore each of these briefly.
Focused stimulation includes

- ■ Arranging the situation to encourage a child to produce communication behaviors, and
- ■ Providing a very high density of models of the target forms within a meaningful communicative context, usually play.

Although a response by the child is not required during focused stimulation, it can still be encouraged and prompted. For example, while rolling a ball back and forth, you might repeat "Push ball" and gesture push when requesting the ball and describing the child's action. The child's pushing gesture can become a gestural request in response to "What next?" or "What do you want?"

Vertical structuring is more appropriate for children using symbols and is a version of expansion in which the adult responds to the child's incomplete utterance with a contingent question, which is used by the adult to build a longer response. For example, if the child requests something with a requesting gesture, the adult might respond, "Want. What do you want?" When the child indicates an object, such as a plush bunny, the adult responds, "Want bunny." In other words, the adult takes the pieces and expands them into a more complete utterance. The child is not required to imitate this expansion. The resulting structure—e.g., *Want bunny*—provides a model for the child of her or his own intended utterances in a more mature form. As you can see from the format, vertical structuring is primarily designed to target early developing language forms but can be used with gestures and signs, along with other augmentative and alternative communication (AAC). Let's look more closely at milieu teaching, an example of a blended functional approach.

Milieu teaching. Milieu teaching is a conversation-based approach to early language intervention using a child's interests and initiations as opportunities to model and prompt language use in everyday contexts. In brief, adults

- ■ Arrange the environment to increase the likelihood that the child will initiate communication,
- ■ Respond to the child's initiations with prompts to elaborate in a manner consistent with the child's targeted skills, and
- ■ Functionally reinforce the child's communicative attempts.

Functional reinforcement may include providing access to requested objects, continuing adult interaction, and providing feedback in the form of expansions or confirmations for the child's communication attempts. These approaches enable the adult to use imitation, prompting, and cueing during the course of naturalistic activities, which, in turn, show the child how the behaviors work to accomplish his or her communicative ends. Variants of milieu teaching will be discussed in more detail later in the chapter.

Prelinguistic milieu teaching (PMT) is designed for children with very limited or nonexistent symbol use who may even be having difficulties with production of nonlinguistic communicative acts. Embedded within ongoing social interactions in the child's natural environment, PMT directly teaches gestures, vocalizations, and coordinated eye gaze behavior. Not surprisingly, gains made by children are positively related to responsiveness of caregivers.

Responsive education/prelinguistic milieu training (RE/PMT) is a parent-oriented intervention in which parents are taught to comply with and verbally map or "put into words" a child's verbal and nonverbal communication. RE/PMT is effective in changing parental behavior and in increasing overall use of intentional communication by children (Fey et al., 2006; Yoder & Warren (2002). This approach will be discussed in some detail in Chapter 9.

Finally, enhanced milieu teaching combines parental responsiveness and modeling (ASHA, 2008b). These or similar intervention techniques are found in many ECI approaches. Parental responsive interaction strategies include

- Following the child's lead,
- Balancing turns so that neither partner dominates,
- Maintaining the child's topic,
- Modeling appropriate language,
- Matching the child's complexity level,
- Expanding and imitating the child's utterances, and
- Responding to the child's verbal and nonverbal communication.

In practice, these strategies are combined in a naturalistic, play-based intervention approach. Included in these strategies are other milieu techniques such as mand-model, expectant delays, and incidental teaching. Taken as a whole, these components are effective in expanding communication behaviors in young children (Hancock & Kaiser, 2002; Kaiser & Delaney, 2001; Kaiser et al., 2000). Let's explore each briefly.

Mand-model has been shown to be an effective direct language-teaching approach. The adult arranges the physical environment in a way that encourages a child to communicate. For example, some very tasty looking cookies could be placed in a clear plastic jar just out of reach. The adult waits until the child shows interest and then "mands" or requests that the child communicate in some way, as in "What do you want?"

If the child responds with the desired communicative behavior, such as a requesting gesture, he or she is praised and offered an appropriate response, such as obtaining the cookie. If the child does not respond or responds inappropriately, the desired communication behavior is modeled for the child. After modeling, the adult waits a short time for the desired behavior. If a behavior is still not forthcoming, the adult may use a prompt to aid the child.

Expectant delays have been used successfully to cue children to communicate in response to environmental stimuli rather than to verbal prompts. Thus, expectant delays create opportunities and reasons for a child to use communication behaviors that are already in her or his repertoire. The environment is arranged so the child will require assistance.

Expectant delays work best in predictable routines. For example, when playing with a wind-up toy, the adult typically winds it up and then gives it to the child to operate. The routine is broken if the adult does not wind up the toy. Instead, the adult sits near and orients toward the child but remains silent for a predetermined period of time. At the end of that interval, the adult gazes at the child with an expectant facial expression. If the child uses the required communicative behavior, such as a request to wind the toy, the adult responds appropriately and complies with the child's request. If the child does not ask in the expected manner, the adult models the appropriate behavior.

During intervention, parents who routinely anticipate their child's needs and fail to pause so that she or he may request might be helped by recorded or videotaped examples of the opposite behavior. This can be followed by a discussion with the SLP of the benefits of withholding assistance and waiting for the child to initiate. New practices can be role-played as a further learning aid.

Incidental teaching is one of my favorite techniques, which, depending on its form, may include several of the methods described so far. In incidental teaching, everyday events are used as the vehicles for intervention. As mentioned throughout this text, bath time, snack, play, dressing, and the like can all be adapted to support communication intervention. For example, instead of just dumping all the child's floating toys into the tub, the parent can wait or prompt for them to be requested.

Parents are invaluable as sources for incidental teaching ideas. I usually brainstorm with parents to find the best situations in which communication naturally occurs or has the potential to occur. Then, together, we decide the best way to elicit and prompt communication within that situation. The possibilities are endless.

 This video provide an overview of intervention with the nonverbal child.
https://www.youtube.com/watch?v=fmHcdbA0n00

Evidence-Based Practice (EBP)

According to EBP, six treatment strategies have been used successfully to facilitate speech development in young children with developmental disabilities, including children with ASD. These evidence-based strategies for eliciting speech-like vocalizations include (De-Thorne, Johnson, Walder, & Mahurin-Smith, 2009):

- Providing access to AAC
- Minimizing pressure to speak
- Imitating the child
- Using exaggerated intonation and slowed tempo
- Augmenting auditory, visual, tactile, and proprioceptive feedback
- Avoiding emphasis on nonspeech-like articulator movements and instead focusing on functional communication

Let's explore each in detail.

Before we begin, we should note that although these intervention strategies show promise according to evidence-based research, they also represent only those strategies that have been researched. In other words, these are not the only strategies that show promise. We only get answers for the questions we ask.

AAC AND THE PRESSURE TO SPEAK

AAC can facilitate speech development by enhancing children's ability to build relevant semantic and syntactic networks. In addition, voice output devices provide a consistent acoustic model of target sounds and words that children can select as needed (Millar, Light, & Schlosser, 2006). We'll discuss AAC, and more specifically the Picture Exchange Communication System (PECS), in much greater detail later.

AAC may also facilitate speech in part by reducing pressure to speak in the traditional sense. In contrast, high-pressure communication situations can have a negative impact on oral motor performance (Hardy, Mullen, & Martin, 2001). This said, both higher-pressure techniques, such as direct requests for imitation, and lower-pressure strategies, such as modeling, enhance word learning outside the treatment setting to an equal extent (Kouri, 2005).

CONTINGENT IMITATION

Being imitated may teach a child to imitate in turn, a useful strategy in learning to use spoken language (Masur & Eichorst, 2002). When a child sees someone perform a familiar action, the child's *mirror neurons* fire, in turn activating the child's motor neurons. An adult's imitation of a child's speech also triggers mirror neuron firing, thus serving as a form of involuntary rehearsal by the child (Oberman & Ramachandran, 2007). Even if a child does not imitate in turn, focusing on a child's spontaneous activity within the natural environment is likely to

- Be more engaging for the child,
- Facilitate generalization of elicited speech sounds, and
- Simplify the speaking task by using a familiar form to elicit an unfamiliar function, imitation (Velleman, 2006).

Children exposed to imitation demonstrate significant increases in vocalizations over time when compared to children simply invited by an adult to play (Field, Field, Sanders, & Nadel, 2001). In fact, there is a strong correlation between the frequency with which mothers imitate their children and the frequency with which their children imitate.

An adult's imitation of a child might include both verbal and nonverbal actions. SLPs and other adults can imitate a child's spontaneous vocalizations and add meaning by treating them as words. Thus "ba" becomes *ball*. Imitation becomes an opportunity to model the adult form of the word.

Intense contingent imitation by adults, even for brief periods of time, increases a child's social interest, even in those with ASD who have little or no functional speech. This leads to a significant increase of both touching and looking at another person and an increase in imitation by the child (Heimann, Laberg, & Nordøen, 2006).

EXAGGERATED INTONATION AND MODIFIED PROSODY

Exaggerated intonation is a commonly used intervention technique. It is possible that the neural mechanisms involved in processing intonation can be used to "bootstrap" or provide a framework for speech production because of overlapping neural networks (DeThorne et al., 2009). In addition, prosodic features may facilitate speech intelligibility. Even if exaggerated intonation does not help with a child's accuracy or fluency, it may highlight important features of the speech signal, thereby increasing intelligibility. Exaggerated prosody can be used with any meaningful word or phrase, and frequent two-syllable phrases can be presented with exaggerated two-tone patterns.

FEEDBACK

Sensory feedback, especially proprioceptive, plays an important role in establishing new speech behaviors (Clark, Robin, McCullagh, & Schmidt, 2001). Children with speech and language difficulties may be less able to process and use typical sensory feedback than TD children. For production, these children may need augmented sensory input to be able to develop internal models that associate motor movements with their sensory consequences (Brass & Heyes, 2005; Iacoboni, 2005; Iacoboni & Wilson, 2006).

Auditory input may be enhanced with slight amplification through headphones or talking into an echo microphone, a section of PVC pipe, a mailbox, or any chamber that creates an echo to attract a child's interest to the words or sounds. Visual feedback can be promoted by face-to-face interaction, mirror work, and gestures. A puppet with a movable mouth can provide visual input for speech in a less threatening way than being asked to attend directly to an adult (DeThorne et al., 2009). Tactile and proprioceptive feedback might include touch-pressure cues, such as a light tap on the clinician's or child's lips while modeling bilabial plosives (Bleile, 2004). Stimulation brushes and cotton swabs and snack foods have been used in intervention to draw attention to articulator locations.

AVOIDANCE OF NONSPEECH ORAL MOTOR EXERCISES

Lastly, some of the most commonly used oral motor activities include blowing, tongue wagging, and smiling. These exercises are not directly related to speech sound production (Lof, 2006). Studies related to the effectiveness of such nonspeech activities have generally not supported their use for facilitating speech. Instead, evidence supports targeting speech movements per se. Although the same muscles may be used for speech and nonspeech oral motor acts, different muscle fibers may be employed in markedly different ways depending on the task (Iacoboni, 2005; Iacoboni & Wilson, 2006). Lof (2003), who represents the current professional opinion on oral motor exercises, finds that disengaging oral movement from speech has little theoretical or clinical justification as a motor speech intervention.

Getting Started

Now that we have the broad outlines of an intervention program, let's begin. As part of the intervention team, you'll develop a plan for services and supports based on information gathered by team members during the assessment process. Ideally, the plan reflects information about the whole child and the concerns, priorities, and resources of the family. Your communication assessment and analysis will be integrated with that of other team members.

The exact design of intervention tasks and procedures is individualized to reflect the child, the family, and their interactive style and desired level of involvement. In some settings, such as an EI classroom, an SLP may be the only professional or one of only a few professionals on site. In these cases, the SLP or another professional should coordinate with the family and professionals to create a collaborative plan that includes other services being provided to the child and family.

One caution is due here. It can be easy to lose sight of the primary ECI goal of enhancing communication and to spin off into other aspects of development, especially if training in those areas is going well. It is important for the SLP to remember that training eye contact within ECI, for example, is not an end in itself and is important only to the extent that it furthers a child's ability to communicate.

Enhancing Communication

The purpose of ECI is to enhance a family's ability to support and sustain their child's development of effective communication (ASHA 2008b). To do this, the child and family's communication system should be addressed where and as it occurs. Collaboratively, the caregivers and the SLP identify high communication situations or potential situations and ways to create additional contexts in which communication can occur. Within these contexts, the child is encouraged to communicate through a variety of techniques while the adult language facilitators attempt to enhance and expand the child's communication attempts.

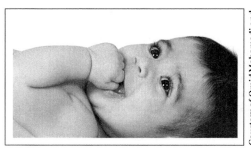

Courtesy of Omid Mohamadi and Mehdi Amiri.

Table 6.1 presents a possible hierarchy of intervention in support of this goal. Let's begin our discussion in the neonatal intensive care unit (NICU) or special care nursery (SCN) and then move to the best environment to set communication in motion.

IN THE NICU OR SCN

One of the initial goals of ECI may be helping the family interpret signals from their preterm infant. Babies let us know when they're ready for stimulation and when they're not, and when they are overstimulated and possibly in distress. Signals fall into three categories:

- Approach signals, which indicate relaxation and readiness to interact or feed, include cooing, smiling, and mouthing
- Coping signals, which signal a desire for stability or the status quo, include sucking a pacifier, holding something, or bracing a leg against something
- Avoidance signals, which express agitation, include finger-splaying, tongue-thrusting, facial grimaces, and later crying

With avoidance signals, infants let caregivers know that they need a change in the level and/or type of stimulation. Parental anxieties can be reduced if an alert SLP helps the family understand the child's signals.

TABLE 6.1 **Possible Hierarchy for Enhancing Presymbolic Communication**

GOAL	TECHNIQUES (IN NO PARTICULAR ORDER)
Establish eye contact with partner's eyes and with objects.	Tempt the child with brightly colored, sound-making objects and bring to your face ("Juan, look at teddy!").
	Move your face into child's central vision.
	Call child's name ("Zack! Zack!").
	Gently turn child's face toward you.
Increase the frequency and spontaneity of eye gaze.	Use objects in which child has expressed an interest. ("Here's your ball!")
	Place looking at object within a requesting routine. ("I see the baby. Where's baby? Want baby?")
	Provide a desired object when the child looks at you. ("Natalia wants brush. Natalia! Oh, Mommy get brush. Brush hair.")
Establish reciprocal routines as a context for communication.	Use contingent imitation.
	Interrupt an established pattern of child behavior with your own, then wait for the child to resume. ("Alyssa dance. All done? Mommy jump.")
	Perform a behavior that the child finds amusing, stop so the child can laugh, then resume. ("Tickle tummy! You laughing? All done. What?")
	Complete an established routine by performing the behavior needed. ("Nico throw ball. That was a big one. Daddy get ball.")
Communicate back and forth with others.	Establish reciprocal play routines through contingent imitation, such as peek-a-boo.
	Hand objects back and forth, add sounds as you do. ("Here's more blocks. Give to Mommy. Here's more.")
	Establish vocal play routines through contingent imitation ("Now Daddy sing like Erik.")
	Play anticipatory games with the child, such as "I'm gonna get you."
Increase the frequency of nonverbal vocalizations.	When child vocalizes while focused on an object or event, use the name of the referent in reply and interact with the object and the child
	Child: *Buh.*
	Adult: *Ball. Roll ball.*
	In sound-making play, respond with sounds in the child's vocal repertoire and introduce new ones.
	In sound-making play, model sounds and syllable structures that approximate real words, as in /bɔ/ for *ball.*
	Imitate child vocalizations and "stretch" them beyond the current repertoire of sounds and syllable structures.
	Child: *Beebee*
	Adult: *Beebee . . . Baby*
	Use vocal contingent imitation.

continued

TABLE 6.1   **Possible Hierarchy for Enhancing Presymbolic Communication** (*continued*)

GOAL	TECHNIQUES (IN NO PARTICULAR ORDER)
Establish communicative intent with movements, sound, and gestures.	Create a need to communicate within a routine, such as request to roll the ball within a ball rolling routine.
	Provide child with a desired object when the child uses a gesture or equivalent behavior.
	Ask "What do you want?"
	Pretend to be confused, "Who wants a cookie?"
	Ask child to be more specific by requesting more information, such as "Show me what you want" or "Which one do you want?"
	Tell the child to gesture, as in "Show it to me."
	Model a gesture, as in pointing while saying "Look at doggie!"
	Respond to all gestural-vocal communication.
Increase frequency, spontaneity, and range of nonconventional and conventional gestures.	Wait expectantly for the entire message from the child; try not to finish it for the child.
	Child runs to door.
	Adult: *What?*
	Child points.
	Adult: *Yes, I see kitty.*
	Verbally model the message for the child.
	Child pushes away cup.
	Adult: *All done juice.*
	Comply with the child's expressed intention.

Sources: Owens, 1982; Rossetti, 2001; Warren et al., 2006.

Sometimes the obvious or typical behavior is counterindicated with preemies. For example, we instinctively pat or rock an infant who is in distress and crying. A newborn preterm infant may become distressed from too much stimulation and our patting or rocking may add to the overstimulation. Likewise, rocking a child while singing may be too much stimulation for a premature infant.

The SLP can help parents to increase stimulation gradually as the child develops the ability to tolerate more and more. This can help to decrease parent feelings of helplessness or failure.

Infants in the NICU are touched, prodded, and poked continuously by the nursing staff in the course of their duties. A child may develop an aversion to touch, which is an early form of parent-child communication. Here again, the SLP can help parents to increase pleasurable touching gradually as a child's tolerance increases.

Parents can also sequence stimulation rather than heaping it on all at once. For example, instead of talking while massaging a preemie's limbs, a parent might tell the infant what is about to happen and then remain silent while the massage takes place. Gradually, soft humming may be introduced, then soft singing, and finally whispering and talking.

In addition, the SLP can help to enhance nursing staff interactions with a newborn through consultation and in-service training. Figure 6.1 presents a list of suggested behaviors for enhancing the communication with both infants and caregivers.

FIGURE 6.1 Enhancing the Communication in the NICU or SCN

Intervention with Caregivers/Parents

Explain roles of all persons working in the NICU/SCN and be a source of information.

Be an advocate for parental rights and needs.

Help parents

- Identify their infant's changing states,
- Adapt to their infant's changing condition, and
- Respond to early attempts by the child to notice and respond the environment.

Teach parents early feeding and swallowing techniques to use with their child.

Assist parents to establish early bonding and attachment.

Explain the importance of early communication and continued communication development.

Answer questions about the child's long-term communication development.

Assist with discharge planning and transition to home and be a resource for community services if needed.

Demonstrate appropriate ways to communicate with their infant.

Intervention with the Infant

Assist in oral/motor feeding and monitor nutritional issues.

Demonstrate appropriate positioning and handling.

Monitor the effect of speech and attention on the infant's state.

Guide socio-communicative interaction of the child and caregivers.

Provide appropriate visual, auditory, tactile, and vestibular-kinesthetic stimulation.

Provide appropriate communication intervention services.

Intervention with the Staff

Increase awareness of the NICU/SCN environment (noise, touch, light, procedures).

Explain communication development and demonstrate how to respond to infant behaviors.

Identify infant signals upon which communication can be built.

Help staff maintain developmentally appropriate interactions with infants.

Help staff enhance the role of caregiver/parents.

Source: Information from Rossetti, 2001.

I would be doing you a disservice if I didn't add a word of caution here. Intensive care is what it says it is. Infants are often medically fragile and their conditions are volatile, meaning they can change in a flash. In this type of environment, passions among the professional staff run high, so collaboration is essential. In addition, skills in aiding feeding and swallowing in infants are critical because compromising an infant's breathing can mean the difference between life and death. The NICU is not for everyone.

 The NICU or SCN is not for everyone. If you want to take a peek, you might be interested in this video from inside a newborn intensive care unit.
https://www.youtube.com/watch?v=OP5104pwRfl

ESTABLISHING EARLY COMMUNICATION

It should be obvious from your language development course, this text, and your own experience that a newborn will not demonstrate intentional communication for several months. This does not stop parents and caregivers from interacting with the infant or interpreting unintentional communication behavior. An infant glance might signal interest, a reach means "I want," and crying signals distress. With a preterm or medically fragile infant, parents may be unsure how to respond to their child. As an SLP, you can assist by commenting on these behaviors and responding appropriately. Routines such as changing and feeding and, after a few months, turn-taking activities such as early social games, will help an infant feel secure and begin to interact more. Look for signals such as becoming excited when seeing a nursing bottle or anticipating being picked up. Add sound-making, but don't expect imitation. Remember that a TD infant does not imitate until around 6 months of age.

Some children, even those approaching age 1 or older, will seemingly have no functional communication system. Others will exhibit little in an assessment that suggests even a need to communicate. For still others, parents or teachers may report that the child doesn't communicate. In these cases, the ECI team will want to explore establishing an initial communication system.

Children learn early to associate a behavior with an outcome. If the infant cries, someone comes. The crying is not a planned means to this end. That comes later. But an infant can learn a very general rule that "My behavior makes things happen even when that's not my goal." You may recall that a child learns early about these *stimulus-response bonds*. Let's use this naturally occurring behavior to build an initial communication system.

One way to accomplish initial communication is through the use of a technique called behavior chain interruption, in which a favorable activity, such as rocking together, listening to music, or eating a treat, is interrupted and does not resume until the child signals for this to happen. An adult request that requires the child to insert another behavior into the sequence enriches this ongoing interactional sequence (Carter & Grunsell, 2001).

Let me illustrate behavior chain interruption with an example. One Thanksgiving not long ago, I was sitting on the floor with my then almost 2-year-old grandson Dakota who, at the time, had few easily recognizable communication behaviors. I was feeding him miniscule amounts of pumpkin pie on a plastic spoon. That's the *behavior chain*. He obviously loved the taste. After several miniscule tastes, I stopped feeding him (*interruption*) and waited until he began to become agitated. That was a signal that he wanted more, so I took his arm and physically touched my hand as I said "More." I followed this with another small taste of pie. Then I waited again. He fussed some more, and I prompted again. After several trials, he got the idea. It was extremely basic, but we had a primitive communication system based on nonconventional gesturing. He could now request more, albeit in a primitive manner, by touching my hand. It's a beginning.

The key is finding something that a child enjoys enough to want it to continue. If Dakota had disliked pumpkin pie, I would have been at a dead end. From here, we can branch out to requesting other desired objects or actions and to having him initiate the request rather than responding to my prompt for "More."

Let's step back and generalize this discussion a bit, focusing on the technique itself. Assume that a child's favored activity is rocking while cradled by an adult.

- *Behavior chain*. I might rock the child while talking about rocking.
- *Interruption*. I stop and wait.
- *Signal*. If the child enjoys the activity, then he or she will likely signal to continue by pushing side to side.
- *Prompt*. At that point, I prompt a signal that differs from the rocking motion and can be generalized as a request to continue other behaviors, such as eating or listening to music. If I had been satisfied with just sideways pushing, then it might generalize to become the child's request to continue with any object or action. This is an odd gesture if the request is for more pudding or music. In other words, I want to train a request that is separate from any one behavior and generalizable to other types of requests.
- *Response*. Once the child imitates my signal, the behavior continues.
- *Generalization*. When the child can reliably signal "More" for continued rocking, I would attempt to have the child generalize this request with some other desired object or action.

I once worked with a 22-year-old man with profound intellectual disability (ID). He had severe cerebral palsy (CP) and no obvious communication system. Using a small amount of vanilla pudding, he and I were able to set up a requesting system in less than two hours using only his eyes. That may not seem like much until you look at it from his perspective. For 22 years, this young man had no way to influence his world except to refuse to cooperate. He has now turned that completely around and is able to influence his world in a proactive positive way. In a similar situation, using rocking with a 14-year-old boy, we established communication in 20 seconds. This is not because I'm a great therapist. It is because of the strength of his being able to influence his environment.

One note of caution is needed. The technique, like most intervention techniques in ECI, does not work with every child. I have had my share of spectacular failures, including one instructional demonstration before a roomful of other SLPs. Without going into the grim details, suffice it to say that I needed to go to the hospital for a tetanus booster when I was finished. See, I did warn you that there was no one-size-fits-all methodology!

FUNCTIONAL EQUIVALENCE AND CHALLENGING BEHAVIORS

When an SLP attempts to replace or modify a challenging behavior that she or he believes has a communicative function, the result is that the child now has two or more behaviors, the original and the one being trained. The behaviors are said to be *functionally equivalent*. In this situation, the child is likely to choose the response that he or she perceives to be most efficient in procuring or maintaining reinforcement. The communication option that results in the greatest reinforcement for the least amount of work is likely to be the more frequently used one. As SLPs, our role is to figure out how to make the acceptable or replacement behavior the child's more desirable option.

Here, the beauty of the team approach is evident. The team's behavior specialist can help the SLP and family design and implement a behavioral plan.

Before we can attempt to replace or modify communication behavior, we need to know whether or not the current behavior has a function or a purpose. It's critical that we understand the underlying message (Bopp, Brown, & Mirenda, 2004). A method for doing this was discussed in Chapter 5.

Once the function has been identified, the challenge becomes teaching new or modified communicative forms to better express this existing function. For example, with a child who communicates "More juice" by throwing her cup, the SLP will attempt to establish a more socially acceptable alternative, such as reaching toward the juice container, holding her cup aloft, or signing "More."

In combination, the five factors mentioned in Chapter 4—response effort, schedule of reinforcement, immediacy of reinforcement, quality of reinforcement, and history of punishment—will determine which behaviors occur in any particular situation. For example, the amount of physical or response effort required to produce the alternative behavior should be equal to or less than that of the older one (Richman, Wacker, & Winborn, 2001). All five factors should be considered when selecting which new behavior to teach a child and which responses to teach the communication partners.

Dealing with challenging behaviors is a multistep process involving the entire ECI team, especially parents (Johnston, Reichle, & Evans, 2004). The process includes

- Agreeing on the need to replace the present behavior,
- Conducting a functional behavioral assessment,
- Defining a communicative behavior more efficient than the current one,
- Developing a strategy to sufficiently reinforce approximations of the new alternative in the presence of stimuli that evoke the current behavior,
- Minimizing reinforcement for the current behavior while maximizing it for the new alternative, and
- Training all team members for consistent responding.

As you may recall, a functional behavior assessment, discussed in Chapter 5, is a systematic data collection process using a variety of techniques (Lucyshyn, Kayser, Irvin, & Blumberg, 2002). The purpose of the assessment is to collect information about what precedes, influences, and maintains the behavior. Ideally, the end result is the development of one or more hypotheses describing variables that affect the behavior. The hypotheses can be tested by manipulating what precedes and follows the behavior and observing the results.

When a form of communication already exists and an SLP determines that another method is possible, such as a verbalization replacing a vocalization or an acceptable behavior replacing a challenging one, the newly learned form and the original form share the same function. Specific types of intervention are needed to make the new form more desirable for the child than the one being replaced.

Intervention with Functional Equivalence

Once the underlying communicative purpose of the behavior is understood, intervention planning and implementation can begin in order to replace it with a more acceptable one. Ideally, the challenging behavior decreases as the functionally equivalent communication behavior increases. Even with nonchallenging or appropriate but immature forms of communication, issues around response equivalence are still important. For example, children with very limited expressive communication may have functionally equivalent AAC and gestural messages with the same intent.

Of upmost importance is a *response match* between the old behavior and the new communicative behavior. In other words, the communicative function of the behavior identified during the assessment and of the new alternative behavior must be the same. When an older behavior has more than one function, the equivalents for all functions may need to be taught before the behavior decreases significantly (Kennedy, Meyer, Knowles, & Shulka, 2000). For example, if self-injurious behavior is used both to protest and to attract attention, alternatives for both must be sought.

It is important to build on skills that are already in the child's repertoire and to teach throughout the day, with a variety of people, and within a variety of natural routines and environments. For example, if the child already makes eye contact and can shift his or her gaze, or if the child uses pictures to communicate in some situations, these could be used as replacement behaviors.

The best time to teach is when the child is not exhibiting challenging behavior. If, for example, the child requests at other times and only exhibits challenging behaviors at snack time, training should begin in the nonchallenging behavior settings while ignoring the challenging behavior or attempting to prompt the replacement behavior during snack.

The alternative can be modeled by the SLP or caregiver and then prompted from the child in the form of an imitation. If the child does not imitate, he or she can be physically assisted to perform the communicative behavior. This should be accompanied by a verbalization by the adult, such as "Want X," which adds meaning to the action.

Ideally, a prompt or cue will elicit the desired behavior, so selecting the right prompt to match both the learner and the behavior being taught is very important (Bopp et al., 2004). Once the behavior is learned, which means that it consistently occurs following the cue, the intensity of the cue is reduced or faded over time.

The goal of fading is elimination of the prompt entirely, enabling the child to perform the behavior independently. For example, if I want the child to request independently, I need to fade the cue "What do you want?" Otherwise, the child will only request in response to my question. She doesn't have any control over her environment if she is dependent on my prompt. Sometimes fading is as simple as touching a child's arm rather than physically manipulating her hands to form a sign or reducing the loudness of a verbal prompt to a whisper. In the final step, all prompting would be removed.

In order for two behaviors to be equivalent, they must result in the same response. Communication partners need to respond appropriately to the new alternative. Failure to do so may strengthen the older behavior, especially if it still results in the desired caregiver response. Even a short delay between a child's presenting the new alternative and a reinforcing response may result in the child's reverting to the original behavior. One slip—a classroom aide is tired and gives in to cup throwing—can undo days and days of intervention with the alternative.

Reinforcement for the replacement behavior should equal or exceed that for the challenging behavior. A nonresponse to the challenging behavior should discourage its use by making it no longer effective.

Alternative behaviors that require high effort by a child will not be sustained unless they are strongly reinforced by all individuals in the child's environment. It should be obvious that just as there are several factors that have supported the unacceptable behavior by the child, similar factors have supported the family's response. Family members have been reinforced in the past, possibly by ending the behavioral outburst, for responding as they did in the past. In other words, response equivalence is working here too.

The team should evaluate the effectiveness of the plan on an ongoing basis and be prepared to make changes as needed. Of interest are an increase in the use of the replacement behavior and a decrease of the previous one, along with changes in the child's overall social and behavioral competence, and generalization of the new behavior to other contexts.

Positive behavior support. When working with children who exhibit severe challenging or self-injurious behavior, practitioners may want to use a method called positive behavior support (PBS) to help a child acquire new communication skills (Buschbacher & Fox, 2003; Fox, Dunlap, & Buschbacher, 2000; Horner, 2000; National Research Council, 2001). PBS attempts to expand a child's behavior repertoire by supporting acceptable behaviors and by redesigning the child's living environment to minimize problem behavior (Carr et al., 2002). PBS seeks to reduce the problem behavior while creating opportunities for more appropriate behaviors to emerge.

The goals of PBS are

- To reduce a child's challenging behavior,
- To enhance a child's more conventional communication skills, and
- To provide a child's caregivers with skills for continuing to support the child's behavioral development.

Ideally, these goals would be addressed across multiple routines and activities within a child's natural environment.

Let's look at an example of PBS. In one study, a 3-year-old child with ASD became aggressive during mealtime (Koegel, Steibel, & Koegel, 1998). Analysis indicated that the aggression was triggered by a combination of factors, including the child's baby sister making noise on a metal high chair tray, the crying of the baby sister, and the mother's lack of attention as she prepared the children's meals. The child with ASD engaged in aggression such as hitting, yelling, and pinching her 8-month-old sibling. Intervention included

- Substituting a plastic high chair tray to reduce noise;
- Teaching the child with ASD to respond to the crying by saying, "(Baby's name) needs help" or "(Baby's name) is talking," or providing a pacifier that the preschooler could offer her infant sister; and
- Having the mother prepare the meal before bringing both children to the table.

Implementation resulted in both reduction of aggression and an increase in the spontaneous use of acceptable behavior.

As those who know the child best, the family is vital to the success of PBS (Fox et al., 2000). Without family participation, intervention strategies used in school or another intervention setting are less likely to generalize to the home and community. In one intervention, I was successful in modifying a child's behavior in the classroom, but lacking parental support, I was unsuccessful in changing it at home.

The team develops a comprehensive behavior support plan. The plan should

- Use multiple intervention strategies,
- Be applied throughout the day in multiple contexts, and
- Be consistent with the values and resources of the child and the persons providing the support.

The goal is to create conditions that make the problem behavior unnecessary and ineffective. The key elements of a support plan are presented in Figure 6.2.

FIGURE 6.2 **Elements of a Positive Behavioral Support Plan**

- Form a hypothesis about the behavior that includes the context of what comes before and after the behavior and the possible communicative function of the behavior.
- Devise long-term support strategies to assist the child's overall social/communication interaction.
- Manipulate what occurs prior to the behavior to reduce the likelihood that the behavior will occur.
- Devise strategies that fit the natural routines and structure of the home and classroom.
- Replace the current behavior with acceptable, effective alternative forms of communication, which should decrease the original behavior.
- Outline carefully how others should respond to the alternative forms of communication.
- Stress that others should not respond to the original challenging behavior.

Source: Information from Buschbacher & Fox, 2003.

As you might imagine, the training requires that the team develop a systematic intervention plan. The plan must "fit" the personal, cultural, and structural values and contexts of the child, family, and classroom. In this way, those persons implementing the plan will be comfortable doing so. If teachers and family members are uncomfortable or find the intervention cumbersome or objectionable, they are unlikely to implement it consistently or support it wholeheartedly.

A note on the use of punishment. Behavior change can occur through a combination of ignoring the child's old behavior and prompting the new communicative one. Unfortunately, some self-injurious challenging behaviors are too severe to be ignored and must be punished to protect the child from injury. We simply cannot allow children to continue to bang their heads or gouge their eyes. At the same time, the team should be reinforcing incompatible behaviors.

I hesitate to even discuss punishment, but we should at least mention it. I've had to use it occasionally in severe cases of self-abuse, but it is my last resort and my least favorite methodology. The term *punishment* has a negative connotation, but in our discussion I'm using it to mean simply *a behavioral consequence that decreases a behavior.*

In your everyday life, "punishment" may be as simple as someone saying, "I appreciate the coffee, but next time could you not add so much sugar." The consequence is that you'll add less. It worked!

Punishment, if used, need not be harsh and often takes the form of a simple time-out. During this period, there is no opportunity to be reinforced (Fisher, Thompson, Hagopian, Bowman, & Krug, 2000; Peck Peterson, Derby, Harding, Weddle, & Barretto, 2002; Perry & Fisher, 2001). This may sound more terrible than in actuality. For example, one child with whom I worked would hit his head with his fist. Teachers responded with a verbal reprimand "No hit" and placed him in time-out, which meant he had to sit away from the class while his hands were restrained so he would not hit himself. Meanwhile, he could see the other children playing.

As it turned out, for this child the hitting behavior was a form of request. When the time-out ended and after a very short pause, he was permitted to request desired objects with an alternative method.

Possible punishments may include

- Time-out
- Overcorrection, or providing assistance to a child to repeat a specific action several times in a row, such as following the command "Hands down";
- Response cost, which is the removal of a preferred action or item.

SLPs and caregivers must be extremely careful in the use of punishment, and decisions to use this method of behavior change must be weighed carefully by the entire EI team, including the behavioral specialist. One potential problem is that there is no way to control the consequences of punishment. I recall a child who had been hitting himself. He was punished and then began to bite himself.

Let's go back to that cup of sweet coffee for a moment. One unintended consequence may be that you decide never to get coffee for this ingrate again. Likewise, a well-intended aide or teacher can become a *punisher* in the child's eyes. And how would you treat a punisher? You'd avoid interacting with that person. This is not the best of circumstances for encouraging communication.

Punishment is a last resort, only to be used

- When the problem behavior can cause physical harm to the child or others,
- After less intrusive consequences have been shown to be ineffective,
- After careful discussion and agreement by the entire EI team, and
- Following training by all team members who interact with the child.

To be maximally effective, either punishment or ignoring of the behavior must be paired with reinforcement of the new alternative behavior. Ignore the tantrum or punish the self-injurious behavior and reinforce an acceptable alternative.

Interfering Behaviors: Self-Stimulation

Some children engage in persistent and seemingly meaningless behaviors such as rocking, grinding their teeth, spinning objects, flapping their hands, or making sounds. I've worked with children who did all of these. At the very least, these behaviors, collectively called *self-stimulation*, provide some level of perceptual input for the child.

For whatever reason, self-stimulation is extremely reinforcing to the child. Possibly rocking provides vestibular stimulation and hand-flapping stimulates the visual cortex. We honestly don't know.

Whatever the pleasurable consequence for a child, self-stimulation interferes with learning. In order to enable the child to focus elsewhere, self-stimulation should be reduced.

Traditionally, self-stimulation has been punished. Increasingly, professionals are realizing that the power of self-stimulation can be used to teach other behaviors. This change mirrors the changing attitude toward echolalia, which was previously viewed as an interfering behavior and is now thought in some cases to signal agreement or is used to aid receptive processing.

If a child is not allowed to self-stimulate in the classroom or at home, as is often the case, then the SLP, with team approval, can permit self-stimulation to occur but only after the child complies with SLP desires. For example, if a child flaps his hands, the teacher may restrict him for doing so. The teacher may prompt compliance by saying "Hands down."

When I sit with the same child, I would begin with that command. I might then ask the child to do something more communicative, such as focus on a toy or request a snack. When the child complies, I would praise the child, play briefly with the toy or give a tiny portion of the snack, and allow the child to self-stimulate for a very short period of time. The self-stimulation always occurs last. In this way, the reinforcing power of self-stimulation is gradually transferred to the verbal praise.

In sequence, the intervention may look as follows:

- SLP says "Hands down" and may prompt this with a hand over the child's.
- SLP holds up a toy bear and says "Where's Teddy?"
- Child looks or points.
- SLP makes the bear dance and says "Yes, you found the bear!"
- SLP releases the child's hands.

Some SLPs worry that through this process self-stimulation will be reinforced. This is incorrect. We are using self-stimulation as a reinforcer, not reinforcing self-stimulation itself. Once the SLP has taught the child several different behaviors, the need for self-stimulation may decrease. Although it may not disappear, it has helped us get past a hurdle in intervention. As with every methodology in ECI, the SLP will need to individualize the approach and collaborate with team members.

I once worked with a 3-year-old child who rocked incessantly. Nothing seemed to penetrate. The team decided to begin punishing the child with time out for engaging in this self-stimulation while reinforcing him for sitting still and focusing.

We had a large rocking platform in the room. After conferring with the team, I decided to use the platform because it could conceivably give him similar stimulation but it differed from self-rocking. I began by drawing the child's attention to my face. I quickly moved to interesting toys near my face. If he looked, we would rock on the platform and play with the toy. When I was able to have the child attend to toys, we began to learn to play with them, and the need for the platform disappeared, as did his self-rocking. My voice and the toys had become sufficiently reinforcing.

Another child was being punished for hand-flapping by both the teacher and the classroom aide, who would place their hands over his. After working with me, he learned that I would let him hand-flap when he performed as I asked. He would see me looking his way or approaching him, and he would instantly respond by putting his hands in his lap. As with the other boy described, this child and I worked on expanding his repertoire of play with toys. Although he still tried to sneak in a hand-flap whenever he could, he was much more responsive to others and to objects. He began to develop some rudimentary exploration and play skills.

ESTABLISHING GESTURES

Learning to effectively influence people's actions is one of the most powerful lessons a child learns about communication. The most basic communication between a parent and child is physical, such as a child's movements, and through this young children come to understand the communicative potential of their own body (Cress, 2001, 2002). Successful communication through other means, such as signs or words, implies experience with earlier physical means.

Teaching gestures has two goals. The first is to enhance communication with a new mode of interaction. Second, the intentions established through gestures will be later used as the vehicle within which to train single words or symbols.

Gestures fulfill multiple communication functions. An SLP may need to establish the function prior to or at the same time as she teaches the gesture. The following discussion will focus on specific functions and gestures. Again, the SLP will need to individualize the teaching of gestures. The targets will vary with each child's needs and ability.

While there are several ways to think of gestures, developmentally gestures move from proximal to more conventional distal types. Proximal gestures include

- Touching an object with the hand
- Giving an object to an adult
- Reaching for an object
- Moving an object toward an adult
- Pantomiming an action

In proximal gestures, hand movements are highly contextual. More conventional distal gestures include

- Headshaking
- Waving
- Pointing to a distant object or action
- Requesting by reaching for a distant object
- Turning the palm up to signal "Give me"

If a child is not producing any gestures, early proximal gestures could become a target of intervention (Crais, Watson, & Baranek, 2009). Natural movements, such as reaching for an object, can be treated as a request or a signal of interest. Ideally, SLPs help establish a strong base of gestures and other means to communicate intentionally before moving to either representational gestures or joint referencing.

Early games of back-and-forth turn-taking with objects such as a ball can be a fun way to help develop the idea of sharing an object and drawing attention to it. Pulling objects or toys from a bag or box can be a way to share attention. Later, the same type of activity could be performed but with objects that require an adult to manipulate, to help find missing pieces, or to repair broken parts.

For a child who only uses contact gestures, the team may consider early distal gestures, such as reaching to pick something up, as targets for intervention. The typical developmental progression is for requesting to precede pointing. In addition, reaching to signal a request is relatively easy to teach.

For a child who is using some early deictic gestures but no representational ones, social games that include these types of gestures, such as peek-a-boo or pat-a-cake, may be appropriate. In addition, targeting early functional play acts, such as stirring or drinking, through modeling and social play may enhance the child's play as well as the use of representational gestures.

I worked with a child and we often played peek-a-boo. For whatever reason, hands over the face became her greeting whenever I appeared. I treated the gesture as a greeting and a request to play the game. Gradually, I introduced a new form of greeting. We now had two communication intentions.

The more we can incorporate behaviors that are already present in a child's repertoire, the easier the learning task. Enhanced natural gestures (ENGs) are intentional behaviors that are present in a child's motor repertoire or can be easily taught based on a child's motor skills and are easily recognizable and interpretable. Distal in nature, ENGs do not require physical contact with entities or interactional partners. Examples of ENGs (Calculator, 2002) include:

- Reaching for an object to signal "I want it,"
- Pushing away with the hand to communicate "I don't want to eat that,"
- Stroking sideways with the hand to indicate "I want to pet the dog,"
- Tapping the lips to signal "I want to eat,"
- Touching the door handle to indicate "I want to go out," and
- Rocking back and forth to communicate "Push the swing."

You may have noticed that some of these gestures are similar to the signals that could have been used in behavior chain interruption.

Some children will have difficulty learning gestures because they do not typically use adults as models for their behavior. This may be one of those places in training where the SLP would want to teach motor imitation as a prerequisite skill. More will be said about these prerequisite skills later in the chapter.

In a seeming paradox, once a child begins to produce intentional communicative behaviors, parents tend to reduce their response to all behaviors. Instead, they prompt for more initiation from their child. Even when a child's behavior is intentional, parents tend to continue to take responsibility for initiating and maintaining conversations (Cress, 2002). It's an unintended consequence to which we should be alert. Gestures need to be treated as meaningful communication. Let's look at how we might teach specific early intentions through gestures.

Requesting

Requesting is one of the easiest gestures to teach because it is a natural extension of reaching and has a naturally reinforcing consequence, the receipt of whatever is requested. The behavior chain interruption techniques mentioned previously can be used within well-established turn-taking routines, such as rolling a ball or pushing a toy car back and forth. Keep in mind, however, that this type of requesting is for something to continue, not begin. We can't neglect initiating requesting.

If a child already reaches for desired items, these entities can be used in request training by placing them just out of reach and encouraging the child to request with "What want?" or "What do you want?" and possibly providing a model. One mistake adults sometimes make is to take an object a child has just reached for and obtained and then immediately place it out of reach and try to train a requesting gesture. This process may frustrate the child by punishing reaching. The child's reach indicates desire. Use the item at another time to train a requesting gesture.

Children with ASD may have a very limited range of desired items. With one 18-month-old child with ASD, his only expressed desire was for his iPad. In this situation, the team will want to explore other objects, foods, and toys in an effort to enlarge the number of entities.

Teaching requesting gestures. Requesting can be signaled by a hand gesture accompanied by a vocalization and eye contact with a communication partner. These behaviors are separate and can be trained through modeling and imitation. Children with CP may indicate desire by eye gaze or changes in body posture, and adults should be alert and respond appropriately.

If a child does not respond to a verbal cue ("What do you want?") in the expected manner, an adult can provide assistance. Adult prompting may come in the form of

- Directing the child's gaze and breaking the task into steps, or
- Providing a model to be imitated.

Requesting behavior has not truly generalized until a child uses it in both a cued ("What do you want?") and a spontaneous mode.

Spontaneous requesting might be prompted with "Look at this" or "See what I have" to attract a child's attention to a favorite object just out of reach. Then the adult waits.

Although requesting is highly desirous, an SLP might want to place some restriction on the behavior to forestall constant requesting. It only frustrates a child if continual requests for a cookie are met with noncompliance by adults. This is easily rectified if such training is confined to snack time and cookies are out of sight at other times.

Once requesting has generalized to other items and is performed spontaneously, it's fine to respond with "Yes, Diego want cookie, but we have to wait for snack." While the adult response does not comply with the child's request, it does acknowledge it.

Occasionally, a child will obsess on one entity or learn to use a general request, such as *want*, as a specific one, such as (*want*) *juice*. Initially, this is not a problem, but the team will want to expand the use of request to other objects to give the gesture more utility for the child.

Rejecting

Rejecting is defined as the use of behavior to enable a speaker to escape from or avoid objects, activities, or social interactions through the mediation of a listener (Sigafoos, O'Reilly, Drasgow, & Reichle, 2002). In contrast to requesting, a rejection is reinforced by removal or withdrawal of an object or postponement or cessation of an action.

Unfortunately, children's tastes are often as fickle as our own. It's important to recognize that just as desired objects and activities change, so do nondesired. For example, previously desired actions, such as playing with certain toys or eating a favorite food, can change from preferred to nonpreferred, especially if overused, and then move from a requested to a rejected item.

For some children easily frustrated by attempts to communicate, rejecting behaviors may help a child eliminate the need to rely on challenging behaviors such as self-injury to express avoidance (Sigafoos, Arthur, & O'Reilly, 2003). Self-injurious behaviors sometimes occur when a child is frustrated or feels threatened in some way. Unless more socially appropriate forms of rejecting are taught, a child is likely to persist in self-injurious or other problem behaviors.

The goal in teaching rejecting is to provide the child with an effective and socially acceptable strategy for escaping and avoiding nonpreferred objects and activities. The SLP will need to consult with a child's family to determine if a prelinguistic form of rejecting is acceptable and effective. For example, if the behavior is acceptable but used inconsistently, it may help to provide opportunities for repeated practice and reinforcement. If acceptable but difficult for others to interpret, the behavior might be enhanced by pairing the old form with an additional form that will increase the likelihood of a correct interpretation.

Given the number of choices we each make every day—These jeans or those? Big Mac or Quarterpounder? Study or play?—the natural environment provides an excellent location for such training. There should be many naturally occurring opportunities for incidental teaching of rejecting throughout the day.

Teaching rejecting gestures. Rejecting gestures might include shaking the head side to side, turning away, or using a defensive hand gesture, such as the hands extended as if pushing something away. Whatever a child's mode of responding, the SLP can follow steps similar to the following (Duker, Didden, & Sigafoos, 2004):

- Conduct an initial preference assessment to identify nonpreferred items or those not selected by a child when they are offered. Nonpreferred items used in training should always be harmless for the child on the odd chance that the child requests the item.
- Move a tray containing nonpreferred items toward the child while asking "Want one?"
- If the child produces the rejecting gesture, remove the tray.
- If the response does not occur, offer one of the nonpreferred items and when the child shows resistance, physically prompt the rejecting response.
- Over successive teaching opportunities, fade physical prompting gradually as the learner's performance improves.

If a rejecting gesture can be taught using a variety of objects, it should generalize enough to become a generic rejection response.

A danger exists that such an effective gesture might become a generalized response to all offers of objects or actions—or worse, to you. It's important, therefore, that highly desirable items be introduced once the rejecting behavior is learned. This should result in some requests and some rejections.

Natural consequences are best. A rejected item is a rejected item even if the SLP recognizes that rejection is not the child's intent. Once this occurs, the SLP can recue with "Want X?" and then reply positively, such as signing or saying "Yes" without requiring this behavior by the child. The item can then be placed within reach of the child. The SLP models the correct response when necessary to prompt a request or correct an error.

To forestall being rejected personally, the SLP should remain positive and a reinforcer herself or himself. I've been met with a rejecting gesture on occasion. I respond, "Okay, for a little while, but then we have to work." This is positive, gives the child some control, and also asserts my role. I've even followed my response by setting a timer in plain view and waiting until it chimes.

Just as with requesting, the situation can occur in which a child rejects everything out of hand, even required activities, such as bathing. As with any child, there are times when all of us just have to do things. As your parents used to say, "This is for your own good." A child doesn't get to choose whether to take seizure medication. To forestall such situations, adults should establish conditional use of rejecting by including both positive and negative teaching examples. A positive example is when the rejection works and the item or activity can be avoided. A negative occurs when the item cannot be avoided.

In the latter situation, a "response inhibition" procedure might be used to teach a child to refrain from making a rejecting response. In this procedure, the child is prompted to refrain from making the rejecting response in the presence of certain entities, such as seizure medication, and is reinforced for not rejecting. Gradually, the child will identify certain objects with nonuse of rejection.

That said, all of us recall our daily morning tantrum as a child when asked to take a vitamin even though we knew the inevitable outcome was swallowing the pill. Likewise, your ECI clients will test you. No one, even you, is 100 percent angelic. Sad to say, but as mentioned, I've had children begin signaling rejection the moment they saw me. *Yuck, here comes that guy who makes me work!*

One way to prompt initiating of rejections is to give items to the child that the child has just rejected or to give nondesired items when others are requested. Either may result in tantruming. Wait it out, and then prompt the rejection response.

FIGURE 6.3 **Principles for Teaching Rejection to Children with Severe Disabilities**

- Identify the current prelinguistic rejecting behaviors of the child. These indicate the child's motivation to communicate in this manner.
- Collaborate with caregivers to decide if there is a need to replace the existing prelinguistic form. The team may decide to accept or enhance the current behavior.
- Accurately and objectively describe the new and more symbolic form of rejecting in measurable terms to be taught. For example, when presented with a nonpreferred object, the child can reject it by selecting the *DON'T WANT* symbol on her communication device.
- Based on functional equivalence, the new rejecting form should be easier to perform than the current method and lead to more consistent and immediate responses. Responding consistently is extremely important. The form to be replaced should be ignored.
- Implement instruction at times when the child is clearly motivated to reject. Offer things that are nonpreferred and disliked.
- Create sufficient and frequent need for the behavior to occur, ensuring that the child receives enough instruction in the new form of rejecting.
- Require the new desired communicative form, even prompting it, during each instructional opportunity to promote learning.
- Reinforce the new form consistently.

Source: Information from Sigafoos et al., 2004.

From the studies on teaching communicative rejecting to children with severe disabilities, several basic principles underlying successful intervention procedures have emerged (Sigafoos, Drasgow, Reichle, O'Reilly, Green, & Tait, 2004). These are presented in Figure 6.3. For more in-depth information, I recommended that you read the excellent tutorial by Sigafoos and colleagues (2004) from which I have taken many of the items in this section.

Choice-making. If requesting has been taught previously, the child will be expected to both request and reject items and actions according to his or her desires. Choice-making, in which one highly desired and one nondesired object are presented, can also foster discriminating choices of rejecting and nonrejecting.

In training a child to signal both *yes* or *want* and *no* or *reject*, it is best to begin with one gesture exclusively. SLPs should expect that introduction of the second sign or gesture will usually result in a decrease in correct responding with the initial one trained. With more training, there will usually be an increase in correct responding with both responses.

A word of caution is in order here. Although use of *yes* and *no* is highly efficient, enabling a child to request or reject a variety of items in response to a question such as "Want X?," it is a responsive behavior that may not generalize to requesting or rejecting in the absence of being asked. In other words, a child may not initiate requests or rejections on his or her own. In addition, without further training, a yes/no response is unlikely to generalize to more general questions, such as "Is this your hat?"

Whether using a yes/no request/rejection strategy or more specific requests, such as gesturing or signing "Want," a child can be taught to repeat the original response when presented with the wrong item, rather than simply accepting that item or tantruming. For example, if a child gestures "Want" but is given a nonrequested item, he or she can be prompted to reject the wrong item and to repeat the initial request. When this occurs, the wrong item is removed and the request is prompted again.

Pointing or Signaling Notice

In general, we point to draw attention to both novel and unusual items and events as a method of establishing joint attending. Later, pointing may be used for establishing a topic, called joint or *shared referencing*. As such, pointing is a form of *proto-declarative*, an early form of conversational comment or reply. True declaratives occur when words are used. The importance of this communicative act was discussed in Chapter 4.

Possibly prior to teaching pointing for directing attention, adults can use the gesture within daily routines, such as pointing to where things go during cleanup. Other possibilities include indicating where puzzle pieces go, touching pictures in a book, and identifying where Elmo or some other fun toy is located. This is not receptive language training, so don't expect a child to respond to symbolic labels. Stick to known objects at this point.

Proto-declaratives occur naturally in situations of joint attending and can be modeled by an adult. Children tend to use them to communicate primarily with individuals with whom they already have an established positive relationship.

Teaching pointing gestures. Pointing, whether the physically easier whole hand type or the single finger variety, can be taught through imitation, assuming that the child can attend jointly. A training sequence can begin by the introduction of a highly interesting object or unusual event. If a child notices something of interest and looks, the adult can prompt a point by asking, "What do you see?" or simply "What see?" If the child does not respond, the adult can say, "Show me what you see" or "Show me." A still unresponsive child may need an imitative model or even a physical assist.

Verbal reinforcement should be in a form that furthers the exchange, such as "Yes, that's Elmo. [Remove Elmo] Uh-oh! I wonder where he went?" or "That Elmo. All gone." The behavior can be extended by having Elmo return and saying, "Now show Mommy what you see." This gives the child a second opportunity to be successful.

Another possible teaching task is to have a child's pointing guide you to a desired treat or toy placed in plain sight or "hidden" under a cloth cover. In order to be successful in the hiding task, the child will initially need to see the item when it is hidden. But recall that the purpose of our teaching task is not hide-and-seek, but pointing to signal that you notice something of interest.

VOCALIZING

Making sounds in order to communicate is not essential, but it sure is nice to have. After all, while speech is only one method of communication, it is the primary route for most folks and has a wider application in the real world than other methods such as signing. This does not relieve you of the responsibility to consider and to alert and educate the family if there is a possibility that AAC may be needed in the future. Unless the family objects, you can begin early to use sign or pictures when communicating with a child.

My grandson Zavier who had apraxia of speech initially responded to and produced some signs and pictures but with continuing intervention for speech was able to begin to speak many words intelligibly. He is no worse off and most probably ahead of where he might be because of this limited introduction of sign. We'll have lots more to say about AAC in the next two chapters.

I like to tell my own students that "Young children become communicators because we treat them that way." In other words, adults anticipate that a child will communicate. It's important that the team, especially the family, have a similar expectation for a child experiencing some difficulties with speech.

Beginning from birth, a child should be encouraged to vocalize. Adults can treat these vocalizations as meaningful communication by replying to and commenting on the child's attempts. For example, a vocalization made when an adult approaches might be responded to as "Oh, you're happy to see me," "Hello to you, too," or simply "Hi!"

The team can identify situations that result in the most child vocalization and show the family how to maximize these situations. Adults can imitate the child's vocalizations and attempt to elicit more.

Vocal Turn-Taking

Imitation of a child's behaviors, called *contingent imitation*, can be a first step in teaching vocal imitation by the child in turn. In fact, I find contingent imitation to be an excellent way to interact with a child, especially in those awkward moments when we're first becoming acquainted. As the saying goes, imitation is the sincerest form of flattery, and it can be fun too. The child makes a sound, I imitate, then wait. If nothing happens, fine. I wait for another sound or make my own. In either case, once the child makes a sound, I repeat it. I do not expect imitation of the exact sound at this point. We're just establishing the parameters of vocal turn-taking. Soon it will be difficult to know who initiated the behavior.

Initially, the child may engage in vocal turn-taking with little attempt to imitate or produce the same sound as the adult. That's fine at this point.

Sound Imitation

Once turn-taking is a well-established routine, adults can attempt to get specific sounds from the child by making sounds that the child has produced spontaneously on previous occasions. A word of caution is needed here, because much early sound-making by infants is random. It's important, therefore, that you pick sounds that the child has produced repeatedly and attempt to have the child imitate these. Teaching new sounds will come later.

Some children play silently. Adults can also model sound-making during play. This demonstrates for a child that making noise is desirable. Sound-making comes in many varieties and can include animal sounds, vehicle noises, or slurping and grunting sounds. Some children find it great fun to make loud eating noises while munching.

For most children, vowel sounds are easier to produce than consonants. The grunt sound "uh" helps to move a child that much closer to words such as *up* and can easily be incorporated into play. Just as actions can be repeated, so can vowel sounds, as in *ay-ay-ay*. Repetitions can lead to easier production of some consonants. For example, a string of *oh-oh-oh* can facilitate later production of /w/ which naturally occurs between the vowels.

With speech sounds, it is important to keep the stimulus model simple. Although "buh-buh-buh" (CVCVCV) may give a child repeated input, it may also be presenting a model impossible to reproduce for a child who is capable of vocalizing only single consonant-vowel (CV) syllables. For some children with CP and limited breath control, single syllables may be the limit of their production capabilities for now. You can approach CVCV production by shortening the interval between successive CV syllables, such as saying "Buh" every time you clap hands.

From development of TD prelinguistic infants, we know that parents respond more frequently when they perceive their infants to be "really talking" (Yoder & Munson, 1995). For parents, real talking includes syllabic vocalizations, more specifically *canonical syllables*, which are a consonant and vowel sequence (CV) that is produced with adult-like speech timing. In response to these vocalizations, parents are more likely to provide a linguistic input for subsequent language development (Gros-Louis, West, Goldstein, & King, 2006).

For children with ID, daily early intervention for canonical syllabic communication is more effective than weekly training (Woynaroski, Yoder, Fey, & Warren, 2014). This increase, in turn, can elicit more parental linguistic input, providing support for spoken vocabulary development (Goldin-Meadow, Goodrich, Sauer, & Iverson, 2007; Masur, Flynn, & Eichorst, 2005; Tamis-LeMonda, Bornstein, & Baumwell, 2001).

When a child is imitating sounds from his or her repertoire, two intervention targets seem appropriate. First, the SLP can try to elicit these sounds in repeated syllables, initially as successive imitations, as in "Muh" followed by "Muh," and then in a two-syllable vocalizations, as in "Mama." For example, successive imitations may be elicited with no reinforcement between them as in the following

> Adult: Muh. (Or "Say 'Muh.'")
> Child: Muh.
> Adult: Muh.
> Child: Muh.
> Adult: Yes, "Mama!" Here's Mama. [Point to the parent]

Two-syllable imitations are usually easier for a child to produce if the syllables are the same, but a similar technique can be used when attempting to have the child imitate two different syllables. This topic will be explored more in Chapter 9.

BOX *6.1*

Progression of Vocal Imitation and Shaping

Hierarchy of Prompts

Begin at the most appropriate level.

Cue/prompt

Consequence

Step 1
Produce an easy-to-say consonant-vowel combination, then say "(Name) say x."
("Sammy do it.")

Successful: Success is imitation of desired sound. Reinforce and try with other sounds.
Unsuccessful: Go to step 2.

Step 2
Produce an easy-to-say consonant-vowel combination, then say "(Name) say x" followed by the sound again.

Successful: Reinforce and go to step 1.
Unsuccessful: Go to step 3.

Step 3
Produce a previously child-produced consonant-vowel combination, then say "(Name) say x."

Successful: Reinforce and go to step 2.
Unsuccessful: Go to step 4.

Step 4
Produce a previously child-produced consonant-vowel combination, then say "(Name) say x" followed by the sound again.

Successful: Reinforce and go to step 3.
Unsuccessful: Go to step 5.

Step 5
Have the child look at your mouth, then produce a mouth posture, such as pursing the lips in preparation to say a sound, and say "(Name) do it."

Successful: Reinforce and go to step 4.
Unsuccessful: Go to step 6.

Step 6
Have the child look at your mouth in a mirror. Produce a mouth posture, such as pursing the lips in preparation to say a sound, and say "(Name) do it."

Successful: Reinforce and go to step 5.
Unsuccessful: Go to step 7.

Step 7
Have the child look at your mouth in a mirror. Produce a mouth posture, such as pursing the lips in preparation to say a sound, and say "(Name) do it." Provide a physical assist.

Successful: Reinforce and go to step 6.
Unsuccessful: Go to step 8 unless you feel the child is actively resisting. If this is the case, find a stronger reinforcer, try another facilitator, change the behavior being trained, or investigate if child is tactilely defensive.

Step 8
Change your criterion and accept any sound, not only the correct one. Produce a previously child-produced consonant-vowel combination or single vowel sound, and say "(Name) say x."

Successful: Success is production of any sound. Reinforce and go to step 7.
Unsuccessful: Go to step 9.

Step 9
Perform a motor and vocal combination and say "(Name) do it."

Successful: Success is producing both parts or the vocal only. Reinforce and go to step 8.
Unsuccessful: Go to step 10.

Step 10
Produce a facial movement and say "(Name) do it."

Successful: Success is physical imitation of facial movement. Reinforce and go to step 9.
Unsuccessful: Child may need more work on physical imitation.

continued

BOX *6.1 continued*

Possible Behavior Targets

The specific behaviors are not important, but learning to follow others is.

CV, VC, and V Words

Bye	Da (Dada)	Eat	Eye	Go
Hi	Key	Ma	Me	No
Out	See	Tea	Toy	Up

Motor-Vocal Behaviors

Blow out cheeks and make "popping sound"   "Bye" with wave
"M-m-m" with rub tummy   Move car while saying "Vroom!"
Raspberries while pushing car   "Uh-oh," knocking something over
War whoop with hand at mouth   "Whee" with bounce
Barking while playing with stuffed dog

Oral Motor Behaviors

Blow bubbles   Lick lips
Move head up and down or side to side   Open-close eyes
Open-close mouth   Pucker/kiss
Puff cheeks   Smile
Stick out tongue

A second target will be the introduction of new sounds. In general, a good place to begin is with

■ Labial sounds, which are visible and therefore easier to teach, and
■ Back consonants, such as /g/ and /k/, if the child has a growl in his or her repertoire.

Both types of sounds develop early in TD children.

It is essential as an SLP that you keep detailed records of the sounds and syllable structures a child can produce, both spontaneously and in imitation. These data will be invaluable in planning the child's initial lexicon, or personal dictionary.

If a child does not imitate sound-making, the SLP may wish to drop back and work on imitation in general, beginning with gross motor imitation, such as clapping hands, and progressing to oral and later sound imitation. This is a good illustration of focusing on communication while introducing presymbolic skills as needed to strengthen communication goals. A progression for teaching vocal imitation is presented in Box 6.1.

Let's face it. It's not much fun to just say sounds. I do two things to make it more enjoyable and to increase communication. First, I pair sound imitation with motor imitation in a game format similar to "Follow the leader." Some children will also benefit from specific hand shapes for each sound. In this way the child can imitate the hand shape and the sound together.

Second, I try to place the sound into a meaningful word and put it to good use. Here's an example,

Adult: [Holding ball] Say "buh."
Child: Buh.
Adult: Yes, "buh." Ball. Here comes the ball. Buh. Ball.

While it may be jumping the gun here, I have had a number of children begin to use the sound, such as "buh," as a word. If they don't, what have we lost? I had a beautiful video, now lost, of the first time a little boy with Down syndrome who was signing but not making any sounds, formed "buh" repeatedly with his lips as he requested I roll the ball toward him. He didn't make a sound, but we were on our way.

 In this video, an SLP describes some principles of ECI.
https://www.youtube.com/watch?v=HX9fzXoYXMw

Language Stimulation: Talking to a Young Child

Communication stimulation has a long and uneven history in intervention. At one time in the 1950s and 1960s, stimulation was the primary method of intervention with minimally communicating children and adults. It was eclipsed by behaviorism, which in turn was replaced by other more sociolinguistic methods. It was believed initially that sufficient stimulation would result in increased communication. Unfortunately, some early practitioners neglected the very essential item of *communication need*. Without a need to communication, there is little motivation to do so.

Communication behaviors flow to and from each partner. A failure of either partner to respond means that the communication process has broken down. It's important, therefore, that parents and caregivers learn to respond to and encourage a child's attempts to communicate. Remember that children become communicators because we treat them that way. Guidance for parents and other caregivers is presented in Figure 6.4.

It's important not to overwhelm busy parents by heaping all these suggestions on them at once. Instead, you can offer these behaviors one at a time and demonstrate, role play, and critique a parent's performance. Naturally, as a child develops, more specific interactive techniques should be tailored to the child's behavior. Suggested adult behaviors based on the child's level of functioning are presented in Figure 6.5.

In general, within adult-child interactions, we should be seeking balance, responsiveness, contingency, consistency, and a nondirective style (Rossetti, 2001). Balance is achieved when neither partner dominates and when communication occurs at the child's level. The adult responds to the child's communicative behaviors in ways the child can imitate, shows the child how next to communicate, and then waits for the child's response. These behaviors can help to sustain joint attending.

Responsiveness requires that the adult reply at a level that reflects the child's interests, pace, and communication skills. Some parents will need guidance to identify when their child is attempting to communicate, especially if the child has motor difficulties. Examples of communication behaviors of children with neuromotor dysfunction are presented in Figure 6.6.

Contingency, you'll recall, is the timeliness of the adult responses to the child's communicative behaviors. In general, the more immediate the response, the more powerful it is in teaching a child to attempt communication again. The manner of the adult response is also important and should be positive, animated, and communicative in nature.

FIGURE 6.4 **Suggestions for Talking to a Young Child**

- **Be animated.** Use exaggerated facial expressions, voice variations, and movement to help the child attend.
- **Be positive.** The tone of your voice conveys a lot of information.
- **Communicate at eye level.** Being at the same level enables a young child to read the messages in your face and to learn the value of face-to-face communication and of paying attention to others. Face-to-face communication is more egalitarian and interactive.
- **Listen, take turns, and know when to stop.** Knowing how to listen is just as important as being an enthusiastic and responsive conversational partner. Listening shows that you are interested in what a child is saying, even if it's not words. The best conversations with young children include a combination of quiet listening and simple talking, with each of you taking a turn in a natural, easy manner. It's important to strike a balance.
- **Provide rich input.** Varied activities, comprehensible language, educational play, and rewarding interactions provide challenging, fun, and interesting experiences. Stay on the edge of the curve so that the child is neither bored nor overwhelmed. Challenge a child to stretch her or his vocabulary by staying one step ahead. Talk about what's happening in your immediate surroundings to enhance the child's comprehension.
- **Pick the best time to communicate and get the child's attention first.** The best interactions with a child occur when the child is awake, alert, and quiet or making noises. Watch for a child's cues, such as eye contact, that he or she is open to communication, indicating I'm ready to engage in play or a chat. When a child shows interest in something, slide into the activity and talk about it. Before beginning your own interaction, get the child's attention first. Sharing attention with another person is a precursor to sharing topics in conversation.
- **Always respond.** Whenever possible, respond to *all* vocalizations and verbalizations. In general, good responses
  - Affirm that you're paying attention.
  - Reinforce the child's efforts.
  - Clarify the child's intentions.
  - Provide evaluative feedback.
  - Model longer or more adult-like phrases.
- **Speak in short two- to four-word phrases.** Children on the cusp of talking understand one- or two-word phrases best. Longer utterances exceed their memory. Once children begin talking in single words, they can usually understand short two- or three-word phrases. Although some experts believe in the use of telegraphic speech with young children with communication difficulties and others favor more mature input, empirical findings on the best type of speech are weak. The majority of the intervention studies showed no difference in language comprehension based on type of input (van Kleeck, Schwarz, Fey, Kaiser, Miller, & Weitzman, 2010).
- **Speak slowly, pause between words, and keep your vocabulary small.** Children's vocabularies begin to grow slowly. Use words that describe things that the child encounters most frequently, that are part of her or his world.
- **Repeat words, but vary your language slightly.** Repetition helps language processing. One or two repetitions should do the trick, and comprehension improves when the words represent something present, visual, and interesting.
- **Focus on one topic, and follow the child's lead.** It's confusing for a child to talk about more than one thing at a time until he or she is about 18 months old, so keep your conversations focused. Early communication is always most effective when focused on an object or action or event that's happening in front of you. Let the child indicate an interest in something by looking, reaching, or picking something up, and then talk about it. If the child says a word, turn that word into a topic of conversation.
- **Gesture and sign to aid comprehension.** Gesturing is a natural accompaniment to and enhancement for spoken language. Natural gesturing holds a child's interest, enhances your message, and helps a child understand your words. The simpler the gesture is to do, the more likely a child will be able to copy it and use it to communicate.

Be consistent; that also helps. Signs can also be used like natural gestures. Children pick up sign language when they're exposed to it, just as they do natural gestures. A few other guidelines:

- Don't overwhelm the child with signs or gestures.
- Speak at the same time you gesture.
- Sign and gesture in context.
- Offer repeated exposure.
- Encourage imitation.
- Sign and gesture only important words.
- **Limit your questions.** Besides requiring an answer that a child may not know, questions are more difficult to process than statements because of the grammar. In general, *what* and *where* type questions, such as *"What's that?"* and *"Where's doggie?"* are relatively easy for toddlers who are using single words.

Source: Information from Owens, 2004.

FIGURE 6.5 **Specific Language Stimulation Suggestions**

Talking with young children is an art. And it's portable. You can take it with you and do it anywhere. To be really good at it, you need to not be self-conscious. Forget who may be observing you out of the corner of their eye. Be an actor and have fun. It's actually one of the best features of working with young children. The suggestions are given in three-month blocks (Owens, *Help Your Baby Talk*, 2004).

1–3 Months

- Accentuate your facial movement and expressions. Put on a good show. Exaggerating your facial expressions and making changes in your voice will keep a child's interest.
- Treat the child's movements or sounds as meaningful. Remember, at this point in development, children do not have an intention to communicate. That said, their behavior still has meaning. They cry when they're uncomfortable or hungry. It's your job to interpret that behavior for both of you.
- Imitate the child's noises and movements. If the child coos when eating, coo along too. Taking turns is one of the first communication skills infants learn.

4–6 Months

- Spend more time playing and talking.
- Convince the child that he or she wants to talk by making conversations fun and pleasurable. Use exaggerated intonation and facial expressions.
- Talk to the child throughout the day.
- Treat the child's movements and sounds as meaningful.

7–9 Months

- Show you understand by responding to behavior, such as pointing, that seems to communicate a message.
- Keep your own speech simple as the infant gets close to saying that first word: short utterances, easy words.
- Repeat words in context, varying the order a little or adding new words here and there.
- Treat the child as a real communicator.
- Mimic the child's reduplicated babbling—e.g., *bababa*.
- Use real word models in conversations, remembering the basic building block of CV syllables and CVCV combinations.
- Respond to gestures; they're the first purposeful communication of an infant.
- Use consistent words for things so the child has a reliable model.
- Gesture and/or sign too.

continued

10–12 Months

- Be a good role model. Use short words and phrases plus gestures.
- Don't interrupt when the child is practicing sounds.
- Expand the child's world with quality experiences that you mediate with simple language.
- Don't expect the child to get it right each time she or he names something. Always respond positively and gently redirect with the right word.
- Try not to be critical of the child's speech.
- Use appropriately simple and useful words that reflect the child's interest at the moment.
- Imitate word-like vocalizations.
- Use the child's name when referring to him or her as you/me can be confusing.
- Encourage the child to initiate communication by manipulating the environment, such as sealing tasty treats or fun toys in clear plastic containers or putting tempting objects just out of reach while the child is watching.
- Respond appropriately and immediately by imitating, expanding, or extending.
- Take advantage of pointing and vocalizing by supplying an appropriate word.
- Sing simple songs at bedtime or other quiet times.

13–15 Months

- Now that the child understands much of what you say, real, albeit limited, dialogues are more possible. Talk about what will happen in the immediate future, as well as what's happening now. Discuss things in your immediate environment that the child can see, feel, smell, and hear; tell her what you're doing as you do it; and expand upon her words.
- Take turns. Allow the child to have a chance to be in a real conversation, and respond to what you think he or she is trying to tell you.
- Teach the child new words by saying them and asking her to say them after you. Don't overdo it—just a few times per request. Try to pick words that incorporate sounds the child already makes, and be sure these words are relevant to your immediate surroundings.
- Expand the child's action verb vocabulary by having her act out the actions named.
- Pulling toys or other objects out of a chest or a bag one at a time is a terrific way to introduce new items. Be sure to say the name for each item *several times* as you introduce it, and to use the objects in their intended way.
- Give the child a space of her or his own to decorate. Stick some Velcro on the back of small reinforced pictures or use fridge magnets. Chat about the pictures, and help her update the art gallery regularly.
- Pick books that depict familiar everyday events and objects, and enjoy shared book reading.

16–18 Months

- Model two-word phrases. Repeat yourself so that the child has a couple of chances to hear the word combination.
- Provide words for all the things that are of interest to the child, especially when the child asks "*Wassat*?" But don't stop here. Explore the object with him and talk about it.
- Sing "favorite" songs adapted to allow the child to fill in the missing word.
- On a walk, collect "treasures" along the way, such as stones, leaves, twigs, flowers, or other nature items, and talk about each one as you add it to your collection.
- Gesture less. The child is relying more on words to communicate so no longer needs extensive signing or gesturing.
- When serving a snack, only give the child a small amount and wait for him or her to request more.

19–24 Months

- Respond to the child's talking by expanding what the child says into longer, more mature sentences. Don't correct, and keep it positive. The trick is to stay a step or two ahead of the child. Use short adult sentences—five or six words max—when you talk with her or him.

- Take advantage of ALL language opportunities.
- Have real conversations. Talk about what you both are doing, comment on sounds you hear, ask questions, and answer hers with enthusiasm. Reply to attempts to communicate, and comment on what the child says.
- Sing social songs in which the child can participate. Pick simple, repetitive songs, or make up your own about everyday activities.
- Be silly. Children love to correct adults. Call things by the wrong name.
- Provide opportunities for language growth. Encourage the child to stretch her or his uses of language—give chances to make requests, ask questions, and describe things.

FIGURE 6.6 **Possible Communication Behaviors in Children with Neuromotor Dysfunctions**

Examples of Early Behaviors

- Widen eyes in response to a novel stimulus.
- Assume an atypical postural pattern in response to being upset or startled.
- Change facial expression in response to a familiar face or voice.
- Increase postural tone when excited or anticipating a familiar game or routine.

Intentional Behaviors

- Open mouth and vocalize to attract attention.
- Attempt to look toward the adult while vocalizing and reaching for an object. This may result in an abnormal movement pattern that prevents the child from redirecting his or her visual orientation to the desired toy.
- Increase postural tone to convey excitement to recreate an enjoyable event, plus look at adult with expectation.
- Look at the adult and then turn toward desired item.
- Vocalize to adult with a concurrent increase in postural tone in an attempt to communicate the child has something to show or tell.
- Hit item with hand to convey interest.
- Increase the volume of vocalizations while continuing to look at the adult when ignored.

Consistent responding increases the likelihood of the child's behavior occurring again. In addition, different communication intentions can be strengthened. For example, if the adult responds consistently to the child's requests, it reinforces requesting and the form, such as a reaching gesture, in which the child signals this intention.

Finally, nondirectiveness is fostered when the adult engages the child more for socializing than for accomplishing some task. Caregivers are much less directive in more open-ended situations such as play that is not goal directed. Adults can also follow the child's lead so the child is allowed to share in directing the interaction. Adults can learn to comment rather than use questions or commands.

Most professionals realize that in and of itself, stimulation will do little to improve communication skill for most children. Combined with the other techniques discussed in this chapter, however, stimulation may provide additional input and a variety of activities for home or classroom. Appendix G presents a long list of communication stimulation activities based on the functioning level of a child. These activities can be incorporated into an intervention program one at a time, following explanation and demonstration for parents and teachers.

BILINGUAL FAMILIES

Just as each family must decide how to communicate with their TD children, parents of children with communication impairment (CI) must make the same decision for their child. These caregivers may quite naturally be concerned that speaking their heritage language could confuse the child or cause further delays in language development (Wharton, Levine, Miller, Breslau, & Greenspan, 2000). SLPs are in a unique role for addressing their concerns.

Although there is little research on bilingual families of children with CI, the information available would suggest that it is unwise to advise a family to speak only English (Dyches, Wilder, Sudweeks, Obiakor, & Algozzine, 2004; Kremer-Sadlik, 2004). When parents are free to use their heritage language, they talk more with their children, who in turn display more affect.

Children with CI exposed to two languages do not demonstrate additional delays when compared with monolingual children (Hambly & Fombonne, 2012). For example, bilingual and monolingual children with ASD demonstrate similar language performance scores, and bilingual children have larger expressive vocabularies (Petersen, Marinova-Todd, & Mirenda, 2012). When compared by the severity of ASD, there appears to be no difference in monolingual and bilingual receptive and expressive language and functional communication (Ohashi et al., 2012). These findings would seem to belie the notion that bilingual exposure is detrimental to the language development of children with CI.

Even so, parents may be reluctant to use their heritage language, believing that it hinders development of English and makes language-learning more difficult (Yu, Scheffner Hammer, & Wilkinson, 2013). Unfortunately, this same view of bilingual development may be reinforced by some professionals.

In some situations, parents may not speak English. Alternative EI strategies may be helpful, including involving siblings or others, using more structured interactions or group settings for language treatment, and using direct training techniques that are consistent with the family's culture (Wing et al., 2007).

Presymbolic Skills

Although presymbolic skills are not the main focus of ECI, an SLP may need to target these if a child is having difficulty increasing the level of communication. In the following section, we'll discuss three behaviors that can sometimes serve this purpose: establishing joint attention, imitation, and means-ends.

SLPs must be careful to keep the role of presymbolic skills, such as imitation, in perspective. Behaviors such as motor imitation are important only insofar as they serve to enhance communication or to increase a child's ability to learn to communicate better. It is all too easy, especially if an SLP is being successful in teaching a presymbolic target, to forget the overall goal.

ESTABLISHING JOINT ATTENTION

Joint attention refers to engaging another person's focus in order to share enjoyment of or interest in objects or events. Sharing joint attention means both partners' observing and interacting with the same object or event. To accomplish this, adults can introduce novel objects or use familiar objects in novel ways. The adult can attract the child's attention by (Arntson, 2009)

- Exaggerating movements,
- Exaggerating and varying voice,
- Pausing before saying words,
- Extending the length of some sounds,
- Giving objects to the child, and
- Gradually increasing the time spent in object interaction.

In a similar fashion, old actions, such as clapping, can be extended to novel locations.

Joint attention can be either simultaneous or sequential and can be demonstrated in many ways, such as

- Responding to a spoken word and/or a gesture referring to an object or event,
- Shifting gaze from an object to a person,
- Showing an object to a person, and
- Giving an object to a person.

For children using augmentative or alternative communication (AAC), refer an adult to an object or event using a sign, picture, or other representation. Children can both initiate and respond to joint attention bids by (Mundy & Thorp, 2006)

- Inviting others to attend,
- Looking at objects placed before the child,
- Following a line of visual regard, and
- Following the pointing gestures of others.

During joint attention activities, caregivers of TD children usually provide rich verbal input. They label objects or events that are the focus of a child's attention (Goodwyn, Acredolo, & Brown, 2000). This caregiver behavior enhances the child's early language acquisition. We want to accomplish the same thing with children who have communication impairment.

Teaching Joint Attention

There are many ways to try to establish joint attending through intervention. These include

- Introducing silly or out-of-place events/objects into typical routines to evoke a response,
- Putting a high-preference item and your face in the child's line of vision to evoke gaze responses, and
- Following a child's lead so the adult focuses on whatever the child is attending to.

Most of these procedures teach a responsive behavior, but do not necessarily teach the child either the purpose of joint attending or that social interactions can be interesting and reinforcing. These lessons can be learned from the responses of the adult, as in "You see doggie. I see doggie, too. He goes 'wuff-wuff.' He's a big doggie. A brown doggie."

Note all the input here. The adult is telling the child that he or she can see the dog that is big, brown, and goes "wuff."

The initial step is establishing the presence of adults as a generalized reinforcer (Jones & Carr, 2004). This can occur by having an adult present a variety of highly preferred items repeatedly or by contingent imitation of the child.

Once physically close to an adult, a child can choose items to be used in teaching by simply showing interest in these items. Highly desirable items might be edible treats or objects that move, light up, or make a noise. The adult should use a variety of items and incorporate novel items that are likely to sustain attending by the child.

To have a child attend to an adult's face, the SLP can place highly desired items before the child but deny access until the child looks at the adult who can smile and nod in return. Only following the SLP's nod and smile can the child have the treat. In turn, this social expression becomes a reinforcer because it is paired with the item. Once established, these social reinforcers can be used to teach other useful behaviors. None of this will occur if the treats are either not desired by the child or not visible initially.

To direct the child's attention to an interesting event or object, the adult can turn, look, point, and make an exclamatory verbalization about the object or event, such as "Wow, it's X!" Ideally, the child will look at the focus of attention, glance at the adult, and then look back at the event or object. This can be prompted by

- Calling the child's name to get her or his attention,
- "Drawing" a line from the adult's face to the object,
- Bringing the object to the adult's face and slowly moving it away, or
- Gently turning the child's face toward the object or event.

These prompts can be reduced or faded over time. Box 6.2 presents additional ideas for teaching joint attending.

BOX *6.2*

Progression of Joint Attending Intervention

Hierarchy of Prompts for Transferring Eye Gaze from Object to Person

Begin at the appropriate step. When the child is successful, be sure to spend some time sharing the object.

Cue/prompt

Step 1
Place an interesting object before the child and when he/she looks at it, call the child's name and/or ask the child to look at you.

Step 2
Place an interesting object before the child and wiggle you fingers near it. When the child looks at the object, call the child's name and/or ask the child to look at you.

Step 3
Place an interesting object before the child and move the object toward your face. When the child looks at the object, call the child's name and/or ask the child to look at you.

Step 4
Break the task into two sequential behaviors. Place an interesting object before the child and call the child's attention to the object by shaking and naming it. When the child looks at it, reinforce the child, then call the child's name and/or ask the child to look at you.

Step 5: Train the missing piece
Eye contact with a person: Sit before the child, call the child's name and ask child to look at you.
OR
Eye contact with an object: Place an interesting object before the child, call the child's name and ask the child to look at it.

Consequence

Successful: Success is transferring eye gaze and establishing eye contact with the adult. Reinforce and refer back to object.
Unsuccessful: Go to step 2.

Successful: Success is transferring eye gaze and establishing eye contact with the adult. Reinforce, refer back to object, and go to step 1.
Unsuccessful: Go to step 3.

Successful: Success is transferring eye gaze and establishing eye contact with the adult. Reinforce, refer back to object, and go to step 2.
Unsuccessful: Go to step 4.

Successful: Success is transferring eye gaze and establishing eye contact with the object and then the adult. Reinforce each behavior separately. Go to step 3.
Unsuccessful: Go to step 5.

Successful: Success is establishing eye contact. Reinforce and go to step 4.
Unsuccessful: Go to step 6.

Step 6: Train the missing piece
Eye contact with a person: Sit before the child, place an interesting object next to your face, call the child's name and ask child to look at you.
OR
Eye contact with an object: Place a noise-making object before the child, activate it, call the child's name and ask the child to look at it.

Successful: Success is establishing eye contact. Reinforce and go to step 5.
Unsuccessful: Go to step 7.

Step 7: Train the missing piece
Eye contact with a person: Sit before the child, place an interesting object next to your face, call the child's name and ask child to look at you, then gently guide the child's chin so the child faces you.
OR
Eye contact with an object: Place a noise-making object before the child, activate it, call the child's name and ask the child to look at it, then gently guide the child's chin so the child faces you.

Successful: Success is establishing eye contact. Reinforce and go to step 5.
Unsuccessful: Find stronger reinforcer, more interesting object, or another partner.

Hierarchy of Prompts for Transferring Eye Gaze from Person to Object

Begin at the appropriate step.

Cue/prompt

Consequence

Step 1
Attract child's attention to your face by noise or movement and when he/she looks, direct child's attention to object by saying "(Name), look at X."

Successful: Success is transferring eye gaze and establishing eye contact with the object. Reinforce and refer to object.
Unsuccessful: Go to step 2.

Step 2
Attract child's attention to your face by noise or movement and when he/she looks, wiggle fingers near your face and move them to object while saying "(Name), look at X."

Successful: Success is transferring eye gaze and establishing eye contact with the object. Reinforce and refer to object. Go to step 1.
Unsuccessful: Go to step 3.

Step 3
Attract child's attention to your face by noise or movement and when he/she looks, wiggle object near your face and move it slowly away while saying "(Name), look at X."

Successful: Success is transferring eye gaze and establishing eye contact with the object. Reinforce and refer to object. Go to step 2.
Unsuccessful: Go to step 4.

Step 4
Attract child's attention to your face by noise or movement and when he/she looks, reinforce. Wiggle object near your face and move it slowly away while saying "(Name), look at X." When the child looks at it, reinforce.

Successful: Success is transferring eye gaze and establishing eye contact with the object. Reinforce each behavior separately. Go to step 3.
Unsuccessful: Go to step 5.

continued

BOX *6.2 continued*

Step 5: Train the missing piece
Eye contact with a person: Sit before the child, call the child's name and ask child to look at you.

OR

Eye contact with an object: Place an interesting object before the child, call the child's name and ask the child to look at it.

Successful: Success is establishing eye contact. Reinforce and go to step 4.
Unsuccessful: Go to step 6.

Step 6: Train the missing piece
Eye contact with a person: Sit before the child, place an interesting object next to your face, call the child's name and ask child to look at you.

OR

Eye contact with an object: Place a noise-making object before the child, activate it, call the child's name and ask the child to look at it.

Successful: Success is establishing eye contact. Reinforce and go to step 5.
Unsuccessful: Go to step 7.

Step 7: Train the missing piece
Eye contact with a person: Sit before the child, place an interesting object next to your face, call the child's name and ask child to look at you, then gently guide the child's chin so child faces you.

OR

Eye contact with an object: Place a noise-making object before the child, activate it, call the child's name and ask the child to look at it, then gently guide the child's chin so child faces you.

Successful: Success is establishing eye contact. Reinforce and go to step 5.
Unsuccessful: Find stronger reinforcer, more interesting object, or another partner.

Suggested Items to Use
Puppets, dolls, action figures, remotely operated or wind-up toys, a flashlight or other lighted object, keys, a ball, a toy car or truck, pull toys, bubbles, a jack-in-the-box, picture books, a pinwheel or other spinning object, food, brightly colored pictures or objects, and live animals.

A natural consequence of joint attending is a social interaction about the entity observed. This might include play and a verbal social response by the SLP (Jones & Carr, 2004). Each adult has his or her own way of responding, including verbalizing a loud "Wow," making a funny face, or delivering gentle touches or tickles. In general, I avoid phrases such as "Good looking," preferring instead to comment on the focus of attention, as in "Yes, you like raisins" or "Yum, raisins taste good." At first, these responses may not reinforce the child's behavior and will need to be paired with another response, such as a taste of the edible treat, in order to become reinforcers.

It is difficult to teach initiation of joint attending by the child without teaching gestures such as pointing. At this level of instruction, it may be best for the adult to follow the child's lead and focus on whatever interests the child at the moment. Some children will resist adult interruption, so initially the adult should go slowly and ask gently to join the activity. The adult should comment on the child's focus of attention, smile if the child establishes face-to-face interaction, and look back to the object or event.

IMITATION

Young children seem to naturally love repetition and familiar objects. Teaching imitation is not a direct goal of ECI but rather an indirect one in support of enhancing communication. If, for example, a child does not gesture or vocalize and does not seem to understand imitating others, then the ECI team may decide to target imitation as an intervention goal.

Intervention might begin with recognition of imitation in the form of contingent imitation of the child by an adult who imitates the child's actions with toys, gestures, and vocalizations. Contingent imitation, mentioned previously, encourages responsivity to being imitated. Children seem to follow a pattern of behavior when their own movements are imitated. First, they are just imitated and may respond minimally, if at all. Then, in turn, they begin to imitate their behavior that was imitated by the adult. They will then imitate behavior by the adult that they previously produced spontaneously.

The adult can intersperse contingent imitation with requests for the child to imitate the adult's behavior. Whether imitating the child or modeling a behavior to be imitated, the adult should accompany each action with a verbal description, such as "Push car."

Once the child will imitate behavior in his or her repertoire, the adult can attempt to expand these behaviors by eliciting these behaviors with different objects, in different locations, and with different people. For example, you can push a ball, a car, or a balloon. The child can be assisted by the adult's placing a hand over the child's hand. Adding sounds, such as *hi* or *bye-bye*, to motor imitation will help stimulate the child and make training interesting, even though a child is not able to imitate sounds.

Next, the adult should try to get the child to imitate novel actions. These can be mixed with familiar actions, objects, and locations to facilitate imitation. For example, from pushing the ball we could move to throwing it. It's important not to change too much too quickly, such as modeling a novel behavior with a novel object. Finally, both familiar and novel actions can be modeled with the same and different toys.

Box 6.3 presents a possible hierarchy for teaching imitation. The SLP would begin at the appropriate level and work toward the highest one.

BOX *6.3*

Progression of Motor Imitation Intervention

Hierarchy of Prompts

Begin with behaviors already in the child's repertoire and at the appropriate step.

Cue/prompt	*Consequence*
Step 1 Cue child with "(Name) do this" or "(Name) clap hands" and perform act.	*Successful*: Reinforce and try with another motor behavior. *Unsuccessful*: Go to step 2
Step 2 Cue child with "(Name) do this" or "(Name) clap hands" and perform act. Gently use a partial physical prompt, such as lifting child's hands for clap hands.	*Successful*: Reinforce and return to step 1. *Unsuccessful*: Go to step 3

continued

BOX *6.3 continued*

Step 3
Cue child with "(Name) do this" or "(Name) clap hands" and perform act. Gently use a physical prompt to help the child perform the action.

Successful: Reinforce and return to step 2.
Unsuccessful: Go to step 4

Step 4
Gently physically manipulate the child through a simple motor behavior and name the behavior as you do this.

Successful: Reinforce and return to step 3.

If a child resists physical assistance, the cause may be

- Lack of a strong reinforce,
- Inappropriate behavior chosen for imitation,
- Child does not understand the task, or
- Child is tactilely defensive, responding poorly to task.

Investigate these causes and return to contingent imitation of the child.

Possible Behavior Targets

The specific behaviors are not important, but learning to follow others is.

Bodily Movements

Clap hands	Crawl	"Dance"
Hop	Jump	Lie down
Open and close hand	Pat objects	Raise arm or leg
Raise hands	Roll over	Shake hands
Sit down	Stand up	Stretch
Swing arm or leg	Take a step	Tap foot
Touch body parts	Wave	

Imitation with Objects

Some children respond better with objects that can provide additional cues to the desired behavior.

Draw with crayon/marker	Build two-block tower	Drink juice
Drop objects into	Eat with a spoon	Fold paper
Hit bell (drum, xylophone)	Pick up, give, take, hand	Push toy car or other vehicle
Put objects into objects	Put on hat	Ring bell
Roll play dough	Roll, kick, or throw ball	Shake, rattle, or noisemaker

One way to encourage imitation is by teaching within games, such as "So big" and "Do as I'm doing." Other possibilities are hand-play, such a pat-a-cake, and action songs. Both types of activities are very appropriate for children at this stage of development. The child can imitate the movements of the song and can be encouraged to participate in "singing" as well but without the words. By moving his or her hands, the child is part of the activity, which becomes repetitive and routine. Once the child can imitate the movements to a song, it will be easier to learn to imitate some of the words within that format.

MEANS-ENDS

In order to gesture, a child must understand the necessity of devising means for accomplishing his or her ends. For example, if you want a cookie that is just out of reach but resting on a napkin that is not, pull the napkin. Likewise, if you desire something that you cannot reach in any manner, ask for assistance by gesturing. This cognitive skill, discussed previously, is called means-ends and is highly correlated with development of gestures.

Although some children will learn forms of gestural communication with no difficulty, others will struggle with the connection between the gesture and some outcome or with generalizing gesture use beyond specific teaching tasks. In these situations, a child may need to work briefly on means-ends. Several tasks and toys can be used in this training,

- Toys that can be obtained or operated by pulling a cord;
- "Busy boxes" or kiddie gyms in which various motions, such as turning a knob or pushing a switch, result in figures' popping up or making a noise;
- Musical or talking toys that require operating a lever or switch to be activated; and
- Jack-in-the-boxes.

As cautioned before, such prerequisite skills as means-ends are not significant in and of themselves but are important to the extent they further the goal of enhancing communication.

 Nonsymbolic children need plenty of verbal input and encouragement to speak. To see this in action, watch this video on pairing words with reinforcement for children with ASD.
https://www.youtube.com/watch?v=fkO1pORWgro

Monitoring Intervention

One of the biggest challenges in ECI is recordkeeping. Because young children may change very rapidly, and families respond differently to a child at various periods in development, periodic assessment of progress and adjustment of goals are needed. As a consequence, SLPs need to monitor intervention results and progress on a continuing basis, revising or establishing new outcomes as appropriate.

As an SLP, you are helping a child and family construct a communication system. This requires intimate knowledge of the communication behaviors of the child and family. For example, as a child moves toward more symbolic communication, the SLP will want to track sounds, syllable structure, and early meanings and intentions in the child's repertoire.

Monitoring serves three broad purposes (Wolery, 2004):

- To validate the conclusions from the initial evaluation/assessment;
- To develop a record of progress over time, including consistency, frequency, and intensity of intervention (Sandall, McLean, & Smith, 2000); and
- To determine whether and how to modify or revise intervention plans.

Monitoring includes attention both to the child's intervention goals and to overall development, including play and social interactions, as well as challenging behaviors. Progress-monitoring may be in the form of narrative descriptions, direct observation, and parent and other caregiver reports (ASHA, 2008b).

Conclusion

We've identified a wide range of teaching and intervention strategies to use in presymbolic ECI. Many of these techniques, such as expansion and extension, are equally applicable to symbolic intervention as well. This means that techniques used to train presymbolic skills, such as motor imitation, can also be used for vocal and verbal training. This provides an advantage for the child who does not have to learn all new intervention routines while focused on beginning to learn language and symbol use.

Not every child will be able to produce speech as a means of communication. While this doesn't negate the need for targeting intentional communication, it does refocus the emphasis on sound and word production. For this reason, we'll consider augmentative and alternative communication (AAC) in the next two chapters before going to symbolic communication.

 Click here to gauge your understanding of the concepts in this chapter.

7

Augmentative and Alternative Communication: Introduction and Assessment

When you have completed this chapter, you should be able to:

- Describe the different types of augmentative and alternate communication (AAC) and considerations with each.
- Explain how evidence based practice informs AAC intervention.
- Explain the elements of a thorough AAC assessment.

Terms with which you should be familiar:

AAC system
Aided AAC
American Indian Hand Talk (Amer-Ind)
ASL
Assistive technology
Augmentative and alternative communication
Automatic scanning
Centering
Circular scanning
Direct selection
Directed scanning
Dynamic display

Inverse scanning
Linear scanning
Representative symbol systems
Row-column scanning
Scanning
SEE$_1$
SEE$_2$
Signed English
Speech generating device
Step scanning
Tangible symbols
Unaided AAC
Voice output communication aids

Some children need extra assistance to be able to communicate more effectively, to play, to eat, or to move more freely. An essential part of early intervention for these children is assistive technology (AT), consisting of adaptations and devices that enable a child to function more independently. Adaptations and devices form a continuum from readily available, off-the-shelf, lower-cost devices to complex, specialized devices designed to address an individual child's particular needs and abilities. Some items used by all young children are readily available and include car seats, strollers, and other baby equipment that is considered low tech. These items may be used as is or adapted slightly for a child. More specialized devices, considered higher tech, include power wheelchairs, computerized toys and communication devices, and other resources not readily available for the general population.

Team involvement includes both

- Assessment to identify appropriate adaptations and devices, and
- Intervention to teach children and families to use them.

With many low-tech adaptations and devices, such as special spoons, children and families may need little training. Usually, however, even with these low-tech interventions, some professional guidance is necessary (Long, Huang, Woodbridge, Woolverton, & Minkel, 2003).

Augmentative and alternative communication (AAC) is a form of AT and an intervention approach that uses other-than-speech means to complement or supplement a child's communication abilities. As such, AAC may include a combination of existing speech or vocalizations, gestures, manual signs, communication boards, and speech-output communication devices. Although AAC use is appropriate for all ages, we'll be focusing on beginning communicators who are 0–3 years old.

You can see from this description that AAC is a multimodality ECI strategy that enables a child to use every mode possible to communicate. An AAC system consists of an integrated group of components used by an individual to enhance communication. Early access to multiple forms of AAC is essential for early communication development in young children.

It must be stressed that the use of AAC does not mean that speech is ignored. Speech is a component of most multimodal AAC systems. In this way, a child makes optimum use of vocal and verbal skills for communication as part of a multimodal AAC system.

Most children with developmental disabilities will acquire functional spoken communication skills during childhood (Abbeduto, 2003). Children who do not develop speech are a relatively small but no less important group. Those who cannot speak face both significant frustration because of their inability to communicate and social and educational isolation. In these cases, the use of AAC is mandated in Part C of the Individuals with Disabilities Education Act.

The breadth of communication behaviors involved in AAC has the potential to enhance communication skill overall. AAC can promote communication development in infants and toddlers by (ASHA, 2008b)

- Enhancing both input and output,
- Augmenting existing vocalizations and speech,
- Replacing socially unacceptable behaviors with a more conventional means of communication,
- Serving as a language-teaching tool (Romski & Sevcik, 2005), and
- Facilitating a young child's ability to more fully participate in daily activities and routines.

Although AAC typically serves as an output mode for communication, other uses, including receptive communication, may be equally important for the very young child beginning to develop communication skills (Romski & Sevcik, 2005).

AAC can be a tool that fosters language development regardless of whether the child will eventually talk or not. In other words, it is never too early nor is it inappropriate to use AAC with young children with communication impairments whether or not this becomes a primary means of communication.

By some estimates between 2.5 and 6 percent of all children who receive special education services are potential candidates for AAC. A higher percentage of younger children may be in need. Results of one statewide survey indicated that approximately 12 percent of preschoolers receiving special education services require AAC (Binger & Light, 2006). Given these findings, there is a critical need for all speech-language pathologists (SLPs) to be prepared to provide AAC services for children who require either some alternative or addition to speech (Cress & Marvin, 2003).

In the same survey, approximately two-thirds of preschoolers using AAC were male, reflecting the generally more difficult time young boys have in acquiring language and the higher incidence of most disabilities among males (Binger & Light, 2006). More than one-third of these preschoolers had a primary diagnosis of developmental delay, and another third were classified as having autism spectrum disorder (ASD). An additional 17 percent were classified as speech/language impaired and 10 percent as having multiple disabilities. Among preschool AAC users, more than half were using gestures and picture boards or books. Only 15 percent of these children used voice output devices to communicate.

It's estimated that from a third to a half of individuals with severe ASD do not use speech functionally (National Research Council, 2001). Potentially, many of these children are candidates for AAC, either as a supplement to their existing speech or as their primary method of expressive communication. Interestingly, the use of AAC seems to decrease rates of severe problem behaviors and to increase rates of social interaction among children with ASD (Frea, Arnold, & Vittimberga, 2001).

Effective implementation of AAC intervention with young children is based on the notion that (Romski, Sevcik, Cheslock, & Barton, 2006)

- All children can and do communicate,
- Children can learn language and communication skills in natural environments through services and supports provided through a collaborative team model similar to that presented throughout this text, and
- Language and communication development involve both comprehension and production.

A child's abilities and needs will change over time. As a result, AAC use should change also, modified over time as a child grows and develops (Beukelman & Mirenda, 2005). Many of the techniques described throughout this text, such as prompting natural communication and adapting environments to increase communication opportunities, are essential aspects of successful AAC intervention as well.

Communication partners, whether actual or potential, are an important factor in the success of AAC use. Listener perceptions of and attitudes about AAC use vary widely and are related to several variables, including the listener's gender, age, experiences with individuals with disabilities, and information about the specific nonspeaking partner; the frequency and specificity of communicative cues; voice output; and the perceived similarity in values and activities of daily living between the listener and AAC user (Beck, Bock, Thompson, & Kosuwan, 2002; Beck, Fritz, Keller, & Dennis, 2000; Hustad, 2001; Lilienfeld & Alant, 2002). In general, use of AAC not only helps a child communicate but also has a positive impact on parental perception of the child's language development (Romski, Sevcik, Adamson, Smith, Cheslock, & Bakeman, 2011).

In the remainder of this chapter we'll discuss several issues related to AAC. I'm assuming that you have at least a passing knowledge of AAC, so I'll spend less time on the basics than I might. Even so, as you'll see, there's plenty to discuss on this topic. After some introductory information, we'll explore evidence-based practices and other issues, followed by a discussion of assessment. AAC intervention with little ones will be addressed in the next chapter.

You may have heard of AAC in your classes, or you may have experienced it firsthand with a child with a communication disorder. Either way, it doesn't hurt to refresh your memory. You'll find an easy introduction to AAC in this video.
https://www.youtube.com/watch?v=r3m8_YmTDDM

Types of AAC

AAC systems are typically divided into unaided and aided based on the nonuse or use of external devices, respectively.

- ■ **Unaided AAC** does not require any equipment and relies on the user's body to relay messages.
- ■ **Aided AAC** incorporates the use of communication devices in addition to the user's body.

Unaided forms consist of gestures, facial expressions, body language, and manual signs. Obviously, gestures and signs require both the adequate fine motor coordination skills to make distinctive hand shapes and communication partners who understand these movements. Aided forms of AAC require some additional external support, such as

- ■ A communication board with visual-graphic symbols, including photographs, line drawings, symbols, or even printed words, that stand for, or represent, what a child wants to express, or
- ■ A computer or other electronic device that generates speech, either synthetic or recorded, and/or a graphic display.

In general, AAC, whether aided or unaided, has the potential to improve lives, especially for those nonsymbolic individuals with severe disabilities.

AAC users often communicate through a combination of unaided and aided systems, in addition to vocalizations and verbalizations, depending on the context and communication partner. For example, John, a 6-year-old boy with ASD, communicated using natural speech, pointing and conventional gestures, a communication book, and a Macintosh PowerBook with a speech synthesizer (Light, Roberts, Dimarco, & Greiner, 1998).

UNAIDED AAC

Unaided AAC systems use the body's own devices to communicate and include signs and gestures in addition to vocalizations and verbalizations, even if unintelligible. Possible sign systems include American Sign Language (ASL), Seeing Essential English (SEE$_1$), Signing Exact English (SEE$_2$), Signed English, and American Indian Hand Talk (Amer-Ind). Other manual systems, finger spelling, and Cued Speech are used infrequently, if at all, with infants and toddlers.

Let's dispel one belief. It has sometimes been argued that manual signing is preferable to aided communication because there is an existing community of manual signers, primarily people who have deafness. This notion may be unrealistic given the unlikelihood that hearing children using sign will be exposed to or embraced by the Deaf Community just because they are able to use a few signs. In addition, the learning demands that signing places on potential communication partners, such as teachers, parents, and other care providers, make it highly unlikely that these individuals will possess more than an extremely limited sign vocabulary. None of these comments should discourage us from using signing with a child if appropriate.

Sign Systems

ASL is the sign language used within the Deaf Community. Unlike most of the other systems, ASL is its own language and not English in a signed form. Initially, in AAC's infancy, ASL was used extensively in AAC intervention with young children whether they were hearing or not. As its own language, ASL has a unique grammar. Because many individuals who used ASL signs did not use ASL grammar, the result was a sort of pidgin ASL.

Both SEE$_1$ and SEE$_2$ are artificially created English-based sign systems. SEE$_1$ or Seeing Essential English, sometimes called Signing Essential English, was developed in 1966 with the intention of teaching English grammar along with or through sign. In SEE$_1$, morphemes are usually formed as separate signs and there are well over 100 obligatory affixes. As you might imagine, it can be difficult for some beginning signers, especially very young ones, to learn the hand shapes and multiple symbols used to express a single concept. SEE$_2$ or Signing Exact English, an offshoot of SEE$_1$, is intended for use with young children and contains approximately 70 affixes to be used with primarily ASL signs plus additional signs for pronouns, plurals, possession, and the verb *be*.

In part as a response to the difficulty in using SEE$_1$ and SEE$_2$ and with young children in mind, Signed English was developed at Gallaudet University, the primary U.S. institution of higher learning for those with deafness. Signed English is simpler to learn than the SEEs because, although it follows English word order, a child does not need to include the 16 optional morphological endings. Although most signs were taken from ASL, many were simplified for young hands. Signed English is the sign system used most frequently in schools with nonspeaking and nonsymbolic children.

American Indian Hand Talk (Amer-Ind) is a form of gestural communication consisting of 250 conceptual signals, most of which can be performed with one hand. The vocabulary is the equivalent to approximately 2500 English words because the signs have multiple meanings. Telegraphic in nature and lacking an exact grammar, Amer-Ind is easier to learn than English. Approximately 40 percent of the signals are intelligible to the untrained eye, making Amer-Ind extremely guessable.

AIDED AAC

Aided AAC can range from low technology to high. Low-tech devices may be electronic or nonelectronic. Electronic low-tech devices may consist of a static or nonchanging display or a single-message single-switch device. In contrast, high-tech devices offer dynamic or changing displays, are usually computer based, and usually require more training to learn to use.

Memory and recall are minimized with aided AAC because representations or symbols are presented, requiring only recognition from among an array of symbols offered. Word finding is accomplished through recognition rather than retrieval from memory as in signing.

Communication Boards

Nonelectronic in nature, *communication boards* are portable, readily accessible, and very adaptable. Although there can be an infinite variety to fit individual needs, most communication boards contain pictures that are selected by pointing. Boards vary in size, shape, and construction, in the symbols used, and in their arrangement and organization.

For young children, using simple communication boards, digital photos, scanned images, and/or color line drawings covered with clear contact paper and backed with Velcro seem appropriate initially. The Velcro allows the symbols to be detached from one location on the communication board and moved to another that may be more appropriate for any ongoing activity.

Electronic Devices

Electronic means of AAC are extremely varied and can consist of commercially available AAC devices, individually designed AAC equipment, or adaptations to existing computers. These range from simple inexpensive single-switch devices, such as the Big Mac, to complex systems that permit access to sophisticated language and literacy skills. Prices are commensurate, ranging from under $100 to over $10,000. Several devices are presented in Figure 7.1.

Devices differ primarily by input mode, control electronics, and output or display. Let's discuss these characteristics.

Input. Input modes vary from simple pressure switches, operated by a touch with virtually any body part, to touchscreen devices and on to position switches, such as a mouse, that direct a cursor.

FIGURE 7.1 **A Range of Aided AAC Electronic Devices**

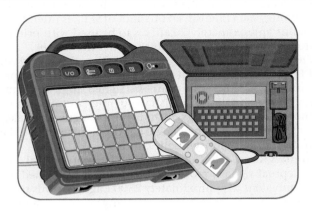

Although simple single-action, single-message voice output devices, such as the Big Mac or Talking Picture Frame, may seem limited in function, they can be easily reprogrammed, making them extremely flexible in use. Activated by depressing the input "switch," these devices might be used to ask for "Help" in a variety of contexts or to attain someone's attention, to greet, or to request "more." In addition, repetitive turns in games or finger plays, lines in songs, and phrases in books can be recorded to enable a child to participate in these activities.

In the past, more high-tech computer-based AAC devices have often been used only with children who have more typical cognition. In part, this was a reaction to the expense of such equipment. In addition, earlier AAC devices often required a fairly sophisticated set of cognitive skills. Technological advances have now made a broad range of AAC options available. As technology has advanced, prices have fallen.

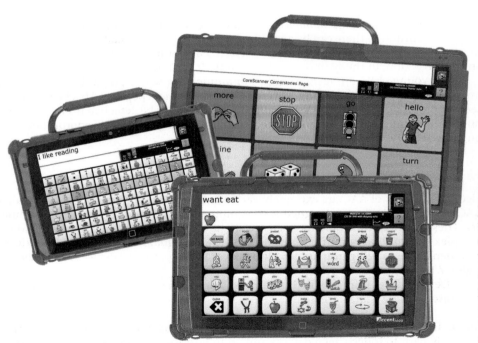

Courtesy of the Prentke Romich Company.

Portable direct selection devices using pictures offer an AAC option for some children.

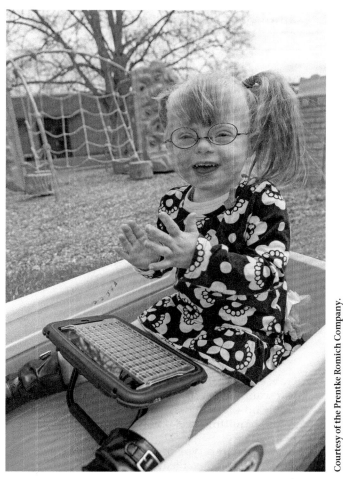

Courtesy of the Prentke Romich Company.

Portable AAC devices can accompany a child throughout the day and be programmed for different daily environments.

Mode of Selection. Input or access to aided AAC may be via direct selection or scanning. In direct selection, a child indicates his or her selection by pointing in a variety of ways, including with a finger, hand, head stick, eyes, or even a foot. These selection methods go by various names, such as eyegaze, in which a child uses his or her eyes to control icon selection, and headtracking, in which a reflective dot on the forehead controls movement and selection.

There is a one-to-one correspondence between cursor movement and switch activation. Single-action, single-message devices, mentioned earlier, would also be examples of direct selection.

In scanning, the message elements are presented in sequence to a child who then makes his or her choice as each element is presented (Beukelman & Mirenda, 2005). The user need only stop or start the scan, compensating for an inability to accurately select directly.

Scanning can take many forms. In circular scanning, the simplest of the scanning patterns, individual items are displayed in a circle and are electronically scanned one at a time in a clock format until the AAC user stops the scanner and thereby selects an item. The AAC user is required only to initiate and stop the scan. Obviously, this type of scan is limited by the user's ability to accurately stop the scan. The circular pattern also limits the amount of information available for communication.

In linear scanning, items are also presented sequentially, but one at a time in a row or rows as the cursor moves through the display. An example is presented in Figure 7.2.

FIGURE 7.2 **Example of a Direct Selection Device**

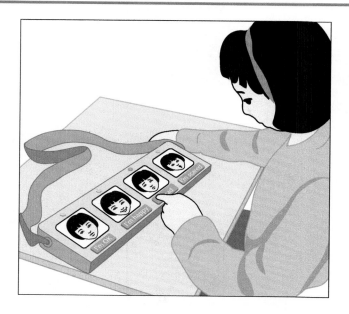

A cursor advances across each symbol in turn until the child indicates the desired one. Relatively simple, linear scanning requires that a child only activate or deactivate the cursor. This requires a simple on-off switch. As you might imagine, linear scanning symbol selection is relatively slow, requiring several pulses before the desired symbol is indicated (Beukelman & Mirenda, 2005).

Circular and linear scans are a type of preset or automatic scanning in which the scanning indicator moves in a predictable, predetermined pattern that is controlled by the electronic scanning device, and a child activates a switch to select an item when it is highlighted by the cursor. In a variation, called inverse scanning, a child holds down a switch that highlights items sequentially until an item is reached and the child releases the switch to select the highlighted item. Obviously, the rate of scan will need to be set for a child's motor abilities, and a child must understand the scanning sequence.

Patterns of scanning may be either one-at-a-time or grouped in either a row-column or block scanning format in which sections of the display are highlighted prior to individual symbol selection. Row-column and block scans usually use step scanning, which allows the user to advance one step at a time with each activation of the switch. Finally, directed scanning, which is under the control of the user, enables the user to move the scanning indicator up, down, left, right, or diagonally, directing it toward a target. Let's say a bit more about a few of these scanning methods.

In either block or row-column scanning, the cursor systematically advances or steps through groups of symbols until the user selects the group containing the target symbol. The cursor then presents each item sequentially within the selected group. For example, in row-column scanning, the cursor indicates rows in sequence until a row has been selected and then highlights individual symbols in that row in sequence. Efficiency is increased as multiple symbols are scanned simultaneously in each row (Beukelman & Mirenda, 2005). Theoretically, undesired symbols can be skipped, and fewer pulses are required to reach the desired symbol (Petersen, Reichle, & Johnston, 2000).

Let's see how this works. Remember that this is a scan and not direct selection. Suppose I have 100 symbols arranged in 10 rows of 10. If I desire the 95th one, in an automatic scan I must wait until the device pulses through all 95. In a row-column scan, I would scan 10 rows, stop on the last, and then pulse across that row five spaces to the 95th symbol. Instead of 95 pulses and the time it takes to wait, the selection has been reduced to 15 pulses and less than one-sixth the time.

FIGURE 7.3 Directed Scanning

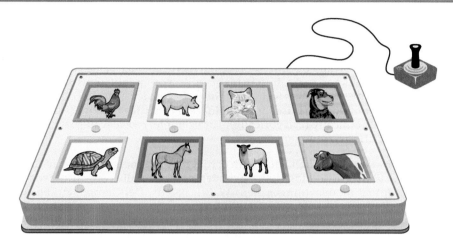

In directed scanning, a multifunction switch, such as a joystick similar to a car gearshift, controls the direction of the cursor movement. Usually, the cursor begins in the center of the symbol array so that the number of movements required to reach a symbol is minimized. In this way, directed scanning may significantly increase selection rate compared to other scanning techniques. As with direct selection, directed scanning, presented in Figure 7.3, gives the child more selection control, although it takes better motor abilities and requires the child to coordinate and monitor the relationship between the cursor and the target (Dowden & Cook, 2002). The child must locate the desired symbol and then subsequently plan and execute a scanning path to reach that symbol.

Whatever the method of selection, after a symbol has been selected, the cursor may remain on the selected symbol or mark it and return to some other location. For example, in centering, the scanning indicator automatically returns to the center of the display after each selection. In other displays, the cursor may move to the beginning of the display. The cursor is now ready to begin a new search.

Organization of the display. AAC systems use either static or dynamic displays. In static displays, mentioned previously, each representation is visible to a child at all times. With a dynamic display, selection results in a new array of graphic symbols. In other words, all representations are not visible at all times. Frequently, categories are visible with representations placed within these categories and requiring a second selection. The child must first remember which category or scene to activate in order to access the word because only a portion of the pictures are available and visible at any one time. Dynamic displays have the advantage of fewer symbols on display at one time while still allowing access to a larger vocabulary set.

Use of a dynamic display technology requires the ability to (Drager, Light, Speltz, Fallon, & Jeffries, 2003; Reichle, Dettling, Drager, & Leiter, 2000)

- Understand that other graphic symbols are accessed via the system, even though they are not visible,
- Recall the correct page where an item is located, and
- Determine the correct selection process to access the desired symbol.

A menu page offers different vocabulary selections. As might be expected, both preschool and early school-age typically developing (TD) children and those with cerebral palsy (CP) make more errors on dynamic displays than on static ones (Hochstein, McDaniel, Nettleton, & Hannah Neufeld, 2003).

If a child has only a few symbols, all may be displayed on the screen in a static or unchanging display. More typical is a categorical display in which symbols are located within various groupings.

Possible organizational designs for symbols include a taxonomic grid, schematic grid, schematic scene or visual scene display (VSD), and iconic organization. All four organizational designs are presently used in aided AAC systems. In the taxonomic grid, vocabulary items are typically organized on different vocabulary pages or screens by part of speech, such as nouns and verbs. In schematic grids, vocabulary items are organized by different events or contexts, such as food or clothing. In iconic displays, icons or line drawings (*knot* to represent "not") are used in combination to retrieve a single word. Icons are often arranged taxonomically (categorically). For example, *people* (category) + *boy* (item) are used in combination to represent "boy."

Schematic Organization. Although adult conceptual models, such as semantic categories, can be successful with older children, these models are not totally compatible with young children's conceptual models (Binger, Kent-Walsh, Berens, Del Campo, & Rivera, 2008; Binger & Light, 2007; Drager et al., 2003; Light & Drager, 2002; Nigam, Schlosser, & Lloyd, 2006). More traditional displays, such as nouns and verbs, may impose cognitive, sensory perceptual, motor, and linguistic constraints on young children by removing symbols from their communication context (Fallon, Light, & Achenbach, 2000; Light & Drager, 2007; Shane & Weiss-Kapp, 2007). In contrast, elements in a scene are depicted in relation to a contextual environment.

Schematic scene organization in VSD uses integrated scenes with items represented within context. For example, a representation of a house may, when selected, yield vocabulary used at home. In another example, a photo of the mother and child playing may contain the words *mommy*, *play*, *me*, and the names of toys seen in the picture. Concepts embedded in a scene free a child from the constraints of rows-columns and abstract semantic categories.

Scene displays offer several possible advantages over traditional grid displays for younger nonsymbolic children. Scenes can (Light & Drager, 2007)

■ Represent familiar events or activities, maximizing the meaningfulness of the symbols;
■ Present symbols in context, providing support for children's understanding;
■ Organize language schematically according to event experiences, a strategy congruent with young children's organization of language concepts; and
■ Preserve the relationships between symbols that occur in life, such as location.

VSDs are not without possible drawbacks, however, especially in generalizing symbol learning to other, nonpictured contexts.

Although older children perform better with VSDs than younger children on initial opportunities, younger children can learn to use VSDs with relatively few instructional opportunities (Olin, Reichle, Johnson, & Monn, 2010). This suggests that VSDs can be used with children as young as 2 years of age.

Output. Output can range from picture highlighting to either synthesized or prerecorded speech, possibly accompanied by printed words, although some form of digital speech comes closest to typical communication and will be more meaningful for a young child than other forms such as printed words. Some devices enable the SLP to record voices, such as a child of similar age, to be activated when a symbol is chosen. While it is important that individual symbols be represented, the SLP should not neglect other messages that foster interaction, such as a favorite song or reciprocal game.

Children with limited vocalizations or restricted vocal control may find that voice output or another auditory signal can effectively gain the attention of others. Partners may also find voice output easy to interpret and understand (Hustad, Morehouse, & Gutmann, 2002). In addition, such systems can communicate across distances more effectively than more subtle behavioral messages such as a gesture.

As an added benefit, a speech generating device (SGD) provides a model of a child's messages that may, in turn, enhance his or her language learning (Romski, Sevcik, & Adamson, 1999). An unfamiliar symbol might provide receptive language input of novel vocabulary.

SGDs or voice output communication aids (VOCAs) can come in the form of portable electronic devices or less mobile designs. To activate the device, a child uses a finger, hand, or some other means to select a graphic symbol from the SGDs display. In addition to speech output, messages may also be displayed graphically.

Multimodality aided communication systems, whether electronic or not, provide communication flexibility, especially when combined with vocalizations, verbalizations, gestures, and/or signs. In some situations, low-tech systems such as pictures may be more direct and simpler than elaborate electronic devices. There is some evidence that children find even simple electronic devices difficult to use in some communicative situations. Because, ideally, AAC use involves multimodal communication, it is not necessary for SLPs to frame system choice as one between total reliance on high- or low-tech systems.

Symbol Systems

We cannot realistically discuss aided AAC use without also discussing the symbol systems used with AAC devices, whether electronic or nonelectronic. Symbol systems range from real objects on communication boards to printed words or letters on both communication boards and electronic devices. In our discussion, we'll progress from actual objects to more abstract representations. Written symbol systems seem well beyond the cognitive abilities of very young AAC users and will not be discussed.

Actual objects are typically very iconic, meaning they look like what they are. Although a chocolate chip cookie can stand for "cookie," for a young child it may represent only that type of cookie and not generalize to other cookies. By its nature, as you can see, this type of system may be very concrete and, therefore, may be difficult to expand beyond this one-for-one representation. Most children do not need to begin at this level unless they are extremely low functioning.

Pictures, photos, line drawings, and miniature objects are called representative symbol systems because they are not the actual object but represent or stand for the object. Several systems are presented in Figure 7.4 for comparison. Color, such as a green car similar to the family vehicle, often helps recognition but may also limit use to communicating only about cars that are green or even to only the family car, so there is the same danger of lack of generalization as with real objects.

Tangible symbols include three-dimensional objects and two-dimensional photographs and line drawings (Rowland & Schweigert, 1989). The type of symbol used should fit the sensory and cognitive abilities as well as the experiences of the individual child. Three-dimensional symbols can either be constructed from materials identical to those of the actual object or be replicas of the object. As with actual objects, such iconic representations as objects, photographs, or line drawings may also represent specific objects, people, or activities for the child rather than more generalized concepts. A continuum of levels of tangible symbol representation is presented in Table 7.1.

Compared to more abstract symbols, tangible symbols make relatively low demands on a child's cognitive abilities. Tangible symbols can be manipulated by a child and can be held, handed to a partner, or placed next to the referent. Because a tangible symbol has an obvious perceptual relationship to its referent, only minimal demands are placed on a child's representational skills.

Tangible symbols are a viable alternative for many individuals who may not be able to acquire abstract symbols readily. As such, they can serve as either a transition or a means of communication. Longitudinal research with school-age children indicates that tangible symbols allow some children to overcome the restrictions of gestural communication, while others progress beyond tangible symbols to use abstract symbol systems, including speech (Rowland & Schweigert, 2000).

Boardmaker is a software program that can be used to create communication boards and electronic device overlays with *picture communication symbols* (PCS). Voice, sound, animation, and video can be added to Boardmaker materials on a computer to enhance the communication experience. PCS has a core vocabulary of approximately 5,000 symbols that are highly transparent or readily guessable.

Rebus and PICSYMS are more abstract symbol systems than PCS. *Rebus*, originally designed to help young readers, uses pictograms to represent symbolic sound, as in a picture of a bee to represent the verb *be*, and is a precursor to the development of spelling.

FIGURE 7.4 **Examples of Representational Systems**

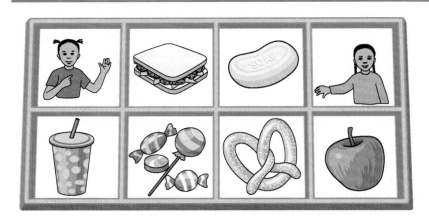

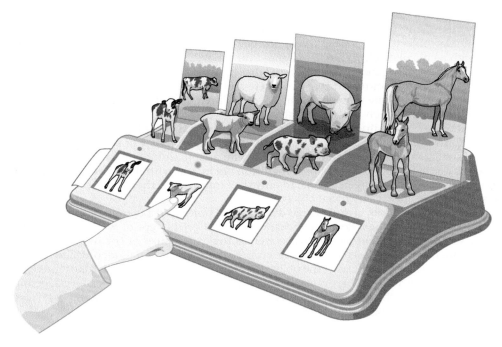

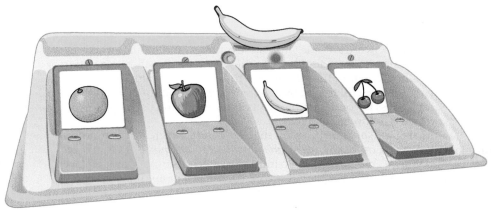

TABLE 7.1 **Levels of Tangible Symbols**

REPRESENTATION	REFERENT	SYMBOL
Identical item	Raisin	Raisins glued to communication board
Partial or associated object	Shoe	Shoelace
	Car	Car keys
Shared features	Pretzel	Styrofoam or plastic pretzel
Artificial association	Cafeteria	Reproduce wooden apple on cafeteria door

Symbols consist of a combination of line drawings, stick figures, and arbitrary symbols, such as check marks and question marks, which are combined to form words. For example, the word *son* is formed by combining *s* with the symbol for *on*. Obviously, considerable cognitive skill is needed to use this graphic system.

PICSYMS, or Pictograph Ideogram Communication Symbols, consist of over 1,800 line drawings of pictographs and ideographs that are accompanied by text labels. These symbols are similar to Boardmaker's representations, but their somewhat more abstract character makes them more conceptually difficult for some children to learn.

Finally, *Blissymbols*, originally conceived as an international language, consists of three elements: pictographs; arbitrary symbols, such as "+" which means either *and* or *too*; and Bliss-created symbols, such as "^" to signal an action. The approximately 100 elements in Blissymbols can be combined in various ways to create a large variety of symbols that are abstract representations of concepts.

Before we move on, I would be remiss if I didn't acknowledge the Picture Exchange Communication System (PECS; Bondy & Frost, 1998, 2001; Frost & Bondy, 2002). PECS is a visual form of communication using pictures, primarily with children with ASD. It is more a holistic approach than a symbol system and will be discussed in the next chapter when we consider AAC use with children with ASD.

The choice of symbol system or systems requires extensive assessment and trial-and-error experimentation. The success of AAC use may hinge more on the symbol system chosen by the SLP and family than on all the gadgetry of the device on which it is used.

 AT and AAC require special adaptations for children in EI. Watch this video for a discussion of communication assistive technology.
https://www.youtube.com/watch?v=ApG0ahrgipw

Evidence-Based Practice

It must be admitted from the outset that our empirical or experimental data on AAC use is thin, especially with very young children, making evidence-based practice a challenge. A review of research articles in peer-review journals since 1980 finds that most studies are single-subject, making comparisons to diverse clinical populations difficult (Campbell, Milbourne, Dugan, & Wilcox, 2006). Although there is some evidence on the efficacy of AAC intervention for infants, toddlers, and preschoolers with a variety of severe disabilities, more studies are desperately needed (Cress, 2003; Romski, Sevcik, & Forrest, 2001; Rowland & Schweigert, 2000).

Single-subject studies compare a subject's performance during intervention to her or his performance before intervention and after intervention is removed. In contrast, group designs frequently compare those who have received intervention with those who have not. In part, the number of single-subject studies of AAC is a reflection of the unique nature of each child in need of AAC and the relatively small population available to a researcher in a geographic area. In one case, a colleague and I worked with a client with the unique characteristics of legal blindness, intellectual disabilities, cerebral palsy, and challenging behaviors (Robinson & Owens, 1995). Matching her with similar subjects for a group study would have been extremely difficult.

Empirical articles on early AAC since 1980 have focused on the specific areas of selection, use, and training. Here are some of the major findings of a review of these studies (Campbell et al., 2006).

- ■ *Switch interface use.* Studies provide relatively strong evidence that infants with a variety of disabilities can be taught to operate switches to activate toys or create other reinforcing outcomes. Importantly, this is facilitated when switch activation uses a previously existing movement, such as head turning or touch.
- ■ *Computer use.* Although there are numerous examples of young children quickly adapting to electronic technology that does not require complicated movements or intricate symbol systems, no studies directly addressed computer use by infants or young toddlers. The small number of studies conducted with preschoolers resulted in inconclusive evidence about the effectiveness of computer use.
- ■ *AAC devices.* Only one study exists on teaching children functional use of an AAC device within the context of typical activities and routines. It does not provide sufficient information to be definitive.

As can be seen, there is a strong need for research to guide evidence-based decision-making (Schlosser & Raghavendra, 2004).

Only recently has it become recognized that AT-enhanced performance can provide a means for infants and young children to participate in everyday activities and routines (Campbell, Milbourne, & Wilcox, 2008; Mistrett, 2001, 2004). Sadly, as we've seen, empirical studies of instructional programs that incorporate the use of aided AAC are extremely rare (Mirenda, 2003).

A meta-analysis of 50 studies across various age groups and populations—not just children—found that although there may be an initial learning advantage for unaided AAC over aided, there is little difference between the two in generalized communication over time (Schlosser & Lee, 2000). Few studies directly compare the two techniques. A second meta-analysis of 24 studies found no evidence to suggest that either signing or aided techniques are more likely to lead to natural speech development (Millar, Light, & Schlosser, 2000). Although research suggests that manual signing or total communication (speech and sign simultaneously) results in faster and more complete receptive and/or expressive vocabulary acquisition than does speech alone, almost all of these studies involve labeling in response to questions such as "What's this?" rather than development of spontaneous communications, such as requesting, asking questions, or making comments.

Obviously, manual signs are more portable and more readily used at a distance from the listener, especially when compared to graphic symbol displays with no voice output. The possible vocabulary size with manual signing is limited by learner variables, such as memory and fine motor ability. In contrast, aided AAC display variables, such as size of the symbols or the display, may be limiting factors.

Ideally, evidence-based practice (EBP) along with individualistic assessment data will guide decision-making by SLPs. Yet, as just noted, there is little clinical research to guide clinical decisions (Schlosser & Raghavendra, 2004). This is changing slowly. In this absence, SLPs potentially are open to the dangers of following fads and highly publicized intervention approaches. Parents may be a factor, especially when they are influenced by Internet hype and chat room advice.

DANGERS IN IGNORING EBP

Several years ago, a new AAC method called "facilitated communication" (FC) was introduced into the United States from Australia. In short, it was a method that used a keyboard and hand-guiding to enable some clients to communicate via computers by typing their message. So far it sounds fine and it can be helpful, especially for some clients with motor control deficits. Some SLPs adopted FC without considering the available research, which was slim at best.

All of a sudden, it seemed as if every nonspeaking individual in the United States was on FC. Children with ASD and severe intellectual disability (ID) began to communicate in words and sentences. Even when it was revealed through research that facilitators were influencing both the typing and the content, FC continued to be used as an intervention strategy in part because it did seem to work for some individuals.

During the frenzied rush toward FC, I happened to visit a school and, while waiting to observe intervention by one of my students, had a pleasant chat seated at the feet of a 7-year-old girl who was waiting for her session to begin. To my surprise, when I observed that session, the SLP had my student teaching this child to use FC. Later, I inquired politely as to why the girl was using FC and was told that it was because she would not communicate with adults, this despite my conversation with her. When I mentioned our chat, I was informed that her phonological errors were so severe that she was unintelligible, something again that had not interfered greatly with our conversation.

I probably need to add that when it comes to talking with children, I'm a very forgiving partner, preferring to focus on the child rather than on the disorder. That aside, when all was said and done, I was left to wonder about the manner in which adults had communicated with this child in the past that had made her so reticent, and about intervention decisions that would place the child on an AAC device rather than simply targeting her phonological problems.

It is essential that you as a future SLP keep abreast of research in our field and learn to read and evaluate this research critically and with an eye toward intervention. Ignoring research findings is not an acceptable professional option.

Unfortunately, I've had to eat crow before and admit that what I've done in the past has sometimes been shown to be less effective than another method. It can be uncomfortable. But the issue is not what makes me comfortable; it's what's best for a child and a family who are depending on me to make the most informed decisions possible.

AAC MYTHS

Although signing has been in use for hundreds of years with individuals with deafness and aided AAC has been used for more than four decades to address the communication needs of both children and adults who cannot consistently rely on speech for communication, some SLPs have been slow to adopt AAC for very young children. This situation may result from "clinical myths" about AAC based on intuition rather than on research data.

Several myths that potentially exclude children from AAC services include (Romski & Sevcik, 2005):

- AAC is a "last resort,"
- AAC hinders or stops further speech development,
- Children must have a certain set of cognitive skills to use AAC,
- Speech-generating AAC devices are only for children with no intellectual disability,
- Children must be a certain age or developmental level to use AAC, and
- There is a developmental hierarchy of symbols.

Although none of these myths is supported by the current research, they are often considered when discussing an intervention plan for a young child. We will discuss each myth in turn as we proceed through the chapter.

Myth 1: AAC Is a "Last Resort"

Approximately 40 years ago, when AAC first emerged as an intervention strategy for nonsymbolic individuals, it was considered to be the last option, something to be tried only when every other method for development of speech had been exhausted. In fact, AAC can play many roles in early communication development and should be introduced before communication failure occurs (e.g., Cress & Marvin, 2003; Reichle, Buekelman, & Light, 2002). Early access to AAC has been shown to be a means for (Brady, 2000)

- Acquiring some necessary prelinguistic and cognitive skills essential for language development, and
- Establishing symbolic communication.

In other words, AAC is appropriate for a young child just developing both communication and language skills in order to prevent failure in these areas of development.

Myth 2: AAC Hinders Speech Development

Despite the documented communication benefits of AAC intervention, some SLPs and many parents still hesitate to adopt AAC for fear that it will impede the development of speech (Romski & Sevcik, 2005). Parents often raise this issue (Beukelman & Mirenda, 2005). They worry that AAC may become a "crutch," negating the need for speech. Furthermore, these same parents and professionals worry that AAC will become a child's primary communication mode and remove the child's motivation to speak. These concerns are not supported by the available research, which actually suggests just the opposite.

As a multimodal communication intervention strategy, AAC attempts to enhance both receptive and expressive communication skills, including any existing vocalizations and verbalizations in addition to gestures, manual signs, and aided communication. Fostering the emergence of intelligible speech, especially in a young child, is an integral part of the AAC intervention process.

Although there are not many empirical studies, the ones we have demonstrate improvement in speech skills after AAC intervention (Beukelman & Mirenda, 2005; Cress & Marvin, 2003). For very young children, the use of AAC appears to enhance the development of spoken communication, although reported gains are often slight (Cress, 2003; Millar, Light, & Schlosser, 2006).

After a systematic review of the professional literature for over 30 years of AAC research and its effect on speech production, researchers report that none of the studies demonstrated decreases in speech production as a result of AAC intervention, 11 percent showed no change, and the overwhelming majority (89%) demonstrated gains in speech (Millar, Light, & Schlosser, 2006). As mentioned, for the most part, the gains were modest. The positive effects of AAC intervention on speech production can occur across children with a variety of disorders and using a variety of intervention methods, from highly structured, clinician-directed instruction to child-centered approaches implemented in play contexts.

It's important to note that spoken word production following the learning of AAC use seems to depend on mastery of verbal imitation at the time of intervention. This factor seems to be more important than either the child's age, IQ, or cognitive skills. Although speech development in conjunction with AAC use is most likely to occur in learners with some speech imitation ability, this outcome is not guaranteed. Nor should this information be interpreted to mean that AAC use should not begin before or in conjunction with verbal imitation training.

Research data clearly suggest that the introduction of AAC will neither cause a child to abandon speech he or she may be using nor prevent acquisition of new spoken words. It has been suggested that a child who learns to use one form of representation, such as AAC, may be predisposed to use another, such as speech, in the same context.

There are several possible reasons why AAC may benefit speech production:

- AAC intervention may reduce the pressure on the individual to speak, thereby reducing stress and indirectly facilitating speech.
- AAC intervention may allow individuals with significant speech impairments to bypass the motor and cognitive demands of speech production and focus on communication instead.
- After clients establish basic communication and language skills, they may then be better able to reallocate resources to improve their speech production.
- Unlike speech, the speed of ACC production, such as activating a switch or even signing, can be slowed without distorting the message, making it more accessible to those with motor impairments.

- When AAC is presented along with the spoken word, and these are followed by a reinforcer, both the AAC mode and speech production should increase in frequency (Mirenda, 2003).
- AAC, especially synthesized or digitized speech output, provides a more immediate and consistent model (Blischak, 2003; Smith & Grove, 2003).
- Being primarily visual in nature, ACC may use other areas of the brain than those used in speech production and reception.

Although the real reason for success may be a combination of these factors or an as yet undiscovered factor, and although speech gains may be only modest, it is important to recall that if nothing else, AAC can provide an acceptable means of communication that was previously lacking for many nonsymbolic children. As the name *augmentative and alternative communication* suggests, for some children AAC will be their primary means of communication while for others it will complement their speech or be a temporary stage in the development of speech.

Myth 3: Needed Cognitive Skills

When AAC intervention was in its infancy, it was assumed that certain cognitive skills were needed in order to learn AAC. There was a rush of professional articles, including one now-embarrassing article by this author, attempting to identify these skills. We now recognize that just as some parents of TD infants and infants with deafness begin signing to their child almost from birth, AAC can be introduced in similar fashion very early in a child's life. Of course a newborn will not communicate at a symbolic level, whether through AAC or speech, until able to do so cognitively, but an electronic device can first be introduced as a toy. Touch the picture and the device talks, just as many "talking books" and toys already do for TD infants.

Although some basic cognitive skills are essential in all children for language to develop, the exact relationship is unclear. In addition, it seems only fair to acknowledge our lack of ability to assess cognitive development in some children, especially young ones. For an infant or toddler with severe sensorimotor problems, it may be extremely difficult to demonstrate his or her cognitive abilities or for professionals to interpret this behavior. This fact calls into question at least some cognitive assessment methods.

Cognition and language interact in a reciprocal manner, and denying a child the means of expression because of the lack of assumed cognitive prerequisites may put the child at a distinct developmental disadvantage. The use of language can affect cognition, and a lack of expressive language skills may hinder cognitive development. In fact, the development of language skills through use of AAC may be critically important to the cognitive growth of many little ones.

In the past, young children with intellectual disability were frequently excluded from AAC intervention because their assessed level of either intelligence or sensorimotor development was not commensurate with those of TD children during early language development. Given that the exact level and type of cognitive skills needed to develop language are unknown, intellectual performance and/or prerequisite sensorimotor skills should not be used as criteria when decisions are made concerning when to begin AAC intervention.

Although it can be argued that some forms of symbolic AAC are beyond the abilities of some children, this fact does not exclude the use of other forms. Primitive signaling systems can be established even with children with profound ID. Likewise, receptive AAC use can begin at any time, in much the same way that parents talk to their infants before the child comprehends speech.

It was previously accepted at face value that computer-based AAC devices should be reserved for children with intact cognition because of the fairly sophisticated cognitive skills needed to operate them. Technological developments in AAC devices have now made a broad range of options available to young children. Many devices require little skill or knowledge of the equipment and can provide an early introduction to AAC, giving a child a means to communicate. I bought my grandson a Big Mac, a single-switch voice-recording and playback device that is easy to use and easy enough for caregivers to program that it can be adapted quickly to any situation.

Discrimination and short-term memory. Rather than overall cognitive skills, it may be that discrimination learning and short-term memory are more important. These two types of cognition interact in an interesting way.

It has been argued that manual signing is easier to learn because it is easier to discriminate signed signals than graphic symbols (Sundberg & Michael, 2001). According to this point of view, in order for a child to request a cookie using an aided symbol display, the child's motivation for a cookie (stimulus #1) and the presence of a symbol *cookie* (stimulus #2) are both required, while in manual signing, the child's motivation for a cookie is the only stimulus required. The child need only form the sign, rather than first scanning and then selecting a specific symbol from an array. This point would seem moot for children in whom discrimination learning and visual-spatial learning are relatively intact.

On the other hand, memory would seem to be a much more important factor in signing than in aided types of AAC communication. Signing requires recall memory for all signs stored in the brain, while aided systems require only recognition memory of the symbols displayed before the child (Oxley & Norris, 2000). Aided systems, therefore, do not require a child to search his or her memory for potential symbols that fit the particular situation. It would appear, then, that recall memory is easier and involves fewer cognitive resources in aided AAC. This presupposes that the graphic symbols are readily accessible. In fact, individuals with memory constraints find learning signs more difficult than learning graphic symbol systems.

Myth 4: Not for Children with ID

It has somehow been assumed by some SLPs that children with ID do not have the cognitive ability to use AAC. This falsehood is in part based on Myth #3. In fact, we find AAC use by children with a variety of disorders. Seemingly more important are the individualization of both the type of AAC and intervention method and the integration of AAC into a child's everyday communication environment. Based on the number of symbols a child with ID produces following intervention, important factors seem to be a child's cognitive development, comprehension, level of play, and nonverbal communication, plus the amount of adult input in the home (Brady, Thiemann-Bourque, Fleming, & Matthews, 2013).

Myth 5: Children Must Be a Certain Age

Intervention practices tend to underutilize ACC in early intervention. In contrast, ASHA (2015) lists AAC as an appropriate communication service for infants.

There is no evidence to suggest that a child must be a certain chronological age to optimally benefit from AAC interventions. Evidence-based practice clearly indicates the benefits of early AAC intervention services for children with a variety of disabilities (Cress, 2003; Romski, Sevcik, & Forrest, 2001; Rowland & Schweigert, 2000).

Usually, professionals do not select ACC options until a child is at least 24 months of age. In other words, some professionals continue to view ACC as a method of last resort. This leads to the introduction of AAC in a negative way that suggests that failure has occurred and the child is somehow at fault.

Instead, we might approach AAC in a positive manner that places the child in the forefront of young children using computers. That sure sounds like a better outlook to me!

Myth 6: Developmental Hierarchy of Symbols

Although a hierarchy of symbols from concrete to abstract does exist, it does not reflect a developmental order. Nor must an SLP proceed with a child through each one in sequence. When given a choice, infants do not seem to prefer one form of graphic representation, such as photos, over others, such as drawings (Da Fonte & Taber-Doughty, 2007).

Data suggest that initial picture symbols need not look like what they represent. In other words, a big "X" may just as easily represent *drink* as a picture of a glass of juice. Initial exposure is where a child learns the purpose of AAC, not the symbolism. That will come.

Notion of a developmental hierarchy can lead to rigidity or the idea that systems can never be combined. In other words, we can't use photos on the same device as line drawings. Or even worse, we can't combine signing with picture communication. This lack of flexibility flies in the face of individualization.

Elements of a Thorough AAC Assessment

All individuals communicate along a continuum from prelinguistic through symbolic to fully linguistic communication. The focus of an AAC assessment is typically not to determine the need for AAC but to explore this continuum and to determine the devices and services that can help a child fully participate in his or her environment (Romski, Sevcik, Hyatt, & Cheslock, 2002).

As we noted in previous chapters, there are a limited number of assessment tools available for use with young children with significant communication impairment. Given that few standardized tests are available and that their use with young children is questionable, informal checklists typically are used during an AAC assessment. Although most checklists have been developed for use with school-age children and adults, they can be adapted for use with young children if developmentally supportive modifications are made.

Given that standardized tests may be of little help in clearly indicating what the nonsymbolic child knows, an assessment should attempt to identify what the child can do successfully and then build on that through dynamic assessment. Of importance is identifying what facilitates and what inhibits communication at each step in the process. Sadly, it's often easier to identify what a child cannot do, although from a practical standpoint, we can only build on positives. The negatives may provide future targets for intervention. In the following section, we'll discuss the major questions to be answered in an AAC assessment.

In addition to a "hands-on" communication assessment, an SLP can determine a child's

- Cognitive abilities,
- Communication methods,
- Physical abilities,
- Self-help activities and routines, and
- Barriers that affect the child's participation.

This can be accomplished through family/caregiver interviews and informal observation of the child interacting with family, friends, and caregivers during natural daily routines and in typical settings. Team members then engage in a problem-solving process to determine the most appropriate devices, adaptations, services, and/or strategies that will reduce or eliminate these barriers and enhance participation. Problem-solving may include trial-and-error usage of a variety of devices and strategies.

> Janice Light and Kathy Drager, professors at Penn State, are real innovative pioneers in the area of AAC and EI. Although I can't provide a direct link because of copyright issues, I encourage you to find and explore their wonderfully creative site. You'll find ideas aplenty and videos of young children using AAC devices. Go to the website for Pennsylvania State University and search for "aackids."

All of the elements of a communication assessment mentioned in Chapters 4 and 5 are equally important in assessing a child for AAC use. Some areas take on new relevance. Keeping in mind that AAC is, or should be, a multimodal communication system, an assessment of a child's abilities should include at least

- Speech and sound making,
- Current modes of communication,
- Receptive language skills,

- Motor skills,
- Visual perception,
- Joint attending,
- Sign/symbol recognition, and
- Child and family preferences.

Let's explore each briefly, then pull it together and end with decision-making.

SPEECH AND SOUND MAKING

Common indicators of future difficulty in vocal speech development include

- Birth or developmental conditions indicating a child is at risk for difficulties with vocal development,
- Feeding difficulties or continuing oral/motor control problems,
- Delayed onset of vocalization and/or speech, and
- Neuromotor difficulties relative to speech and language development.

Remember, however, that children's motor systems develop in ways that cannot always be predicted. Almost all children who can vocalize will use sounds in some way to communicate. Early AAC intervention should be paired with speech intervention that provides practice in controlling and diversifying a child's vocalizations and increasing a child's potential range of vocal signals that can be used for intentional communication.

Although the jury is still out, late onset of consonant-vowel babbling may be one predictor of later disorders in both speech and language (Oller, Eilers, Neal, & Cobo-Lewis, 1998). The ability to vocally imitate may also be of special importance developmentally.

Overall, the best predictors of speech and language for children with developmental disabilities under age 3 seem to be (Yoder, Warren, & McCathren, 1998)

- Five or more conventional words in a 5-minute interaction with a parent,
- The rate of protodeclarative use, and
- The ratio of number of words used to number of words understood.

Protodeclaratives, you'll recall, are gestures, such as pointing or reaching, and vocalizations that direct the conversational partner's attention to particular referents. The rate is determined by dividing the number of protodeclaratives by the length of the sampling session in minutes. In general, one or more protodeclaratives every 2 minutes, or a rate of .5/minute, is considered to be a positive sign for continued growth of speech and hearing.

Using a parent report form similar to the *McArthur-Bates Communicative Development Inventory* (CDI; Fenson et al., 2006), an SLP can quickly calculate the ratio of words used to words understood. The ratio is calculated by dividing the number of different words the mother reports that the child says by the number of different words (NDW) she reports that the child understands. For example, let's assume the mother reports that her child says 20 different words and understands 25, including all 20 that are spoken. Our ratio is calculated as follows:

$$\frac{\text{NDW spoken}}{\text{NDW spoken and understood}} = \frac{20}{25} = .8$$

Some children may produce words but seem not to understand them. Suppose that the same 20 words are spoken but that only 15 are among the 25 understood words. In other words, the child speaks 20 and understands 10 more. The spoken and understood total is 20 spoken plus 10 more understood but not spoken or 30.

$$\frac{\text{NDW spoken}}{\text{NDW spoken and understood}} = \frac{20}{30} = .67$$

The closer the ratio is to 1.0, the better a child's chances of developing speech and language.

At the very least, an SLP should attempt to describe a child's speech and sound-making as thoroughly as possible. This might include the child's

- Response to speech;
- Oral structures and functioning;
- Range of sounds, sound combinations, and syllable structures; and
- Ability to imitate oral movements, sounds, and words.

The presence of eating difficulties may indicate oral anatomical or physiological problems.

The more severe a child's motor limitations, particularly initiating and controlling oral and vocal movements, the more likely that the child will experience continued difficulty controlling the movements necessary for speech. That said, the same child may have a wide range of functional sound-making that is not linguistically based but nonetheless significant (Cress, 2002).

CURRENT MODES OF COMMUNICATION

A difference exists between exposing a child to AAC and expecting that same child to use an AAC system effectively to communicate. Successful expressive use of AAC devices implies experience with more basic communication strategies, just as we see in TD children's communication development (Cress, 2002). High-tech voice output, electronic, or picture systems are most likely to be successful if a child already uses basic communication tools such as facial expression, vocalizations, or gestures volitionally and appropriately. While none of these are prerequisites, they sure are nice to have!

Describing how a child communicates at present will be important for future AAC use. Ideally, you'd include these modes of communication in the multimodal system used by the child. As an SLP, you can note the child's responsiveness to other people's attempts to communicate and the child's indications of a desire to communicate with others. As carefully as possible, note the ways in which the child currently expresses various messages.

Occasionally, a mode of communication is message specific. For example, the child may tantrum for only one reason, such as "I want X." I've also seen children who become self-abusive to let us know that they want something, although the "something" is not always obvious.

For a child not using intentional gestural communication, expressive communication intervention might begin at this point and then introduce other forms of AAC. When communicative intent is absent, the acquisition of large numbers of graphic symbols is probably unlikely. The child who does not reach to pick up desired objects will most likely have difficulty learning to hold out or touch a symbol for these same objects.

If a child is unsuccessful with nonsymbolic communication, adding symbols may simply add complexity while increasing cognitive learning demands and decreasing the child's communication success (Light & Drager, 2000). For example, a child must understand that an AAC system, especially an aided one, represents his or her own communicative message. This recognition requires cognitive skills beyond simple gestural or behavioral forms of communication (Cress, 2001). That said, lack of success is not a foregone conclusion.

Experiencing communicative success with a voice output or picture-based system may help an infant learn the effect of his or her behavior on others (Rowland & Schweigert, 2000). Obviously, the relationship of nonsymbolic to symbolic communication is a complicated one. Describing that relationship requires careful monitoring of a child's behavior.

Receptive Language Skills

Receptive understanding of speech is not a prerequisite to AAC use. In fact, AAC may be used as a receptive mode of communication. It is important, however, to know what a child comprehends when initiating expressive communication intervention.

Before beginning intervention, an SLP will need to assess a child's level of meaningful symbolic representation. This can be accomplished informally or with an instrument such as the *Levels of Representation Pretest* (Rowland & Schweigert, 1990). Using a matching format, this tool probes a child's ability to associate various types of symbolic representations with highly preferred referents. On a less formal basis, an SLP can assess receptive language as outlined in Chapter 5.

Children ages 12–42 months of age with severe expressive impairments have better receptive language scores than expected for either their cognitive or overall development, as measured on both the *Battelle Developmental Inventory* and the *MacArthur Communicative Development Inventory* (Ross & Cress, 2006). Receptive language measures may provide a better estimate of a child's mental age than cognitive scores, which can be limited by motor disabilities.

Appropriate symbols can be created or adapted, using materials meaningful to the child. As mentioned throughout this text, vocabulary selection should be individualized and include items highly motivating to a specific child.

MOTOR SKILLS

It would appear from research data that when given the choice, children will use the method of communicating that they find most efficient and that this may vary even by individual symbol (Richman, Wacker, & Winborn, 2001; Sigafoos & Drasgow, 2001). While these data do not provide a definitive answer, they do suggest that SLPs should not impose restrictions that artificially make AAC use physically difficult, such as placement of graphic symbols in inaccessible areas of a wheelchair tray or requiring difficult methods of interfacing with an AAC device.

Not surprisingly, individuals with motor coordination problems experience difficulty in learning to sign (National Research Council, 2001). Motor difficulties affect both manual sign vocabulary size and the accuracy of sign formation. While it may be appropriate to teach children with poor fine motor skills a limited number of simple, functional signs (e.g., *eat, more, want*), they will probably require aided communication techniques as well. All of this suggests that for many children a combination of AAC systems is appropriate.

With the help of a physical therapist and/or occupational therapist, an SLP can document a child's

- ■ Manner of ambulation,
- ■ Fine motor skills, including range and consistency of motion, and
- ■ Motor imitation skills.

The manner of ambulation, or the ability to move about from place to place, may be important in AAC system selection and design. Some children will require a stationary system, while others will need a light, even malleable, one that travels with them.

Fine motor skills will be extremely important in determining the AAC system or systems to attempt with a child. Assessment can include a trial run with various systems to find one or more that seem to best fit a child's abilities. Good fine motor skills might indicate that signing is appropriate. Of importance are the consistency and reliability of desired movements.

One important question to answer for a child with neuromuscular difficulties is whether the child can cross the midline reliably. Some children have great difficulty executing movements when a limb, such as an arm, passes into the plane of the opposite side of the body. The ultimate design of the AAC system and the method of interfacing with the device may depend on such considerations.

The range and consistency of movement are important when determining the placement of a device or of individual symbols. For example, when I think a wheelchair tray is an appropriate location, I set objects or a grid on the tray and map the child's consistency in touching various locations. Using a play format, I look for the child's ease and reliability touching objects in various locations. From this information, I make some tentative decisions on the shape of the communication board or electronic device and the size of symbols, which may vary by location.

VISUAL PERCEPTION

It may be difficult for a child with vision problems to identify various representations or symbols. The size of these representations and the manner of selection may, in part, be determined by visual acuity. For example, I worked with one client with extremely poor vision and for whom signing was not a viable AAC mode because of neuromuscular difficulties. The team decided to use black-and-white drawings of a very large size which the client selected from individual cards worn on a clip on her belt. She would bring each picture close to her face for identification and then hand her partner the desired one.

Because SLPs are not qualified to perform formal vision testing, this is best left to optometrists, but an SLP can determine the minimum size at which clients can discern difference and match images. With very young children, trial and error is best.

JOINT ATTENDING

A child should be able to attend, even if only momentary, to both people and objects to learn to use AAC other than receptively. We've discussed the importance of this ability previously in Chapter 4. Even for children who do not attend, AAC can be used receptively, and training can begin using switch-activated toys. There is also value in a child's activating an SGD even if the intent and meaning of the message are not understood by the child. Learning to participate and to have a turn are valuable steps in learning to communicate.

SIGN/SYMBOL RECOGNITION

In assessing sign/symbol recognition and selection, an SLP might consider the following (Schlosser & Sigafoos, 2002):

- The role of iconicity and realism,
- Language comprehension of various referents,
- Concreteness of the referents,
- The reinforcement value of the referents, and
- Correspondence between the symbol and the referent.

Iconicity is an association that a child forms between a symbol and its referent based on a recognized physical link between the two, such as the degree to which a symbol visually resembles its referent or some aspect of its referent, or on any individualistic association made by the viewer. In contrast, opaque symbols are ones in which such association is not made easily.

Iconicity can influence symbol acquisition and use. Research-based findings suggest that iconic symbols can be learned in fewer trials than more opaque symbols. Iconicity may be trumped by usefulness, however, and a sign for a highly desired object may be easier to learn even when it is opaque. When the intervention target is learning to request, the desirability of the objects or activities seems to be more important than iconicity.

The best way to assess sign/symbol recognition is by trial and error. To which signs or symbols does the child respond best? Naturally, these considerations will differ with specific AAC systems.

Unaided AAC

It's easy to mistakenly assume that signing is easier because signs are highly iconic. In other words, signs supposedly look like the concepts they represent. For example, although it varies with the sign system, the sign for *drink* is usually performed by miming drinking from a glass. This sign is highly iconic. Unfortunately, only a small fraction of signs are iconic, and many signs included in children's initial AAC lexicons do not fall into this category. It has been estimated that only about 20 percent of signs are iconic in nature.

Iconic signs, such as *book*, made by opening the hands in imitation of a book opening, are often easy to teach. In the case of *book*, a child's book can be placed in the hands and opened and closed as the SLP repeatedly says "book," and then removed and repeated with only hand movements and the spoken word.

Although most signs are not iconic, many are said to be *transparent*, or easily guessable. The ease of deciphering is often based on adult responses and not those of young children. For example, the sign for *milk*, which is often made by miming milking a cow, is only guessable if you know where milk comes from and how it is extracted. A better way to know if an AAC sign/symbol system is appropriate for a child may be to give it a "test drive." Teach a few signs or symbols to a child and see how readily the child learns them.

In order for communication to be functional, it must be easily understood by communication partners (Mirenda & Erickson, 2000). In this regard, manual signs may impede communication with partners who do not sign. This can be overcome by teaching signing to parents and other caregivers. This would seem an essential aspect of intervention, given our emphasis on the child's communication environment.

Aided AAC

Iconicity in aided AAC varies between the pictures for the concrete nouns, such as *apple* and *dog*, and abstract nouns, such as *love* and *need*. By their nature, pictures used for concrete nouns have high iconicity and are highly related to those words. Abstract nouns, on the other hand, cannot be represented as well with pictures and thus have lower iconicity and are not as highly related to the words. Simply put, the association between a vocabulary item and the picture is more difficult for abstract nouns. In general, symbols with high iconicity are initially identified more readily and are recalled better than symbols with low iconicity.

Keep in mind that ideally a child's communication will be multimodal in nature and will change as the child's abilities change. For example, a child who begins with objects on a communication board may progress to pictures and on to written words in the future. During initial phases of AAC intervention, it may not matter whether a child uses abstract or iconic symbols because for the child beginning to explore AAC all symbols may be abstract (Romski & Sevcik, 2005).

Again, it's important for the family to have a say. If an AAC system seems too exotic, some families or family members may not use the device.

CHILD AND FAMILY PREFERENCES

Within reason, an SLP can give the child and certainly the family a choice of their preferred methods of communication. If the family is not comfortable with an AAC device, they may not use it at home. Nothing is sadder than a potentially life-changing AAC device being abandoned.

Several studies have demonstrated that positive results with AAC are critically tied to a family's participation in both assessment and intervention (Angelo, 2000; Goldbart & Marshall, 2004). This requires a thorough exploration of family needs, preferences, and priorities. It is important to remember that tastes change, but more importantly, abilities change, and a child or family may opt for another system in the future.

One of the best ways to know if an AAC system is a good fit is to try it. If possible, a device on loan may help families adjust to this new technology. The choice of an AAC system should be determined by the extent to which that system enhances a child's interaction with people in the child's environment.

Your sales abilities will be important here. A family needs to be convinced of the value of using AAC. Always bring it back to the family's concerns. For example, if a family member says, "Why do we need to use another way to communicate when we understand her already most of the time," reply, "Good, and we won't take that away. Our goal is to make her understood all the time."

Although preliminary research results suggest that graphic representations or pictures have greater intelligibility for potential communication partners, aided symbols must be selected carefully to match environmental demands and listener capabilities. In addition, SGDs are not always the most effective or intelligible type of AAC communications, especially if the speech output quality is poor.

Output technologies are an important factor, especially for potential partners of the AAC user. For example, although older child partners (4- and 5-year-olds) perform better than younger ones with a partner using an SGD, they both perform less accurately when interpreting synthesized speech compared to recorded speech (Axmear, Reichle, Alamsaputra, Kohnert, Drager, & Sellnow, 2005). In addition, although older preschool children do better than younger children on interpretation tasks, neither do very well with single words in isolation, whether the mode is synthesized or digitized recorded speech (Drager, Clark-Serpentine, Johnson, & Roeser, 2006). In short, 3- to 5-year-olds are less accurate in comprehending digitalized single words than single words in natural speech (Drager, Ende, Harper, Iapalucci, & Rentschler, 2004). As might be expected, children's accuracy increases with repeated exposure (Pinkoski-Ball, Reichle, & Munson, 2012). In addition, the intelligibility of both digitized and synthesized speech in environments with considerable background noise, such as a classroom, is difficult, suggesting that other preschoolers may be reluctant to communicate with children using these devices (Drager, Clark-Serpentine, et al., 2006).

Interpretation can be improved when words are used in context or placed within longer messages. Although intelligibility of sentences is better, use of sentences doesn't seem to foster novel word combinations by users, thus limiting ongoing communication as a method for generalizing novel words.

Given that most adults do not understand manual signs, there are inherent advantages in using printed words, graphic symbols, and/or high-quality SGD speech when the intended communication partners are literate (Mirenda, 2003). When the intended partners are young children or those with poor reading skills, SGDs or graphic symbols with a clear visual relationship to their referents would seem more appropriate.

DECISION-MAKING

To be optimally effective, an AAC system needs to (Light & Drager, 2005)

- Have versatile uses in everyday environments,
- Be appealing to the child,
- Be easy to learn and use, and
- Be dynamic and changing with communication needs.

Versatile systems meet a child's communication needs in a variety of situations and contexts and provide the potential for growth. As mentioned, you should not overlook the use of multiple modes of communication. A dynamic systems approach is capable of changing and growing as a child learns new skills and matures.

Selection of the best system or systems is based on many factors. For example, children with Down syndrome (DS) would seem to be good candidates for sign and simultaneous spoken language, given their strong use of gestures. The use of naturalistic teaching would also seem to be beneficial, given the social strengths of children with DS. The only real way to know, however, is to thoroughly assess both the child and the environment.

With aided AAC, there are several specific issues to be addressed. These include the symbol system, the method and rate of symbol selection, and the organization of symbols. It's important to remember that as an SLP, you are attempting a difficult task. Fitting a child and family to a communication system that meets their complex needs is not easy. You will make mistakes. No one can fault you if you have assessed the child and family thoroughly and systematically.

Symbol System

As with many clinical decisions, the system selection process should be based on evidence-based practice and on an individual child's and family's abilities and needs (Schlosser & Raghavendra, 2004). The research literature should be evaluated based on the clinical decisions to be made in each specific case. In selecting a graphic symbol system or systems, SLPs are faced with the difficult task of determining which type(s) of symbols to select from several possible choices, ranging from representation alone to words and letters with no pictorial representation, although the latter are most likely inappropriate for very young children.

Professionals often suggest that children can only learn symbols in a representational hierarchy that begins with real objects and passes through photographs to line drawings, then on to more abstract representations, and finally to written words or traditional orthography. In other words, concrete symbols are easier than abstract. Among 13- to 18-month-olds, however, early symbol learning does not seem to be specific to any predetermined model of representation (Namy, Campbell, & Tomasello, 2004).

As mentioned previously in Myth 6, at the onset of language development, iconicity does not affect the ability to learn symbol-referent relationships. Most likely, a child simply matches a representation, whatever it may be, with an entity, much as the TD child matches an abstract word with its referent. Although preschool children with severe intellectual disabilities and language delays may have difficulty linking a symbol to its referent, the visual complexity and iconicity of a graphic symbol does not seem to affect the ease of initial symbol learning, despite conventional wisdom to the contrary (Barton, Sevcik, & Romski, 2006). In real practice, therefore, an *X* can symbolize "I want" or "mommy" without greatly affecting initial learning.

Interestingly, concrete-abstract representational distinctions do make a difference by the time the typically developing child is 26 months old, suggesting that learning has moved beyond the simple matching of symbol to referent seen in earlier learning. In other words, during early phases of development, it may not matter if the child uses abstract or iconic symbols because to the child they all function in the same manner. Only later, as vocabularies are expanding and a child begins syntactic learning, does the level of abstractness become a factor.

In all honesty, we don't know how young children conceive their world. Although young children can learn a variety of AAC symbols, many of these symbols are not immediately transparent to young children, and thus their representations may differ significantly from those designed by adults for AAC or other uses (Light, Worah, Drager, Burki, D'Silva, & Kristiansen, 2007). Young children's concepts do not seem to exist in abstract isolation, but rather are part of familiar events and contexts.

This discussion would seem to negate all that was previously said about the level of abstraction and iconicity. This is not the case because although individual symbol representation does not greatly affect initial symbol use and recall, it is likely to have a great effect on later learning. As an SLP, you cannot limit your intervention goals to the immediate needs of the child. It is important to have a vision and a plan for later AAC use in which you cannot ignore the iconicity of symbols and the abstract nature of the concepts they represent.

Symbol Selection: Input

The actual method of individual symbol selection is critical. For children using electronic AAC devices, effective communication relies, in part, on the accuracy and efficiency of the symbol selection process (Reichle et al., 2000).

The most common symbol selection methods are direct selection and scanning, discussed previously. With direct selection, a child may use a variety of methods, including pointing directly at or touching a symbol on the display using a finger, optical or other head pointer, or directed eye gaze. With most types of scanning, the child starts and stops the cursor, which moves through a predetermined path.

The input interface can make or break intervention success with aided AAC. Simply put, systems that require difficult or complicated actions by the child will most likely not be used. For example, navigating with a mouse may be beyond the abilities of many young children, while using a touch screen is not. Use of touch screens simplifies access, and there is a direct relationship between the action and the result. Choice of a symbol system or systems should be based on ease of use and on expected user independence.

Unfortunately, not all children can use touch screens, especially those with motor impairments. Children with severe neuromuscular problems typically use scanning, although this is a difficult means of access to learn (Petersen et al., 2000). In scanning, as explained earlier, a person or device presents choices or groups of choices sequentially to a child, who then signals when the desired item is reached. Scanning performance may be related to a number of factors, such as the child's motor, sensory, perceptual, and cognitive skills, and to the method of symbol selection and the characteristics of the array, such as the size of the array and of individual items.

Although children 30 to 50 months of age have more difficulty planning and executing timely selection using row-column scanning than linear scanning, they make significantly more errors in linear scanning when selecting symbols requiring only a small number of cursor pulses (Petersen et al., 2000). In one study, TD preschoolers who were instructed to select line-drawn symbols from a 36-symbol display configuration were more accurate using directed rather than group-item scanning (Dropik & Reichle, 2008). Although they required a greater number of pulses with group-item than with directed scanning, no differences in actual selection time were apparent, indicating that directed scanning did not afford a relative advantage in children's selection efficiency. This may not be true of children with motor impairments, for whom the additional movements needed for directed scanning may require great effort.

For young children, it seems particularly difficult to attend to and monitor the cursor during scanning and then to activate the switch only when the desired item is highlighted. Scanning involves three essential components (Grodzicki, Jones, Panek, & Parkin, 2006):

- Offer of the item within an array,
- Selection of the item by the child, and
- Feedback provided to the child upon selection.

It's difficult for young children to understand the requirements of each component. Although children with severe motor impairments often have difficulty with direct selection, scanning as an alternative means is difficult for young children to learn because of the design of current scanning techniques. Often scanning

- Does not explicitly identify the array of items available from the selection array, and
- Does not provide explicit feedback after switch activation for target item selection.

The result is that even TD 2-year-old children have difficulty learning to use scanning techniques.

In contrast, enhanced scanning, including making both the offer of items and the feedback upon selection more explicit through the use of speech output with appropriate intonation, increases accuracy by as much as 100 percent (McCarthy, Light, Drager, McNaughton, Grodzicki, Jones, Panek, & Parkin, 2006). Unfortunately, despite the promising outcomes of redesigned scanning techniques, access continues to be very slow.

The rate of selection is, in part, influenced by the method of selection. Rate can be a barrier to communication for children with severe motor challenges. One way for a communication partner to increase the rate is for the partner to attempt to finish the message for the child. Depending on a child's age and abilities, some AAC users are offended or frustrated by this practice while others appreciate being saved both effort and time (Mirenda & Bopp, 2003). In either case, the role of the communication partner is more active than we find in typical face-to-face communication.

A less partner-active system can be found in a device that predicts multiword utterances. Use of this technology requires that the child have the ability to recognize and confirm these predictions.

Organization

Navigating a system or moving about a device to find a target symbol can pose a particular challenge for young children. A child must remember the symbol while trying to recall its location. Organization and layout of symbols can either facilitate or impede the accuracy and efficiency of a child's ability to locate, select, and functionally use those symbols.

Potentially important factors that may influence learning and use include grouping and arrangement of symbols, color, background, borders, shape, pattern, texture, size, position, and movement/animation (Beukelman & Mirenda, 2005; Scally, 2001). For example, if young children organize concepts by events and context, it would make sense to organize symbols on an aided device in that manner (Shane, 2006). On the other hand, if an SLP does not consider the cognitive functioning of a child using AAC, the introduction of these technologies may actually present additional barriers to language development rather than be a potential means for a young child to use and develop language and interact with others.

Decisions on arrangement and color of symbols often occur in the absence of an evidence base for such decisions, even though such decisions may influence a child's performance. In practice, most aided symbol displays are created by clinicians or purchased as part of prepared commercial packages. Current computer-based AAC technologies are based on the conceptual models of adults and may not be compatible with conceptual models of young children (Light & Drager, 2002).

Arrangement of symbols. The arrangement or organization of vocabulary should, as much as feasibly possible, reflect the organizational preferences of the child as well as the child's motor, sensory, and perceptual abilities. Vocabulary arrangement in AAC systems for young children often reflects what seems the most logical to SLPs and other team members and/or a child's visual and motor capabilities. It's entirely possible that adult-generated vocabulary arrangements do not reflect the cognitive organization of young children who require AAC.

When preschool children are given the choice, they purposefully arrange approximately 40 percent of vocabulary items (Fallon, Light, & Achenbach, 2003). The remainder are seemly arranged randomly or "because I like it there." Concrete items, such as nouns and verbs, tend to be organized in pairs (*juice-cup, juice-drink,* or *drink-cup*) or small groups (*playground-slide-I*) according to event schemes—e.g., *juice* goes in *cup* and you *drink* it. Common pairs are *juice-cup, cry-sad,* and *pizza-yummy.* Groupings tend to be small, two to four items, which may suggest that large groups of vocabulary items make selection more difficult. Young children have greater difficulty organizing abstract items, such as prepositions, than they do concrete words (*cookie*). Joint creation of categories by the SLP and the child may facilitate more effective and efficient vocabulary access.

Dynamic displays that enable a user to easily move from categories, such as *food,* through various subcategories, such as *snacks* and *fast food,* to individual symbols, provide more independence and flexibility. With young children, however, semantic organization based on categories may be difficult. Organization based on word order, such as "eat" followed by various food options, may be more practical.

Three-year-old TD children perform significantly better with a contextual scene or schematic format in which foods and utensils are presented in a kitchen scene rather than a grid format based on separate semantic categories such as foods, utensils, and actions (Drager, Light, Carlson, D'Silva, Larsson, Pitkin, & Stopper, 2004). In contrast, 2½-year-old children have great difficulty regardless of the format of the display, although contextual embedding is easier (Drager et al., 2003).

In a contextual scene format, the children may be able to take advantage of decreased working memory demands by chunking together vocabulary symbols represented together within a scene. In the contextual scene format, the scene on the menu page may serve as an external reminder of the operation and structure of the system, making the design more transparent and decreasing the memory demands on the user.

Scenes are most helpful when they are displayed initially so that a child may select a scene and then locate the desired symbol (Drager, Light, et al., 2004). For example, in a playground scene the child can touch the *swing* or the *slide* to indicate these items. Actions can be selected by touching children performing these actions. A car parked in the background indicates how the child gets to the playground. If a photograph is used, the child and significant others can be included so the child can select *daddy* and *me.*

Four- and 5-year-old children can more accurately locate vocabulary in the taxonomic grid, schematic grid, and schematic scene displays than in an iconic encoding condition (Light, Drager, et al., 2004). In iconic encoding, icons such as line drawings with a semantic association are used in combinations as codes to retrieve single words or phrases. In the four conditions, the word *baby* might be accessed as follows:

- ■ Taxonomic grid: people page, then *baby*
- ■ Schematic grid: going to the page for the home, then *baby*

- Schematic scene: going to the living room page and selecting the crawling *baby*
- Iconic encoding: selecting *people* and *love*, then *baby*

More iconic coding, such as a picture of a knot to represent *not* based on the sound of the word, may also be confusing because the underlying meanings are very dissimilar. Although conceptually clever, such encoding does not fit the more concrete thinking of children and is more appropriate for adults using AAC.

Use of color. Color affects a number of functional outcomes, such as initial response time, immediate recall, long-term retention, and categorization of stimuli, and can be used in background or page displays or in the symbols themselves, called symbol-internal colors. We do know that for adults with severe intellectual disabilities, background color can attract attention and focus visual attending to an object. In fact, several professionals have recommended color coding the background of symbols or page displays by categories of concepts or word types almost from the inception of AAC intervention (Beukelman & Mirenda, 2005; Wilkinson & Hennig, 2007). For example, all food symbols might be on a yellow background where they are gathered together.

With symbol-internal coloring, individual food items may have a yellow background or be colored yellow but be scattered throughout the board. Still, clustering symbol-internal color images by color facilitates the speed of locating the target (Wilkinson, Carlin, & Thistle, 2008). For younger preschool children and those with Down syndrome, symbol-internal color clustering facilitates search accuracy. Older TD preschool children are able to locate line drawings featuring foreground or symbol-internal color faster than drawings featuring only background color (Thistle & Wilkinson, 2009).

For some children, a symbol whose internal color is consistent with that of its referent, as in yellow bananas, may be more readily matched than symbols whose color is mismatched or black and white (Stephenson, 2007). This seems especially true when matching a picture with an object, but less so going in the opposite direction. For typically developing children, color, whether individual symbol color or category distinct colors, increases both accuracy and speed in learning to locate graphic symbols (Wilkinson, Carlin, & Jagaroo, 2006).

Responses are significantly faster and more accurate when the target of search is the only one of its color (the only blue symbol in the array, for example) than when all symbols are the same color. This advantage also holds when subsets of symbols share a color, such as when four out of eight symbols are blue. This would be the case when different categories of words have different colors.

Conclusion

Identifying appropriate and effective means of communication is critical. Ideally, the communication system used by a child is flexible, capable of expansion and growth, and multimodal in nature. Although a very young child may have difficulty with sophisticated electronic devices, a device can be made simpler through appropriate representations, organization of these representations, the interface between the child and the device, and device output.

 Click here to gauge your understanding of the concepts in this chapter.

8

Augmentative and Alternative Communication: Intervention

Although children and adults with developmental disabilities have used AAC systems to develop language skills and functional communication, infants, toddlers, and young preschool children have often been considered too young or too prelinguistic to benefit, and therefore not introduced to AAC until certain prerequisite behaviors were in place. Recent research, as noted in Chapter 7, has challenged this notion. It is now recognized that AAC can be a useful tool for teaching communication roles and behaviors and functional communication use.

AAC intervention can begin when a child's earliest communication behaviors are difficult to interpret, unconventional, inconsistent, or too subtle to be noticed by most caregivers, or when a child begins to fall behind developmentally. You'll recall from your language acquisition course that communication starts at birth when children produce behaviors that are interpreted as communicative by someone in their environment. The child's behavior is given communicative significance.

Children's natural actions and behaviors are the only prerequisites needed for AAC (Cress & Marvin, 2003). In fact, many augmented methods of signaling can precede the development of more formal and symbolic strategies. The earliest AAC intervention is not necessarily concerned with switches and type of output or complicated computer systems. Instead, as in much that we have said in this text, speech-language pathologists (SLPs) focus on existing communication through gestures, sounds, and shared actions and on the caregivers' adapting of their responses to their child's communication signals (Dunst & Lowe, 1986). Learning skills such as intentional communication or operating a switch are a part of AAC intervention but should not preclude a child's receipt of AAC services.

AAC does not depend either on controlling complicated systems and devices or on attainment of a list of prerequisite skills. In fact, AAC use can foster development in these areas. In the rest of this chapter, we'll focus first on introducing AAC to a child, move to child-based intervention, intervention issues such as vocabulary selection, and intervention methods, and end with special considerations for some children.

Getting Started

As an SLP, you can monitor a child's development carefully to decide the appropriate time to introduce AAC, especially more complex systems. We do not have to wait for a child to fully develop motor, language, and communicative skills before introducing electronic devices, but we should do so gradually and then slowly expand both the range of device features and the communication purposes for which they are used. For example, a multi-picture display might be limited at first to one or two representations. The complexity of modes of input can be increased gradually as a child's motor control improves.

One of the first steps in intervention is to identify meaningful daily contexts that can promote AAC communication and social interaction by providing opportunities for these to occur. If we expect a child to learn a new communication skill, we need to provide opportunities to use that skill. Several enjoyable child-parent routines, such as songs, books, interactive toys, and games, can provide multiple turn-taking opportunities. These types of fun activities are motivating and age appropriate. As we know, young children learn well in simple joint activities such a book-sharing.

Routines have predictable patterns. Our brains look for patterns and changes in those patterns. Patterns of interaction are learned through experience. Once a child has learned a routine, such as passing a toy back and forth, changes in the routine, such as ceasing the activity, elicit attending. Learning occurs when an unexpected or novel pattern is compared to an existing one. Moderate changes in routines can provide opportunities for learning by encouraging curiosity. Changes can then be related back to the expected pattern.

The trick is to balance novel and known information to keep interest and not cause boredom. SLPs and other adults can set up activities in which a child can use a combination of applying previous knowledge and learning new information.

The SLP can help parents identify high-interest child activities. It's important to begin small, choosing only one or two contexts in which to begin. Parents will need help and practice adapting their communication to this new form. New contexts and activities can be added gradually, with parents taking more and more responsibility for intervention.

Initially, it will be difficult for most young children to coordinate attention to a partner, an AAC system, the context, and themselves (Light & Drager, 2005). The child can be helped in part if the conversational partner is positioned for maximum communication and if the context and the AAC system are integrated. For example, Velcro-backed symbols can be infused into an activity by detaching them from a communication board and bringing them into an activity.

When aided AAC systems are not integrated into children's lives, the device tends to sit to the side and be used as an afterthought, if at all. When outside of its natural conversational context, language is decontextualized, making it more difficult for the child to learn and use.

It's easy for adults to focus on an AAC system or device at the expense of the individual child. In addition, children such as those with ASD may become fascinated with the communication device itself to such an extent that it interferes with using that device for communicative interactions (Mirenda, Wilk, & Carson, 2000). I worked with a young child with ASD who was fascinated by his iPad but not with using it to communicate. In this case, every effort to reinforce iPad use to communicate strengthened his obsessive focus on the device.

In the last analysis, technology is just a tool. Ideally, intervention focuses on the interaction between a child and an adult or between a child and other children, and success is measured by the child's ability to interact and communicate appropriately in these contexts using his or her AAC system.

Similarly, the use of multiple modes to communicate is far more powerful than the use of any single system. Reliance on one or more systems is dependent on the context and on the participants. Remembering that communication is the goal, an SLP can honor the communication system a child chooses as best for a particular situation. This does not prevent the SLP from demonstrating other ways to convey the same information.

As an SLP, it's important not to inadvertently limit a child's communication by focusing only on one AAC system while neglecting speech sound making, gestures, eye gaze, and the like. Instead, it is important to enhance all methods of communication.

INITIATING COMMUNICATION

Even AAC does not guarantee that a child will initiate communication. Initiation is a complicated behavior that depends on the opportunities and support for communication and on an individual's motivation and communication skills. Phrases such as "She's not motivated" or "He doesn't want to communicate" are signals that intervention methods need to be reevaluated and most likely redesigned.

Motivation is highly context dependent. As in any type of early communication intervention (ECI), if a child is not initiating communication, the characteristics of the environment and the communication partners' responses should be evaluated.

An SLP may need to consider the kinds of structured interactions used in intervention that may elicit primarily responsive communication from the child. Understanding a symbol is very different from knowing how and when to initiate that message. Increasing the size of a child's receptive vocabulary does not promote communication development if the child does not initiate. In short, if the outcomes of a child's self-initiations are not consistently prompted and reinforced, there will not be enough environmental support for initiations, and the frequency of initiation attempts may decrease.

ACTIVE LEARNING

Active learning is preferable to passive participation. It's easy for children with special needs to become passive, especially when their needs are anticipated by those in the environment. By thinking outside the box, parents and teachers can create participation opportunities within daily activities. Active participation is increased by creating opportunities for children to exert control and to make meaningful choices. When adults follow a child's lead, they are ceding some control to the child.

Drill and practice foster rote learning but not necessarily useful communication skills. We learn to communicate by actually doing it. Language is learned through broad experiences that provide multiple repetitions of concepts, vocabulary, and conversational conventions. This situation provides a scaffold from which children can construct language. In addition, learning in functional situations facilitates generalization.

Features of Child-Based AAC Intervention

Most aided AAC systems reflect adult thinking, making them potentially less appealing to infants and toddlers. AAC systems can be made more appealing by (Light, Drager, & Nemser, 2004; Light, Curran, Page, & Pitkin, 2007)

- Using bright colors and decorations;
- Incorporating
  - Sound effects, such as laughter, music, and songs, and
  - Popular movie, book, or television characters;
- Including the devices in
  - Motivating, interactive activities, and
  - Favorite activities and routines;
- Allowing a child to make choices; and
- Making use fun and rewarding.

Let's face it, we all like doing something that we enjoy and that reflects our desires.

Ease of learning is fostered by reducing the learning demands. This can be accomplished by the

- Representations of language concepts;
- Layout, organization, and navigation;
- Selection techniques; and
- Output (Light & Drager, 2005).

Let's take a moment to explore each of these.

REPRESENTATIONS

Representations of language through the AAC symbol system(s) may reflect adult thinking, not children's. Symbols that seem very concrete to an adult may, in fact, seem very abstract to a child.

Some commercially available representations or pictures are not designed with a young child in mind. It's important that the representations used reflect a child's perspective. Decisions about symbol systems may force the team to think about how a child experiences the concept being represented. For example, the concept *push* may be represented by a picture of a person pushing something heavy. For a child, however, pushing may be associated with a ball and may need to be represented in that way. It's important to remember that a child's initial meaning of a symbol may be very context specific. A picture of *eat* that includes the use of a fork may not conform to the meaning of *eat* for a child who uses finger feeding.

ORGANIZATION

As noted in Chapter 7, organization of the symbols being used, whether on a communication board or electronic device, can either facilitate or unnecessarily complicate system use. Some children will benefit from visual schematic scenes depicting daily experiences, such as preschool, with vocabulary embedded within. This type or organization reflects a young child's world more than adult categories of nouns and verbs or abstract groupings such as pets or utensils.

Young children's concepts are often embedded in familiar contexts. The amount of time a child needs to learn and use a symbol may be significantly decreased if representations reflect young children's understandings. For example, symbols can be placed within photos of familiar events, as mentioned in Chapter 7, and actually taught within those contexts (Fallon, Light, & Achenbach, 2003). Food items can be taught within an eating activity that takes place in the family kitchen. Likewise, symbols could be placed within or next to a photo of that same location. As previously discussed, these visual scene displays (VSDs) capture events in an individual's life, are less abstract than semantic categories such as *foods*, and offer contextual support for communication interactions (Capilouto, 2005). For young children, specific context, such as a photograph of the family kitchen, is easier than a generic contextual picture.

The typical semantic category layout reflects adult organizational notions of grids and boxes. I would suggest that a child's world is somewhat messier. The adult model may distort spatial relationships that are essential to the thinking of some children by placing *eat* with actions and *cookie* with foods. You may recall from your language acquisition course that semantic categories, such as food, seem to be more closely aligned with the thinking of school-age children and adults, not infants and toddlers.

SELECTION

For children with neuromotor difficulties, size and location of symbols may depend on motor abilities. More frequently used symbols can be placed in easy-to-access locations. Individual symbol size depends on a child's indicating abilities once he or she has arrived at the desired symbol location. These considerations would seem to negate similar-size visual symbols all placed in the nice neat columns and rows preferred by adults.

OUTPUT

Although output often focuses on device output, vocabulary output may be even more important. What does the child want and need to talk about?

New vocabulary should be modeled regularly in context. As stressed throughout this text, vocabulary should be individualized, functional, developmentally and culturally appropriate, and motivating and fun, and should support overall language learning (Light & Drager, 2005).

THE CHILD'S COMMUNICATION SYSTEM

Despite the potential communication benefits of AAC, these outcomes don't occur automatically. In aided AAC, a child must learn

- To operate the equipment, which may be a sophisticated computer-based device;
- To recognize and use the symbol system, such as pictures or drawings; and
- To use the technology in communicative interactions (Light, 1997).

Typically, an AAC device is just one part of a child's AAC system. It is not uncommon for children to also use signs, gestures, vocalizations, and speech approximations in different situations with different communication partners (Beukelman & Mirenda, 2005).

 Before we get too deeply into intervention, you may find it useful to watch this video overview of AAC and evidence-based practice (EBP).
https://www.youtube.com/watch?v=XzT2Bq5F2O4

Issues

AAC intervention is multifaceted and raises several issues. Some of these are discussed in the following sections. You may notice that some of these have been mentioned before. Keep in mind that AAC is just one strategy within our overall ECI approach.

FUNCTIONAL EQUIVALENCE

In Chapter 6, Presymbolic Early Communication Intervention, we discussed functional equivalence, which occurs when two or more behaviors achieve the same end. One of the factors that determines equivalence is response efficiency. Any of the four positive components of response efficiency—response effort, rate of reinforcement, immediacy of reinforcement, and quality of reinforcement—may have an effect on a child's use of AAC (Johnston, Reichle, & Evans, 2004). In reality, these four components interact to affect the probability of a child's engaging in AAC use or another behavior. Let's briefly address response efficiency and reinforcement as they apply to AAC.

Response Efficiency

Response efficiency is a vital consideration when developing AAC intervention for a beginning communicator. Response effort includes both the physical effort required to produce a communicative act and the cognitive effort required to recall or use symbols or a communication system. For example, holding up an empty cup to request more juice may be both physically easier than activating an electronic device and cognitively easier than locating a symbol in an array. Although SLPs may be greatly concerned with the physical demands of communicating with AAC, they may neglect to consider such cognitive challenges as inattentiveness resulting from the inherent slowness of scanning selection or the difficulty in locating and selecting symbols in larger arrays.

For many young children using electronic means of communication, direct selection, as in a touchscreen display, facilitates AAC use. As vocabulary increases, storage may be a problem, leading to other potentially more difficult selection methods, such as scanning and organizational schemes in which symbols are not initially seen on the screen but are accessed through categories or scenes.

Although various traditional instructional methods can be used to teach young children to scan, a significant amount of instructional time may be required. One way to decrease the time required to teach scanning is to redesign scanning techniques to facilitate learning. Examples might include:

- A simplified video game in which a hand or other device catches an animal or other symbol as it crosses one of several boxes or spaces
- An enhanced animated array in which the selected item appears to move from the array to a more prominent position in the front and center of the screen, while the original array remains in the background minus the selected item
- Accompanying speech output, delivered with a flat intonation ("Dog"), confirming item selection

Changes such as these can increase a child's attending, speed of learning, and accuracy (Grodzicki, Jones, Panek, & Parkin, 2006).

If a child does not possess the motor behavior required to activate a switch, a simple training procedure consisting of systematic prompting and prompt withdrawal techniques may be used. Prompting and assistance are gradually decreased from hand-over-hand physical guidance through a physical prompt to a verbal-only cue.

As mentioned, these variables usually do not function in a vacuum, but interact with each other. Just as you decide whether to note something with a word, vocalization, gesture, or combination of these, an AAC user has to determine the most efficient response for the message he or she wishes to send. A natural gesture may be more efficient than selecting a picture symbol. In other situations, the specificity of the picture may make it the more efficient choice.

The notion of efficiency depends on the demands of the communicative context. Ideally, efficient use would support the training of multiple ways of communicating so that different options are available to a child. Think of yourself. At a fast-food restaurant, you just tell the counter person your order. When ordering in a Thai restaurant, however, you may point to the menu items or use a number, unless you speak Thai, because of the difficulty of pronouncing your order. Children need the same types of communication options.

Remember that AAC use may be a novel method of communication for a child. Response efficiency is a very important factor in influencing the communication behavior of AAC users. These variables may also influence a communication partner's perceptions regarding interactions with AAC users.

Intervention should be designed after examining the role of response efficiency for both the child and caregivers. The first step is collecting information on the efficiency of a child's current behavior. The variables related to response efficiency are then incorporated into the intervention program. This may mean adjusting the rate, quality, and/or immediacy of reinforcement as well as the response effort.

Reinforcement

Reinforcement rate is particularly important if responses are functionally equivalent and the SLP is attempting to move a client from one behavior to another, especially if the older behavior has a history of reinforcement. Assume, for example, that a child has been given a treat when he reached and whined. In an attempt to expand the child's repertoire of requests, you, as the SLP, require the child to point to a picture of the treat. This behavior has no reinforcement history. You and the caregivers will need to reinforce the new behavior while simultaneously ignoring the older one. Manipulating the rate of reinforcement in response to a child's communicative behaviors has been shown to influence his or her subsequent use of those behaviors.

Reinforcement is never as simple as new clinicians imagine, and the latency between producing a communicative act and the delivery of a reinforcer can also influence a child's use of AAC. Reinforcement may be external, such as a caregiver's offering praise or a requested item, or internal, such as a device's voice output itself, which is more immediate.

Immediacy of reinforcement would suggest that aided communication devices be present and available for use by children throughout the day. If not, children may simply ignore a communicative opportunity rather than tolerate the delay in reinforcement resulting from finding and using the AAC device. Imagine the frustration for a child who gestures to request a cookie at snack time but then must sit and wait while his device is located, turned on, and the appropriate scene located.

When moving from single-symbol communication, such as signing "Want," to two-symbol communication, such as "Want cookie," immediacy of reinforcement can become a factor. Previously reinforced after signing only "Want," the child must now wait as reinforcement is delayed until both signs are produced. This may require a two-tier reinforcement system in which the adult responds verbally to "want" but with verbal reinforcement and delivery of the treat only following "cookie."

Reinforcement quality relates to the desirability of the reinforcer. Simply put, when one event or object is preferred over another, the preferred one has a higher quality of reinforcement.

VOCABULARY

AAC systems offer increased communication opportunities within activities in the home, school, and community for nonsymbolic children with communication impairment. While that statement is true, without the appropriate vocabulary, these systems will not be effective (Fallon, Light, & Paige, 2001). An initial vocabulary for a young child needs to be functional or useful, individualized, meaningful, and motivating; be appropriate to the child's age, gender, background, personality, and environments; and be able to support a range of communicative uses and intentions.

Vocabulary selection should reflect a child's

- Current language and communication abilities,
- Changing communication needs and contexts,
- Individual needs, and
- Interests and motivation.

This necessitates a detailed understanding of the child's most frequented contexts, the communication expectations of those settings, and an appreciation of each child's own style of communication. As you can see, determining the appropriate AAC vocabulary depends on multiple sources of information.

Core and Fringe Vocabulary

When selecting vocabulary, an SLP may want to consider two types of words:

- A core vocabulary of words commonly used in a given situation, such as common verbs and greetings, and
- A fringe vocabulary of words specific to an individual or activity, such as the SLP's name, song words for preschool circle time, and favorite treats at home.

Effective vocabulary selection requires multiple techniques to ensure that both types of vocabulary words are included (e.g., Beukelman & Mirenda, 2005).

Core vocabulary is generally stable across people and contexts and generative in nature so that symbols can be combined into longer utterances. Several potential core vocabulary lists exist and can be accessed easily by typing "core vocabulary" into your laptop's search engine. Even so, core vocabulary should be adapted to the individual child. Possible core vocabulary symbols might include *eat, Mommy, more,* and *no.*

Fringe vocabulary is activity specific and infrequently used in other environments and contexts. Examples of fringe vocabulary might include action words such as *paint, dance,* and *pull* and object symbols such as *toothbrush* and *crayon* that only occur in certain contexts.

Although both core and fringe vocabularies are important, children tend to use their core vocabulary more frequently. Core vocabulary words such as *that* or *the* are more difficult to teach and to represent graphically than nouns, but they can be used to fulfill a variety of syntactic, semantic, and pragmatic functions through AAC devices. For example, the symbol *that* combined with a gesture could signify "Look at that," "I want that," or "What's that?" In this case, *that* can substitute for all the words that could take its place while the child is learning to form two-word utterances.

Words that are difficult to represent can be taught to young children by modeling use of these words within activities. The key is consistent pairing of seeing the picture or symbol with hearing the word, uttered by the partner and/or preprogrammed into the device.

Combining core (*want*) and fringe (*juice*) vocabulary symbols increases the frequency of AAC use. A child can get plenty of "mileage" from a well-constructed core vocabulary, especially when combined with fringe vocabulary.

Vocabulary Selection

There are three main approaches to selecting vocabulary for children: developmental, environmental, and functional, none of which are mutually exclusive. A developmental approach involves the use of vocabulary lists developed from studies of typically developing (TD) children. Be cautioned that such lists may not be wholly appropriate for children with developmental disabilities. In contrast, an environmental approach is based on an ecological inventory, in which words are identified for specific communication environments. Finally, a functional approach is pragmatic in nature, with words identified based on expressed communication functions such as requesting. Although these are three different approaches, they can be combined creatively.

Developmental considerations. Children get a lot of mileage out of a few words. The most frequent words occur over and over again. Think of how often you've heard a young child say *more, no, up,* and *wassat* (What's that?).

Nine words were used most frequently by the 24- to 30-month-old TD children in one study: *I, no, yes/yeah, want, it, that, my, you,* and *more* (Banajee, Dicarlo, & Stricklin, 2003). Other common words included *mine, the, is, on, in, here, out, off, a, go, what, some, help,* and *all done/finish.*

Despite the paucity of nouns among the most frequently used words of the young children in these studies, SLPs and other team members typically select nouns as first symbols for AAC systems. According to clinicians, nouns are easier to teach and assess and are of considerable functional use. We should also note that the 24- to 30-month-olds mentioned in the previous paragraph were somewhat more advanced than children using AAC and just beginning to produce symbols. Although nouns seem a good place to begin building a vocabulary, adults cannot ignore other words, especially those that may form a core vocabulary and can be used to build longer utterances, such as *more, no, eat, drink,* and *see.*

Environmental considerations. Children using AAC both in preschool and at home have similar vocabulary use patterns in each setting (Marvin, Beukelman, & Bilyeu, 1994). Approximately one-third of the words are produced only at home, one-third only at preschool, and another third are used across both home and preschool contexts. Frequently used words in the home and preschool are listed in Figure 8.1. Typically, vocabulary is selected for inclusion by others who are familiar with the child and her or his communication contexts, and/or is based on age-appropriate vocabulary for young children.

FIGURE 8.1 **Frequently Occurring Home and School Content Words**

airplane/plane	cereal	feet	key	peepee	stinky
all	chair	finger	kiss	phone	stop
all gone	cheese	fish	knee	pig/piggy	stove
apple	chicken	fix	leg	pillow	sun
arm	chin	flower	light	pizza	swing
baby	choo-choo	food	little	plate	teddy bear
bad	church	foot	look	please	teeth
ball	clap	french fries	love	potty	telephone
balloon	clean	girl	lunch	pretty	thank you
banana	clock	glasses	mama/	pretzel	there
bath	coat	gloves	mommy	puppy	thirsty
bathtub	cold	go	man	purse	throw
bear (teddy)	comb	go bed	marker	push	thumb
bed	come	go bye-bye	McDonald's	radio	tired
bee	cookie	go night-night	me	read	tissue
big	cough	go out	meat	ride	toast
bike	cow	good	milk	rock	toe
bird	cracker	grandma	mine	run	toothbrush
blanket	crib	grandpa	mirror	school	towel
block	cup	grapes	money	see	toy
boat	dada/daddy	gum	monkey	shhhh	train
booboo	dance	hair	moon	shirt	tree
book	dark	hamburger	more	shoe	truck
boot	diaper	hand	mouth	show (me)	tummy/belly
bottle	dirty	happy	nap	shut/close	TV
bottom/butt	doctor	hat	night-night	sing	uh-oh
bowl	dog/doggie	heavy	no	sink	under
boy	doll	help	nose	sit/sit down	up
bread	don't	here	nugget	sky	walk
breakfast	done	hi	off	sleep	want
broken	done (all done)	horse/horsie	old	slide	wash
brush	down	hot	on	snack	water
bubble	dress	hot dog	open	sneaker	wet
bug	drink	house	orange	snow	what
bunny	duck	hug	out	so big	what's that
bus	ear	huh?	own name	soap	woman
bye/bye-bye	eat	hungry	pajamas/	sock	wow
cake	egg	I	jammies	soda/pop	yes
candy	eye	ice cream	paper	soup	you
car	face	in	park	spaghetti	yucky
cat/kitty	fall down	juice	pattycake	spoon	yum/yummy
catch	feed	jump	peekaboo	stick	zoo

We cannot automatically assume that a child using AAC has communication functions and topics similar to those of TD children. One study found that the communication of a 6-year-old child using AAC and her parent mostly concerned the immediate context, either directly or tangentially. In contrast, an age-matched TD child and parent conversed on a variety of personal topics beyond the immediate present (Ferm, Ahlsén, & Björck-Åkesson, 2005).

Several ecologically sound and individualized methods can be used by SLPs for fringe vocabulary selection. These may include

- Conducting an ecological survey of the environments and activities in which a child needs to communicate,
- Compiling a list of words and phrases thought to be potentially useful to a child,
- Observing a child's attempted interactions, and
- Completing a caregiver vocabulary selection questionnaire similar to that for other nonsymbolic children. A fine one is presented in an article by Fallon, Light, and Kramer Paige in the *American Journal of Speech-Language Pathology* (2001).

No one technique is sufficient to identify all potentially important vocabulary items. The thorough vocabulary selection process includes two important components:

- Multiple vocabulary selection techniques, and
- Multiple informants, such as a child's parents and teachers.

At best, the vocabulary selection process is cumbersome and time-consuming and likely to result in redundant lists. But there are some savings of time and effort across children as words identified across several children begin to form a generic core vocabulary list that reflects children's lives in your area.

We ensure maximum usefulness of an AAC system for a child and caregivers when we individualize a child's vocabulary. It should be obvious that the cultural background of the family is extremely important. While *Kimchi* works in a Korean American home, *arepa* will not. In turn, *arepas* may be served in a Latino household but not in a Vietnamese American family. Of course, there are exceptions, and nothing substitutes for a thorough environmental assessment. This is the beauty of having the family as team members.

Functional considerations. Children are most apt to communicate if they have vocabulary that allows them to do the things they want to do. In other words, they need to be able to request and discuss things they enjoy, including foods, games, and toys. The ECI team should focus on those situations in which the child is trying to communicate currently and on the most likely messages in those contexts.

Potential words should be selected based on the extent to which they enable a child to talk about the things in his or her environment and to use each symbol to express a variety of intentions. Remember that young TD children are able to answer, question, reply, describe, state, and call, to name just a few potential communicative intentions.

Appropriate vocabulary or content can go beyond single words and include short phrases such as "What's that?" and "All gone," plus sounds such as giggling. Some words and phrases are contextual, and this should be reflected in the organization of these in the device.

It is important, however, not to rely entirely on preprogrammed phrases, such as "How are you?" and "I love you," unless the phrases can be easily integrated with more flexible single symbols. "Can I please have?" can be combined with numerous desired items. While stock phrases can increase the speed of communication, they may decrease accuracy and precision. For example, if a child has a phrase such as "My cat's name is 'Fluffy'" but no other way to refer to her pet, she has great difficulty building utterances to talk about her cat.

I once met a young man with severe cerebral palsy (CP) who had an augmentative device on his wheelchair tray. When I introduced myself, he activated the device which reeled off a two-minute preprogrammed solo including his name, address, phone, and interests. While this was intended to provide as much information as possible with a single-switch device, it was awkward, interrupted real communication, and left him without AAC for any subsequent utterances he wished to produce. Even as someone who has worked with both children and adults using AAC, I was left momentarily speechless as I searched for my reply. I may be wrong, but I sensed by his unease that even he felt that this introduction was inappropriate.

Appropriate and Individualized Vocabulary

You'll recall that early intervention (EI) is required by law to be culturally appropriate and individualized. This is true whether learning speech or AAC. SLPs can work closely with the family to select vocabulary and contexts that reflect the family's culture. For example, eating utensils may be inappropriate for some Ethiopian American children while *injera*, a doughy flatbread used to bring food to your mouth, may not.

The vocabulary selected should reflect food, clothing, and celebrations from the child's world, such as Muslim or Buddhist holidays. Pictures should also depict the child's cultural background in skin color, facial features, and clothing, to mention just a few. For example, it's inappropriate for an African American child to have pictures that depict only European Americans.

In your busy schedule as an SLP, it will be all too easy to use a program that already has vocabulary. I discourage this practice. While well-intentioned, it is not individualized. My own grandson was being taught animal names with little relevance to his communication needs. In fact, he could live his entire life and not need to use the symbol for *penguin*. There is a flip side to this. He should not be limited to "survival" vocabulary—*hungry, tired, hurt*—either. While Dakota's language is limited, he does have interests, including his bike, music, trampoline, and certain toys and foods.

In part, the words we each use to communicate reflect our individual nature. Think about the choice to swear or not. The ECI team can select vocabulary that enables a child to express that unique personality as well. Some children, even as infants, are more social, while others prefer to interact with toys and objects.

A viable AAC system changes with a child. This change also includes the vocabulary available to the child. Young children using AAC can only learn new words if parents and teachers introduce new vocabulary regularly. One way to help a child learn new vocabulary is to give the child a method of asking questions, such as "What's that?" When this message is activated, the adult should provide the sign or symbol and the verbalization for the new word.

Canned lists of symbols or adult-selected vocabulary may have little real relevance to the individual child. It is also all too easy for parents and professionals to select symbols that are of interest to them but not necessarily to the child. A child's speech should be childlike not miniaturized *adultspeak*.

It is occasionally assumed that the high-usage words *yes* and *no* are simple concepts that can be introduced first into a child's AAC system. In part, this assumption is based on uncomplicated communication aids that enable adults with acquired communication disorders to make *yes/no* responses (Garrett & Kimelman, 2000). Adults who have previously acquired language are not children still learning it. Using *yes/no* questions to prompt responses only works if the respondent already has a stable understanding of *yes/no* concepts. Even adults may use this strategy incorrectly in difficulty communication processing tasks (Garrett & Kimelman, 2000).

I can attest from firsthand experience that teaching *yes* and *no* is complicated. I worked with a teen who had severe brain damage from encephalitis, a brain infection. The team decided to go for a "quick fix" with *yes/no* responding. With no seeming understanding of the terms, the young man took three weeks in twice daily one-hour sessions to learn to accurately respond to simple factual questions such as "Is this a window?" In retrospect, choice-making and requesting would have been better, more functional, and presumably easier to learn.

Young children with limited experience do not use *yes/no* responses with as much success as adults. Answering with a *yes/no* response is a communication skill that develops between 18 and 36 months for TD children. These words can have a wide variety of meanings and results, depending on the vocabulary used and the intent of the question asked (Owens, 2012). A TD child's ability to use conventional words or head gestures to indicate *yes/no* does not stabilize until well into the second year of life after a child has had considerable experience with using language for a variety of other purposes.

The specific meaning conveyed by a *yes/no* response depends upon the question asked. A child answering the question using AAC has only limited control of the communicative message, and the conversation tends to involve more speaker turns and control, even when the individual using AAC is skilled. The AAC user may become an infrequent initiator, because *yes* and *no* are not useful for initiating messages.

MULTIMODALITY AND DEVELOPMENT

In designing an expressive AAC system, it is important to provide a mode or modes that can grow with a child. Each child needs a communication system that can facilitate crucial transitions from one level of linguistic complexity to another. If these transitions are not inherent in an AAC system, a child cannot expand his or her communication abilities.

Speakers typically rely on multiple modes of communication to meet their needs (Blackstone & Hunt-Berg, 2003). Young children using AAC need the same (Binger & Light, 2006; Light & Drager, 2005). The choice of modes should relate to a child's skills, communication contexts, partners, tasks, and intent (Blackstone & Hunt-Berg, 2003).

A child should be encouraged to use as many modes of communication as available, possibly using different modes for different messages. Waving while saying "Bye" or vocalizing a similar sound seems a natural way to communicate. More complicated messages may require use of another mode. Although children can learn to use multiple communication strategies across different activities, SLPs should be cautious, introducing only one new element at a time so as not to overwhelm the child's ability to learn and to adapt.

Although there is evidence of the positive impact of individual unaided and aided AAC systems, there are only limited data on the comparative effectiveness of various systems (Bartman & Freeman, 2003; Charlop-Christy, Carpenter, Le, LeBlanc, & Kellet, 2002; Johnston, McDonnell, Nelson, & Magnavito, 2003; Romski, Sevcik, Adamson, & Cheslock, 2006; Sigafoos et al., 2004). In part, this lack of data reflects the number of factors involved, including those intrinsic to an individual child, and extrinsic factors, such as partners, context, and present and future needs (Mirenda, 2005). In practice, most nonspeaking preschoolers use a combination of gestures, vocalizations, and nonelectronic communication boards or simple AAC technologies with digitized speech output. Few use advanced AAC technologies that might offer greater communication options (Binger & Light, 2006; Hustad et al., 2005).

Unfortunately, in many cases, AAC systems have insufficient capacity to provide for language and communication development. As a result, a young child's development may be limited by those technologies or methods. For example, parents may have only limited knowledge of signing (Light & Drager, 2005). An AAC system or systems can be chosen with an eye toward future communication growth and development. Likewise, limiting a child to using only one system exclusively may limit communication experiences. If AAC systems are modified frequently to accommodate a child's changing needs and abilities, the child's language and use grow accordingly.

For some children, AAC will be the avenue to functional speech production, but that requires planning and forethought by adults. When infants and young children with language delays are presented with a spoken word, such as "cookie," repeatedly paired with a desired item, such as a cookie, they begin to produce an approximation of the spoken word (Yoon & Bennett, 2000). If AAC symbols or signs (*cookie*) and spoken words ("cookie") are presented together and followed by a reinforcer (a cookie), both the symbol/sign and the spoken word increase in frequency.

GENERALIZATION: ROLE OF THE ENVIRONMENT

While intervention seems to be more effective with unaided systems than with aided in general, there is no evidence for a difference in generalization. The intervention data may reflect the need to facilitate the use of aided systems through continual redesign and update and the more physically and cognitively impaired status of most individuals recommended to aided systems.

Although there are some data on generalization from a large number of studies, most involve single subjects and only a small percentage include children under age 5 (Schlosser &

Lee, 2000). This said, analysis reveals that training using multiple exemplars, such as several examples of cup along with a symbol for *cup*, or training of a symbol within multiple intentions, produces higher levels of generalization than programming common stimuli only. Similarly, the use of multiple exemplars also produces better maintenance of intervention targets. The most effective teaching strategies seem to be mand-model mentioned in Chapter 6, graduated guidance, and a combination of prompt strategies. Graduated guidance, also mentioned in Chapter 6, attempts to provide fewer cues and prompts as a child requires less in order to be successful.

The Everyday Use Environment

One of the biggest concerns, an issue I have stressed throughout this text, is generalization of newly learned AAC skills to different use environments. In order for generalization to occur, it must be actively promoted from the onset of the intervention process rather than as a later add-on. Short of this, SLPs are left with a "train and hope" approach in which, unaware of the variables that affect generalization, they "hope" that it will occur.

Research data indicate that intervention most often focuses on changing the behaviors of AAC users rather than that of partners (Schlosser & Lee, 2000). This occurs despite the importance of working through families, based on the concept that communication is a transactional process.

Language development proceeds as a result of a complex interaction between biology and the communication experiences of a child with caregivers and other significant people in the child's environment. Children, even those with similar individual characteristics, can display quite different rates and patterns of use with AAC. More important than the individual characteristics of each child, however, is the communication context and its influence on family-child interactions (Olsson, 2005).

The language development of children using AAC is different from the implicit learning typical in spoken language development (von Tetzchner & Grove, 2003). For example, explicit teaching plays little or no role in typical language development. In AAC intervention, teaching of language is often explicit.

In the everyday world, we communicate primarily through speech. Modifying the environments for a nonsymbolic child learning speech is one thing, but modifying that same environment for AAC requires changes to the very context for communication. The success of that change depends on several variables across the communication partners, the family, and the school.

Communication Partners

Through interactions, a child comes to learn the means of communication and the cultural knowledge of language use. Even the simple act of asking for more juice requires that both communication partners share common underlying competencies. For children learning AAC, both the mode of communication and the acculturation process are altered.

It seems reasonable to assume that in order for a child to develop communicative competency via AAC, there must be individuals in the environment who are more competent than the child in understanding and using the child's AAC system. Unfortunately, many children who use AAC systems have a restricted input in vocabulary and grammatical structure and limited communicative experiences outside of structured intervention situations.

For children using AAC, most communication partners may have only marginally higher, if not lower, AAC competency than the child. This results in a situation in which the educational needs of a child developing AAC competency may coexist with similar educational needs among professionals, staff, and caregivers.

The effectiveness of an augmentative communication system depends on the commitment of all communication partners. SLPs must consider not only the needs and abilities of the child with communication impairment (CI) when designing an AAC system but also the needs, preferences, and interactional styles of these communication partners. The congruence between an intervention and variables such as the child's and caregivers' characteristics and needs is called contextual fit.

Ideally, a good contextual fit results from the most efficient AAC system for a given context. We might reasonably assume, for example, that communication partners will be more likely to initiate and/or maintain interactions with a child if using AAC speeds up exchanges, makes the exchange more understandable, or lessens the need for the partner to act as an interpreter (Johnston, Reichle, & Evans, 2004).

Unfortunately, the behavior of some communication partners may not effectively support positive communicative interactions. In general, communication partners tend to

- Dominate communicative interactions,
- Take the majority of conversational turns,
- Provide few opportunities for an AAC user to initiate conversations or to respond,
- Ask primarily yes/no questions,
- Interrupt frequently, and
- Focus on the AAC device or technique instead of the child or the child's message.

In response, AAC users respond by

- Assuming a passive role, initiating few interactions and responding only when required to do so;
- Producing only a limited range of intentions, such as answers to yes/no questions; and
- Using restricted linguistic forms, such as one-word responses.

This situation is less than optimal and works against language and communication development for a young child.

The relative slowness of most AAC methods can influence a child's or partner's use of AAC to communicate. Often, speaking partners use more directive speech and take more turns in interactions with children who use AAC than in interactions with speaking children. These same partners tend to speak too fast to enable the child using AAC to take a turn. The result is that children who use AAC are likely to demonstrate more limited communicative intentions than speaking partners and to be reduced to a responder role. For a child with limited expressive abilities, this may mean adopting a passive interactional role (Cress et al., 2000). Unfortunately, learning to communicate is not a passive act.

As TD children move from gestural-vocal communication to single words, there is a huge increase in the frequency of their communication. This increase is important for development of a range of intentions. Sadly, AAC users often experience preemption of their messages by listeners who finish the message for the child. As a result, opportunities to express intentions are curtailed.

An SLP can work to encourage parents and caregivers to actively foster communication and reinforce communication attempts. With more frequent meaningful communication, a child's message complexity also tends to increase.

Obviously, the key to changing a child's role to a more active one is changing the behaviors of a child's communication partners. In part, the more active role by adult partners flows from parents' and therapists' perceiving their role as promoting language development through instructional and directive behavior. Interaction strategies that respond to a child's attempts to communicate tend to facilitate language development better than more didactic and directive teaching strategies.

We have discussed interactive strategies with children who do not use AAC. The child's partners can naturally prompt initiation of a frequent behavior, such as reaching, and then model a new behavior for completing the action, such as touching a picture for the desired item. In this way, touching the picture becomes a request in a situation that makes sense. Likewise, the time to introduce *more* is when a child reaches for a second cookie after consuming the first one.

It's obvious from these examples that successful AAC communication requires training for both parties (Beukelman & Mirenda, 2005). For a child's partners, this means learning to facilitative interactions and to use strategies to better support the communication of the child using AAC. Four interactional skills have been identified as intervention targets for the communication partners (Kent-Walsh & Light, 2003):

- ■ Modeling AAC system use in both
  - ▪ Responses to the child's communication attempts, and
  - ▪ Initiations of communication with the child
- ■ Extending conversational pause time or expectant delay by initiating and holding eye contact with the child to provide enough time to enable the child to use the AAC device and to build an expectation that the child will respond
- ■ Being responsive to a child's communicative attempts in a timely manner
- ■ Using open-ended questions to enable the child to offer real answers and make real choices rather than responding simply with *yes* or *no*

Following instruction, communication partners can learn to lessen conversational dominance and to provide more turns for the child using AAC. In turn, conversational participation, turn-taking, and the range of communicative functions of child AAC users increase.

An excellent model for communicative partner training is *strategy instruction*, in which partners are taught a series of multistep procedures for supporting AAC communication in a wide variety of contexts (Kent-Walsh & McNaughton, 2005). Figure 8.2 presents an overview of five suggested steps of caregiver instruction. Training does not occur in isolation, and parallel instruction would occur with the child using AAC in order to maximize use of the interaction strategies. Specific training targets would vary, depending on the needs of the communication dyad of the child and partner.

FIGURE 8.2 **Suggested Steps of Communication Partner Instruction**

SLPs must be careful not to overwhelm parents with a long list of communication strategies to use with a child. It's important, therefore, to introduce such strategies one or two at a time. The steps below provide a model for accomplishing this task.

Commitment to the Plan for Intervention

Agree on the goal and methods for achieving it.

Introduce the new teaching strategy and the training procedure to both the child and communication partners.

Strategy Description and Demonstration for the Communication Partners

Describe the new teaching strategy and steps and the component skills.

Discuss the expected impact of implementing the new teaching strategy.

Solicit partners' opinion of the new teaching strategy and obtain their commitment to using it.

Model use of the teaching strategy and give explanations of and rationale for the steps involved.

Verbal Practice of Strategy Steps

Have communication partners practice all steps in implementing the teaching strategy.

Practice and Feedback

Help communication partners practice implementation in controlled environments.

Provide instructional feedback.

Help communication partners practice implementing the teaching strategy in multiple situations within the everyday environment with the child.

Gradually fade instructional prompting and feedback.

Generalization and Commitment to Long-Term Strategy Use

Document and review communication partners' mastery of the teaching strategy.

Elicit feedback on the impact of the teaching strategy.

Assist communication partners in generating plans for maintenance and generalization of the teaching strategy.

Have communication partners practice use of the teaching strategy across a wide range of settings.

Source: Information from Kent-Walsh & McNaughton, 2005. See the original source for a wonderful, more in-depth discussion.

Unfortunately, because long-term data on sustained behavior are unavailable, we don't really know if new partner behaviors continue to be used over time. Nor do we know from research the best instructional methods to use with these partners beyond modeling, direct instruction, and role-playing.

Families

If we hope for a child to use AAC, it is essential that we establish an atmosphere of AAC that supports such use. One aspect of that AAC atmosphere is parents' using AAC in everyday activities with the child at home. When a parent uses AAC, pointing to a symbol as he or she speaks, it demonstrates for the child how AAC can enhance communication. There is also research to suggest that such receptive AAC use increases understanding and recall for the child AAC user. It seems reasonable to suggest, therefore, that parents be taught to touch a symbol or to sign simultaneously with speaking.

For many children, especially those with neuromuscular disorders, AAC communication will be a time-consuming task. It is important that parents and family members be coached to wait and allow time for a child to complete her or his message. In addition to providing additional time for the child to communicate, pausing and waiting clearly indicates to the child that the parent expects communication and has provided an opportunity for it to occur. Some children may need help initiating a message and may have difficulty, especially with the give-and-take of conversation.

Although research data are sparse, in general, the effects of AAC intervention on the language and communication behaviors of both children and their parents in home settings are positive (Romski & Sevcik, 2005). In-home intervention is not without its problems, however, and parents report concerns with the following (Granlund, Björck-Åkesson, Wilder, & Ylven, 2008):

- Influencing the selection of AAC systems
- Selecting appropriate vocabulary
- Guiding the child to develop strategic and social competence

In general, for a variety of reasons, parents report having problems influencing intervention decisions and learning intervention skills from professionals (Campbell & Sawyer, 2007). Unfortunately, in clinical settings, family members report that they are mostly passive observers. This begins with selection of intervention goals.

Intervention goals. There is little research into who actually decides on the intervention goals for families with children who require AAC. In focus groups, parents express concerns that professionals lack interest in involving them in the decision-making process (McNaughton et al., 2008). This can result in goals that do not reflect the priorities of the family, and AAC systems that do not fit the family's lifestyle. Simply stated, when AAC intervention does not match family priorities or lifestyle, it places an extra burden on families that can be stressful. In contrast, when treatment recommendations from professionals take into account the routines and patterns of family life, families are more likely to carry out the recommendations. It's important for professionals to remember that outcomes of AAC intervention extend beyond the primary impact on a child and affect the entire family (Blackstone & Hunt-Berg, 2003).

It may be especially important that parents perceive that they have well-functioning formal and informal long-term emotional supports in order to have the strength and energy to implement recommendations (Moes & Frea, 2002). In families in which support is perceived as limited and intervention recommendations viewed as disruptive to family functioning, levels of intervention implementation are low.

Intervention goals related to participation or involvement in life situations are more directly related to a child's communicative functioning in the family than are goals that are focused on execution of an AAC task such as using a new scanning technique (Granlund, Björck-Åkesson, Wilder, & Ylven, 2008). In other words, operating a device successfully is not nearly as important to the family as learning to communicate spontaneously in family interactions in the home. In general, outcomes of AAC intervention that focus on executing a task, such as touching a symbol when asked, tend to be more specific and short term than goals related to participation in interactions with the family. Participation in family life requires broader-based, longer-term AAC intervention.

As professionals, we must focus on both short- and long-term intervention goals. The key is providing a child with a means of communicating at home while at the same time teaching basic responding techniques. Now, it should be obvious why an SLP should consider a range of means of communication.

It is sometimes assumed that more immediate goals, such as improving intelligibility of AAC system use, will affect overall participation in interactive contexts. In fact, outcomes in one area of AAC intervention do not necessarily affect other areas of functioning (Lund & Light, 2006). In other words, better ability to select a given symbol doesn't mean a child will use it at home.

If we hope to improve participation within family life, we should directly target this area of functioning and not just hope it will occur. In general, children with better AAC outcomes tend to have more supportive family environments than those with less positive outcomes (Hamm & Mirenda, 2006).

Challenges. Parents report that their greatest challenges in supporting their children in using AAC technology are (McNaughton et al., 2008)

- Their own lack of skills in dealing with technology breakdown,
- Selection of vocabulary, and
- Ability to support their children in the creation of sentences using available vocabulary.

For these and other reasons, parents indicate that ongoing support from SLPs and family members is important for intervention sustainability (McNaughton et al., 2008). Abandonment of AAC technology by a family may be related more to loss of professional support than to rejection of the technology (Fager, Hux, Beukelman, & Karantounis, 2006).

It's important for an SLP to understand how and to what extent AAC devices will affect the family, because parents are the key to achieving positive outcomes in AAC. In short, when caregivers are supportive of AAC, children are more likely to experience the benefits of these devices (Beukelman & Mirenda, 2005). Thus, SLPs need to assess and monitor the impact of AAC devices and methods on the family.

As noted, when families are not supported, devices are simply abandoned and not used. The most common reasons for abandonment have to do with

- Failure of a device to enhance independent functioning,
- Limited access to a device, such as one kept at school,
- Difficulty in programming or maintaining a device,
- Questionable reliability of the device, and
- High levels of assistance required by the child to use the device.

Any one of these variables can compromise the anticipated benefits. This, in turn, can lead to family stress and frustration.

One survey of more than 100 families of both children and adults using AAC (Angelo, 2000) found generally favorable opinions toward AAC use by both caregivers and users. That said, parents, particularly mothers, reported increased roles, responsibilities, and demands on their time because of AAC. If anything, these data should highlight the importance of including AAC in everyday routines rather than requiring more formal instruction by families.

Roles. Over time, children using AAC become dependent on one or two skilled interactional partners within the family, usually the mother (Wilder & Granlund, 2015). Children become less apt to interact with a range of partners within the family's social network. This pattern of isolation may be reinforced if a child learns to use AAC but his or her family members do not develop sufficient skills in using that mode. For example, a child who uses manual signs might be isolated from the family or extended family when only teachers or the mother know sign language (Joseph & Alant, 2000).

Knowing the roles caregivers play in AAC use is important for sustaining family involvement and supporting those roles as they evolve. Because caregivers already experience considerable demands on their time related to parenting a child with special needs, it's important to fully explain to families the anticipated commitment with AAC devices. Information specific to particular devices, such as technical programming, should be discussed early in the assessment process.

Parental concerns. Within a family, it's important for an SLP to identify possible sources of negativity toward AAC devices and technology in general. SLPs can identify cultural values affecting attitudes toward both disabilities and technology. Early identification of potential problems and culturally sensitive interventions can increase the likelihood of positive outcomes.

Although, as we've seen throughout this text, parent-implemented language intervention is complex, early AAC language intervention may be even more so (Kaiser & Hancock, 2003). Both parental perceptions about communication and parental stress may play even larger roles in AAC intervention.

Although many parents may not be afraid of technology because of extensive use of computers and smartphones in daily life, an SLP's understanding of how to capitalize on this knowledge, given the often hectic pace of modern life, is a challenge. In addition, as a consequence of Internet use, parents may be surprisingly knowledgeable about AAC devices and options. SLPs cannot expect all parents to be ignorant on this topic, although parental attitudes will vary widely.

An SLP can inform parents up-front that successful AAC outcomes are related to the time commitment of family members. A portion of the assessment process can be devoted to identifying time commitments, constraints, and the potential level of involvement of each family member (Angelo, 2000). In some cases, it may be helpful to recruit and train others, such as extended family members, community volunteers, teachers, and school peers. Retired grandparents may prove to be excellent communication partners with the time to devote to their grandchild's AAC training.

Parents also express a need for informational supports about AAC device options. This is important not only for their own child but because knowledgeable, well-informed parents can become invaluable resources and support networks for other families. In support of this outcome, an SLP can become a source of information and referral.

For both professionals and parents, some sources of evidence carry more weight when making critical intervention decisions (Rycroft-Malone, 2004; Rycroft-Malone et al., 2004). Data suggest that the closer the evidence is to the family's situation, the greater is the probability that it will affect the family members' motivation to implement intervention. It is important, therefore, for families to meet with other families in similar situations, possibly through group meetings, and to have access to examples of successful intervention.

Given the importance of AAC use in all communication environments, it is extremely important for an SLP to monitor the extent to which children communicate at home with AAC devices. This is critical given the reported underuse of devices in the home and community. Parents need family-sensitive training on integration of AAC devices across all communication environments.

Not surprisingly, parents identify the key measure of success in AAC intervention as their child's ability to use an AAC system to communicate independently. In order to be successful in the use of AAC, it is important for a family to be active members of the intervention team (Parette, Huer, & Brotherson, 2001). This said, there is only limited information on parents' perceptions of the learning and use of AAC technologies (Goldbart & Marshall, 2004). Parents participating in an online focus group format identified several areas of concern (McNaughton et al., 2008). These are presented in Figure 8.3.

While this is a formidable list of parental concerns, parents were not without suggestions for improving AAC training and use (McNaughton et al., 2008). These included teaching strategies such as

- Independent exploration ("fooling around"),
- Imaginary or role play,

FIGURE 8.3 **Parental Concerns**

Program Issues

Lack of parental input or true collaboration

Intervention often focused on related skills rather than functional communication

AAC system not meeting family's and child's needs

Lack of flexibility or lack of a dynamic nature to the programming

Difficulty identifying appropriate core and specific vocabulary and helping children form units of communication beyond single words

Need to use a variety of modalities (e.g., eye gaze, vocalizations, facial expressions, and sign language)

Need for strategies to deal with conversational breakdowns

Child's need for a means of attracting attention

Child's need to learn different communication functions, such as asking questions

Content focused on colors and size rather than what their child wants and needs to express

Device Issues

Little or no parental input in selecting a device

Need to become competent in use of and programming for their child's device

Physical effort required of children with cerebral palsy to operate the device

Difficulty in receiving funding for the device

Generalization

Lack of support for AAC use in other environments such as the school

Extended periods of nonuse because of technical problems with the device

Difficulty introducing the AAC system to others and instructing them not to finish messages for the child

Lack of professionals, especially teachers, trained in AAC, frequently resulting in delayed or inappropriate interventions

Need for constant and consistent access to the devices in order to develop competency

Problems developing communication opportunities in a variety of environments given the negative attitudes toward children who use AAC and the reactions from their child's peers

Sources: Hurd, 2007; McNaughton et al., 2008; Smith & Hustad, 2015.

- ■ Structured drill and practice with family members, especially when the classroom teacher is reluctant to be involved,
- ■ Learning from peers who use AAC,
- ■ Technology supports built into AAC devices, such as icon prediction programs, and
- ■ Manufacturers' trainings and technical assistance.

In the same online forum, parents also recommended educating society about AAC use and preparing a child for the negative reactions they might experience. Parental recommendations to professionals included the following (McNaughton et al., 2008):

- ■ Be sensitive to the specific needs of each child and family.
- ■ Know the basic technical operation of an AAC device.
- ■ Teach and inform others, including parents and teachers.

Parents are advised to take a leadership role in obtaining services and to become experts in both AAC technology and highly motivating instructional programs. In short, parents are not only caregivers but must also become partners and teachers, technical support personnel, and advocates.

Supporting a child's communication. Parents and other family members can be taught techniques to support their child's communication. These include (Light & Drager, 2005)

- Collaborative planning with the SLP on ways to integrate the AAC system into the natural environment,
- Identifying communication opportunities within each context,
- Modeling AAC and speech for the child,
- Learning to wait and to anticipate the child's communication, and
- Responding to the child's communication attempts in meaningful ways.

As mentioned in other chapters and still true with AAC, meaningful responding is contingent and timely and fulfills the child's communication intent. The caregiver can expand on the child's communication while replying in a conversational manner that models communication for the child.

Beginning with the caregiver's current strengths, an SLP can gradually introduce new knowledge and skills through a combination of explanation, modeling, practice, monitoring, and feedback. It's important to be mindful of family needs and comfort level and not to introduce too many new things at once.

The last thing a family needs is a time-consuming burden, such as endless drills involving AAC. A review of the family's routines can assist an SLP in determining how AAC use can enhance a child's participation.

Book-sharing. Shared storybook reading is a rich context in which to support language-learning and emergent literacy skills (e.g., Justice, 2006; van Kleeck, Stahl, & Bauer, 2003). Parents can learn to implement interactive strategies using children's books. Training parents to interact with their children using AAC within a book-sharing task can improve parent-child interaction patterns and facilitate communicative expression and turn-taking in their children (Kent-Walsh, Binger, & Hasham, 2010).

Given the predictable vocabulary, characters, and actions in a story encountered in repeated reading of books, SLPs and parents can preprogram a child's AAC device. For example, visual scene displays that depict whole scenes from the storybook can be programmed into a device, which may generate voice output when the child touches particular images on the screen (Light & Drager, 2007).

Classrooms

Preschool or other ECI group settings are important language-learning environments for many children, a place to learn to communicate with other adults and children. The quality of any language-learning environment directly depends on the match between the abilities and limitations of a child and the language and communication in that environment. While educational settings in which all children use AAC provide more supportive language environments, these settings may provide children with fewer opportunities for enculturation. In a more inclusive classroom in which children with disabilities and those without are educated in the same setting, there is more typical use, although training is required of all children in the class in order to maximize interactions (Guralnick, 2001; Mulvihill, Shearer, & Van Horn, 2002).

Preschool inclusion can provide a context for learning age-typical communicative interactions, but this does not occur automatically. Teachers, aides, SLPs, and parents working with children using AAC need to understand the characteristics of a child's AAC system and know how to promote its development. Otherwise, professionals may unintentionally limit a child's development and severely restrict AAC use. If, for example, an AAC device is used in the classroom only for requesting at snack time, then we fail to consider AAC use as a part of regular activities and social communication (McNaughton, 2003).

While inclusive preschool settings have the potential to encourage AAC use, the language environment of the class must be sufficiently adapted to the abilities and limitations of each child and supported by the communicative practices of adults and children in these preschools (von Tetzchner, Brekke, Sjøthun, & Grindheim, 2005). In order to maximize use, the intervention team should attempt to identify daily activities and the best use of a child's AAC method within those activities.

Peers. One factor in the classroom is the interaction between children. Although children with limited speech tend to have less social interaction with peers than children with better spoken language skills, inclusive preschool settings can offer a variety of communication experiences for children using AAC (Harper & McCluskey, 2002). In order for this to occur, the speaking children need to become competent AAC users too. This only occurs when AAC becomes part of the everyday communication in that classroom. For example, if speaking children never use sign when speaking to a child who does, or if speaking children reduce the signing child's participation to answering *yes/no* questions, then the environment is not supporting the signing child (Clarke & Kirton, 2003; Smith, 2003; von Tetzchner & Grove, 2003).

Although there is little research on young children, studies with school-age children indicate that children's attitudes toward peers who use AAC can be influenced positively through a combination of information about AAC and the opportunity to role-play being nonspeaking (Beck & Fritz-Verticchio, 2003). Results are more positive than when children are provided with information alone. Role-playing may be an especially powerful teaching method.

Inclusion requires the creation of a shared language environment. Professionals can facilitate not only caregiver-to-child interactions but also child-to-child in order to promote communication, especially in inclusive settings. One way to ensure that these interactions occur is to teach AAC to all staff and children, even speaking peers. If only some staff members use AAC, and only when communicating with the child who depends on it, then speaking children in the class are unlikely to use AAC. I recall one teacher who had a huge communication board that dominated one wall of her classroom. She touched symbols as she talked and had speaking children respond similarly.

Simply providing an AAC system is not enough to ensure use by a child. In one study, three preschool children with ASD were taught to use a graphic symbol representing "Can I play?" to request entrance into play in a naturalistic strategy that included (Johnston, Nelson, Evans, & Palazolo, 2003).

■ Creating communicative opportunities,
■ Providing a model of the desired behavior,
■ Prompting the child to engage in the desired behavior through prompting and waiting, and
■ Providing natural consequences for appropriate responses.

Intervention occurred within ongoing play activities in the classroom.

Although teachers and SLPs cannot directly plan the interactions of children who are using AAC and those who are not, techniques to encourage communication between peers might include (von Tetzchner & Grove, 2003; von Tetzchner, Merete Brekke, Sjøthun, & Grindheim, 2005)

■ Reinforcing TD children for using AAC devices, when invited, to talk with their friends;
■ Including communication in classroom routines or devising routines, such as greetings;
■ Adapting movements easy for a child with motor deficits into prized or special behaviors, such as "Timmy's special wave bye";
■ Establishing acceptable nonverbal procedures for the classroom;
■ Encouraging story-sharing during snack;
■ Having shared playtime or shared toys or books; and
■ Establishing a routine by which AAC users can invite other children to use their devices.

While these peer interactions will not replace direct instruction in AAC, they do reduce the social isolation of children using AAC, aid in enculturation and development of language, and increase generalization.

One caution: We are not trying to turn speaking peers into "little teachers." If staff uses only a teaching-oriented style of interaction with children using AAC, this behavior has the potential to further isolate these children. Speaking children may also adopt such a style, going so far as to praise nonspeaking children for AAC use, thus reducing the natural quality of communication (Smith, 2003). Of more value is teaching speaking peers to attend to, wait for, and prompt AAC use. A functional intervention strategy in which caregivers use real conversations can model the type of interaction desired from peers.

NEUROMOTOR CONSIDERATIONS

Children with neuromotor dysfunction, such as CP, may have difficulty accessing AAC devices. Obviously, AAC device selection will be extremely important. Learning requires multiple exposures to the device and to responsive partners. Unfortunately, simple practice with remote switch toys may not translate directly into communicative uses of the same switch.

The addition of a voice output to the activation switch on an AAC device may produce a more recognizable signal to which others can respond more consistently and help the child associate a behavior with an environmental response. Once others are alerted, the child can proceed with a message.

Positioning is extremely important for children with AAC. Electronic devices should be child size and located for best access. The child's body needs to be supported and the upper trunk, neck, and head aligned. If the child is in a chair, he or she should be firmly against the back of the chair for lower back support, with both feet flat on the floor or supported flatly on an elevated block or a stool. Knees and ankles should be flexed at 90° with good thigh support. A physical therapist can help you get this "just right" for maximizing a child's performance.

 Introducing AAC takes some skill, as you can see in this video of a first session with a 2-year-old child.
https://www.youtube.com/watch?v=hrQclfxmRsE

Intervention Methods

There is sometimes an assumption that ECI using AAC is devoid of all the other aspects of early communication. The communication base within which language develops is just as important in AAC as in speech. The device is not a substitute for early communication but may act as an aid.

For very young children, aided electronic devices may be introduced simply as an interesting object that causes things to happen. Push the "button" and there's a response, such as a voice, from the device. Introducing language or even communication at this point may be too complex, except for receptive use by the child.

Relatively inexpensive, single-switch devices such as the BigMac, which can be easily programmed for new messages, may be used within routines to aid a child's participation even when the child does not understand the message. Think about very young TD children who participate in "singing" by vocalizing with intonation although they do not comprehend the words.

An additional interactional component is for those in the child's environment to also respond to the signal coming from the device. In this way, the child learns that his or her behavior has an effect on adults even when that is not the child's intention. Recall that the early crying of TD children is not intentional but is interpreted as meaningful by adults in the environment.

EARLY COMMUNICATION INTENTIONS

Early AAC intervention should include the same intentions as spoken communication. This often begins with behavior regulation or controlling someone else's behavior, often through requesting. These wants and needs may first be expressed by body postures, gazes, vocalizations, gestures, or other actions or physical behaviors. As children develop, more of their communication involves sharing information, commenting, or continuing social interaction routines. Some children may find it difficult to express joint attention or word labels without intervention.

There is a danger that children with restricted communication intentions, such as simple requests, will become "stuck" at this level without increased emphasis on promoting others (Cress, 2002). Requesting alone does not lead to conversational interaction and tends to be limited to the adult cueing the child with "What do you want?," the child responding, and then the adult giving the desired item.

Many intentions, such as greetings and protests, can be fulfilled by other means and do not require deliberate intent by the child if they are easily recognized by communication partners (Sigafoos et al., 2000). For example, a child may initially turn away from an unwanted activity. Later the child may learn a gesture or shake her or his head side to side as a more deliberate protest. Similarly, waving "bye" is learned as part of a routine, long before the child learns about signaling departure.

Communication that begins as random behaviors or signals can help a child learn the meaning of messages within different interactional contexts. Even children who do not demonstrate intentional communication can learn from contingent responses of others to use these behaviors to communicate. Even random activation of an AAC device can be reinforced by adult compliance with the message produced.

By structuring the interactional environment, an adult can ensure that a child's spontaneous behaviors have a reasonable likelihood of initiating a message without adult prompts. As the child's production of the target behavior becomes more deliberate, contextual cues can be reduced. This fosters independence in initiating communication. For example, rather than prompting a request with a question, such as "What do you want?," a caregiver may look at a desirable item and then look at the child expectantly.

Initially, parents ignore messages that are ambiguous. With consistent feedback, however, a child can advance from partner-perceived communication to intentional communication. A child learns to associate meaning to a behavior through adults' interpreting that behavior as meaningful.

Although responding to adults is important, it can limit a child's participation. Interactional approaches that teach children to respond solely to adult initiations promote passive interactions. A child may learn to comply with adult expectations at the expense of expressing his or her own communicative messages. In such adult-directed communication situations, a child may demonstrate learned helplessness or dependence on others in order to communicate. In contrast, teaching parents and teachers to reduce their conversational dominance facilitates greater child initiation in conversations.

By introducing a child to the active role of communicator and reinforcing communication initiations, parents can help a child learn to become a true conversational partner before a passive role is well developed (Cress & Marvin, 2003). Children do not have to understand the meaning or intention of their own behaviors fully in order to learn from the experience of using those behaviors in ways that are interpreted as communicative by conversational partners.

TRANSITIONING FROM NONSYMBOLIC TO SYMBOLIC

Young TD children transition from vocalizations to meaningful symbolic communication and subsequently from single word to multiword utterances. Although typical development provides some guidelines for designing AAC systems, there is no guarantee that development will proceed according to a parallel route when in an alternate form or mode of communication such as AAC.

The transition to symbols can be fostered by building onto a mode of communication that a child is using spontaneously. For example, if a child is already using some gestural communication, signs might be introduced. *Molding-shaping* is an effective method for teaching signs, especially when the hand shape of the sign suggests the referent or action it represents, such as placing a book in a child's hands while opening and shutting both in imitation of the sign *book*. A similar procedure can be used with a cup for *drink*. Subsequently, the object is removed while the hand shape is maintained.

Transition from prelinguistic to linguistic forms of communication is also affected by the types of symbols used. There is a belief among some professionals that initial AAC systems need to consist solely of easy-to-learn iconic symbols, even though individuals with severe intellectual disabilities (ID) have demonstrated an ability to learn abstract symbols for augmented communication. We sometimes forget that TD children at 12 months learn to use very abstract symbols in the form of words to communicate. More abstract symbols may in fact form a good foundation for transition to multisymbol messages, but of course the real test is how well the symbol works for the child.

RECEPTIVE USE

Among the factors that predict preschool children's success in learning AAC is the amount of parental language input. Other factors are intrinsic and include a child's nonverbal cognitive development, language comprehension, communication complexity as measured by the child's combined means of communication, and level of play (Brady, Thiemann-Bourque, Fleming, & Matthews, 2013).

The amount of AAC communication that occurs is very important, even before a child begins to sign or use an aided device. Think of the amount of language a TD child hears before making her own attempt to talk. For several reasons, whether they are using speech or AAC, children do not choose to produce all the words they hear. Communication increases the symbols an AAC user hears and sees, so he or she can pick and choose which ones to express. For this reason, adults need to stay ahead of a child's production and regularly introduce new words. In short, adults should not sign only the words the child signs.

Traditionally, AAC intervention has focused on enhancing expressive communication. AAC can also augment communication input during both communication interaction and instruction in AAC use. For example, an adult's spoken message can be augmented by elaborating with visual and verbal AAC techniques. To optimize the use of this component in a way that supports AAC, the partner needs to confirm that the message is understood by the child. A communication partner can help the child associate symbols with their referents by showing, pointing to, or producing the symbols with relevant items or events.

As noted, typically developing children learn to comprehend and produce words that are frequently spoken to them. Similarly, AAC intervention should try to incorporate language input strategies into teaching new symbols because these same processes contribute to learning to comprehend and produce graphic symbols. It is quite possible that spoken language input may aid a child in associating meaning with a graphic symbol or sign. Spoken language input might come from a speech-generating device (SGD), a communicative partner, or both.

To aid understanding and use, at some point the AAC user will need to connect the symbol to its referent. There is an expectation that a child will eventually begin to use the symbol expressively. Unfortunately, it seems that communication partners infrequently provide simultaneous input, such as touching the AAC symbol while saying the word.

Although there is little research on young children, adolescents with severe disabilities and various levels of language comprehension will begin to comprehend symbols and then use them on their AAC systems expressively without direct instruction. This would seem to indicate that receptive intervention supports the learning objective of expressive communication by providing a model for the use of AAC as a viable communication mode. In addition, receptive use teaches the meaning of the symbols the child may later use expressively. Learning will require multiple opportunities to experience the symbol in different contexts.

Many children who use AAC are able to learn or "fast map" new symbol meanings. As with TD children, fast mapping uses language input to promote rapid symbol acquisition. The child forms a hypothesis of the meaning and then tries it expressively. To do this, the symbols must be available to the child.

Receptive use may also facilitate the AAC user's recall of a message by providing a concrete representation of the idea. In visual systems, the graphic symbol is present on the display and may assist recall.

One approach is to have conversational partners point to symbols on the learner's communication display in conjunction with ongoing language directed toward the child. Although the AAC device may or may not be activated to speak, the conversational partner should point to symbols while speaking. This method has been shown to effectively teach both receptive and expressive language use (Harris & Reichle, 2004). Some children may benefit further by the partner's using the SGD as a supplement to speech. Unfortunately, we don't have enough data to compare the outcomes of the two methods definitively, and results may vary with individual children.

TD children often learn new vocabulary items within the conversations surrounding everyday events and activities. This is the perfect vehicle for introducing new symbols in AAC as well. Children learn words or symbols by seeing and hearing others use the words in conversation.

It is difficult to determine what concepts or vocabulary a child, especially one who does not speak, actually understands because judgments must be made on the basis of the child's performance, which may or may not reflect underlying competence. Judgments are complicated by the type of partner input, use or nonuse of voice output, and demands of the language comprehension tasks used (Sutton, Soto, & Blockberger, 2002).

EXPRESSIVE USE

SLPs can severely limit a child's use of AAC if they wait for the child to demonstrate full comprehension of a concept before targeting production of the associated symbol. Children with symbolic skills can learn new concepts as they explore their use via various AAC methods (Cress & Marvin, 2003). Through interpreting of a partner's prompting cues, a child can infer or "fast map" symbol meanings.

Even among TD children, expressing new words and combining these words with other linguistic features for various communicative purposes is an essential part of refining both meaning and use. Use of words or symbols does not have to wait until a child fully understands the concepts underlying them. Full comprehension of a symbol is a gradual and sometimes extended process for all children. Continued social use, especially accompanied by adult feedback, and subsequent cognitive development aid a child's lexical maturity.

AAC intervention with young children should include teaching new concepts and words by actually using them. We know from TD children that words are often learned within routines and scripts that provide a supportive environment for early production of words and phrases that a child may not fully understand. By experiencing a word within a routine, the child forms an activity-based concept to which the label may be attached. This is one aspect of *fastmapping* a word onto a child's existing vocabulary.

TD children usually learn early words or symbols during routines in which the child matches messages to functional goals within the interaction. Gradually, the child applies these messages toward additional communicative goals. The same is true for children using AAC, and SLPs can plan for such generalization. Restricted use of single words or symbols by children using AAC may be related more to limited communicative functions or uses, such as using symbols solely to request, than to the child's limited vocabulary. Therefore, it is important to be flexible with uses of a symbol and to recognize various meanings (Cress & Marvin, 2003).

Keeping AAC simple enough for a young child can be a challenge. It's important not to flood the child with too many new symbols. New symbols can be introduced as a child indicates a desire to communicate about things in the environment. If a child sits passively and watches an object or activity, an SLP may need to entice the child to respond or to request "more" by using a behavior chain interruption technique as we discussed in Chapter 6.

As TD children expand their spoken word use beyond familiar routines, they may initially make semantic errors, such as overgeneralizations of word meanings. You'll recall from your language development class that a child may call all men *Daddy* or all four-legged animals *doggie* until she settles on a more conventional meaning. Children with more restricted vocabularies may cling to these overextensions longer than do TD children. This may occur because these children

- Do not experience as many communicative functions for individual messages because of physical or social restrictions, and
- Do not receive as much meaningful feedback about their errors.

It's important, therefore, that a child have adequate opportunities to play with the vocabulary, to explore new uses, and to experience meaningful combinations in a trial-and-error fashion. Adult modeling and feedback are critical (Cress & Marvin, 2003).

By experiencing different responses, a child can gradually learn the consequences of varying messages and the strategies for repairing ambiguous messages through alternative strategies. In this way, children learn the power and meaning of communication by observing its impact on those in their environment. One way a TD child explores the appropriateness of communication is by making mistakes. A child with limited communication needs similar opportunities.

Even acceptable communicative behavior is not appropriate at all times. For example, signing "cookie" to obtain one at snack time is fine, but doing so while on the school bus is not and will not result in obtaining one. Learning when not to produce a particular communicative act involves conditional use.

Without specific instruction, some AAC users have a difficult time using their new communicative behaviors conditionally. Conditional use requires that a child be able to evaluate potential communicative opportunities to determine if communication will "work" in a given context and if so, the relative efficiency of available alternatives. For example, a child might be taught to request a snack by reaching toward the plate of snacks on the table and in response to the question "What do you want?" At other times, when not asked the question, the reaching would be ignored.

Teaching conditional use becomes more difficult when no verbal prompt, such as a question, is used. This would occur when the goal is spontaneous use rather than responsive communication. Spontaneous use can be taught by reducing the verbal cue and using a visual cue, such as the desired object, to elicit the request.

Requesting

During the initial stages of AAC intervention, a child is often taught to request as a means of gaining and maintaining access to preferred objects or events. Several reasons exist for targeting requesting as an initial communicative objective with AAC. In short, requesting

- Is one of the earliest communicative functions to emerge in TD children,
- Provides the learner with a means to gain and maintain access to reinforcing objects and events, and
- Enables a child to exert some degree of control over his or her environment.

Interestingly, the critical element in maintaining requesting behavior with AAC devices is not the device but the presence of something highly desirable to request (Sigafoos, Didden, & O'Reilly, 2003). While this may seem self-evident, it can easily become lost in the concern for teaching a child to activate a device.

Requesting can be learned easily by interrupting a child's reach for an object. As the child reaches, the SLP places a picture before the child's hand. When the child touches the picture, even by chance, the adult supplies the requested item. In this way, the child learns to touch the picture to request the item. Gradually, the item is moved from a location behind the picture to another location out of reach. This occurs gradually as the child begins to see the pictorial representation as symbolizing *want* or the specific object.

Generalized requesting, such as *want*, has the advantage that it can be used to request several desired items. There is always the possibility, however, that the child will interpret the symbol as representing a specific item. It's important to use the symbol with several desired items in order to forestall its becoming item specific. The same is true of signing *want* as well.

If a child persists in using a generalized *want* sign or symbol for a specific request, you have two choices. First, you can acquiesce and begin to teach specific signs or symbols for other specific requests. An alternative is to require the child to identify the specific request—*Want? Want what?*—thus maintaining the generalized meaning of the *want* representation.

A generalized *want* sign or symbol can easily be expanded into the two-symbol message "Want X." A possible method for doing this is presented in Box 8.1.

BOX *8.1*

Hierarchy of Prompts for Expanding from Single Sign/Symbol Requests

Cue/prompt	*Consequence*
Step 1 Place highly desirable object before child and look at child expectantly.	*Successful*: Reinforce and try with another object. *Unsuccessful*: Go to step 2.
Step 2 Place highly desirable object before child and cue with "What do you want?"	*Successful*: Reinforce and return to step 1. *Unsuccessful*: Go to step 3.
Step 3 Place highly desirable object before child and cue with "What do you want?" Model "Want X" and wait expectantly. An alternative is to have someone else model a response and receive the desired item.	*Successful*: Reinforce and return to step 2. *Unsuccessful*: Go to step 4.
Step 4 Place highly desirable object before child and cue with "What do you want?" Model "Want" and look at the child expectantly. If the child performs the sign or touches the symbol for *want*, immediately point to the desired object while looking at the child expectantly. An alternative is to point to the desired object after the child performs *want*.	*Successful*: Reinforce only after the second sign/symbol and return to step 3. *Unsuccessful*: Go to step 5.
Step 5 Place highly desirable object before child and cue with "What do you want?" Model "Want" and look at the child expectantly. If the child performs the sign or touches the symbol for *want*, immediately model the second word.	*Successful*: Reinforce only after the second sign/symbol and return to step 4. *Unsuccessful*: Go to step 6.
Step 6 Place highly desirable object before child and cue with "What do you want?" Model "Want" and look at the child expectantly. If the child performs the sign or touches the symbol for *want*, reinforce the child and then model the second word.	*Successful*: Reinforce after each sign/symbol and return to step 5. *Unsuccessful*: Go to step 7.
Step 7 Place highly desirable object before child and cue with "What do you want?" Model "Want" and look at the child expectantly. If the child does not perform the sign or touch the symbol for *want*, gently assist the child, reinforce, and then model the second word. If the child does not perform even with a physical assist, he or she is likely resisting you. Try a more desirable object and ensure that the child can perform a single symbol request.	*Successful*: Reinforce after each sign/symbol and return to step 6.

Two-symbol requests should only be attempted with words the child has previously used spontaneously in single-symbol requests.

Explicit requests can be taught by having the child touch or sign *want* and then touch the desired object. On subsequent trials, an SLP can substitute more representational symbols or signs, such as *cookie*. More representational visual symbols might consist of pictures or product containers/logos. With logos, the SLP might increase the representational nature by gradually changing the size and deleting colors. For example, Cheerios might be requested by using the package front, then simply the word in color, and finally just the word in black and white. With signs, the SLP may need to improvise in order to be explicit. The sign for cereal may not be explicit enough if a child has several favorites.

There is always the danger of opening Pandora's box when we teach requesting, resulting in the child's continually doing so. In this case, as with children using speech, adults need to specify situations in which requesting is acceptable and others in which it is not.

When intervention centers primarily on requests, the focus is on the preferred item, not on the social interaction. After the child receives the requested item, the interaction often ends. As a result, a child has few opportunities to learn to participate in social interactions. It is important, therefore, that communication partners engage the child in conversation throughout and following the requesting process.

Rejecting

Rejecting can be elicited by presenting an undesirable or nonrequested item. If the child rejects the item by pushing it away, turning away, or tantruming, the SLP can present a general rejection sign or symbol for the child to imitate. The response can be physically prompted by hand-over-hand modeling. Once a child has both requesting and rejecting responses, the SLP or adult can begin to offer meaningful choices.

As with requesting, adults will want to plan intervention and everyday interactions so the child can use these behaviors to both initiate and reply to communication. Otherwise, the child is left to respond to "What do you want?" or "Do you want X?" Of importance is being able to convey "I want/don't want X" and "I want/don't want more" as well as "I want something else" and "I want to stop doing this." Imagine the possibilities in a feeding situation when the choices are small pieces of hamburger, French fries, and a soda!

Commenting

The teaching of commenting can build on the techniques mentioned in Chapter Six. You might want to review these if you've forgotten them.

You'll recall that we point to draw attention to novel and unusual items and events as a method of establishing joint attending. Adults can model pointing for a child. If a child notices something of interest and looks but does not point or is unable to do so because of motor difficulties, the adult can prompt a response by asking "What?" and physically prompting the child to touch a generalized comment representing "Look!" The adult then looks where the child is looking and makes some relevant comment or begins a discussion on the item of interest.

Once the child is using the *look* representation or sign reliably to attract attention, the SLP or other adult can prompt a second, more specific response by asking "What do you see" or simply "What see?" If the child does not respond, the adult can say "Show me what you see" or "Show me" while forming the hand shape of the sign or holding the appropriate picture before the child. Two-symbol responses ("Look doggie") can be taught as shown in Box 8.1 for requesting.

Here again, it is important that the child not just respond to the adult. If the child only responds to specific requests, the adult can play stupid and look at the child when he or she signals "Look." This may nudge the child into being more specific.

Training Multiword Utterances

Children who use AAC often experience difficulties expressing multiword messages, relying instead on single symbols to communicate. The movement from single- to multiword messages is an important developmental step that marks the emergence of syntax and the onset of generative language. Any number of factors may contribute to the predominant use of single-symbol communication by children using aided AAC (Binger & Light, 2007). These are presented in Figure 8.4.

FIGURE 8.4 **Factors Contributing to Single-Symbol Communication by Children Using Aided AAC**

- Inherent nature of AAC systems, such as a lack of communicative efficiency, that encourages single-symbol messages
- Co-constructed messages in which the communication partner, in an attempt to speed up the pace, completes the message
- Symbols (*Juice*) that represent multiple concepts (*Want juice*) for a child, negating the need to point to additional symbols
- Communication partners asking questions that require one-word or *yes/no* answers
- Asymmetry between the multiword spoken language input from others and AAC output, giving a child few opportunities to experience models of multisymbol AAC messages

Source: Binger & Light, 2007, with support from Light, Binger, & Kelford Smith, 1994; Sevcik, Romski, Watkins, & Deffebach, 1995; Smith & Grove, 2003; Sutton, Soto, & Blockberger, 2002; Loncke, Clibbens, Arvidson, & Lloyd, 1999.

Both a lack of communication opportunities and the types of opportunities that do occur may contribute to a lack of multisymbol AAC production. Unlike typically developing children, those using AAC may not spontaneously combine symbols and may need instruction in doing so.

Caregiver instruction. Caregiver instruction is also important. Caregivers can be taught to be patient and wait for a child to finish a message, to prompt longer messages, to ask process questions ("What/how did you ...") rather than product questions ("What's that?"), and to provide linguistic modeling via both speech and AAC input to the child.

Simply put, modeling is the use of speech while pointing to and labeling appropriate graphic symbols on an AAC device. Suppose, for example, that a child points to the symbol *juice* to signify "I want more juice." The adult can respond by saying "More juice" while pointing to *more* and *juice* (Harris & Reichle, 2004; Johnston, McDonnell, Nelson, & Magnavito, 2003; Johnston, Nelson, Evans, & Palazolo, 2003; Kent-Walsh, 2003).

Adding voice output to signing can enhance learning of single words and multiword communication. This could be as simple as an adult saying the word as either the child or adult signs.

Vocabulary. Expressive multiword AAC communication requires simultaneous access to vocabulary that can be combined to express new concepts and functions. Unfortunately, without careful planning by the intervention team, messages on AAC devices may represent only a behavior regulation function, such as requesting or rejecting. This comes at the expense of other functions, such as commenting or making conversational replies.

It is difficult to express more mature functions and symbol combinations without vocabulary that is used to create these types of messages. Ideally, AAC systems would contain symbols and concepts that are easy to combine in simple semantic relations. This requires that SLPs plan potential vocabulary that includes other words and functions beyond nouns and naming.

As in the Deaf Community, signing can be used to express complex concepts in several ways, including syntax, morphology, modified signs, or a combination. Syntactic modifications include multisign utterances and word order, as in *Mommy + eat + cookie*. Morphological modification involves the use of morphological markers such as plural *-s*, as in *cookie + s*. Modified signs are subtle changes that indicate changes in meaning, such as signing *cookie* twice to indicate more than one, or plural. Syntactic word order modifications seem difficult for many children with ID, who seem unable to induce word order easily from the language they hear (Grove & Dockrell, 2000).

Interestingly, some children will modify signs spontaneously to indicate changes in meaning, such as making a one-hand sign with both hands to signify plural. This behavior is consistent with signing in the Deaf Community, in which the sign's meaning is modified by other actions. For example, the sign *sick* can mean anything from the sniffles to bubonic plague, based on actions associated with the sign. Likewise, the sign *big* can be modified by extent to indicate difference in *slightly larger* or *massive*.

Although few young non-deaf children who use manual signs for expressive communication progress beyond a level of basic sign combinations, young school-age children with ID are capable of expressing complex meanings consistently by modifying the form of their signs in subtle ways (Rudd, Grove, & Pring, 2007). Unfortunately, evidence suggests that their patterns of use are more characteristic of a gestural system than a linguistic one, but such modifications are used spontaneously by these children.

Transitioning. As a child moves from single-symbol communication to symbol combinations, some of the strategies used by TD children can provide guidance. For example, TD children use successive one-word utterances or word and gesture combinations as a transition to two-word utterances. This transitional behavior may reduce both the cognitive and the motor programming load required for production. For example, a child might request (*want*) through a grasping gesture followed by pointing to a picture of the desired item (*ball*).

Multisymbol messages may initially be produced as a series of single messages or successive one-word utterances. These can be prompted by questions with reinforcement held until the final symbol is produced. This process, called **vertical structuring**, builds a longer utterance from its parts. For example, a child is shown a picture or objects demonstrating a certain semantic relationship, using individual words that the child already uses on his or her communication device or via sign.

Let's assume that the picture shows a cat sleeping in a chair. The utterance "Cat chair" might be constructed as follows:

Adult: What's this? (Points to picture of *cat*)
Child: Kittie. (Points to picture on device or signs)
Adult: Yes, kittie sleeping. Where is the kittie? (Points to pictures)
Child: Chair. (Points to picture on device or signs)
Adult: Yes, Kittie chair. Kittie sleep chair. (Selects symbols on device or sign).

In this way, a child is shown how to create longer utterances in sequence from the symbols already in her or his repertoire. I would go one step further and while touching *cat-sleep-chair* would add "The cat is sleeping in the chair" and then begin a discussion on cats or sleeping.

It is important to make sure that single words have a variety of semantic functions so they can be combined into longer utterances. Verbal and concrete visual feedback about the meaning of the message is important.

In one study, four of five preschoolers with developmental disabilities learned to consistently produce multiword AAC messages within play and to generalize use of symbol combinations to novel play situations (Binger & Light, 2007). Within play scenarios, such as washing a baby or playing, adults model agent + action, action + object, and agent + object combinations, such as *boy drink*, *drink milk*, and *boy milk*, respectively. The adult modeled symbol combining as follows:

- Label each of the two symbols while touching each on the child's AAC system (*Boy, Drink*), and then
- Provide a spoken model of a more mature form of the utterance (*The boy drinks*).

For example, in fast-food restaurant play, a child might pretend that the pig spilled some milk. The adult would select the symbols *pig* and *spill* while saying "Pig spill" and then provide a spoken model, such as "The pig spilled the milk!" Several factors may account for the success of this method, including the contextual support provided by the play, the use of simplified AAC speech input followed by an expanded speech message, and the slower input inherent in the adult's use of AAC.

I encourage you to explore the wonderful Penn State website of Professors Janice Light and Kathy Drager, where you'll find great ideas and videos. Go to the website for Pennsylvania State University and search for "aackids," then click on the intervention steps in the left margin.

Children with Deafness and Blindness

Infants and toddlers who have deaf-blindness require learning support that goes well beyond that needed by typical infants. Families are rarely informed and equipped sufficiently to provide that support on their own. For these reasons, EI is extremely important. If families are going to be primary contributors, they will require systematic and intensive support from service providers.

Initially, parents will need to be impressed with the importance of early attachment and bonding as supports for overall development. Deaf-blindness may seriously compromise the infant's ability to bond with caregivers.

Early educational opportunities should occur in natural settings, often in play-based activities, where incidental learning is key to the interaction. Play-based situations should be structured to ensure that the activities are more natural yet systematic. Daily activities, such as feeding and bathing, can be structured to provide tactile communication and the development of nascent communication patterns that may involve a number of communication modes. Methods must be highly individualized, with a communication facilitator who is familiar with the child's unique communication needs and methods of learning.

Parent and family education are a vital component in promoting learning among young children with deaf-blindness. Because of the need for consistency between the home and educational settings, the SLP should provide the family and teachers with cueing strategies to be used with the child in multiple contexts. Through in-service training, caregivers can learn methods to use in structured learning environments as well as teaching techniques that are instructional and supportive of their interactions with their child. It is important that home-based educational events be balanced with other normal family functions if parents are to be fully participating team members.

The different forms of communication with and for nonsymbolic children can range from contextual cues, such as touching and exploring an item, through gestures and signs, to vocal language or high-tech AAC devices (Stremel, 2000). Cues may take the form of tangible symbols or objects, such as a cup to signal a drink. The selection of communication methods depends upon a child's current functioning. Factors include the present method of communicating, the degree of hearing and visual impairment, and physical or cognitive limitations.

With a dual sensory impairment, there is an urgent need to optimize audition. The first step in intervention is usually the fitting of personal hearing aids by a pediatric audiologist. The introduction of consistent hearing aid use and EI beginning before 6 months of age optimizes long-term speech and language development for children who are deaf or hard of hearing (Moeller, 2000). Frequency modulated (FM) systems, by selectively amplifying an adult's voice while not amplifying background noise, provide a clear speech model for the child. Directional microphones selectively amplify sources of sound in front of the listener, providing a significant listening advantage. All methods of hearing aid fitting require the expertise of a pediatric audiologist.

For a child whose hearing loss is so profound that hearing aids will not provide adequate speech audibility, cochlear implantation may be appropriate. Even implantation does not ensure that a child will be able to use audition effectively, and EI services will still be needed even if only for the short term.

Children with ASD

Some children with ASD seem to benefit from the use of AAC, either as a bridge to verbal communication or as a primary method of communication. Although EBP is limited, some methods, discussed below, demonstrate communication gains for these children.

Although many nonspeaking individuals with ASD use manual signs, it's rare to find a child who learns to sign fluently and flexibly (National Research Council, 2001). Signing may, however, facilitate a child's understanding of communication in general.

Most of the studies reporting the effectiveness of signing with children with ASD are single-subject designs, calling into question the generalization of the results to other children. A meta-analysis of seven single-subject studies of the use of signing with older children (ages 4–14) with ASD found moderate positive treatment effects for both sign-only and sign-plus-speech methods (Schwartz & Nye, 2006). By comparison, speech-only intervention was less effective. Only three of the studies reported generalization of the newly learned skills to other environments. It should be noted that none of the studies found the use of sign or sign and speech to be detrimental.

AIDED AAC

Evidence strongly suggests that with appropriate opportunities and instruction, children with ASD can learn to use aided techniques for functional communication (Mirenda, 2003). For example, individuals with severe ASD have been taught to request desired items or activities using nonelectronic aided symbol displays such as real or partial objects, photographs, line drawings, or other types of pictures (Keen, Sigafoos, & Woodyatt, 2001; Mirenda, 2001; Rowland & Schweigert, 2000; Sigafoos, 1998; Stiebel, 1999).

A growing body of research suggests that the use of aided AAC techniques may also facilitate speech development and production in children with autism (Broderick & Kasa-Hendrickson, 2001; Charlop-Christy et al., 2002; Kravits, Kamps, Kemmerer, & Potucek, 2002; Mirenda, Wilk, & Carson, 2000; Rowland & Schweigert, 2000). Although the extent to which output from a speech-generating device (SGD) contributes to speech development is unclear, the consistency of spoken words provided by SGDs immediately following symbol selection may have had a positive effect.

SGDs also have the potential to facilitate natural interpersonal interactions and socialization for children with ASD. For example, preschool children with ASD and little or no functional speech can be taught to make requests, respond to questions, and make social comments using SGDs plus line drawings that represent simple messages, such as "I want a snack, please" (Schepis, Reid, Behrmann, & Sutton, 1998).

Most intervention studies using AAC focus on teaching simple requests (Brady, 2000; Sigafoos & Drasgow, 2001; Wendt, Schlosser, & Lloyd, 2006). Sadly, for some individuals with ASD, requesting and rejecting are the extent of the intervention (Mirenda, 2008). Although children with ASD and limited speech actually produce more spontaneous communication than elicited communication using unaided AAC, these children are more likely to communicate for requesting purposes (Chiang, 2009).

Most methods of teaching AAC to individuals with ASD use systematic instructional techniques that include providing communicative opportunities, various types of prompts to elicit responding, systematic fading or decreasing of prompts, and both reinforcement and error correction strategies (Sigafoos, Arthur-Kelly, & Butterfield, 2006). Gains tend to be modest and involve requesting preferred items or activities, rejecting or terminating undesired items or events, and repairing communication breakdowns (Beukelman & Mirenda, 2005).

While the research is slim, it suggests that less structured natural aided language techniques can be used productively in AAC intervention with individuals with ASD (Cafiero, 2001). A technique referred to as aided language modeling (ALM), consisting of providing models of AAC symbol use during naturalistic interactive play, has shown positive results (Drager, Postal, Carrolus, Castellano, Gagliano, & Glynn, 2006; Romski & Sevcik, 1996).

As suggested throughout this text, naturalistic teaching techniques—such as child-preferred stimuli, natural cues including expectant delays and questioning looks to elicit communication, and nonintrusive prompting techniques—can be used during natural play and/or snack routines in the classroom. While there is growing evidence that both SGDs and computers with communication software can be used effectively with children with ASD in school settings, there is a paucity of data on the use of these technologies in home or community settings (Mirenda, 2003).

My experience from teaching is that students have a keen interest in trying to understand ASD. Although it is somewhat dated, I recommend looking at the professional journal *Focus on Autism and Other Developmental Disabilities*, volume 16, issue 3, from 2001 for a discussion of many of the issues concerning AAC use with individuals with ASD.

PICTURE EXCHANGE SYSTEM (PECS)

The Picture Exchange Communication System (PECS; Bondy & Frost, 1998, 2001; Frost & Bondy, 2002) teaches children to make requests by handing a picture of a desired item to a recipient. PECS, which uses laminated drawings and a binder containing pictures, is a low-tech AAC system, requiring no electronic devices. Handing the picture to the adult shows coordinated attention to both the object and the person. It is also intentional communication.

In the training, a second adult, positioned behind the child, physically prompts the child to pick up the picture and give it to the partner when the child reaches for the item of interest. These prompts are gradually faded to encourage independent picture exchange.

A meta-analysis of the efficacy of use of the Picture Exchange Communication System (PECS) with children with ASD found preliminary evidence that PECS is readily learned by most participants and provides a means of communication for individuals with little or no functional speech (Preston & Carter, 2009). While data suggest some positive effect on both social-communicative and challenging behaviors, these data are extremely limited.

PECS instruction is designed to teach children to request desired items. According to its developers, PECS, unlike other approaches, does not result in children producing prompt-dependent, nonspontaneous speech (Schreibman, 2006). In contrast, PECS relies on child-initiated communication and minimizes prompt dependence through systematic fading.

Unlike sign language or speech, PECS provides concrete visual reminders in the form of pictures and requires that children use only a small number of simple motor movements rather than the complex, abstract, and varied fine motor movements of sign or speech. In addition, PECS requires few prerequisite skills.

In one study, nearly 60 percent of children with severe ASD began using speech to communicate within a year of PECS training (Bondy & Frost, 1994). PECS may facilitate spoken communication for several reasons (Yoder & Stone, 2006a,b):

■ Coordinated attention elicits parental linguistic input to preschoolers with developmental delays (Yoder & Munson, 1995; Yoder & Warren, 2001a,b).
■ In Phase IV of PECS (sentence strip exchange), the interventionist uses a cloze procedure ("I want ___") to elicit the child's production of the key word.
■ Linguistic mapping, or putting the child's request into words, is used consistently after every picture exchange.

Mostly secondary and anecdotal reports claim that PECS increases expressive language through pictures alone and pictures in combination with speech (Kravits, Kamps, Kemmerer, & Potucek, 2002; Stoner et al., 2006).

PECS training consists of six phases (Frost & Bondy, 2002).

■ Phase 1: Teaching the child to exchange a picture/line drawing with a communicative partner for a preferred item. In close proximity to two adult trainers, the child learns to hand one communicative partner a picture, initially prompted by a second trainer who is sitting behind the child, and to receive an item corresponding with the picture.
■ Phase 2: Expanding picture exchanges to a variety of communicative partners and across expanding distances. Phase 1 is extended so that the child learns to travel to

his or her communication binder, 5 to 10 feet away, retrieve a picture, bring it to the communicative partner, and receive the desired item.

- Phase 3: Learning to distinguish between several visual images, preferred and non-preferred items, and eventually between numerous preferred items. First, the child is taught to discriminate between a preferred and a nonpreferred item. Then the child is taught to discriminate among up to six preferred items.
- Phase 4: Teaching the child to form sentences using PECS pictures to make requests. The child is taught to place the sentence starter picture "I want" on a sentence strip, put a picture of a preferred item on the strip, and give it to the trainer. The trainer then verbally models the words written on the sentence strip, using backward chaining to teach each step (Cookie; Want cookie; I want cookie). Following mastery, the trainer uses time delay to provide the participant the opportunity to say the words before being given the verbal model.
- Phase 5: Learning to answer "What do you want?"
- Phase 6: Expanding on previously learned skills, such as answering "What do you see?"

Throughout each phase of training, the communication partner provides a verbal model of the words printed on the pictures the student exchanges.

In general, PECS has been shown to be effective with participants across a variety of ages, including preschoolers (Magiati & Howlin, 2003; Stoner et al., 2006; Yoder & Stone, 2006a, 2006b). In addition, use of PECS reportedly results in decreased tantrums and other problem behaviors, increased requesting, improved social interactions, and improved skill generalization (Charlop-Christy et al., 2002; Frea, Arnold, Vittimberga, & Koegel, 2001; Ganz, Sigafoos, Simpson, & Cook, 2008; Marckel, Neef, & Ferreri, 2006; Stoner et al., 2006).

A meta-analysis review of the current empirical evidence for PECS found that PECS is a promising but not yet established evidence-based intervention for facilitating communication in children with ASD (Flippin, Reszka, & Watson, 2010). Although the data report small to moderate gains in communication, gains in speech are small to negative.

Although some children with ASD master PECS quickly, the outcomes vary with the unique characteristics of the participants (Ganz, Simpson, & Corbin-Newsome, 2008). For example, even pictures may be too abstract for some children who do better if actual objects are used. In addition, while PECS use can result in a functional communication system, the jury is still out on whether it significantly increases expressive speech and if changes can be maintained over time.

Conclusion

Although the positive effects of AAC intervention have been documented, development of AAC technologies has not kept pace, especially for young children. Most current AAC technologies reflect the priorities of the nondisabled adults who design them (Light & Drager, 2007).

To be truly useful, AAC technologies will need to be redesigned to increase their appeal, expand functions, and reduce the learning demands for young children (Light & Drager, 2002). For example, the appeal for young children might be increased by (Light, Drager, & Nemser, 2004)

- Integrating play into both AAC design and intervention,
- Providing meaningful fun contexts for interaction and intervention,

- Expanding output options to include voice or animation,
- Enhancing aesthetics to resemble toys in color and design, and
- Providing options for personalization

When given a choice, older children prefer AAC technologies that they consider "cool" and that enhance their self-esteem and social image (Light, Page, Curran, & Pitkin, 2008). Functions can be expanded by designing technologies that interface with current electronic devices, such as cell phones, tablets, and video games (DeRuyter, McNaughton, Caves, Bryen, & Williams, 2007).

These modifications cannot be accomplished at the expense of ease of learning. At present, learning AAC systems is extremely challenging for young presymbolic children, especially given the need to attend to and interact with communication partners at the same time (Light, Parsons, & Drager, 2002). Add to this the dynamic nature of communication, and you get some idea of the challenge for a young child with communication impairment. You may recall that it is the very joint attention needed here that is the crux of the problem for some nonspeaking children.

While redesigning AAC devices will aid some, rethinking use can also be helpful. The more technolo-gies are integrated into existing activities, the easier use becomes. In addition, different technologies may be adapted for different activities, such as a simple pressure switch, one-message device for participation in group book-reading in which children repeat one line over and over, as in books such as *Good-Night Owl!* (Hutchens, 1990) in which the last line of each page is "and Owl tried to sleep." Similarly, individual symbols attached to a communication board with Velcro can be removed and brought to any activity.

Useful Websites

Several very wonderful and informative websites exist. Among the best is the Pennsylvania State University site, accessed by typing "aackids.psu" into your search engine. The "aacintervention" website offers tips and tricks, while the University of Nebraska–Lincoln site, accessed by typing "aacunl" into your search engine, has an extensive bibliography. Other websites can be accessed by typing "aacinsti-tute"; "communicationmatrix" for an online version of the Communication Matrix, which helps SLPs detail communication profiles of children; and "lindaburkhart" for simplified technology. Finally, the Assistive Technology Law Center, accessed by typing "aacfundinghelp" into your online search engine, offers information on funding of AAC assistive technologies.

 Click here to gauge your understanding of the concepts in this chapter.

9

Early Symbolic Intervention

LEARNING OUTCOMES

When you have completed this chapter, you should be able to:

- Provide guidelines for early symbolic intervention
- Describe general symbolic intervention techniques
- Explain techniques for specific intervention targets
- Explain how to involve parents, teachers, and other adults in symbolic intervention
- Describe two examples of early verbal communication intervention

Terms with which you should be familiar:

Telegraphic speech

Although the division of intervention into presymbolic and symbolic levels is helpful for teaching soon-to-be speech-language pathologists (SLPs), it is somewhat arbitrary and does not reflect the reality of working with nonsymbolic children. At what point, for example, can we say that my grandson with apraxia of speech became symbolic? He seemed to comprehend single words and short phrases early on, but his production of words in speech lagged many months behind. In addition, how do we reliably date his early comprehension? During typical development (TD), adults will use symbols when they interact with a child, as in saying "Wave bye," well before the child seems to comprehend the meaning.

The TD child hears "doggie" as an adult points to the family dog, pets it, feeds it, bathes it, and invites the child to touch it. Over time, the sequence of sounds that forms the word becomes associated with the family dog. When the child turns to look or points upon hearing the word, he or she is transitioning to a symbolic level of communication. Research would suggest that this is a gradual process, not an "Ah-ha!" moment.

It is probably incorrect to think of the transition to symbols as an all-or-nothing phenomenon. It usually occurs over time with words that are heard frequently by a child and refer to entities of interest to the child. A TD child usually begins to make a limited number of these associations around 7 months of age.

For our purposes, I'll consider the transition to symbolic communication to occur when a child responds to the consistent pairing of a symbol or a word with its referent or meaning. There are many ways to demonstrate that pairing.

In this chapter, we'll discuss teaching a young child to use symbols. We'll begin with some guidelines such as selecting symbols, move to techniques to use in intervention, then discuss specific targets within single words and longer constructions, and end with a look at two sample programs, the Hanen Early Language program and Responsive Education/Prelinguistic Milieu Teaching.

Early Symbolic Intervention Guidelines

Symbolic intervention can go in several directions at the same time. Here again, accurate recordkeeping is essential. Let's consider the following four areas:

■ Selecting new symbols
■ Expanding the range of intentions
■ Teaching symbols in different semantic categories
■ Combining single-symbol utterances into longer ones

None of these areas of intervention is as simple as the one-line entry above would suggest. For example, adding single symbols for expression should be preceded by ensuring that a child has the concept and understands the symbol receptively, plus has the ability to produce the appropriate sounds and syllable structures. Let's briefly explore each of these directions for intervention separately.

SELECTING NEW SYMBOLS

There are no rules for how to add new symbols or words, but some guidance is available. Initial vocabularies are extremely individualistic. I've worked with children whose first words would even embarrass me, making me wonder what is said in the home. Suggestions for possible first words are presented in Figure 9.1. It's important to keep in mind, however, that first words come from the interests and sound-making skills of the child and not from a general list. There is no list of words that all children use. Note as you peruse the words listed in Figure 9.1 that there is an overabundance of nouns. While nouns are important, an SLP cannot neglect action words and words such as *more, no,* and *big* that go across other words.

FIGURE 9.1 Possible First Words

Possible first words are based on ease of production and the words of TD children. Each child differs, and for some this list may be inappropriate. At best, it's a list of suggestions, nothing more. To the list, add the names of family members, pets, friends, teachers, aides, and yourself.

Apple	Crayon	Hurt	Push
Baby	Cry	In/out	Puzzle
Ball	Daddy (Dada)	Juice	Read
Bed	Dance	Jump	Ride
Bell	Dirty	Key	Ring
Bib	Dish or bowl	Kick	Roll
Big/little	Dog	Kiss	Run
Bike	Drink	Kitty	See
Block	Drop	Lego	Shoe
Boat	Ear	Light	Sit
Book	Eat	Look	Sleep
Box	Egg	Milk	Soap
Broke	Eye	Mine	Sock
Brush	Fall	Mommy (Mama)	Stand
Bus	Fast	More	Table
Bye	Foot	Mouth	Teddy
Cake	Gimme	My	Throw
Candy	Gum	Night-night	Toy
Car	Hand	No	Truck
Chair	Hat	Nose	TV
Chip	Head	Nut	Up/down
Clap	Hear	'Nuther	Walk
Climb	Hi	Old	Wash
Coat	Hit	Open/close	Watch
Comb	Horse	Pencil	Water (wawa)
Come/go	Hot/cold	Play	Yucky
Cookie	Hug	Pop or soda	

The SLP and caregivers should select a few words initially. The words should have the following characteristics:

- Words or concepts that occur in daily routines
- Words that occur often at home in adult language, especially language used when addressing the child
- Words that contain sounds and syllables the child can already produce
- Words that the child understands
- Objects or actions the child likes or has an interest in or concepts, such as *No*, that the child is already expressing through gestures, such as a head shake

Only by careful data collection can you and the caregivers select appropriate words to target. If, for example, a child can produce /p/ in repetitive syllables, as in /pʌpʌpʌ/, looks at the new dog whenever it's around, and wants to pet it and play with it, then puppy

(/pʌpi/) is an obvious choice. Not every selection is so easy. As just one example, the family may wish for the child to say "Papa" even though the child seems to have little motivation to do so. Here's where your negotiating skills come in.

For most children, words for objects (*cup, shoe*) are easier to learn than other types of words, such as those for actions (*eat, throw*), negatives (*no*), and descriptions (*big*). You may choose to wait and add action words and descriptors after a child knows several object names. It's these other non-noun words that will enable you to begin teaching word combinations (*no cup*).

Occasionally, you'll make a mistake and decide on a word that may not be best. I've done this plenty of times. When you do, remove the word and set it aside for later teaching. Of importance is the child's communication, not my pride.

I've also had parents or other caregivers suggest words in which the child has little interest and will most likely not say or that will be extremely difficult to teach or elicit from the child. For example, *thank you* has some difficult sounds and clusters and no immediate referent. It can be taught as part of a routine of handing objects and although it sounds polite, it has very little other functionality for a child. It's not where I would choose to begin, but I have included it with other words just to keep parents motivated. After all, we can't ask for parental participation and then ignore it when it does occur. If the parents aren't wedded to the idea of teaching *thank you*, I somehow "forget" that it was mentioned while eagerly accepting other suggestions. I'm old; I forget lots of things . . . some more conveniently than others.

Phonemes and Syllables

Meaningful speech requires the production of phonemes in various syllable formations. The TD child by 10 months of age has honed his or her sound perception to those phonemic contrasts found in the language to which the child is exposed. These sounds and the patterns they form in words become a template or model for the words the child will say. To the best of the child's ability, the child attempts to match his or her sound production to these templates. Figure 9.2 offers some helpful advice on expanding a child's sound production prepared by two very knowledgeable colleagues.

Among TD children, the phonemes /p, b, w, m, g, k, h/ predominate in first words, as do the consonant-vowel, or CV, and VC, CVCV-reduplicated, and CVCV syllable structures. From an accurate list of a child's sounds and syllable structures, an SLP can begin to construct a possible vocabulary for a child. It may require some creativity to match a child's interest and knowledge to the words that can be created by these sounds and syllables. Remember, it's more important to have the child using speech symbols than to have perfect articulation. Most TD children do not say "ball," but rather an approximation sounding more like "/bɔ/." Good enough for me!

Isolated speech sounds produced by a child in imitation can be used by an SLP to help the child form words or approximations of words. If a child is having difficulty pronouncing a word, modeling may help. For example, if a child produces a CVC word such as *dog* as CV, or /dɔ/, the adult can repeat the word in a positive manner emphasizing the final consonant, as in "Yes, do**g**." It may also help some children if the word is repeated multiple times, as in "Yes, that's do**g**, bi**g** do**g**, do**g**." This sequence of behaviors may or may not be accompanied by augmentative and alternative communication (AAC).

If the child produces /g/ in the initial position in words, the SLP might model "do**g** **g**one" in an attempt to get the /g/ to migrate to the final position in "dog." For this to make sense to a child, a stuffed dog would need to appear and disappear, hence "dog gone."

If a child is having difficulty with an initial consonant but can produce the sound in the final positions as with the final /p/ in *up*, VC syllables can be produced in a series so that the ending consonant becomes the initial one. In this example, repeated production of up as in *up-up-up* results in production of *pup* within the series.

Consonant clusters can be taught in a fashion similar to initial consonant learning. The first sound in the cluster is placed in the final position in the first word and the second sound in the cluster is placed in the initial position in the following word. If, for example, an SLP is attempting to have the child produce the /sm/ cluster, words such as mouse and mess produced in a series, *mess-mess-mess*, will result in a /sm/ combination. Assuming that a child can produce two-symbol utterances, short phrases, such as *ice milk* and *bus man*, can accomplish the same goal.

FIGURE 9.2 **Stimulating Speech Production in the Young Child with Minimal or No Speech Production**

Use the vocalizations and/or verbalizations that the child already demonstrates and build additional syllable shapes.

- Stimulate vocalizations and speech sound productions using environmental sounds such as car engines, sirens, whistles, and windy audible air sounds. To elicit consonant-vowel (CV) combinations use animal sounds such as *bah, moo,* and *neigh.*
- Stimulate for meaningful vowels and vowel combinations such as *oooh, ahhh, uh-oh, ah-ha* (yes), and *ah-ah* (no). Include appropriate prosodic features and body movement to convey meaning.
- Demonstrate and withhold tempting and enticing toys/flip books in order to encourage imitation of simple VC, CV, or CVC combination such as *up, in, out, go, no, boo,* and *me.*

Focus on movement patterns rather than isolated sounds.

- Once a syllable pattern (VC, CV, CVCV, or CVC) is established, use repeated trials and errorless learning.
- To increase speech sound production, use a multimodal approach to incorporate visual, auditory, tactile, and kinesthetic stimulation. For example, encourage gestures, signs, picture assists, tactile prompts, and sound-naming strategies.
- Teach oral movement positions such as *mmm* to facilitate production of bilabial stops (*bee, pa*), *ooh-ee* vowel movement (we) and *ee-oo* (you).
- Use touch, tapping, hopping movement activities to reinforce production of two-syllable CVCV combinations such as *baby, Mommy, Daddy,* and *doggie.*

Embed prosodic features throughout treatment to reduce equal stress and increase meaningful productions.

- Repeat commonly used phrases when in a natural context such as *uh-oh* combined with exaggerated intonation, facial expression, and hands-up gesturing.
- Read books with repeated phrases and words using cloze technique to encourage productions. Some examples include Eric Carle and Sandra Boynton books.
- Use singing and clapping rhythm games and activities to stimulate syllable awareness and prosody—for example, "Old McDonald," clapping to *e-i-e-i-o.*
- Provide realistic home practice ideas that can be accomplished during activities of daily living—for example, the *Big Book of Exclamations* by Teri K. Peterson (Chatterbox Books, Inc., 2008).

Source: Prepared by Barbara Hoffman and Elizabeth Baird, College of Saint Rose.

The basic building block is the canonical CV syllable. Two similar syllables (/kʌkʌ/) can be expanded into syllables with the same consonants but different vowels, as in *cookie, puppy,* and *baby.* Eventually, the SLP can introduce different syllable sequences, as in *doggie* and *ducky.*

Although words such as *ducky* may seem immature, recall that young TD children begin with these constructions because the basic canonical CV building block can be easily adapted to a CVCV structure. Every child is different, and syllable structure will vary depending on the sounds involved. For example, my grandson with apraxia of speech had few CVC words but, much to my joy, found *Bob* to be extremely easy to produce. It's certainly easier than "gran'pa."

Children can be prepared for production of final consonants by lengthening the vowel sound in CV syllables. Figure 9.3 presents a list of possible CVC words, although actual selection depends on the sounds a child can produce and the child's interests.

Some children, especially those with childhood apraxia of speech (CAS) will have greater difficulty. I, for one, don't hold out for an exact replica of my spoken model. In these cases, approximations are fine. We'll fine-tune production later. It's more important to get the "word" into use so it works for the child. Both language production and communication use are our goals.

FIGURE 9.3 **Possible CVC Words**

back	chip	goal	like	pool	soar/sore
bad	coat	goat	line	poop	sock
bag	coke	goes	lip	pop	song
bake	comb	good	log	pot	soup
ball	come	goose	long	pour	sub
base	cook	gull	look	puck	sun/son
bat	cool	gum	loon	(hockey)	tack
bean	cot	ham	loose	pull	tag
bear	cow	hat	lot	push	tall
beat/beet	cut	hair	love	rag	tan
bed	deer	have	mad	rain	tear
beg	dig/dug	head	mail/male	rake	tell
bell	dish	her	make	rash	thick
bib	dog	hide	man	red	thief
big	doll	him	map	rib	thin
bike	duck	hip	mash	ride	thing
bin	fall/fell	hit	mix	ring	tight
bite	fan	home	moon	roar	tin
boat	far	hop	mop	roll	toes
book	fat	hope	more	room	tool
bow	feed	hot	mouse	root	tooth/teeth
bug	feel	house	much	rope	top
bull	fib	hug	mule	rough	tub
bun	fig	jar	nail	rub	tug
bus	fight	jet	name	rug	wag
butt	fill	juice	nap	run/ran	wall
buzz	fish	kick	night	sad	watch
cage	fit	kiss	nose	seat	well
cake	five	kite	note	sheep	what
call	fog	knees	nut	shell	wheel
can	foot/feet	knife	pain	ship	where
car	four	lake	pal	shore	wing
cash	fun	lamb	paw	shot	wipe
cat	fur	laugh	pet	shove	wire
cave	fuzz	leaf	phone	sick	wish
chair	'gain	leg	pick	sing/sang	wood
cheese	game	lick	pig	sip	yell
chick	get/got	lid	pill	sit/sat	zip
chin	give/gave	light	pipe	soap	

Comprehension

A guide for production is the child's comprehension. What does the child seem to understand? At this point in development, comprehension boils down to association of a symbol with a referent, and we should not expect a young child, even those developing typically, to have either adult comprehension abilities or definitions. Symbol-referent links can be taught through comprehension intervention similar to the dynamic assessment techniques presented in Table F.1 in Appendix F. Remember that functional use, where appropriate, is also part of early meanings and may be very specific. A ball may only be associated with pushing.

Unfortunately, there are few studies on effective receptive language interventions for very young children (Law, Garrett, & Nye, 2004). Most research has been with children older than 36 months and has focused primarily on children with expressive language difficulties (i.e., Gibbard, Coglan, & McDonald, 2004). Few studies have examined receptive language outcomes following intervention for children with both expressive and receptive language impairment (LI) (Glogowska, Roulstone, Enderby, & Peters, 2000). Available studies suggest only that early intervention may affect auditory comprehension abilities (Flax, Realpe-Bonilla, Roesler, Choudhury, & Benasich, 2009). We do know how important receptive abilities are for long-term language development. Preliminary data do strongly suggest that parent-implemented interventions are effective treatments for children with both expressive and receptive LI (Roberts & Kaiser, 2012).

The paucity of data on the effectiveness of receptive language training and my own clinical experience suggest to me that we use receptive language as a brief waystation on the road to speech production. It is not an end in itself. Even if a child seems to enjoy finding objects named, don't get stuck there. Use that game as reinforcement for sound and word production.

Child's Interest

A child's interests are a powerful indicator of the direction of vocabulary growth. I never would have guessed that "engine" would have been one of the first words I targeted for a young child. This particular little boy with autism spectrum disorder (ASD) was extremely interested in trains, so that is where we began. Because of his good speech skills, we expanded to "caboose" and so on. Eventually, the train goes into the station, so we were able to expand his vocabulary to include all the people waiting for the train and the items associated with them, such as *car, sit, hat, in, coat,* and so on. The people exiting the train eventually went home, offering another opportunity to add new words, such as *drive, house,* and *dog.*

If a child is not interested in the referent—and this sometimes means we need to help a child develop that interest—he or she will most likely not talk about it. This is sometimes difficult with a child with ASD who seems to be absorbed in narrow interests. In this case, early communication intervention (ECI) may also include helping a child explore the world more and, hopefully, develop new and broader interests.

EXPANDING THE RANGE OF INTENTIONS

Single symbols are often taught through imitation, a logical strategy given that most children have the ability to imitate at some level, such as physical imitation, by this time. This method of teaching can be accomplished within a variety of intentions. This would seem to be a good strategy given that first words fill the intentions previously established through gestures.

Often the first speech production taught is in response to "What's this?" I would suggest that it may be more appropriate initially to teach symbols within a child's preexisting intentions where the symbols are most likely to be useful.

If an SLP desires for a symbol to generalize to the everyday use environment of a young child, then the symbol must "work" for the child in accomplishing those intentions the child expresses in a nonsymbolic way. You know from your own attempts to expand your vocabulary that unused or seemingly useless words are forgotten over time. The early intentions of TD children are presented in Table 9.1.

As noted in Chapter 6, although some intentions are easy to teach, such as requesting, they do not seem to be as important as declaratives and comments in furthering our goal of communication development. In fact, one of the primary distinguishing characteristics of children with ASD is the low frequency of declaratives. In contrast, children with intellectual disability produce declaratives at a higher rate. Some psycholinguists have theorized that the attempt to share the contents of one's mind, evident in declaratives, may be one of the primary motivating factors in learning to speak.

TABLE 9.1 **Intentions of Young Children**

Typically developing (TD) children express a range of intentions in their single words. These intentions are typically those expressed in gestures and vocalizations prior to the production of single words.

INTENTIONS	EXAMPLES
Responsive (Following verbal request)	
Answering	*Horsie* (In response to "What's that?"); *juice* (In response to "What do you want?")
Repeating/practicing	*Cookie, cookie, cookie* (In repetition of self); *Mommy* (Following request to "Say Mommy.")
Spontaneous (Not cued by a verbal request)	
Demanding/requesting/commanding	*Cookie, More, Want, Help*
Protesting	*No, Stop, Yucky*
Content question	*What's that?* (*Wassat?*)
Hypothesis testing	*Doggie?*
Declaring/making statements (Describing)	*Eat, Throw, Fast*
Replying	*Eat* (In response to adult saying "Dog hungry." Note that no reply is requested or expected.)
Exclaiming	*Uh-oh, oops*
Accompanying play	*Up* (As car rises in wind-up garage elevator); *go* (As car rolls down ramp)
Expressing attitude or state	*Hungry, tired*
Greeting	*Hi, bye*
Calling	*Mommy!*

TEACHING SEMANTIC CATEGORIES

Until recently, psycholinguists believed that children learned words within semantic categories, such as objects, locations, and recurrence. These categories and their subsumed words were then combined in predictable ways that could account for approximately 70 percent of the two-word utterances of TD toddlers. Most psycholinguists no longer accept that young children combine words exclusively using semantic word order rules. In fact, the categories probably reflect adult thinking rather than that of young children. Nonetheless, the semantic categories offer a conceptual framework within which you may find it easy to teach words and to combine them. If nothing else, these categories offer possibilities for diversifying a child's use of single symbols and early symbol combinations. Semantic categories and early category combinations are presented in Table 9.2.

COMBINING INTO LONGER UTTERANCES

TD children progress naturally from single words to two-word utterances, often to talk about many of the same things they talked about previously in their one-word utterances. According to constructionist theories, children's multiword utterances come in three varieties (Tomasello, 2003):

- Word combinations,
- Pivot schemas, and
- Item-based constructions.

TABLE 9.2 **Semantic Categories of Early Child Speech**

SEMANTIC CATEGORY	EXAMPLES	EXPANSIONS/COMBINATIONS
Negative	*No, allgone*	Negative + X (*No bye-bye*; *Allgone juice*)
Locative	*Here, bed, me*	X + Locative (*Throw me*; *Doggie bed*)
Entity (Name)	*Doggie, horsie*	This/that + Entity (*That horsie*; *This cup*)
Modifier		
Attributive	*Big, little*	Attributive + Entity (*Big doggie*)
Possessor	*Mine, Mommy*	Possessor + Possession (*Mommy car*)
Recurrent	*More, 'nuther*	Recurrent + X (*More up*; *'Nuther cookie*)
State	*Tired, hungry*	Experiencer + State (*Me tired*)
Action		
Action	*Dance, eat, drink*	Agent + Action (*Mommy dance*)
		Action + Object (*Throw ball*)
Agent (Cause action)	*Mommy, boy*	Agent + Action (*Mommy eat*)
Object (Receive action)	*Cookie, ball*	Action + Object (*Eat cookie*)
Dative (Action performed for)	*Mommy*	X + Dative (*Feed baby*; *Cookie Mommy*)

Each offers targets for intervention. As we go through these strategies for combining words, you will notice that some words can be used in more than one type. How a word is learned depends on the individualist style of each young language learner; however, these strategies give us possible ways to expand single-symbol utterances.

Word combinations consist of roughly equivalent words. These words are paired in combination but are not combined with other words. For example, a child may use the single words *Daddy* and *chair*. These can be combined into *Daddy chair* but are not used by the child in combination with other words to form *Daddy car* or *Mommy chair*.

These constructions suggest a place to begin teaching two-word utterances. If you begin combining words in myriad ways, it may confuse a child who is just beginning to use two-symbol constructions.

To increase breadth of use, *Daddy* and *chair* can be taught within the two-word semantic rules X + Location and Possessor + Possessed. In both cases, the utterance *Daddy chair* is the same but signifies very different meaning. This becomes obvious when we add the cue for eliciting each response. We elicit the location with "Where is Daddy?" (or "Where Daddy?") and the possessor with "Whose chair is this?" (or "Whose chair?"). By manipulating your cues as outlined in the following sections, the two-word utterance can fulfill more than one intention while remaining unchanged for now on the surface.

Pivot schemas, the second way of building two-word utterances, show a more systematic pattern than word combinations do. Often one word or phrase, such as *want* or *more*, acts as a carrier phrase for other words. The "carrier phrase" structures the utterance by determining the intent of the utterance as a whole, such as a demand, thus linking the structures to a specific intention. In many of these early utterances, one event word is used with a wide variety of object labels, as in *More cookie, More juice*, and *More apple*. Other words, such as *cookie*, or phrases, such as *go-bye*, fill in the blank or slot, as in *More cookie* or *Want go-bye*.

The use of pivot schemes is a good strategy for producing many two-word utterances from a limited set of constructions and can be a natural progression from word combinations for some utterances. For example, the previously mentioned *Daddy chair*, an X + Location semantic structure, could expand into a pivot scheme, such as *Daddy car, Daddy out, Daddy bed*, and *Daddy home*. The grammar of pivot schemes is flexible, and word order may be reversed.

Children can be taught pivot schemes with different intentions. Possibilities might include:

More _____ (Demand)
Want _____ (Demand)
No _____ (Protest)
Lookit _____ (Directing attention)
Bye _____ (Greeting)
Hi _____ (Greeting)
This _____ (Naming)
That _____ (Naming)

Nor are you limited to these somewhat formulaic constructions. For example, think of all the animals and people who could precede *run*, as in *Mommy run, Doggie run, Horsie run,* and so on. Carrier phrases offer an opportunity to increase the number of two-symbol utterances quickly and easily.

Item-based constructions seem to be following word order rules with specific words. A child's word-specific, word-ordered constructions seem to be dependent upon how a child has heard a particular word being used. Some verbs may be used in only one or predominately one pattern of word order (e.g., *Cut __*), while others are used in more complex forms of several different types (e.g., *Draw doggie, Draw on paper, Mommy draw, Draw for me, Draw here*). Item-based constructions offer the opportunity to combine words, such as Agent + Action (*Mommy eat, Daddy drink, Girl throw*) and Action + Object (*Eat cookie, Drink juice, Throw ball*), which can then be joined to form even longer Agent + Action + Object utterances (*Mommy eat cookie*). Possibilities include:

_____ Eat _____
_____ Drink _____
_____ Throw _____

For example, *drink* might be combined with *Daddy* to form *Daddy drink* and with *juice* to form *Drink juice*, then expanded into *Daddy drink juice*. Similar multiple locations could be found with *throw* and several other verbs. The individual words depend on a child's interests and context.

While these three two-symbol constructions need not be followed strictly in intervention, they do suggest methods for training beyond single-symbol utterances. For example, carrier phrases suggested by pivot schemes and item-based constructions provide a way to increase the number of constructions without greatly increasing the number of vocabulary words. These two goals are often in competition when a child has a limited number of symbols.

 Several videos are available online for parents of early symbolic children. This one offers strategies for encouraging speech and language development.
https://www.youtube.com/watch?v=rvf0KqRx1Jo

General Symbolic Intervention Techniques

The overall design of intervention and many of the techniques described throughout this text will be observed in symbolic intervention. Certainly parents, teachers, and other significant adults are vital to intervention and for generalization of newly learned skills.

Children should be given opportunities within their natural environments to play with and to explore new vocabulary items and structures on a trial-and-error basis. Their meanings will sharpen through the meaningful responses of their communication partners. Through this natural process, errors of overgeneralization will hopefully disappear.

Don't expect perfect performance from a young child, especially when introducing new concepts or new structures. When TD children first use spoken words, they make semantic or meaning-based errors. For example, a child may overgeneralize a word, as in calling all four-legged animals "doggie." These behaviors will appear in children in intervention as well. Among children with somewhat restricted vocabularies, as is the case with many children with LI, these errors may not disappear as quickly as with TD children, possibly because of the children's more limited use and feedback.

Let's explore intervention techniques, including feedback. In general, we can think of categories of verbal strategies as those that

- Model language for a child but do not require a response,
- Model language and require a response,
- Provide feedback but do not require a response, and
- Respond and require feedback.

Effective intervention is the use of these techniques together.

MODEL LANGUAGE BUT DO NOT REQUIRE A CHILD RESPONSE

Children's speech can be modeled in a variety of ways. The most common are

- Self-talk, and
- Parallel talk.

In self-talk, you'll recall, an adult describes his or her actions while engaging in play with the child (e.g., "I'm *putting* the baby in the bathtub. My baby is *splashing*. I'm *washing* the baby. *Washing*."). In contrast, by using parallel talk, the adult provides a model of self-talk for the child's actions, providing a description of what the child is doing. Neither technique requires the child to speak.

It's worth considering at this point the potential problems for some children with the deictic pronouns, *I-you* and *me-you*. Deictic terms such as these can be difficult to interpret because the point of reference changes with each new speaker. A child may know herself as "I" but you're calling her "you." And remember that the auxiliary verb *be* changes with the pronoun change. As adults, we're so familiar with this switch that we do it automatically. Not so for children. Add to this mix, a child with ASD who uses echolalia, and you can begin to see the potential for confusion in some children.

One way around deictic terms is to talk about a third party such as a doll and what she is doing. There's no need to use pronouns at this point. Simply talk about what the doll is doing.

If you feel compelled to use pronouns, one caution is that for some children gender distinctions are equally difficult. Do not expect correct pronoun use with *he-she*. Instead, assume the teddy bear is "he" and the doll is "she" and don't muck it up with female teddies and male dolls for now.

MODEL LANGUAGE AND REQUIRE A CHILD RESPONSE

The most common way to have a child produce a word is by eliciting it with "Say X." While it may induce a child to reply, it is a strategy that does not yield independent or spontaneous production by the child. Other cues such as "What do you want?" are similar.

Verbal scripts derived from favorite picture books, fingerplays, songs, and games can be used for both modeling and cueing production. For example, if a parent has read the child a book repeatedly to the point where the child knows the book by heart, the parent can misread various portions and then await a response or cue one by saying "Did Mary have a little elephant? No! Mary had a little. . . ."

In fingerplays that are part of a child's routine, such as "Where is Thumbkin?," a teacher can purposely hold up an incorrect finger for one part of the rhyme. Cloze techniques in which the child fills in the missing word can also be used in routinized contexts. For example, in *Ring Around the Rosey*, no one falls until the child says "Down." The Internet is bursting with early childhood songs and fingerplays and is an excellent source.

Violations of verbal scripts, whether in books, songs, or play, also can be encouraged as a way to provide a scaffold or framework for moving from a known form to a slightly different or more complex variation. The child is encouraged to "play with" the script of a book, song, fingerplay, or poem once it has been overlearned. For example, in *Ring Around the Rosey*, any action verb can be used in place of "fall," such as "All *jump* up" or "All *drink* juice." The possibilities are endless.

PROVIDE FEEDBACK BUT DO NOT REQUIRE A CHILD RESPONSE

Adults often reply to TD toddlers in ways that model language for the child. The same can be done in ECI but with a conscious attempt to greatly increase the frequency of these responses. These responsive strategies have shown positive results, especially when parents are taught to use them at home. Children with infrequent talking can be helped to increase their rates of communication and their use of specific language targets. Children with higher levels of language show moderate increases in their spontaneous use of targets, in mean length of utterance (MLU), and in standardized test scores. For children with ASD, naturalistic interventions that use direct elicitation of child language report greater short-term gains in the use of expressive language targets, especially prompted requests, than interventions that use more responsive strategies only (Ingersoll, Meyer, Bonter, & Jelinek, 2012).

By requiring no response from a child, these strategies may reduce processing demands on the child. They may also free a child's cognitive resources so the child can compare his production with the feedback. In addition, these strategies may facilitate communication because they occur within an interactive context in which the child attends to the adult's response and is motivated to continue. The shared focus theoretically increases the likelihood of the child's attending to the adult's response.

Responsive strategies are dependent on a child's rate of production. If a child has low rates of communication, there may be few opportunities to respond.

Examples of responsive interaction strategies that model a target communication behavior without requiring a child to respond include the following (ASHA, 2008b):

- Contingent imitation
- Corrective feedback
- Expansion
- Extension
- Buildup and breakdown
- Recast sentence

Many of these techniques were mentioned before with presymbolic behaviors so they will be touched on briefly. These responsive strategies are not mutually exclusive and may be used together as a "package" to enhance the communication of children using symbols (Kaiser, Hancock, & Trent, 2007; Mahoney & Perales, 2005).

With contingent imitation, the adult imitates what the child says. Adults often repeat what TD toddlers say anyway. The technique provides evaluative feedback and confirmation of the child's utterance. In turn, these children tend to imitate the adult imitations, leading to advances in language development (Carpenter, Tomasello, & Striano, 2005).

Corrective feedback is used when the child makes a mistake. In this technique, a correct model is supplied but nothing is required of the child. The adult merely provides the correct word and a possible explanation, such as "Doggie? No, he's too big. That's a cow." The technique can also confirm a child's utterance while providing corrective feedback as when the adult responds to "Tow" (/taʊ/) with "Yes, that's a **C**ow."

Expansions provide a more grammatically correct form of a child's utterance while generally maintaining the child's word order. For example, if a child says "Throw ball," an adult might reply, "Yes, I'm throwing the ball." In general, expansions are credited with grammatical development across a number of structures in children with various communication impairments (Saxton, 2005).

In contrast, extensions are replies in the form of comments that add some additional information to a child's utterance. For example, an adult might reply to the previous example with "Yes, this ball is too big." Such responses are associated with significant increases in children's sentence length.

Typically developing 2-year-olds regularly engage in monologues in which they break down their own utterances into smaller, phrase-sized pieces, and then build them back up into a sentence. These breakdowns and buildups are associated with enhancing language growth in TD children. In a variation on this behavior, an adult can expand a child's utterance and then break it down into several smaller units in a series of sequential utterances that overlap in content. For example, in response to a child's "Doggie bed" an adult might say "The doggie's sleeping in the bed. Doggie sleep. Sleep in bed. Doggie sleep in bed."

Recast sentences expand a child's utterance into a different type of utterance or more elaborate sentence, changing the voice or modality of the child's utterance. In this way, recasts are both expansions and extensions. For example, if a child says "Throw ball," the adult might reply "Where should I throw the ball?" or "Do you want me to throw the ball?" Recasts have been shown to be an effective way to teach grammatical forms to preschoolers with specific language impairment (SLI), but only when they occur in greater frequently than they typically do in conversations with TD children (Proctor-Williams, Fey, & Loeb, 2001).

Meta-analysis supports the use of recasts with children with LI (Cleave, Becker, Curran, Van Horne, & Fey, 2015). Because of the limited number of studies and variation across them, it's difficult to draw conclusions. In general, greater frequency of recasts and more variability in target words seem to have greater effects on morphological learning (Plante et al., 2014).

Both recasts and expansions present feedback that highlights features in the child's utterance that he or she has not mastered. Because the feedback immediately follows the child's utterance, the child may note the difference between the two and subsequently change his or her speech accordingly.

RESPOND AND REQUIRE A CHILD RESPONSE

Responding to a child's verbalization and then requiring a response is very conversational in nature. Look at the following conversation:

Child: Doggie!
Adult: I don't see a doggie. Where's the doggie?
Child: Doggie! [Point]
Adult: Oh, you're right. What's the doggie doing?
Child: Run.
Adult: Yes, he's running. He's chasing a . . .
Child: Ball.
Adult: Yes, he's chasing the red ball.

Several techniques mentioned previously are obvious, such as expansion in "Yes, he's running." In addition, note the use of questions (*What's the doggie doing?*) and fill-ins (*He's chasing a . . .*) that are contingent or based on what the child has said.

Commenting or replying to what a child says and then requiring a reply from the child in turn is called a *turnabout* and is commonly used by parents when talking to TD preschool children. Turnabouts can come in the form of questions, fill-ins, *I wonder* statements (*I wonder why he's running*), corrective feedback requiring a response (*That's not a doggie. That's a horse. Say "horse."*), and requests for clarification when the child is in error (*Is that a doggie?*).

Specific Targets

At the risk of offering a "cookbook" approach in which we devolve into a how-to format, it might be helpful to explore various methods for teaching symbols. I find the production of new symbols in response to the frequently used question "What's that?" to be limited. Why not teach a new symbol and place it in a preexisting intention? Our discussion in this section will focus on teaching words within the semantic and intentional categories presented previously in Tables 9.1 and 9.2.

Possible symbolic intervention targets might include

- Consistently responding to an increasing numbers of words and expanding expressive vocabulary,
- Regularly saying new words and combining words into longer utterances,
- Producing words for a variety of intentions and semantic functions,
- Expressing experiences in words and sentences for communication,
- Taking turns in conversations, and
- Keeping the conversation going.

In the following section, we'll discuss each of these, although within the broader contexts of single words, two-symbol utterances, and longer constructions.

SINGLE WORDS

Even a child who is not talking may be communicating through gestures, sounds, and looks, either naturally or as a result of intervention, and these behaviors form a foundation for language-learning. The SLP and parents should first identify how the child is communicating now and begin word training there. The adult can imitate the child's sounds and/or gestures, adding a word or a sound. If the child gestures, a vocalization or word approximation can be added to enhance communication.

The best time to intervene is when the child attempts to communicate. Through observation, the SLP can help parents identify these moments. When communication attempts occur, the adult can provide a model of the appropriate words to relay the child's message. This can be followed by an attempt to have the child use the word if it is one of the words being targeted.

Occasionally, caregivers attempt to have the child imitate every adult model. This is frustrating for the child and may be counterproductive if the word or concept is too difficult for the child to produce.

When the child uses sounds to communicate, these can be incorporated and modified into words. For example, if the child makes a *buh* sound and enjoys rolling a ball back and forth, the vocalization can be used to signify *ball*, changed to /bɔ/, and finally to "ball."

Modeling and Prompting

As noted throughout this text, daily activities provide the best opportunities for children to learn to communicate through the natural interactions that occur. Assume that a daily routine is bathing. The SLP and adults in the family need to analyze the steps involved to determine which words could be targeted, where they occur in the routine, and how to elicit them. Possible words might include *boat, bubbles, cold, dry, ducky, hot, Mommy, pajamas, shampoo, soap, towel, tub, wash,* and *water,* to name a few. Initially, the parent would talk about the bathing process as it occurs, using the words repeatedly, as in

Mommy make *bubbles*. Put in *bubbles* stuff. Turn water on. Look at all the *bubbles*. Touch *bubbles*. Uh, you have *bubbles* on your nose! Shawna likes *bubbles*.

The adult could also give the child choices, such as "Want *boat* or *ducky*?" When caregivers share experiences in this way, it encourages the child to respond and interact.

Modeling and prompting words does not come naturally to many adults. The SLP will need to help parents identify when and how to speak to their child to maximize input and encourage production. The SLP can model behaviors and have parents practice.

Repeated models of target words are extremely important. In fact, it may take several hundred exposures before a child attempts to produce the word. Think of how often a child hears "Mommy" before producing the word spontaneously. If we go back to our previous example, words such as *water* and *soap* need not be confined to bath time; exposure can be increased by incorporating them into hand-washing, doing laundry, washing dishes and the family car, and bathing the dog. Similarly, *water* is for bathing, cooking, washing, playing in the sprinkler, and drinking.

Throughout this text, we have stressed the importance of joint attending. At the verbal level of intervention, it is doubly important that adults follow the child's focus of attention. Sometimes in their enthusiasm for intervention, adults will jump from activity to activity and miss the child's attentional lead. Most likely, it is the focus of attention that is the focus of the child's attempts to communicate. In addition to labeling what the child is attending to, adults can also describe the objects and actions being performed. Thus, *ball* can be enhanced with "Red ball," "Big ball," "Roll ball," "Push ball," and "Throw ball."

Symbolic production usually begins with imitation. Even here, intervention can be pragmatically relevant if the imitation is placed within a meaningful context in which the imitation "works" for the child and accomplishes some desired end. Here are a few examples:

- When someone leaves or enters the situation, cue the child to imitate "hi" and "bye" while simultaneously waving.
- While playing a repetitive game, singing a repetitive song, or doing a fingerplay, cue the child to fill in the missing word. A jack-in-the-box can be cranked while singing the song, then stopping on the last line and not advancing until the child imitates "Pop."
- During shared book-reading, cue the child to imitate the names of objects, people, animals, and actions in the pictures.
- During snack, cue the child to request more or to ask for a specific food item by imitating your behavior.
- When the child indicates an intention by gestures and/or vocalization, supply the word ("Cookie") or intended request ("Want"), and ask the child to imitate.

Imagine all the intervention situations possible: snack, bath, play, shopping, riding in the car, and so on.

I like to incorporate nonverbal cues as well as verbal ones. For example, I might hold up an object or perform an action and ask the child to "Say ___" as I nod to the child to respond and form the first sound on my lips. Later, the verbal cue can be removed and the nonverbal nod and mouth posture retained as a transition to more independent production of the word. Later, even these prompts will decrease and eye contact can be used, much as we all do, to signal the end of our turn and beginning of the partner's turn to speak.

One method for prompting spontaneous production of a word is to pause and await a response. This is one of the most important strategies for eliciting words without an adult's verbal cueing with a request or question.

Some adults mistakenly assume that the use of questions is the only way to cue the child to respond. Some questions move the conversation and the activity along, such as "What will the doggie do now?" Others, such a repeated use of *yes/no* questions or "What's that?," may have the effect of stopping the interaction or result in a minimal response. Instead, adults can be taught to use comments or questions that show an interest in the focus of the child's attention.

For children experiencing difficulty, pairing an action and a word can facilitate production and can be a bridge to spontaneous production (Arntson, 2009). For example, if a child requests an object by pointing and vocalizing, the adult can retrieve the object but not release it. Next the adult can pull the child's hand to the adult's face, say the name, and then place the child's hand near the child's face. Some children will follow by saying the object name or an approximation.

Some children, especially those with ASD, will echo an adult's productions, including cues such as "What do you want?" To forestall this, it may help to say a word, but before the child can echo, whisper "What do you want?" or "What's that?" In practice, the sequence might be as follows:

Adult: Cookie.
Child: Cookie. [Echoing]
Adult: Cookie. *What do you want?* [Whisper second utterance]
Child: Cookie.

> Adult: Cookie! [Interject] *What do you want?* [Whisper second utterance]
> Child: Cookie.
> Adult: Yes, here's a cookie.

This sequence will, in some cases, lead to a method for eliciting other responses with the same cue. Notice that the last thing said before the child echoes is the cue to elicit that response. This sets up a sequence for the child's response.

Feedback

Even incorrect or inaccurate child verbalizations can provide an opportunity for language learning. For example, when a child uses the wrong word, the adult can respond by providing the correct label. I try to do this in a teasing manner such as "A doggie? Are you being silly? That's a cow!" and to provide additional information as in "Cows live on a farm. Doggies live in the house." Responses of this type give corrective feedback and also reinforce the child with adult attention.

In a similar fashion, mispronounced words can be modeled correctly through feedback. For example, when the child says "baw" (/bɔ/), the adult can respond very positively with "Yes, I see the ba**ll**," emphasizing the corrected portion.

Generalization

To maximize generalization to everyday situations, the SLP can think of all the possible uses for the word being targeted. For example, the word *dog* can be used as a request, question, answer, comment, or call. Multiple uses or intentions increase the likelihood of words' being used by the child. We do a great disservice to children if a word is trained simply as a response to "What's this?" or "What do you want?" Creative intervention occurs by providing a variety of opportunities and reasons for a child to communicate.

Creating opportunities requires first that the child be familiar with a routine. Once a routine is established, an adult can interrupt it in some way and prompt communication. Recall our earlier discussion, in Chapter 7, on *behavior chain interruption*. Adults may also prompt communication by "forgetting" a necessary item or object, such as bubbles for bathing, or skipping a necessary step, such as undressing before getting into the tub.

Although we can't force a child to talk, we can create opportunities through daily routines to encourage a child to use words. For example, the adult can leave a desired object out of reach and wait for the child to indicate a need for the absent item. Too often with children with developmental disabilities, adults anticipate the child's needs and desires. Such behavior by well-meaning adults negates the need for the child to communicate.

I recall one TD 5-year-old who accusingly stated, "It's not fair; you're making my little sister work!" I will plead "guilty" to that charge. Her "work" was requesting what had previously been supplied in seeming anticipation of her every want. We need to help parents and caregivers learn to wait for the child to indicate a desire and then provide the word that complements or completes that need.

Semantic and Pragmatic Categories

Single words and simple word combinations, as noted previously, can be taught within semantic and intentional categories. A word in a particular context has a specific meaning and a semantic category as well as an intention. For practical purposes, this means an individual word has great potential. When intervention is conceptualized in this way, a child is given multiple ways in which to use a word, making the word immediately useful and fostering generalization to several linguistic contexts. Examples of possible target categories are presented in Figure 9.4.

Let's take the word *no*. It can mean rejection or protest (*I don't want spinach!*), disappearance (*It's not here!*), denial (*That's not a cookie!*), or disagreement (*I dislike that proposition!*). The word *no* fulfills the semantic category of *Negative* but may be trained within the intentions of *Answering, Replying, Protesting,* and *Declaring.* Similarly, action words may be taught for answering, replying, declaring, demanding, and hypothesis-testing.

FIGURE 9.4 Possible Symbolic Categories

Semantic Categories	Practice	Answer	Request	Protest	Question	Declaration	Reply	Call	Hypothesize.	Greet
Negative Negative + X										
Locative X + Locative										
Entity (Name) This/that + Entity										
Attributive Attributive + Entity										
Possession Possessor + Possession										
Recurrent Recurrent + X										
State Experiencer + State										
Action Agent + Action Action + Object										
Agent Agent + Action										
Object Action + Object										
Dative X + Dative										

Intentional or Illocutionary Categories

A single symbol or combination can theoretically occur in each block, although some are not as practical or easy to teach with specific words.

Declaratives. As we discussed previously, requesting and protesting are relatively easy to teach relative to declaratives. In part, this is because declaratives are intrinsically self-initiated. Although declaratives can be prompted by novel and surprising objects and events, this is difficult to sustain over time simply because continually producing novelty is taxing for adults. Nor can we sufficiently reinforce the production of declaratives or comments with a child who uses them infrequently or not at all.

It may be easiest to teach declaratives in the form of answers following questions. Although the use of questions by an adult does not result in spontaneous declaratives by the child, questions may be used to advance a conversation by eliciting statements in the form of answers. Adult comments, on the other hand, result in fewer and less complex child replies. Question cues can be phased out later and replaced by nonverbal cues, such as a quizzical look.

If a child already points to request, this behavior can be modified into a declarative in the form of a point or verbal comment. In this way, teaching declaratives builds on what a child can already do and changes its function or intent. The reinforcement would be social in nature in the form of an adult comment. Among children with Down syndrome, nonverbal requesting and the rate of parental responding are important factors in learning declarations (Yoder & Warren, 2004).

Building blocks. Even at the one-word level of communication, the SLP and family need to be thinking about expanding into two-word utterances. This means that the child needs to have words in a variety of grammatical categories that fulfill several functions. Training just nouns in response to "What's that?" is limiting expansion of the child's language.

Although psycholinguists no longer recognize the validity of semantic categories and rules as the organizing principle of early language, these concepts still can provide a framework for intervention, so let's take a look and examine a few ways to train semantic and intentional categories of words. Remember that a single word can fulfill several categories of words depending on its meaning and its use.

In the following discussion, I am assuming that the child can imitate single words, even if the production is only an approximation. At this point, using words, however unintelligibly, is preferable to focusing solely on correct pronunciation. While I'll be primarily discussing eliciting a verbal response, don't lose sight of the importance of adult feedback.

The adult can use expansion to respond, thus building a two-word utterance with the same meaning and intent as the child's utterance. For example, if the child requests "Cookie," the adult can respond "Yes, want cookie. Here's a cookie." In this way, the adult provides a more mature model while not requiring the child to do anything. Occasionally, a child will imitate the adult model, moving us that much closer to producing longer utterances.

Negation. Words that fulfill a negative semantic function are difficult to train without a preceding utterance to elicit a child response. The exception is the use of an empty container that is expected to be full or has recently been emptied in the child's presence. That situation may elicit "No" or "All-gone" spontaneously, although a verbal prompt will most likely be required initially.

Concepts of *yes* and *no* are somewhat difficult for young children, so I would not begin with that contrast. Instead, a word such as *no* can be trained by itself in the absence of *yes*. This can be accomplished using a contrast such as "Juice" vs. "No (juice)."

Believe me, I have tried a variety of cues, and the *X vs. No (X)* model is the easiest to teach and for children to learn. My favorite failure when shopping for an alternative was to ask children to perform an impossible task, such as touching the ceiling, in the hope of eliciting a negative response. I fondly recall one compliant little boy with Down syndrome who repeatedly tried to comply with my request to climb into a sandwich bag. He kept looking at me as if I had a serious mental disorder, but he kept trying and never did tell me "No."

You can place juice or any liquid in a container, and then name the liquid, as in "Water." Upon emptying the container, you can ask "Water?" and reply "No" while shaking your head side to side. The child can be encouraged to imitate the behavior and the word "No." If a child can imitate single words, this should be an easy task. The task has the added enjoyment that children seem to find in filling and emptying things.

It's best if "No" is trained with a variety of containers (cups, glasses, boxes, can) and a variety of fillers (liquids, blocks, balls) to forestall the child's associating the negative word with a specific container and filler. If "No" only means "No juice," it will have little generalization.

In subsequent training, the negative word can be trained within other intentions. Appendix H presents some examples and suggestions on the sequence for expanding negation.

Negative responses are fun to train because they give adults permission to be silly or to play dumb by misnaming objects or actions. In addition, they give a child a measure of control over their environment.

Location. An object name or a preposition or adverb can also serve as a location. Examples include *bed, bowl, box, chair, cup, dish, down, here, in, me, on, outside, sofa, stove, table,* and *up*. These words can fulfill several intentions of early child speech. Appendix H presents a possible order for expanding location into different intentions. Location words offer a challenge to teach within different locations but can also offer the possibility of fun, especially if objects are hidden and found.

One caution: Be careful with the words *here* and *there*. Although these words are often present in the first words of children, it is rare that they designate a location. Instead, *here* often accompanies a giving gesture, and *there* signals that the child is finished. In addition, these word's deictic nature, based on the location of the speaker, makes them extremely difficult to teach.

If, as an SLP, you attempt to teach *here* and *there* as deictic terms—which I would not do at the single-word level of intervention—there is a better chance of success when another person models the correct response for the child. With deictic terms, it is difficult for the same person to be both questioning and modeling the answer.

Entity. Entity is a semantic category in which a name or the process of nomination labels things in the environment. At an imitative level, names of objects can be introduced into several games and activities, such as naming objects before rolling, pushing, or throwing them to a partner or naming objects pulled from a container. Verbal imitation can be worked into other tasks and mixed with physical imitation.

While nomination per se is of limited communication value, it is where many children begin word-learning, suggesting that the semantic category may be easy for young children and a place to begin word-learning. Nomination, or naming an entity, can be trained within several naming games, such as pulling objects from a box and naming each in turn or playing Roger Brown's "Original Name Game." Parents and TD children will ask "What's that?" and the other responds. The danger is that this type of training can be overused, and occasionally SLPs and caregivers forget to move on to the other uses of naming with a variety of intentions. Appendix H presents a possible order for teaching nomination within different intentions.

A few comments are in order. Ultimately, we want a child to initiate communication on her own. This again can be accomplished with nonverbal cues. For example, if you have an established requesting routine in which the child selects a snack or treat, you can perform all the behaviors except the verbal cues ("What do you want?"). For many children, the strength of the routine will be enough to elicit a verbal request. If the child does not request spontaneously, the adult can name the items under consideration and await the child's request with a quizzical look or nod.

Some adults may feel that pointing, making eye contact, and using a quizzical expression to elicit naming is awkward, and yet we do it all the time, usually as an accompaniment to speech. Turns between speakers are often signaled by the speaker's making eye contact with the listener to signal *I'm finished; your turn.*

Spontaneous requesting can also be elicited by the adult's acting silly. For example, within a dressing routine in which the child selects the next item, the adult can offer both an article of clothing that the child already has on and the real choice. If the child selects underwear after previously being dressed in long pants, the adult can respond in a teasing way as in "You want underwear over your pants?" If the child does, who cares; you got your naming request.

Note over time if, when given a choice, the child always selects the last item named. After all, cookie and cake are both equally appealing. In this case, the last item named can be switched to one that the adult knows the child dislikes. Selection will result in not being reinforced by getting a desired item. This is often enough to encourage the child to consider the options seriously. If all else fails, the adult can ask "What do you want?" and limit the choice to only one item.

One aspect of nomination questions ("What's that?" or "Doggie?") that is sometimes overlooked is understanding when to ask a question. The child must first realize that he or she does not know the item's name. I've had some success with this within the "Name Game" format, using items both known and unknown. A child familiar with the routine will respond with item names that he or she knows. Unfamiliar objects often result in the wrong name or no response. The adult can respond by suggesting that someone else may know the name but that the child will have to ask. A second adult then cues the child to ask "What's that?" and supplies the answer. At this point, the child turns and names the item for the first adult. The entire sequence might proceed as follows:

Adult:	What's that?
Child:	Book.
Adult:	Yes, dinosaur book. Let's look for dinosaurs. Okay, your turn.
Child:	What's that?
Adult:	Spoon. Like the spoon for oatmeal. [Adult pretends to eat] What's that? [Hammer]
Child:	No response or "Spoon."
Adult:	[To no child response] That's a new one. Who could help? [Looks toward other adult]
	[To child's "Spoon" response] Spoon? [Teasing manner] You couldn't eat soup with that. It's not a spoon. Who knows? Who could help? [Looks toward other adult]
Child:	[Turning to other adult] What's that?
2nd Adult:	Hammer.
Child:	[To 1st adult] Hammer.
Adult:	Yes, hammer. We use hammer to hit pegs like this. You do it. Hammer. What's this?
Child:	Hammer.
Adult:	Yes, hammer. Damion hits pegs with his hammer.

Although it is not essential to the questioning process, it's an added nicety if the process eventually leads to the learning of a novel word. Wait a few turns, and ask about hammer again. Don't do this too often if the child is becoming frustrated. Notice that the definition of hammer was not an adult one but rather one that related to something the child can do with hammer. An adult definition—*Yes, hammers are used by carpenters to drive nails when building houses*—will not do.

Attribution. Attribution, or the naming of characteristics, is present in the early words of TD children but not in great abundance. Young children are not able to describe many attributes. Colors, for example, do not seem to be particularly salient to young children. In contrast, size in the form of *big* and *little* is salient, as is the temperature word *hot* and seemingly its opposite *cold*, although this is rare in first words. There are few subtleties here, so we can forget *short* and *warm* for now. Other possible words might be *yucky* and *broke(n)*.

As with the other semantic categories, attribution can be expressed through a variety of intentions. The one-word utterances of children can easily be expanded into two-word adult responses while keeping the child's meaning and intent. For example, when the child says "Big" upon encountering a horse for the first time, the adult can reply, "Yes, big horsie." It's important that training occur with a number of items, such as *big doggie, big plane, big truck*. Otherwise, the child will learn that the characteristics apply to only one type of object. Yes, a ball can be either big or little, but so can a multitude of other objects. Although the child is not required to respond to the adult expansion, it nonetheless provides a model when the child is focused on it.

Assuming that a child can imitate words, attribution can be expanded into other intentions. Appendix H presents suggestions for expanding attribution.

Possession. TD children include possession in their first words, identifying objects by their owner. Interestingly, they do not usually associate possession with body parts, making the assumption that if it's attached to you it must belong to you and that it would be redundant to name you as the owner. Children are sense-makers and naming the "owner" of an arm doesn't make sense to children, even if we befuddled adults often forget that point. That said, there are plenty of objects—clothes, sports gear, vehicles, toys, household items—that are associated primarily with one person, and thus there are multiple opportunities to teach and use possession words.

It's important to understand that a young child is not naming a person but identifying a person with an object. Pointing to an empty car while saying "Mommy" is obviously not an attempt to name Mommy. This is a response that would logically follow the question "Whose X is that?" or the statement "I wonder whose X this is."

Avoid teaching words such as *mine* and *yours* because the deictic nature of these terms can confuse young children. As you may recall from your language development course, deictic words change referents with the speaker. When you say "Your book," it's *my* book to me. This has the potential to be confusing, especially if the child uses echolalia.

Along a similar vein, don't expect children to add the possessive -'s ending to the owner's name. The morphological marker is added much later to TD children's language.

Assuming that a child can imitate words, possession can be expanded into several intentions. Appendix H presents suggestions for expanding the uses of possession. Possession words can be worked into several activities, especially cleanup, grab bag, or sorting tasks such as putting away laundry.

It may be easier for a child to name the object rather than the owner, if this has been the routine in the past. It might be helpful to use objects for which the child does not have a name. The adult may have to give an imitative cue until the child understands and responds to the adult request. The cue can come before—"Mommy. Whose sock is this?"— or after "Whose sock do you want? Mommy." It's important that the child connect the adult cue or question with the expected child response.

After a child's verbalization, the adult can expand into a two-word utterance, as in "Yes, Mommy's hat" without requiring the child to respond. The adult can also extend or reply to the utterance with a related remark, such as "Yes, Daddy needs his gloves today. It's cold."

Recurrent. Recurrent words are usually limited to *more* and *'nuther*, although their use spans a number of words and situations. In addition, the word can be used with both objects and actions to continue receiving either. The words can be cued through behavior chain interruption activities and by not providing enough materials for a task.

Although recurrent words are primarily used in requesting, they are not limited to that intention. Initially, a child may be inclined to name the object or action rather than the recurrent word. If this occurs, the adult can prompt the recurrent word by responding, "Yes, cookie, but all gone. Jenna want ____." It may also be helpful, through imitation, to begin with a single object receiving the object name, such as "grape" and a larger quantity receiving the recurrent word. Thus a single cracker is "cracker" and the box is "more."

Assuming that a child can imitate words, recurrent can be expanded into a number of different intentions. Appendix H offers a possible order to this expansion.

State. State words are somewhat limited initially and are used by young children to describe primarily their own state, as in *tired*, *sleepy*, *hurt*, and *hungry*. We've all heard a young child whine, "I hungry." It is only somewhat later, usually around age 4, that the development of *Theory of Mind* (ToM) enables a child to discuss the emotions, feelings, and thoughts of others. Still, a child can be taught to recognize more physical states in others, although the adult may have to overemphasize the obvious signs and use verbal cues such as "Baby wants to go to sleep."

Books such as Eric Carle's *The Very Hungry Caterpillar* might also be helpful. Several children's books address emotions, as do several varieties of emotion-expressing dolls, and photos of sad and happy faces and emoticons can be found online.

Young TD children recognize facial emotions very early, although they cannot name the emotions expressed. For young ones, the range is somewhat limited and includes happy, sad, angry, and surprised, so don't expect subtle emotions to be named.

There are routines, such as feeding a pet, falling down, or taking a nap, in which these words occur naturally. Unfortunately, some events in which these words occur are traumatic, and it may be difficult to elicit a verbalization when the child is crying. For this reason, it may be easier to teach state words with dolls or puppets. Emotions such as happy and sad can also be used, but as mentioned, you should keep in mind the somewhat limited ability of young children to recognize more subtle feelings.

As adults we may be inclined to use a *why-because* format, as in

Why is she happy? Because . . .

Remember that very young or low-functioning children will not have a concept of cause and effect. Instead, the adult can provide the correct state word or use a question-answer format as follows:

Daddy's sleeping. Is he hungry? No, he's not hungry. Daddy's sleeping. Is he tired? Yes, daddy's tired. Daddy is _____."

A one-word "Why?' prompt may be less difficult for a child to comprehend if taught within a routine. For example, one teddy bear might be designated as "Tired Teddy" or "Hungry Huggie," and in play he protests in kind. Still, I prefer cues such as "What's wrong with Teddy?" to "Why is Teddy . . . ?"

Assuming that a child can imitate words, state can be expanded into a number of intentions. Appendix H presents a possible order for expanding intentions.

Action (agent, object). In and of themselves, action words are not difficult to teach. This is somewhat complicated by the TD child's electing to describe an action by the action itself (*Eat*), the agent or person causing the action (*Mommy*), or the object receiving the action (*Cookie*). These three semantic categories of words—agent, action, object—will later become the building blocks for longer utterances, which will eventually become the basic subject-verb-object sentence. To aid children in sorting these words into semantic categories, adults can ask specific questions using words such as *who, what,* and *what happened*.

A child's day is filled with actions, so there will be ample opportunity to cue utterances that describe these events. Possible action words include:

Brush	Cry	Give	Open	Sit
Buy	Dance	Go	Play	Sleep
Clap	Down	Hit	Pull	Stand
Climb	Drink	Hug	Push	Throw
Close	Drop	Jump	Read	Up
Comb	Eat	Kick	Ride	Walk
Come	Fall	Kiss	Run	Wash

Note that not all the words are, strictly speaking, verbs. What makes them action words is the manner in which they are used. "Up," for example, often means *Pick me up*.

Adults can respond in a number of ways, including "Yes, I see throw," "Um-hm, he's throwing the ball," and "Sure, I'll throw the ball." Actions by the child are more likely to elicit action words than describing the actions of others. So roll up your sleeves and get ready for some "active" learning.

Assuming that a child can imitate words, action words can be expanded into a number of intentions. Appendix H presents a possible order for expanding intentions.

Action words can occur within a routine of requesting. Imagine that the SLP and child are throwing balls and each time prior to throwing, the adult asks "What do you want me to do?" or "What next?" while holding the ball and looking expectantly.

Assume that the SLP reaches into a container, pulls out a ball, but does not cue the child. Within a routine such as this, the child may say "Throw" without the adult's verbal cue. At this point, the adult can change the routine so the child requests "Throw" prior to the ball being removed from the container.

Adults can respond to all three types of one-word action-type utterances naturally by expanding into an *agent + action* or *action + object* utterance. If the child imitates, wonderful, but it's not required at this point.

TWO-WORD CONSTRUCTIONS

Typically developing children begin to combine words when they have approximately 50 words in their expressive vocabulary. While this benchmark may be of some developmental significance for TD children, it is not a rigid criterion to be used in intervention. Instead, a child's verbal behavior may indicate when the child is ready to move to longer utterances. As the adult expands a child's single words into longer utterances, the child may signal readiness by attempting to imitate the longer adult utterance. Children may also begin to put a sound before or after a word, such as "da car," "Mommy guh," or "uh doggie." Other children use gestures to expand speech, as in "Mommy" while pointing to car, or may begin to use common phrases as a single word, such as "Idunno," "gobye," "comere," and "wassat?"

In intervention, I have stressed that we need to have a fallback position when the child is unsuccessful. This comes in the form of prompts, as mentioned in dynamic assessment. It's also important to push a little even when the child may be incapable of complying. For example, if the child says "Doggie" spontaneously, I will reply with "Yes, doggie. Doggie eat. Say 'Doggie eat.'" If I just get "Doggie" or "Eat" in response I do not try to prompt more because we are not at that level of intervention yet. Instead, I acknowledge the response as an attempt and continue. "Yes, doggie eat. He's hungry."

No word should be chosen for production in a two-word utterance until it is used reliably as a spontaneous single-word utterance. Otherwise, the SLP is attempting to teach two tasks—new form and new word—at one time. This makes the task more difficult for the child and highlights the importance of continuing to add new words to a child's expressive vocabulary.

When children begin speaking in longer utterances, they don't suddenly cease using single words and gestures. It's important that these continue to be viable communication options for children.

As mentioned, gestures can possibly expand a child's utterances beyond single words. Some gestures reinforce an utterance while signaling the same information as a word spoken simultaneously. For example, saying "car" while pointing to a car conveys the same information. While an important communication skill, this word-gesture combination, called a *reinforcing gesture*, does not indicate readiness to move to two-word communication in the way pointing to the car and saying "Mommy" does. The second combination, called a *supplemental gesture*, may signify possession, as in *Mommy('s) car*; location, as in *Mommy (in) car*; or action, as in *Mommy (go) car*.

Semantic Constructions

Helping children expand beyond one-word utterances is relatively easy and natural. Some semantic categories are easier than others. With negation, location, entity, attribution, possession, recurrent, and state, the semantic function remains the same but the utterance increases in length. In addition, several of these have a predictable word order in English that also remains stable. For example, in negation, the negative word almost always precedes the second word. This formula aids learning for the child. The longer forms of each semantic type are as follows:

- Negative + X (*No juice, No nite-nite, No up*)
- X + Locative (*Kittie chair, Throw me, Come here*)
- This/that + Entity (*This book, That doggie*)
- Attributive + Entity (*Big horsie, Little baby, Yucky peas*)
- Possessor + Possessed (*Mommy car, Baby bottle, My book*)
- Recurrent + X (*More juice, 'Nuther cookie*)
- Experiencer + State (*I tired, Baby hungry, Doggie sick*)

If a child can produce single words in these semantic categories, often adults can provide a model and prompt a longer utterance using a simple question, a gesture, or a facial expression.

I should add some caution regarding words such as *here, there, this,* and *that*. These terms have deictic characteristics, a language concept learned much later. We should not expect, therefore, that our young charges will comprehend this distinction. Also be careful not to confuse the issue by insisting on interpreting things from your own perspective. If a child says "That pen" for one in your hand, don't reply "Yes, this pen." Instead, go with *that* and wait for a few years until the child learns about deixis.

Two-word action utterances are not as easy for children to learn because the format is not as stable. The action word may be at the end, as in *Agent + Action*, or at the beginning, as in *Action + Object*.

Although common in languages with a subject-object-verb sentence structure, such as Korean, two-word *Agent + Object* utterances, "Mommy cookie" and "Daddy ball," meaning possibly *Mommy eat cookie* and *Daddy throw ball*, occur only occasionally among English-speaking toddlers. When this form does appear, it is often a call for directing attention, as in "Mommy, (look at) doggie." In these cases, the intention and the semantic function are quite different from *Agent + Object*.

Because the action word can occur in either the first or last position, it might help some children if the SLP focuses on one structure exclusively and then gradually introduces the other. Introduction can come in the form of expansion, as follows:

Adult: What's happening?
Child: Mommy
Adult: Yes, Mommy. What's Mommy doing? (What Mommy do?)
Child: Wash.
Adult: Yes, Mommy wash. You tell me.
Child: Mommy wash.
Adult: Yes, Mommy wash. Mommy wash car. Do you want to help?

Notice how the adult pushes to the next level but only with a model.

As in the previous section, it is just as important in two-word utterances that the child use these utterances to express a range of intentions and that these longer utterances be used frequently. If the child doesn't have a use for a longer utterance, he or she will not produce the utterance and may eventually lose it.

As a child uses gestures and possibly pairs these with sounds, the way that adults respond helps the child learn words that he or she will eventually put together into longer utterances. One of the easiest ways to help a child build two-word communication is to expand by imitating the child's utterance with an added word. When this is done in the context of the child's one-word utterance, it is relevant to the situation and captures the child's interest because it builds on his or her utterance rather than introducing another. For example, if the child has finished his juice and says "More," the adult can reply "More juice."

Another good strategy is to offer choices, each containing a longer utterance as a model. For example, the adult could ask "Do you want **little ball** or **big ball**?" Similar contrasts could be modeled altering another word as in *more cookie or more apple, throw ball or kick ball*, and *Mommy's hat or Daddy's hat*.

Assuming that a child can say all the words used in expanding to two-word utterances, a simple point and a quizzical expression can be used to elicit the second word. For example, I worked with a child who imitated the last word I would say. If I said "What are you doing?" he would reply "Doing." I changed my cue to "What do you ride?" He replied "Ride." In response, I immediately pointed to his tricycle and looked questioningly. He'd say "Bike" and I'd respond with "Yes, ride bike, Billy ride bike." Over time, he became less dependent on the adult model and when asked "What are you doing?" could respond "Ride bike."

If the more subtle point and look strategy fails to elicit a second word, a question may elicit it. Examples for expanding single-word utterances into two words are presented in Figure 9.5. Don't make this too drill-like, and be sure to follow the child's utterance with a meaningful response. For example, when the child produces a two-word "No juice," the adult can reply, "No juice. Juice allgone. You drank all the juice? Want more juice?"

As mentioned, several two-word forms have only a few words that can be used to express the semantic function. Following the notion of pivot schemes, or carrier phrases, these words can be used as carrier phrases to quickly expand into a variety of two-word utterances, including the following:

More _____   Want _____   No _____
Lookit _____   Bye _____   Hi _____
This _____   That _____

Although action words do not have a location-specific construction, they also offer an opportunity to expand into several two-word utterances. For example, words such as *eat*

FIGURE 9.5 **Examples of Expanding One-word Utterances to Two Words**

Negation. If the child says only "No," the adult can ask "No what?" or "No, there's no _____," and respond, "No, there's no juice. You tell me."

Location. If the child says only the location, the adult can ask, "Who's in car?" (or "What's on table?") When the child names the person (or object), the adult can respond, "Yes, Mommy in car. You tell me."

Entity. The child is most likely to give the entity name rather than saying this or that. The two-word utterance can be elicited by a choice-making routine in which the adult asks "Do you want this cookie or that cookie?" If the child says "Cookie," the adult can ask, "This or that?" If the child says only the demonstrative *this* or *that*, the adult can ask "This what?" or "This _____," followed by "Yes, this cookie. You tell me."

Attribution. If the child names the item, such as "Hat," the adult can recue with "Which one?" or "Big hat or little hat. Which one?" If the child says only the attribution word, such as "Big," the adult can ask "Big what?" or "Big _____." When the child has produced two one-word utterances in the correct order, the adult can respond, "You tell me."

Possession. If the child names the possessor, the adult can ask "Mommy's what?" or "Mommy's _____." If the child names the possession, as in "Shoe," the adult can ask "Whose shoe?" When the child has produced two one-word utterances in the correct order, the adult can respond, "Yes, Mommy shoe. You tell me."

Recurrent. This semantic function is most easily taught within requesting. Use small quantities of a treat, so that the child continues to request *more* without becoming full too quickly. If the child produces only the recurrent word, the adult can ask "More what?" or "More _____." If the child names the action, the adult can respond, "I pushed you. Now you want _____." Respond to the object name with "Yes, cookie all gone. Now you want _____." When the child has produced two one-word utterances in the correct order, the adult can respond, "You tell me."

State. Most likely the child will give you the state word. If the child does, the adult can ask "Who's tired (or hungry or sad)?" If the child produces the experiencer of the state, the adult can ask "How does baby feel?" or "Baby _____." When the child has produced two one-word utterances in the correct order, the adult can respond, "Yes, baby tired. You tell me."

Action. Action utterances are a little more complicated because the child has a few possibilities. If the child produces only the agent, the adult can respond, "Yes, Mommy. What is Mommy doing?" If the child provides only the action, the adult can ask "Who is eating?" If the child produces only the object, the adult can ask, "What's happening to the cookie?" When the child has produced two one-word utterances in the correct order, the adult can respond, "Yes, eat cookie. You tell me."

and *drink* can be combined with an almost endless list of foods and beverages in *Action + Object* constructions (*eat _____*).

Intentions

Although we have moved into semantic constructions, the focus on grammar should not come at the expense of pragmatics. The intentions taught previously can be continued into longer utterances. Routines, such as requesting at snack time or directing during dressing, can be expanded to require more language from the child.

Early questions, such as *what, where, who, whose,* and *which* can be introduced slowly. Children will understand the concepts behind these words if they have the semantic categories of entity (*what*), location (*where*), agent (*who*), possession (*whose*), and attribute (*which*). Questions can often be taught within a guessing routine in which guesses are asked with rising intonation. The adult can ask the initiating question, such as "Whose hat is in the bag?" and the child responds "Mommy hat?" Later the roles can be switched so the child is asking "Whose hat . . .?"

TABLE 9.3 **Combining Two-Word Utterances into Longer Constructions**

Combine These Categories . . .	To Produce
Agent + Action Action + Object	Agent + Action + Object (*Mommy throw ball, Daddy ride bike, Baby eat cookie*)
Agent + Action X + Location	Agent + Action + Location (*Mommy sit chair, Baby sleep bed, Boy play slide*)
Negation + X Action + Object	Negation + Action + Object (*No throw ball, No drink juice*)
Recurrent + X Action + Object	Recurrent + Action + Object (*More eat cookie, More throw ball, More ride bike*)
Possessor + Possessed Action + Object	Action + Possessor + Object (*Ride boy bike, Eat my sandwich, Drink baby bottle*)
Attribution + Entity Action + Object	Action + Attribution + Object (*Kick big ball, Eat sweet candy, Pet little kitty*)

LONGER CONSTRUCTIONS

Once TD children begin to develop two-word constructions, they quickly move to even longer utterances. In ECI, this can occur by combining two-word constructions into longer ones. Table 9.3 presents some possible combinations. The table contains only a few of the possible constructions. When you add to this mix the new words a child is acquiring, the possibilities are nearly endless.

Language should continue to develop gradually. Once a child is reliably producing three- and four-word utterances, the SLP can begin to target other grammatical structures, such as prepositional phrases (*in, on*), progressive -*ing*, pronouns, past tense -*ed*, and plural -*s*.

▶ Before we wrap up communication intervention and move on to feeding and swallowing in the last chapter, you might want to explore this video, which offers some helpful tips for early years practitioners.
https://www.youtube.com/watch?v=joqVklnnPoY

Involving Parents, Teachers, and Other Adults

Everything we've been saying about working with parents and other caregivers is just as important at the symbolic level of intervention as it was at the presymbolic. Let's discuss some related topics: book-sharing, which often begins as TD children begin to talk, and language modeling by parents and other caregivers.

BOOK-SHARING

Shared or joint book-reading offers a particularly effective teaching context because the book can provide many opportunities for commenting, asking questions, and taking turns. These opportunities may not be found as naturally and readily in conversational contexts (Cole, Maddox, & Lim, 2006). Because a large percentage of children with disabilities do not enjoy storybook interactions, adults may need to encourage book-sharing through more active involvement using movement, chants, songs, and action and finger play (Justice & Kaderavek, 2002).

While reading the book may provide some stimulation, it is not enough by itself to be an effective intervention tool and should be accompanied by specific interactive techniques (Hargrave & Senechal, 2000). Shared book-reading means that the child and adult share the experience and the content. Merely hearing the word *bear* in the text is not enough, at least initially. Adults can help the child make the book her own by discussing what a bear is in very simple child language.

What seems most important for children's language-learning is commenting on and discussing the story and pictures, asking questions, responding to the child by adding a little more information, and giving the child time to respond. While reading the book is important, the book better serves as a vehicle for learning language through interaction with an adult.

Initial books need not have a plot. Books with several pictures, such as types of trucks or farm animals, provide lots of grist for early conversations.

Child: [Points to a cow]
Adult: Oh, that's a cow. We get milk from a cow. Do you remember what cows say?
Child: Moo.
Adult: Yes cow says "Moo." We saw a cow when we . . .
Child: Ride car.
Adult: Yes, ride car. We saw lots of cows when we went for a ride in the car. [Points to horse] Do you know what this is?
Child: Doggie?
Adult: It looks like a doggie, but . . .

You get the idea.

As children mature, their books can mature also, with more characters and simple plots. Books can be shared differently too. Children can participate based on the text. For example, some children's books repeat the same lines over and over, and the adult can pause at this point and have the child say the missing line. In *Good-Night, Owl* (Hutchins, 1990), each page ends with the refrain "and Owl tried to sleep." A parent could read right up to that last phrase and wait for the child to finish. Other books have a series of things that occur in the same order, as in *The Little Old Lady Who Wasn't Afraid of Anything* (Williams, 1986), in which the boots go clomp, clomp, the shirt goes shake, shake, and so on. What fun to read and perform the actions together! If, as we read to a child, we relate the story to her or his everyday life, there are many opportunities for language learning and use.

LANGUAGE MODELING

There has been an ongoing debate as to the type of language to use when addressing young language-learning children. We are on safe ground to assume that when SLPs use simplified language with a child, they do so to eliminate possibly distracting elements (Fey, Long, & Finestack, 2003). The question is the effect of this on the child.

Although the evidence on the most beneficial practice is inconclusive, some ECI professionals advocate using speech input that is simplified, sometimes ungrammatical, called *telegraphic*, while others advocate simplified but grammatical input (van Kleeck et al., 2010). While most ECI professionals have been of the opinion that language input to young language-learning children should be simplified, there is little agreement on the degree of that simplification. Many parents use short fragments of speech with their young TD children. These shortened utterances are pragmatically, prosodically, and grammatically complete but are not fully formed sentences, as in "Mommy drink juice" instead of "I am drinking juice" (Cameron-Faulkner, Lieven, & Tomasello, 2003). Word order and meaning are maintained while morphological endings and less content-heavy or function words (e.g., articles, auxiliary verbs, prepositions) may be omitted.

Telegraphic speech is a term from the 1970s that characterized children's earliest word combinations as sounding like old telegrams, in which some components of grammar were omitted to save costs when one was paying for every word transmitted (Brown, 1973).

Examples from child speech include *Mommy eat, Baby bed,* and *Car go bye.* Although these forms characterize much of TD children's early expressive language, the benefit of adult telegraphic input (TI) for children with LI has long been debated. Even the most ardent supporters of the use of TI recognize that such input must change as a child's language changes if the adult input is to remain slightly more advanced than the child's production.

The crux of the debate is whether these changes are necessary and beneficial. It could be argued that learning grammatical morphemes poses a special problem for children with LI and that omitting these forms further complicates this task. Omission or infrequent use of these forms by adults may give the unintended impression that morphological affixes or short function words are optional and unimportant.

Function words and inflections may alert children to grammatical word classes and to underlying meaning that may be missing in shortened forms (Golinkoff, Hirsh-Pasek, & Schweisguth, 2001; Höhle & Weissenborn, 2003). For example, there are prosodic, morphological, and syntactic features in adult speech that provide important clues for children about linguistic boundaries, grammatical classes of words, and possible word meanings. These may be eliminated in simplified speech.

While simplified speech may possibly facilitate comprehension for some children, it may also deprive a child of exposure to more complex linguistic models that are within his or her range of comprehension. That said, the increased pitch variability, increased loudness, and slower rate found in simplified speech have been shown to facilitate word-learning by children with LI. In the end, it may not be just what is said but how it's said that facilitates comprehension (Pepper & Weitzman, 2004). If you wish to pursue this topic in more detail, please read the excellent review of the research in van Kleeck and colleagues (2010).

A HELPFUL WEBSITE

Wilcox, Bacon, and Greer (2005) offer an excellent online guide for training caregivers in a group format supplemented by home visits. The site includes outlines for each of 15 sessions, handouts, and periodic questionnaires to be used in assessing progress. I would strongly recommend browsing the website of the Infant Child Research Programs at Arizona State University, which can be accessed by typing "icrp asu.edu" into your search engine and then exploring the many fine materials available. Sessions generally follow a pattern in which a few interactional techniques are presented and parents are helped to identify everyday situations in which these might be used. In subsequent sessions, these techniques are reviewed and critiqued, and daily records are reviewed.

Similar to the advice I have given throughout this text, parents are introduced to new techniques a few at a time so as not to overwhelm their already busy schedules of childcare. Emphasis is on teaching communication through natural interactions during daily activities. If there is a more formal teaching component, it should occur in short 10-minute sessions each day within activities that encourage the target words.

In the initial session, parents are provided with a general overview of the training. As a group, parents watch videos describing the important role they play in helping their child learn language. This is accompanied by a brief overview of communication and language development, including the difficulty some children encounter. Caregivers are encouraged to review this development and to reflect on what their child is already doing. Words to be taught to each child are determined by the child's parents, and then interactional plans are determined. The importance of recordkeeping in the form of "target word logs" is also discussed. As part of an interaction plan, parents identify daily routines, such as bathing, and are helped to note the steps in the routine, the props needed, the opportunities for target words, and the partner response options.

Two Examples of Early Verbal Communication Intervention

As we conclude this chapter, it might be instructive to discuss two well-respected ECI approaches that take somewhat different paths in attempting to achieve the same goal. Although these two methodologies—the Hanen Early Language Program and Responsive

Education/Prelinguistic Milieu Teaching—are different, you will note several similarities as well. Also note as you read that they incorporate several of the techniques and strategies discussed in this chapter.

With both programs, although the gains are sometimes modest when compared to SLP-only services, there are benefits to training parents to implement naturalistic language intervention strategies at home with their preschool children (Kaiser & Roberts, 2013). These gains seem to persist over time, suggesting greater generalization when parents are trained.

HANEN EARLY LANGUAGE PROGRAM

The Hanen Language Program, outlined in *It Takes Two to Talk* (Manolson, 1992), is a parent-focused language intervention program for young children. *It Takes Two to Talk* reflects a family-centered model of intervention, focusing on the child within that context. A naturalistic approach, the Hanen Program identifies and uses learning opportunities throughout the child's day.

The major goal is to increase a child's social communicative skills by enhancing the quality of adult-child interactions. In addition to learning these general language facilitation strategies, parents are also taught specific interactional behaviors for the more direct communication goals of the child, such as prelinguistic skills. Hanen-certified SLPs train parents through group sessions and individual video feedback sessions.

More specifically, the Hanen Program has three objectives (Girolametto & Weitzman, 2006):

- Parent education in which basic concepts of communication and language are taught to help parents understand their child's needs and the importance of nonsymbolic communication,
- Early language intervention using strategies that facilitate communication development, and
- Social support of the family through group and individual learning and feedback.

In general, parents are taught to use (Girolametto & Weitzman, 2006; Pepper & Weitzman, 2004)

- Parental child-centered strategies, such as waiting and following the child's lead, that encourage child initiations;
- Strategies designed to promote interaction by facilitating and balancing turns and keeping the conversation going, such as asking questions and cueing the child to take a turn; and
- Language-modeling strategies, such as commenting and expanding a child's utterance

Following a child's lead, adults can join the child in play, use contingent imitation to facilitate interaction, interpret a child's messages, and comment on the focus of the child's interest.

Interaction-promoting strategies encourage turn-taking. These include adults' matching a child's turn with one of their own, asking questions, waiting expectantly for the child to take a turn, and using everyday play and routines to make participation easier for the child.

Language is modeled at the child's level by labeling the child's focus or commenting on an event or action. If the child vocalizes or verbalizes, the adult can expand these utterances into words or multiword utterances.

The Hanen Program provides parents with approximately 16 hours of group training, as well as three individual video feedback sessions on how to facilitate their child's language development in naturalistic contexts and maximize the child's daily opportunities for communication development. Parents learn to apply responsive interaction strategies consistently to their everyday interactions with their child. Program content is taught in a highly interactive, experiential manner, with strategies being given concrete, user-friendly names to make them easier to remember and apply.

RESPONSIVE EDUCATION AND PRELINGUISTIC MILIEU TEACHING

The Prelinguistic Milieu Teaching (PMT) technique was developed by Paul Yoder and Steven Warren (1998) at the Vanderbilt University. This technique uses settings, such as the home, and situations in which the children are naturally disposed to employ proto-declaratives (Yoder & Warren, 2002).

Most appropriate for children functioning between 9 and 15 months, responsive education/prelinguistic milieu teaching (RE/PMT) is a hybrid approach that combines parent responsive education with PMT's direct teaching of gestures, vocalizations, and coordinated eye gaze within the ongoing social interactions in the child's natural environment (Warren et al., 2006; Yoder & Warren, 2000, 2002). Based on the assumption that parents may not be appropriately responsive to their children's early communication attempts, RE targets parents' compliance with and recoding of children's verbal and nonverbal acts. Caregiver responsive education, similar to that in the Hanen Program, supports parents in playing with and talking to their children in ways designed to facilitate children's communication and language development. The optimal conversational style is one that fosters reciprocal interactions.

PMT is a child-led, play-based incidental teaching method designed to enhance intentional nonverbal communication. Transactional in nature, the program targets gestures, nonword vocalizations, gaze use, and word use as forms of intentional communication for turn-taking, requesting, and commenting. The development of prelinguistic skills is an important building block in a child's progression to expressive and receptive communication skills. PMT does not focus on making the child talk, but rather builds the child's motivation and awareness of a communication partner (Yoder & Warren, 2001a,b).

The overall intervention model assumes that early communication development is fostered by reciprocal interactions between the child and those in the child's environment. Because PMT is most effective with children whose parents are more responsive to their children's communication before intervention begins (Yoder & Warren, 1998, 2001b), PMT is used in combination with responsive education for parents.

Milieu language-teaching strategies, such as prompting and time delay, are particularly effective for children in the early stages of communication development, such as those with an MLU below 2.0. In contrast, responsive interaction techniques are better suited for facilitating acquisition of higher level morphological and syntactic skills and MLUs above 2.5 (Yoder, Spruytenburg, Edwards, & Davies, 1995 et al., 1995).

There are two reasons why RE/PMT may facilitate language acquisition (Yoder & Stone, 2006a,b):

- Linguistic mapping, putting into words the child's immediately preceding nonverbal message, is in response to a child's communication.
- Milieu Language Teaching facilitates spoken communication through the use of prompts for verbal imitation and questions to evoke spoken communication (Fey et al., 2006).

PMT provides specific opportunities for children to initiate communication, while responsive education maximizes the effects of PMT on a child's interaction skills and habits.

Several studies have documented the effects of PMT on both prelinguistic and linguistic abilities of young children with developmental disabilities (Yoder & Warren, 1998, 1999a,b, 2001a,b, 2002). Even when used minimally with children with developmental delay and few expressive words or signs, RE/PMT can increase a child's rate of intentional communication and generalize frequently spoken communication in children with few vocal communication acts (Fey et al., 2006; Yoder & Warren, 2002). Gains in spoken communication have been maintained 12 months after the end of treatment.

The principal components of RE/PMT are

- Arranging the environment to increase communication opportunities and naturally support the need to communicate,
- Following the child's attentional lead, and
- Building social routines in which both the child and caregiver play predictable roles (Warren et al., 2006).

Taken together, these approaches help create frequent teaching interactions and encourage child engagement. Through environmental arrangement, the adult provides more opportunities for the child to communicate, which in turn results in more adult opportunities to clarify and enhance the child's message. Environmental arrangement, such as temptations or structured communication-eliciting situations, is used to encourage communication. For example, desirable food or toys kept just out of reach provide an opportunity for the child to request, or if a child is struggling to operate a toy, the adults may ask, "Do you need help?"

PMT focuses on two general types of early communication: requests and comments. When prompting requests, an SLP must recognize that some children are disinclined to persist if their efforts to obtain desired objects and services are challenged. For these children, gaze shift alone is initially accepted as an approximation of a request. As children became more proficient, response requirements are increased gradually until children are required to combine gestures or vocalization with gaze shifts between the child's object of attention and the adult.

Comments are social acts in which the child seeks to share observations and experiences with a communication partner. When a child produces a nonverbal vocalization that clearly makes reference to a specific object or event, adults respond by complying with the act and/or by providing the correct verbal label. In other words, if a child says "bebe" in the presence of a doll, the adult might hand the child the doll, say "baby," or do both. Some practitioners may imitate the child's vocalization instead of supplying the verbal label. Both methods have been tried and may be appropriate at different stages of intervention. Parents who receive training comply with and linguistically map/recast more of their children's communication acts than do parents who are not trained.

PMT techniques include prompting, modeling, and providing natural consequences embedded in ongoing child-caregiver interactions. Prompts are used to evoke intentional communication and to encourage more frequent and/or complex communication. Models can support and enhance a child's intentional communication attempts by providing a slightly more complex form of a child's communicative behavior. Finally, responses to nonverbal communication attempts are in accordance with the child's intent. Thus, a clear request is followed by the adult's responding with a requested action or object and verbalizing the meaning of the child's message.

Conclusion

Many of the techniques used in speech mirror those found in AAC. The important factor is teaching a variety of words that can be used across contexts and be elicited naturally within the child's everyday environment. It is important to teach several uses for words and structures taught so that a child will not forget these words and structures because of very limited use. Our goal is to train items that will have utility for the child in natural contexts. This often means constructing interactions so these words and linguistic structures occur. In this endeavor, parents and other caregivers are especially important to success.

 Click here to gauge your understanding of the concepts in this chapter.

10

Feeding and Swallowing

Jessica Kisenwether, Ph.D.
Misericordia University

When you have completed this chapter, you should be able to:

- Describe the role of the speech-language pathologist (SLP) in pediatric dysphagia.
- Name special considerations in pediatric swallowing.
- Describe feeding skills development and explain common etiologies of feeding disorders.
- List and describe the feeding team members
- Describe the assessment and explain basic treatments of feeding disorders.

Terms with which you should be familiar:

Bolus	Micrognathia
Choanal atresia	Nasogastric Tube
Corrected Age	NPO status
Delayed gastric emptying	Patent ductus arteriosis
Diaphragmatic hernia	Pierre Robin sequence
Dysphagia	PO feeding
Enlarged tonsils/adenoids	Septal defect
Esophageal dysmotility	Stenosis
Failure to thrive (FTT)	Stridor
Fiberoptic endoscopic evaluation of swallowing (FEES)	Suck intake pattern
	Suckle intake pattern
Fundoplication	Tracheoesophageal fistula (TEF)
Gastroesophageal reflux disease (GERD)	Tracheomalacia
Gastrostomy	tracheostomy
Glossoptosis	Transposition
Hyolaryngeal excursion	Vallecula
Hypoplasia	Velocardiofacial syndrome
Laryngomalacia	Videofluoroscopic swallow study (VFSS)
Macroglossia	

Throughout the text, we've been discussing communication impairment. The same interruptions in gross and fine motor development that can lead to speech and language delays may also create problems with eating and drinking. A swallowing difficulty or inability to swallow is called dysphagia. Children who have no difficulty swallowing but struggle with the preparation of food for the swallow (chewing, sipping, biting, etc.) have what is called a *feeding disorder*. It is possible to have components of both and this chapter will provide a review of the complications and implications of these disorders.

Overall, children need adequate nutrition and hydration to continue to grow and develop appropriately, achieving the expected milestones you have read about thus far. Unfortunately, a child with dysphagia or feeding impairment will have difficulty maintaining the daily caloric intake expected to attain those goals. Inadequate nutrition can lead to fatigue and have a negative impact on the child's health status, including motor, sensory, and overall development. As a result, feeding and swallowing issues are of serious concern and get much attention in the pediatric population.

For medical professionals like yourselves, the health and development of a child is of the utmost concern and will be outlined in detail throughout the chapter, but it's also important to address the social ramifications of a feeding or swallowing disorder in addition to the health and wellness component. Eating is a social experience, and often a forum for communication with loved ones. Sharing food with others brings comfort and companionship. In fact, for infants, eating is one of the first bonding experiences with the caregiver. As I'm sure you can relate, many of us sit down with family or friends to enjoy a meal and interact with one another; however, the family of a child with a feeding/swallowing disorder may have altered feeding schedules or food choices, limited opportunities for interaction, or stress surrounding the mealtime for reasons outside of their control. As a result, a family approach to therapy is used to assure that not only are feeding and swallowing skills being addressed at home to improve caloric intake, but also that the necessary social and communication elements essential for the child's overall development and well-being are receiving attention.

Background

Pediatric feeding and swallowing disorders are a growing area in the field of speech-language pathology. It is estimated that between 25 and 45 percent of all children, at some time during childhood, are diagnosed with a feeding or swallowing problem (ASHA, 2013a). With improved medical technology and continued early detection, the number of children identified with severe and chronic medical concerns has continued to increase (O'Donoghue & Dean-Claytor, 2008). As a result of intervention, survival rates for these children are much improved (Hamilton et al., 2007). With improved survival, an increase in feeding difficulties and an increased awareness of the need for early intervention to provide children with the best opportunity for success has followed.

Feeding and swallowing intervention may begin shortly after birth in the neonatal intensive care unit (NICU) or in the home through early intervention (EI). Some children are not identified with a feeding or swallowing impairment until they reach the school setting. Regardless of the time frame for initiation of therapeutic intervention, a team of individuals assesses, diagnoses, and provides services for a child having difficulty, not solely the speech-language pathologist (SLP). This team is also responsible for teaching appropriate strategies to the caregivers and professionals the child may come in contact within the school setting.

Although the number of cases is growing and SLPs are the professionals who receive the most training in dysphagia on the team throughout their coursework, they report low self-confidence in treating feeding and swallowing difficulties, especially in the schools (O'Donoghue & Dean-Claytor, 2008). Despite these findings, SLPs are expected to identify and treat this ever-growing population. This adds to the already extensive list of treatment areas in the EI setting, but the Individuals with Disabilities Education Act (IDEA, PL 99-457, 1990) secures the treatment of children with complex medical issues in the educational setting. Consequently, coursework is being incorporated into more and more graduate programs in speech-language pathology to provide students with some background information and practicum opportunities before entering the work environment.

Role of the SLP

The American Speech-Language-Hearing Association (ASHA) states that it is the role of the SLP to diagnose and treat infants and children with dysphagia and feeding disorders (ASHA, 2014). This does not come as a surprise, given the training speech-language pathologists receive in the area of adult dysphagia. The responsibilities are very similar and include the following:

- Conduct an exhaustive chart review related to swallowing function.
- Assess (by determining appropriateness of clinical and/or instrumental evaluation) swallowing and feeding disorders.
- Diagnose abnormal anatomy and physiology of swallowing.
- Detect additional disorders of the upper aerodigestive tract and provide appropriate referrals.
- Provide recommendations to manage identified feeding and swallowing disorders.
- Develop a culturally sensitive treatment plan to manage swallowing and feeding disorders.
- Document progress and determine criteria for discharge.
- Educate families/caregivers and other professionals about swallowing and feeding disorders.
- Provide counseling to families/caregivers regarding dysphagia-related complications.
- Monitor quality of services and identify risk.
- Participate as an interdisciplinary team member through collaboration and consultation, providing referrals when necessary.
- Advocate for individuals experiencing swallowing and feeding disorders.
- Advance knowledge regarding swallowing and feeding disorders through research, and review the current research base. (ASHA, 2014)

Although graduate programs often address children and adults with dysphagia, more extensive education is still needed in the assessment and treatment of dysphagia and feeding disorders in the area of pediatrics.

Special Considerations in Pediatric Swallowing

In addition to the knowledge and skill areas for treating dysphagia listed in the previous section, ASHA (2002) mandates that SLPs working with children must also demonstrate knowledge of

- Embryology,
- The effect of postural changes,
- Etiologies,
- Signs and symptoms of suck/swallow incoordination as well as aspiration,
- Nutritional knowledge and understanding of the consequences in the first few years of life,
- Infant and early childhood development, and
- Appropriate assessment and treatment strategies per developmental age. (ASHA, 2002)

This knowledge may seem specific to newborns, but a thorough understanding of the differences in anatomy and physiology between adults and children, as well as typical feeding development, is crucial when treating children who present with feeding and swallowing problems.

Classroom and clinical background in the area of adult dysphagia is helpful, but children differ from adults in their anatomy and physiology, causes of feeding and swallowing difficulty, communication skills, types of swallowing impairment, and the fact that they are still developing. Children may also have a congenital disorder contributing to their difficulty. For all of these reasons, research and background from the adult population cannot be applied accurately to the pediatric population, and additional treatment strategies and considerations for continued developmental needs beyond that of adults must be implemented. Let's explore some of these differences between children and adults.

DIFFERENCES IN ANATOMY AND PHYSIOLOGY

Children are smaller. This you already know, so it's a good place to begin. Their anatomical structures are underdeveloped and often difficult to see during instrumental evaluation; therefore, it's important to know what structural differences to expect when evaluating a child's swallow.

Young children have a high laryngeal resting position, so little to no superior and anterior movement of the larynx, called hyolaryngeal excursion, will be observed during the swallow. This is presented as A in Figure 10.1. As you can also see in this figure, the child's airway seems more susceptible to penetration and/or aspiration as compared to an adult's. As a result, although there is minimal epiglottic movement to cover the opening to the airway for the child, the pharyngeal wall compensates by moving anteriorly. This action aids to close off the entrance to the airway.

You may have also noticed the absence of an oropharynx and a more gradual turn into the pharynx from the oral cavity as compared to the anatomy of an adult. Overall, because the structures are smaller and there is less distance for the bolus, or soft mass of food or liquid that has been prepared to swallow, to travel, the swallow will be much faster.

Although the anatomical differences between young children and adults are more obvious, there are also significant differences between infants and older children. Some of these differences are outlined in Table 10.1. The stages of swallowing remain the same, but our expectations as clinicians change from infant to school age.

In regard to the physiology of the structures we've reviewed, there are continued differences between infants and school-age children. For instance, drinking patterns are significantly different. An infant will demonstrate a suck/swallow/breathe pattern with specific coordination while drinking. A burst of sucking occurs first (approximately 3–6 sucks) while liquid collects in the valleculae, or spaces between the base of the tongue and the epiglottis. This is illustrated in Figure 10.2. Once the liquid reaches an adequate amount, the infant will trigger a pharyngeal swallow and then briefly pause to breathe. This pattern repeats, varying with the infant's pace. A more adult-like swallow pattern develops over time as the infant grows and achieves success with continued feeding development. For example, a school-age child will prepare the bolus, using anterior-posterior as

FIGURE 10.1 **Child (A) and Adult (B) Lateral View of Swallowing Structures**

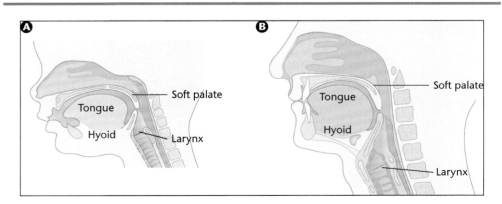

TABLE 10.1 **Structural Differences Between Infants and Older Children**

STRUCTURE	INFANT	OLDER CHILD
Tongue	Fills oral cavity	Tongue moves inferiorly and posteriorly
Mandible	Small, receded	Adult-like in proportion
Teeth	Edentulous	Dentition
Soft Palate	Large and touching epiglottis	Separate from epiglottis
Cheeks	Include fatty pads for sucking	Lack of fatty pads with more muscle activity
Hyoid	High in neck, close to thyroid cartilage	Drops in neck, separate from thyroid cartilage
Pharynx	No oropharynx	Presence of oropharynx
Larynx	Small, high in neck	Larger, drops in neck

Sources: Arvedson & Brodsky, 2002; Swigert, 2010.

well as superior-inferior movement of the tongue, followed by a trigger of the pharyngeal swallow at the base of the tongue, rather than the valleculae.

DIFFERENCES IN ETIOLOGY

Common causes of a swallowing difficulty in the adult population include stroke, traumatic brain injury, and degenerative diseases (ASHA, 2013a). Unfortunately, children are not exempt from these difficulties, but there are additional circumstances that could lead to a swallowing or feeding problem. Some of the more common complications include neurological disorders, prematurity, respiratory issues, craniofacial anomalies, and failure to thrive (Prasse & Kikano, 2009). These disorders will be explained later in this chapter.

FIGURE 10.2 **Lateral View of Infant During Swallowing with Material in Valleculae**

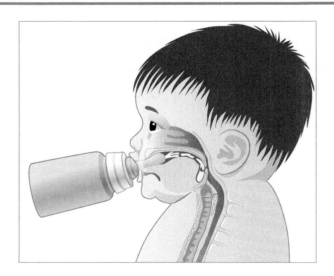

First, we will discuss medical complications and their impact on feeding and swallowing. These difficulties at birth can seriously affect swallowing and, at times, be life threatening. Such complications may require multiple surgeries and the use of ventilators and/or feeding tube placements to maintain an adequate respiratory status or to ensure nutritional intake, respectively. In severe cases, children may receive parenteral feeding (nutrition through intravenous fluids only) or enteral feeding (nutrition through a tube inserted into the mouth, nose, or stomach). Although vital, the use of either respiratory or feeding aids can also lead to a feeding disorder secondary to the infant's lack of experience with sucking, swallowing, and oral play during this time. Additionally, the presence of pain and discomfort during feeding or medical procedures can contribute to a limited exposure to sensory experiences or a negative feeding experience, ultimately stunting the child's development of feeding and swallowing.

Most importantly, unlike an adult, the child with a feeding and swallowing disorder will continue to grow and develop in the presence of this impairment. For the developing child, these abnormal processes and behaviors become part of the child's feeding and swallowing routine. In other words, difficulty feeding or swallowing can result in abnormal patterns being learned and strengthened as the child develops. Unlike an adult who develops swallowing difficulties as a result of injury or illness, the child with difficulty has no experience with typical feeding and swallowing.

DIFFERENCES IN COMMUNICATION SKILLS

Very young children typically cannot communicate their difficulties. Of course, verbal communication is not expected for infants, but even children who are verbal may not have the appropriate vocabulary to express what they are feeling or experiencing. A difficulty with communication will be present for any individual, child or adult, who has a swallowing problem in the presence of a language, speech, or cognitive deficit. In these cases, you will need to rely on nonverbal communication and observation of behaviors during feeding and swallowing to convey a struggle, such as fussiness, coughing, and crying during eating. An intimate understanding of the anatomy and physiology of swallowing in pediatrics, as well as the signs and symptoms of difficulty, will aid with assessment and diagnosis in this population.

DIFFERENCES IN TREATMENT

There are many approaches to treating dysphagia in older children and adults, but unfortunately most cannot be used with young children because they require some level of receptive language skill and independence (ASHA Technical Report, 2001). Young children are often unable or unwilling to follow directions and cannot actively participate in some more common adult treatment options. As a result, compensatory strategies are often used with young children to promote safe eating. For example, it may be necessary to change the bottle system being used during feeding to compensate for aspiration or food or liquid entering the airway.

Treatment will rely on caregiver participation, and as stated earlier, the SLP will provide education and training to the caregiver regarding the signs and symptoms of dysphagia as well as compensatory techniques specific to his or her child. Multiple treatment strategies, in relation to the pediatric population, will be reviewed later in this chapter.

Development of Feeding

As you may recall, feeding and swallowing are multistage processes requiring many different muscles and their coordination at each step. These processes will be described in the following sections, as there are some age-related differences and additional considerations that need to be outlined with the pediatric population. For instance, an infant may encounter challenges to development that require intervention to encourage a more normalizing experience with the hope of enhancing his or her neuromuscular development.

An intimate understanding of the normal stages of feeding development will assist you in identifying normal versus abnormal functioning. Although you may have received this information in a development course, we'll review it briefly if only to help your recall.

Children are expected to move through the feeding stages successively, as each skill relies on the development of a previous one. For example, just as we cannot expect a child to run before he or she walks, we cannot expect the child to chew before he or she can move the tongue side to side. Unfortunately, there are many circumstances that could inhibit a child's progression through the feeding stages.

An issue with one stage of feeding development will easily affect another, resulting in problems such as food refusal, hypersensitivity, or limited oral intake from lack of motor or sensory development. Of course, a child's growth is directly related to his or her success with feeding, and continued development hinges on weight gain (Delaney & Arvedson, 2008). If the child has difficulty with one of the stages of feeding development, the SLP cannot expect the child to eat what is appropriate for his or her chronological age and must consider picking up where his or her developmental feeding progress plateaued. This development is briefly outlined below, but please be aware that there are variations to this timeline because of different beliefs and cultures.

NEWBORNS–3 MONTHS

As you've learned in your coursework so far, newborns are born with the ability to suck and swallow. The suck/swallow/breathe pattern is reflexive and easy to trigger. Once initiated, the child will pace himself or herself independently. It is important to note that the suckle intake pattern dominates until approximately 6 months of age. This is an immature sucking pattern that consists mainly of a forward and backward movement of the tongue with a loose lip approximation around the bottle nipple or mother's breast. An important part of this process includes the relationship between the caregiver and the child, in that the caregiver's responding appropriately to the child's cues for hunger, satiety, and breaks will encourage safe self-exploration with the feeding process in stages to come (Delaney & Arvedson, 2008).

In Chapter 2, we discussed many of the motor reflexes present in infancy. Those associated with normal feeding development include the suck/swallow reflex, the rooting reflex, the transverse tongue reflex (movement of the tongue toward the stimulus inside the oral cavity), gag reflex, and the tongue protrusion reflex. At birth, movements are reflexive and infants rely on external support for proper feeding positioning. A slight recline (approximately 45 degrees) will be most comfortable for the child when bottle- or breast-feeding.

Around 3 months of age, oral play begins. With the introduction of more volitional or purposeful movement (that was encouraged in earlier months with appropriate caregiver response), the child will place fingers and objects in his or her mouth. The gag reflex is very hypersensitive at birth, and this continued oral play throughout development assists with its desensitization. Oral play also helps the child learn the dimensions and configuration of the mouth for future feeding and speech development. These early feeding patterns are linked to the advancement of communication skills (Delaney & Arvedson, 2008). Lastly, better head and neck control develops, and as a result positioning may change. The child can be held more upright while bottle- or breast-feeding, subsequently preparing the child for eventual autonomy.

6–12 MONTHS

As a result of success with the previous stages, a child can sit upright independently for feeding by 6 months, allowing freedom of the hands and more involvement throughout the feeding process. Not only will the child attempt to hold the bottle, but also the introduction of soft solids or pureed textures at this time promotes play and involvement with food. Because this is a new experience, some loss of food from the lips and confusion with opening and closing of the mouth around the spoon is normal. Practice with new textures and new oral motor movements is critical for the continued development of motoric and sensory aspects of feeding.

Over time, with continued practice, the child will begin to learn to close the mouth around the spoon with improved jaw and tongue coordination. Nutritionists and dietitians suggest to caregivers that they present one food item at a time for a few days before introducing a new taste to better identify possible food allergies.

Also at 6 months of age, the suckle pattern transitions to a more mature suck intake pattern. This intake pattern has a firmer approximation of the lips and an upward and downward movement of the tongue during the swallow. This is closer to the adult swallowing pattern, but still includes some forward and backward movement of the tongue. Anatomically, tooth eruption also begins in this stage, which will increase oral motor play and exploration.

Between 9 and 12 months, the child will become more mobile and more active. Children at this age will self-feed, and this is to be promoted. Some parents may continue bottle- and breast-feeds at night, but around this time, cup drinking is usually introduced. Again, until the child becomes more familiar with the process, a learning curve is common, with loss of liquids from the lips and/or coughing and some gagging. Continued use of the cup, rather than the bottle- or breast-feeding, will promote a more adult-like swallow pattern and minimize anterior movement of the tongue or tongue protrusion during the swallow.

Easily dissolvable solids or crunchy carbohydrates, such as puffs, cheese curls, or dry cereal, are usually introduced at this time, as the child will have several teeth. The child will demonstrate a munch-chew pattern with immature up-and-down movements of the jaw but will begin to demonstrate lateralization or side-to-side movement of the tongue and accompanying movement of the chewed bolus to each side of the mouth. Much of this skill is learned as a result of the continued oral play over the past few months with a desensitized gag reflex.

15–24 MONTHS

With continued cup drinking and refined chewing skills that have led to a more rotary movement, children may move toward the use of straws and open cups and the chewing of hard solids, such as meat or raw vegetables, that are not easily dissolvable. There should be very few difficulties noted during feeding. In fact, by 24 months, all feeding skill sets should be in place. Food items that are not eaten are a result of taste preference rather than difficulty (Morris & Klein, 2000). In this stage, an adult-like swallow pattern, without tongue protrusion, is being utilized, and the child is eating independently.

Causes of Feeding/Swallowing Difficulty

You've probably heard the saying "Practice makes perfect." The same is true for early feeding and swallowing. The more successful practice a child experiences, the more the evolving patterns of behavior will assist oral motor and sensory development. Motor development in feeding refers to the growth and maturation of movements associated with the oral structures needed to assist with feeding intake patterns, such as the tongue, jaw, lips, and teeth. Sensory development in feeding refers to the maturation of sensation (or feeling/awareness) of accompanying oral intake patterns that triggers the motor movements for feeding, such as taste, temperature, size, and texture.

Structural abnormalities, physiological boundaries, medical/wellness issues, environmental factors, and/or experience limitations can interrupt development and result in a feeding problem (Morris & Klein, 2000). Often, there is a combination of the above contributing to the child's feeding difficulty. Although the list of causal factors is quite extensive, in this section we'll review the more common difficulties that contribute to feeding issues in pediatrics.

PREMATURITY AND/OR LOW BIRTH WEIGHT

As you recall, a premature infant is an infant born before full-term gestation, or 38 weeks. By 34 weeks, most infants have developed the suckle/swallow skills needed for oral feeding (Arvedson & Brodsky, 2002). In contrast, the premature infant may exhibit immature feeding patterns, with limited development of reflexes, motor skills, and sensory skills needed for safe feeding. An underdeveloped neurological system affects an infant's ability to suck, swallow, and coordinate the suck/swallow/breathe pattern, thus putting him or her at risk for aspiration.

Children who have a low birth weight also may exhibit many of the same difficulties as a premature infant during feeding and swallowing. As mentioned previously, fatigue will result from a limited nutritional status and hinder the child's motor and sensory development as well as the weight gain necessary for continued growth. This lack of growth, in turn, continues to affect nutritional intake, leading to continued fatigue, and a cyclical pattern arises.

For both the premature infant and the low birth weight infant, treatment may include alternative feeding methods. The infant may be placed on tube feedings, which will be discussed later in this section, to sustain nutrition and hydration until feeding skills develop and mature. Prolonged tube feedings or other medical interventions, such as intubation for adequate breathing, may deprive the infant of sensory experiences needed for typical development (Bingham, 2009; Arvedson, Clark, Lazarus, Schooling, & Frymark, 2010).

A loss of experience with feeding and oral play will hinder a child's succession through the stages of feeding development; however, if a child receives oral stimulation, such as that provided by nonnutritive sucking on a pacifier, occluded bottle nipple, or gloved finger while being tube fed, that can provide the necessary sensory experiences to continue to advance (Bingham, 2009). If you're interested in learning more about the effect of oral motor stimulation on preterm infants, read the excellent review by Arvedson and colleagues (2010).

NEUROLOGICAL CONDITIONS

Central nervous system malformations occur in approximately 1 of 3,000 births and are caused by a combination of environmental and genetic influences (Arvedson & Brodsky, 2002). A common neurological condition affecting feeding and swallowing in children is cerebral palsy (CP), which was discussed in Chapter 2. Although physical disability is a main concern, these children are also at risk for delayed and impaired growth and development from limited oral intake (Kuperminc & Stevenson, 2008). In fact, in a study conducted by Burklow, Phelps, Schultz, McConnell, and Rudolph (1998), a review of feeding team written evaluation reports indicated that children with developmental disorders and developmental delay were at a high risk for feeding complications.

Overall, children with impaired motor ability of a neurological origin may demonstrate poor posture and impaired oral and pharyngeal stages of swallowing. Untreated, these difficulties may lead to drooling, reflux, and/or respiratory complications from chronic aspiration. An interdisciplinary approach is needed to address motor and sensory development, nutritional status, positioning, and safe feeding. For an extensive review regarding feeding issues among children with cerebral palsy, read Rogers (2004).

CARDIOVASCULAR CONDITIONS

Approximately 25 percent of all congenital malformations are cardiovascular in nature, meaning they involve the heart and circulatory system (Arvedson & Brodsky, 2002). Some common abnormalities include

- Narrowing of blood vessels, or stenosis;
- Holes in the heart, or septal defect;
- Underdevelopment, or hypoplasia;
- A failure of vessels to close, or patent ductus arteriosis; and
- Blood vessels connecting to the wrong areas, or transposition.

Many of these congenital heart defects, in addition to others, can be found on the American Heart Association website if you're interested in reading more about them.

Children with cardiovascular difficulties often require surgery, resulting in prolonged hospital stays with the placement of a feeding tube. In addition, interventions and repeated testing may be necessary. These can include respirators to maintain an adequate respiratory status or transesophageal echocardiography to evaluate heart function. These procedures can lead to missed feeding experiences and possible dysphagia (Kohr, Dargan, Hague, Nelson, Duffy, Backer, & Mavroudis, 2003).

As you recall, oral play throughout feeding development is necessary for continued progression through the feeding stages. Medical interventions may put oral play on hold, resulting in the possibility of hypersensitivity and speech and language delays. As mentioned when discussing premature infants, intervention that provides nonnutritive feeding experiences is necessary in order to assure continued oral motor and sensory development.

Children with cardiovascular complications can also demonstrate generalized low muscle tone, oral motor/sensory delay, and poor nutritional status. The infant may break the suck/swallow/breathe coordination pattern to take breaths more often because of a faster heart rate. As a result, the child will become fatigued during feeding and demonstrate minimal endurance, resulting in malnutrition. Often, additional services, such as physical or occupational therapy, may be beneficial as they assist with gross and fine motor development and improve tone and stamina.

RESPIRATORY CONDITIONS

An infant's circulatory health depends on adequate respiration (Arvedson & Brodsky, 2002). Both systems are very closely related. Children with respiratory complications will breathe more often, raising their heart rate, again causing fatigue during eating, as discussed in the previous section (see Figure 10.3). As a result, the adult feeder must control the child's pacing externally. The child may appear to need frequent sensory prompts, such as moving the nipple, to continue the suck/swallow reflex if the child ceases often. Because the child's response to continue sucking following prompts is reflexive, one must be careful, as this could elicit lethargy with continued trials. Knowledge regarding this close cardiorespiratory connection will shed light on whether such prompts should be utilized.

Many congenital anomalies can result in respiratory difficulty, ultimately affecting feeding. We'll quickly review a few. A tracheoesophageal fistula (TEF) is a condition in which there is an opening in the shared wall between the trachea and the esophagus. This may be difficult to diagnose because food enters the airway after the swallow and the child does not cough or show overt symptoms. When diagnosed, surgery to repair the fistula is required, and children often resume normal safe swallowing.

Another structural complication of the respiratory system is a diaphragmatic hernia, in which a portion of the digestive system pushes through the wall of the diaphragm encroaching on lung space and negatively impacting breathing. With limited volume to expand the lungs, the child will need to pause more often during feeding to breathe.

Infants are nose breathers, as you may have guessed. Anomalies narrowing or closing off the nasal cavity, such as choanal atresia, a blockage in the back of one or both nasal passages, or enlarged tonsils/adenoids, will cause the child to break his or her seal around the nipple and take frequent breaks while eating to mouth breath. We've all experienced similar discomfort when we have a cold and we are attempting to eat and mouth breathe simultaneously. As a result, eating may become exhausting for the infant and lead to a learned discomfort or fear.

FIGURE 10.3 **Relationship among Oral Intake, Nutrition, and Stamina**

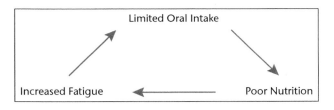

Some respiratory conditions, such as laryngomalacia and tracheomalacia, will result in stridor, or noisy, harsh breathing. Laryngomalacia is a condition in which the walls of the larynx are frail and collapse inward, narrowing the airway, during inhalation. Tracheomalacia is a condition in which the walls of the trachea are frail and collapse inward, again narrowing the airway, but during exhalation. Usually, both resolve later in life without intervention but may lead to discomfort or a lack of coordination during feeding as the infant breaks often to catch his or her breath.

Lastly, micrognathia (small jaw) or macroglossia (a large tongue) can make breathing a struggle. In these cases, positioning, such as placing the infant on his or her back, should be avoided so as not to close off the airway with the tongue slipping posteriorly in the oral cavity.

Severe respiratory difficulties may require medical interventions, such as intubation or a tracheostomy, in which a hole is placed in the neck and a tube is inserted to improve respiratory status. Alternatively, this placement can also lead to additional difficulties, such as infection, aspiration, irritations in the airway, and bleeding (Joseph, 2011). It is also important to note that many children are often discharged with a tracheostomy tube and the caregivers are taught to provide care in the home. Because of the potential negative effects discussed above, this prolonged experience can further affect the development of feeding skills. In fact, 80 percent of children with a tracheostomy also have dysphagia (Norman, Louw, & Kritzinger, 2007). As a result, it is important for the caregiver(s) to receive appropriate education and counseling surrounding this responsibility with a medically fragile infant. For more information regarding tracheostomy care in the home setting, read the great review by Joseph (2011).

Because of the relationship between respiration and cardiac status, children with breathing difficulty will most likely also demonstrate generalized low muscle tone, oral motor/sensory delay, and poor nutritional status. Both cardiovascular and respiratory difficulties result in a circular or downward spiraling pattern of behavior in which oral skills worsen quickly. Again, early intervention is imperative and a multidisciplinary approach is recommended to target oral motor/sensory, gross, and fine motor skills. For a more detailed discussion regarding respiratory complications, read the fine article by Laya and Lee (2012).

TRAUMATIC BRAIN INJURY

Traumatic brain injury (TBI) may also affect oral motor and sensory development and result in atrophy of the musculature and delayed motor ability. For example, as a result of TBI, the child may exhibit paralysis or paresis (weakness) affecting oral motor movements necessary for safe feeding and swallowing. In additional to motor impairment, many children with TBI may have difficulty swallowing because of a cognitive deficit (Morgan, 2010). The struggles they may face can include both oral and pharyngeal stage difficulty with varying severity (Morgan, Ward, Murdoch, Kennedy, & Murison, 2003).

Treatment strategies for children with TBI are very client specific, as severity varies. For example, for mild to moderate impairment, treatment frequently includes compensatory feeding strategies, including diet modifications or changes in texture to prevent aspiration. Although this is not an end goal, it may be necessary to provide safe feeding experiences while treatment ensues to improve the affected areas. Alternatively, children with severe impairment are often in a coma and benefit from continued oral stimulation to protect against decreased strength, range of motion, and coordination of the swallowing musculature as well as loss of experience. In any event, continued exposure to oral motor and sensory experiences will maintain already learned skills and promote feeding and swallowing development if milestones have not already been reached.

FAILURE TO THRIVE

Failure to thrive (FTT) is defined as a negative impact of inadequate nutrition on growth and development (ASHA Technical Report, 2001). FTT can be a result of anatomical, physiological, medical, or psychological difficulty. As you now know, limited nutrition will decrease feeding stamina, ultimately delaying brain and motor development. When a child

TABLE 10.2 **Alternative Means of Nutrition**

	OROGASTRIC	NASOGASTRIC	GASTROSTOMY
Location	Mouth > stomach	Nose > stomach	Stomach
Requires surgery	No	No	Yes
Affects swallowing	Yes	Yes	No
Visible	Yes	Yes	No

is not sustaining nutrition/hydration via oral intake, called PO feeding, alternative feeding methods may be necessary to assure neurological and physiological development. Some children will require feeding via a tube that is placed through the nose into the stomach, called a nasogastric tube, or a tube that is placed directly into the stomach, called a gastrostomy. Alternative methods of feeding are presented in Table 10.2. Ideally, children on continuous tube feedings, which provide small amounts of nutrition all through the day, will be gradually shifted to intermittent bolus feeds, or a predetermined amount of food given every few hours. If a child cannot tolerate bolus feeds, the continuous tube feedings may continue. The issue for both the SLP and the family is that a child on continuous tube feeding will not be hungry enough to shift to eating orally. Another difficulty is that the child may not eat enough orally to reduce tube feeding. Making decisions regarding feeding tube placement and/or changes in feeding team regimen are not in our scope of practice; therefore, a team approach with the physician(s) and dietitian staff will provide the best opportunity to maintain nutritional status as well as a safe progression to oral feeding.

For more information and resources regarding feeding tubes, please visit the Feeding Tube Awareness Foundation website.

Lastly, a more broad spectrum diagnosis, such as either food refusal or FTT, may also lead to a possible tube feeding placement. These conditions can be the result of hypersensitivity, commonly seen in children with behavioral feeding disorders and autism spectrum disorders (ASD). Often, issues with sensory processing, as in ASD, can lead to defensiveness regarding new tastes and textures. These children are not to be viewed as mere "picky eaters" regarding their food refusal. Their condition is a physiological feeding disorder affecting sensory integration.

ESOPHAGEAL COMPLICATIONS

Children who experience gastrointestinal disease may have feeding difficulty due to the effect the esophageal stage of swallowing has on the oral and pharyngeal stages. At first, a child with esophageal stage difficulty may be referred to you, the SLP, because it presents much like an oral or pharyngeal stage difficulty. An understanding of gastrointestinal issues and related signs and symptoms will assist you in determining when to refer the child for a consult with a gastroenterologist.

One of the most common gastrointestinal (GI) diseases among children with feeding issues is gastroesophageal reflux disease (GERD). GERD is diagnosed when stomach contents enter the esophagus, leading to discomfort. The most common symptom in infants and children is vomiting (Rudolf et al., 2001). An infant will also often arch backward during his or her feeding. More subtle symptoms include burping, hiccups, chronic cough, and frequent ear infections. Dental cavities may also indicate increased acidity in the mouth. In more serious cases, a child may develop pneumonia from aspirating reflux.

Dr. Owens's grandson Dakota, mentioned throughout this text, had severe GERD. Backward arching complicated his CP by putting him into an extensor position with arms raised and head back, making it almost impossible for him to accomplish even simple motor movements.

Early in life, infants with severe symptoms may undergo surgery to address their reflux. A procedure, called a **fundoplication**, narrows the lower esophageal sphincter to prevent stomach contents from reentering the esophagus. This surgical management, although helpful for reflux, does not eliminate other GI issues such as **esophageal dysmotility** and **delayed gastric emptying** (Loots et al., 2013).

Esophageal dysmotility is a disorder that affects the movement of food through the esophagus. When there is content lingering in the esophagus, the upper esophageal sphincter remains closed, putting the child at risk for aspiration during the swallow as the food has nowhere to go but potentially into the airway.

Delayed gastric emptying is a disorder in which the emptying of the stomach content into the small intestine is delayed or slowed. This problem occurs after the bolus passes the lower esophageal sphincter or the location of the fundoplication, but the stomach discomfort that follows frequently affects feeding as the child is often nauseous, bloated, or simply not hungry.

Approximately half of the children with GERD will outgrow the disorder by age 1 because of increased mobility, but continued discomfort, which can include nausea, bloating, indigestion, vomiting, constipation, and diarrhea, may lead to refusal to eat and subsequently a diagnosis of FTT. Also, GI issues can quickly lead to negative associations with food and the feeding process.

In the presence of GI complications, the SLP will need to refer to a gastroenterologist as diagnosis and treatment of such disorders is not in our scope of practice. Some approaches to alleviate GI complications may include a change in positioning during feeding, diet modifications, and medical or surgical management. Treatment approaches will be decided in a team approach with the GI physician. Very frequently, when the GI problems have been resolved, the oral and pharyngeal stages of the swallow also improve. In some cases, behavioral feeding disorders or food aversion may result and continued treatment is necessary.

CRANIOFACIAL ANOMALIES

It is no surprise that structural limitations affecting anatomy and physiology can have a negative impact on feeding and swallowing. We have reviewed some examples of this in the cardiorespiratory sections. In addition, any impairment affecting specifically the coordination, strength, or range of motion of the oral structures will make feeding and swallowing a challenging process. Although the list is extensive, some of the more common craniofacial anomalies affecting feeding and swallowing include Down syndrome, cleft lip/palate, **Pierre Robin sequence**, and **velocardiofacial syndrome**.

The most common chromosomal syndrome is Down syndrome, or trisomy 21, occurring in 1 of every 650 to 1,000 live births (International Craniofacial Institute, 2014). Characteristics that may affect feeding ability include an enlarged tongue, low nasal bridge, low muscle tone, cardiac abnormalities, and mental impairment (International Craniofacial Institute, 2014). Children with Down syndrome may experience fatigue while eating, poor lip seal, decreased suck intake pattern, and aspiration, all possibly resulting in weight loss (Lewis & Kritzinger, 2004).

Cleft lip and palate is the fourth most common congenital anomaly of the face (Kummer, 2014). This is a disorder in which the upper lip, hard palate, and/or soft palate may fail to close during gestation, leaving a hole or gap. It can occur in one structure, two structures, or all three. Although the swallow reflex and oral motor and sensory skills are intact, the child is often unable to latch onto a bottle nipple and demonstrate an efficient suck. Without a separation of the oral and nasal cavities, the child cannot develop the negative pressure needed to draw liquid from a bottle, straw, or spoon. Adaptive equipment and special bottle systems may be necessary until surgical intervention. For more information and resources regarding cleft lip/palate, please visit the Cleft Palate Foundation website.

Pierre Robin sequence is a congenital condition including a chain of malformations caused by chromosomal anomalies. The three most common are cleft lip or palate, micrognathia, and **glossoptosis**, which is a posterior tongue position. This combination can result in upper airway obstruction. In addition to the feeding difficulties discussed for cleft lip and palate, children with Pierre Robin sequence will also have difficulty with sucking and swallowing coordination. Again, adaptive equipment, in addition to alternative means of nutrition and postural changes, may be necessary until surgical intervention.

Lastly, velocardiofacial syndrome (VCFS) is a genetic disorder that is highly variable; in fact, more than 180 behavioral and physical features have been portrayed (Shprintzen, 2008). Some of these features include heart defects, facial anomalies, and cleft lip and/or palate (Kummer, 2014). It is one of the most common multiple anomaly syndromes, and rather than identifying by feature, it is best diagnosed by genetic testing to identify the deletion of DNA in chromosome 22 (Shprintzen, 2008). Congenital heart defects with VCFS are common (Shprintzen, 2008), and as you now know, cardiac complications can lead to decreased nutritional status, low muscle tone, and respiratory difficulty. This, coupled with cleft lip/palate, will require ongoing treatment to sustain caloric intake.

Some craniofacial anomalies may be life threatening and require extensive medical attention. By now, you are very well aware of the difficulties that can arise from prolonged tube feedings, multiple surgeries, and intubations, although they may be medically necessary.

It seems prudent at this point to also mention that prolonged oral experiences such as thumb-sucking and extended bottle/pacifier use may also negatively affect feeding and swallowing by altering structures related to feeding. Structural changes, including dental and mandible deformation, can require orthodontia or additional surgical intervention. In these cases, behavioral treatment approaches, which will be reviewed later in the chapter, may be necessary to reduce immature swallow patterns for prevention.

ENVIRONMENTAL CONSIDERATIONS

Socioeconomic status is an additional factor that can affect the growth and feeding development of a child (Morris & Klein, 2000; Kersten & Bennett, 2012). Families in poverty not only have difficulty providing adequate, healthy meals, but they may also struggle to provide consistent mealtimes, which will have an impact on hunger cycles. Parents of children with feeding issues have many additional expenses such as specialized formula, specialized bottle systems/cups, specialized spoons, medical equipment, and specialized seating equipment. In other words, access to healthy food options, a mealtime routine, and specialized equipment may be an additional burden to the family (Kersten & Bennett, 2012).

Children who are not meeting their nutritional needs are at risk for FTT, frequent illness, delayed development, behavioral issues, and increased anxiety (Kersten & Bennett, 2012). In fact, an effect on the child's health can begin in utero as mothers who have inadequate nutrition place the child at risk for low birth weight and birth defects (Kersten & Bennett, 2012). An SLP must also consider the effect of caregiver and child depression on interactions with food, caregiver-child mealtime interactions, and mealtime motivation (Morris & Klein, 2000).

Feeding Team

Regardless of the setting in which you may be working, as an SLP you'll find that pediatric dysphagia and feeding disorders are addressed by a team of individuals. This is in part because many children with feeding and swallowing issues may also exhibit other developmental concerns that require the attention of multiple disciplines (Miller, 2011). This interdisciplinary team allows for a global approach to assessment and treatment (Arvedson, 2008). See the helpful article by Nancarrow and colleagues (2013) regarding what principles constitute a good interdisciplinary team.

As a team member, respect for and collaboration with other disciplines are essential for effective treatment. Although SLPs receive specific education in the area of dysphagia, everyone on the team is also expected to have extensive knowledge regarding the health concerns associated with dysphagia and feeding disorders so as not to add to the problem (Arvedson, 2008). The exact makeup of the feeding team, with the exception of a few common key players such as the SLP, occupational therapist (OT), and dietitian, is determined on a client-to-client basis. You may be working closely with one or several of the following disciplines/individuals:

- *Occupational therapist.* The OT has training in sensory input and integration as well as positioning. An OT can also have additional training specifically in dysphagia.
- *Physical therapist.* The PT also has training in sensory input and in positioning, and may also have additional training specifically in dysphagia.
- *Dietitian.* The dietitian determines nutritional status and growth patterns and provides appropriate recommendations regarding caloric intake for the child to receive adequate nutrition/hydration. This includes oral and tube feeding recommendations.
- *Primary care physician (PCP).* The PCP is often the source of referral. The child may be presenting with chronic health issues that have become a red flag for the PCP. The PCP will make medical decisions for the child, including feeding tube placement. He or she may also need to refer the child to other specialists for continued care.
- *Nurse.* Nursing staff members spend a lot of time with the child, whether he/she is in the hospital setting or the child requires home health services. They are familiar with various signs and symptoms of dysphagia and may serve as a referral point in addition to aiding with treatment recommendations you have provided.
- *Teacher.* He or she may begin to notice difficulty in the classroom or may be asked to provide feedback to the caregiver(s) and/or member(s) of the feeding team to assist with treatment recommendations.
- *Psychologist.* The psychologist may be consulted for feeding disorders with a behavioral component/origin or when suspecting a psychological overlay. This individual may also serve as a resource for child-caregiver dynamics that may be concerning.
- *Specialist physicians (GI, dentist, orthodontist, ear nose and throat, plastic surgeon, neurologist, neurodevelopmentalist, etc.).* Children with structural and/or physiological abnormalities may need to see additional physicians for consultation and treatment.
- *Parent(s)/caregiver(s).* These individuals are the *most* important contribution to the feeding team. They not only know the child better than anyone else, they will carry out your recommendations day to day. They need to learn how to become the clinician.

These are only a few of the feeding team members that may be involved in a child's care plan. As stated, this group is variable and will be case specific. Some of these individuals may be present in an EI classroom or hospital setting. When applicable, it may be beneficial to collaborate with other members of the team during treatment sessions to increase carryover across disciplines.

Assessment Strategies

You've just had a young child referred for a suspected feeding disorder. Now you need to decide where to begin. Your best bet is to gather as much information as possible about what led to this referral.

There is an art and a science to assessment, and both are found in a systematic step-by-step approach. An SLP begins by talking to the child's caregiver(s), teacher(s), and physician(s). It's also important to review the medical and dietary history if available. "Red flags" that indicate the child is having difficulty include some common reasons for the referral:

- Choking
- Coughing
- Wet vocal quality
- Frequent throat clearing
- Gagging
- Vomiting
- Food refusal

- Failure to thrive
- Decreased interest
- Extended time for meals
- Reflux
- Chronic infections
- Spiking temps

As an SLP, you will need to gather medical, surgical, nutritional, and developmental information about the child. Subsequently, you'll want to observe the child and conduct a physical examination in regard to oral motor sensory skills, as well as assess oral, pharyngeal, and esophageal stages of the swallow through an informal and/or instrumental assessment (instrumental assessment can confirm suspected pharyngeal stage issues and is necessary to evaluate esophageal stage issues). Let's go through the process together.

MEDICAL HISTORY

In any swallowing evaluation, whether adult or child, it's good to begin with a thorough review of the medical history. The child's experiences, such as past surgeries, medical complications, or lack of opportunities for feeding, can provide a better understanding of why he or she is experiencing a feeding problem. In the EI setting, an SLP may need to request this history from the caregiver or primary care physician (PCP) prior to the assessment.

If there is no specific issue related directly to the structures or physiology of eating and drinking, the SLP should then examine the medical history for a possibility of lost feeding experiences (there may also be a combination of both). For severely impaired children, life-threatening medical conditions at birth are addressed first, putting the development of feeding and swallowing skills on hold. Aside from experience limitations, an extensive surgical or medical history may signal interrupted feeding development. For example, if the child had cardiorespiratory issues followed by multiple surgeries, you may deduce that the child could have missed opportunities for oral play and oral feeding from a prolonged status of nothing allowed by mouth (NPO status), as reviewed earlier. Another example may be that the child has significant gastroesophageal reflux and feeding has become less enjoyable because of consistent discomfort. Such background information, given your knowledge, can guide you during the caregiver interview as well as assist a dietitian when determining strategies to obtain adequate caloric intake.

NUTRITION/DEVELOPMENT

A consultation with a dietitian is necessary if there is a concern with nutrition, which there often is. Occasionally, such concerns will initiate the referral process for a feeding assessment, but if not, a referral is appropriate for most, if not all, feeding cases.

The dietitian will make recommendations to improve the child's diet if the child is felt to be below average for weight, height, and/or length for his or her chronological age. For children who eat some or all of their meals by mouth, simple suggestions may be provided to increase calories, such as adding butter, sour cream, milk, or heavy cream into many of their snacks and meals. Alternatively, for the child who has limited food and liquid intake, the PCP or dietitian may have expressed concern with the growth and development of the child and feel that feeding skills should be assessed before considering alternative means of nutrition and hydration. In severe cases, it is critical to improve oral and pharyngeal skills, resulting in an increase in PO (by mouth) intake, thus avoiding a feeding tube placement. In many cases, this can seem like a race against time.

A report from the dietitian will typically include the child's average daily caloric intake and his or her weight and length/height as compared to normative data. The dietitian may also have asked the parent to keep a diary recording the PO intake of the child over the last several days. This information should also be included in an SLP's feeding report as it will be very helpful for the SLP to identify patterns of feeding difficulty and to track progress over time.

It's important to remember that our goals as SLPs focus primarily on safety and efficiency of feeding and development. Caregivers will naturally have questions regarding the recommended amount of PO or tube feeding intake. These questions and concerns should be referred to the dietitian or primary care physician, as it is not in our scope of practice to make such decisions.

INTERVIEW

The SLP's review of medical, nutritional, and developmental history will help guide the discussion during the interview process. Remember, no one knows the child better than his or her caregiver(s), who serve as very important members of the interdisciplinary team. This is usually the first meeting with the caregiver, and the SLP should start to build a rapport with the family from the very beginning. If conducted appropriately, an interview with the caregiver will give insight regarding the trouble the family is experiencing and suggest possible strategies for improvement. It will also demonstrate to the caregiver your willingness to help and serve as an additional team member, a process in which they are very much included.

During the interview, you can gather information about the child's difficulty as described by the caregivers, their goals and concerns, the child's likes/dislikes, attempted strategies, current therapies if any, and frequency and duration of difficulty. It's important to also consider the feelings and attitudes surrounding the feeding experience and listen to all concerns. A sample interview questionnaire targeting many of these areas can be found in Appendix I.

OBSERVATION

Information gathered during the interview will supplement the medical and dietary history, but it is not a substitute for directly observing the child during feeding and assessing the child's oral and pharyngeal function. Most young children will not be able to speak for themselves and even the caregivers' description may not adequately describe the feeding and swallowing process. As SLPs, we must rely on signs and symptoms as well as behaviors to determine the best plan of treatment. Table 10.3 describes some of the common signs and symptoms of feeding difficulty you may observe with infants and young children.

For caregivers who find it difficult to describe their child's feeding struggle, it may be easier for them to *show* you, especially if they feel attempted strategies have had little success. To aid in this process, an SLP may want to ask the caregiver to bring items such as food

TABLE 10.3   **Some Signs and Symptoms of Feeding Difficulty**

Infants	Young Children
Crying during mealtime	Tantrums during mealtime
Fatigue and long feeds	Prolonged feeding times
Gagging	Gagging
Upper and lower extremity movement	Turning away or lack of interest
Furrowing of brow	Food selectivity
Wet vocal quality, coughing, choking	Wet vocal quality, coughing, choking
Arching	Fear
Food refusal	Food refusal
Vomiting	Vomiting

and utensils the child likes and dislikes to the evaluation. When possible, the SLP can ask the caregiver(s) to demonstrate exactly what happens in the home. Ideally, the caregiver feeds the child in the usual position with frequently used utensils to mimic the natural feeding environment as much as possible. Of interest are both the child's mealtime behaviors and caregiver responses. If the caregiver is unable to attend the evaluation, obtaining this information prior to the observation will be helpful so you can prepare appropriately.

Throughout the text you've read about dynamic assessment, and as an SLP, you'll want to notice specific areas where the child may be having difficulty and suggest as well as implement different strategies to quickly assess for changes and/or improvement. Quick stimulability tasks, such as changes in position or bottle flow rate, will not only allow for an efficient treatment plan but may motivate the child and caregiver when experiencing success.

PHYSICAL EXAMINATION

As reviewed earlier in the chapter, ASHA has clearly outlined an SLP's responsibilities in regard to assessing, diagnosing, and treating feeding and swallowing problems. This requires a thorough physical examination during the evaluation. Through direct observation, discussed above, an SLP will notice specific oral motor, sensory, or positioning difficulties that provide clues for what to explore in a more formal oral motor assessment.

A good place to begin is by noting the appearance and symmetry in both static and dynamic states of all the facial structures. Of particular interest are any differences in symmetry of oral structures, both at rest and during movement, as well as their development. Are all structures present, of an appropriate size for the child's age, and working as expected? The SLP should also note the presence of teeth and their number as well as be alert for possible drooling while evaluating the strength, range of motion, and coordination of the jaw, tongue, lips, cheeks, and soft palate.

In a more general sense, the child may present with hypotonicity or hypertonicity, which can affect feeding ability. For example, a child with low muscle tone, or hypotonicity, may have facial drooping, decreased lip closure, and consequently the presence of drooling. In contrast, a child with hypertonicity, or increased tone, may have difficulty controlling jaw movements and tongue movements during the oral and pharyngeal stages of the swallow. In other words, any alteration of muscle tone (be it hypo- or hyper-) will also affect posture during eating and drinking. In turn, altered posture can increase the risk of aspiration or feeding difficulty.

As discussed earlier, the physical examination must assess sensory skills in addition to motor skills. A child with hypersensitivity may be defensive with the presentation of food or toys near the mouth. In contrast, a child who is hyposensitive often seeks input and may put a lot of food in his or her mouth when eating. Table 10.4 presents a few signs and symptoms of sensitivity issues affecting feeding safety.

This was a very general overview of assessment, but a more detailed assessment sheet summarizing areas of interest to evaluate feeding and swallowing can be found on the ASHA website listed as "Pediatric Feeding History and Clinical Assessment Form."

TABLE 10.4 Signs and Symptoms of Sensitivity with Feeding

HYPERSENSITIVITY	HYPOSENSITIVITY
Defensiveness	Large bites/sips
Prolonged feeding times	Fast rate
Food selectivity	Drooling/anterior loss
Dislike of toothbrushing	Bulky tongue
Limited oral play	Seeks oral play

When you've gathered your information regarding oral motor and sensory skills, consider what is appropriate for the child's chronological or corrected age. Corrected age is an allowance for the premature child to catch up developmentally. If a child is born prematurely, his or her age is adjusted for developmental milestones. For example, if the child was born two months early and he is currently 12 months old chronologically, his corrected age would be 10 months. A comparison of what the child presents and what he or she is expected to present will help with quantifying a level of deficit and give you a starting point for treatment planning. An SLP must be very familiar with the feeding stages discussed earlier in this chapter to determine appropriate goals based on the child's current ability.

SWALLOW EVALUATION

Although the observation and physical assessment of the swallow can yield information regarding what we can *see* during feeding (specifically the oral preparatory and oral stages of the swallow), the SLP will also need to assess and document the pharyngeal and esophageal stages of the swallow. This is difficult to do without visualization, but learning the signs and symptoms of difficulty can be helpful. Signs and symptoms of aspiration include coughing, choking, wet vocal quality, and throat clearing. Because many children silently aspirate, the SLP must also rely on the child's behavior to give indications of swallowing difficulty. For example, infants will often furrow their brow, demonstrate excessive extremity movement, or become agitated or fussy during feeding. The most common sign of difficulty is when a child simply refuses a particular food or beverage. This is a message to the caregiver that the item is uncomfortable and must not be confused for a taste preference choice. Unpleasant eating experiences from aspiration or choking events can instill fear and generalize to other foods, further affecting nutrition and hydration.

In those situations in which visualization of the pharyngeal or esophageal stages of the swallow is not possible, an understanding of the behavioral signs of difficulty is extremely important. For example, an SLP can also ask about the child's respiratory status and overall wellness to give insight into the adequacy of the swallow. If the child is a chronic silent aspirator, he or she may have frequent spikes in body temperature. These children are also often sick with "colds" or the "flu" which can be confirmed by the caregiver. Although much of this information is helpful, it may be most beneficial to use instrumentation to be sure.

INSTRUMENTAL EVALUATION

As noted, many young children silently aspirate, so as an SLP, you may want to take the safe route and consider instrumental evaluation when receiving mixed signals during the evaluation or question inconsistency during eating/drinking. The most common methods of instrumental evaluation include flexible fiberoptic endoscopic evaluation of swallowing (FEES) and a videofluoroscopic swallow study (VFSS) (Miller, 2011). Working in early intervention, you'll rarely have access to the equipment needed for these tests; however, you can refer to another feeding team or clinic for this type of evaluation. Each method provides visualization of the pharyngeal stage of swallowing, and each has its advantages and disadvantages.

FEES is conducted by an otolaryngologist or ENT in conjunction with the SLP and/or additional feeding team member. Nasal, pharyngeal, and laryngeal structures can be viewed, including tonsils. Using this procedure, presented in Figure 10.4, the clinician can see how well the child is managing secretions, observe the sensory skills in relation to the pharyngeal swallow, evaluate aspects of the pharyngeal swallow, such as hyolaryngeal excursion, and check for penetration/aspiration before or after the swallow.

A major disadvantage of the FEES is that it is invasive. A scope must be passed through the nasal cavity and rest in the pharynx during eating and drinking. This requires compliance and children with hypersensitivity may struggle significantly. In addition, you cannot see what is happening *during* the swallow, only before and after, because of the action of the epiglottis. You also cannot view the the esophageal stage of the swallow. FEES is particularly difficult to use with bottle-feeding secondary to successive swallows. On the

FIGURE 10.4 **Fiberoptic Endoscopic Evaluation of Swallowing (FEES)**

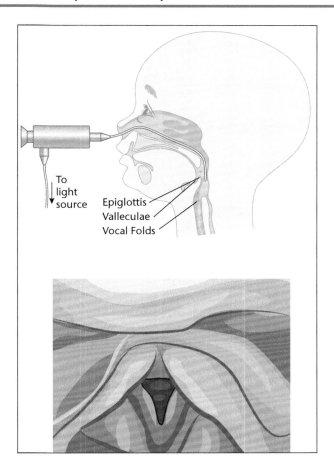

plus side, when using FEES, the child does not need to be exposed to radiation, which is extremely beneficial for medically fragile children in need of multiple procedures. In addition, nothing needs to be added to the foods/liquids in order to visualize the bolus during the swallow; therefore, tastes will not be altered.

Children who have had many hospital visits may be more willing to tolerate a less invasive method, like a VFSS. This procedure is conducted by a radiologist, an SLP, and an additional feeding team member when possible. A VFSS allows visualization of all the stages of the swallow, including the esophageal stage, as well as the timing of the swallow, anterior-posterior transfer of the bolus, coordination of the swallowing structures, hyolaryngeal excursion, penetration/aspiration, and adequacy of strategies, to name a few. Although the clinician can visualize what is happening during the swallow, some disadvantages include barium added to the food or liquid and radiation exposure.

It is important to remember that, regardless of the instrumentation used, results are subjective and professional opinions may differ. In fact, agreement between results from FEES and VFSS is low (da Silva, Lubianca Neto, Santoro, 2010). As a potential referring clinician in the future, you need to understand the advantages and disadvantages of each procedure and ask for a detailed report. Knowing *why* there is a difficulty, in addition to *where* there is difficulty, will be beneficial when determining an effective treatment plan. The two procedures are compared in Table 10.5.

Thorough assessment is fundamental when determining candidacy for treatment as well as an appropriate treatment method. A diagnosis-specific treatment will provide a structured approach to ultimately increase the child's stamina and PO tolerance (Schwarz,

TABLE 10.5   **Comparison of VFSS and FEES**

	VFSS	FEES
View of all stages of swallowing	Yes	No
Invasive	No	Yes
Radiation exposure	Yes	No
Numbing agent	No	Yes
View laryngeal penetration	Yes	Yes
View aspiration	Yes	Yes (but not during the swallow)
Compliance issues	Yes: barium	Yes: passing of scope
Food alteration	Yes	No
SLP and. . .	Radiologist Possibly OT or PT	Otolaryngologist Possibly OT or PT
Use of adaptive equipment	Yes	Yes
View vocal fold movement	No	Yes
Requires training	Yes	Yes
Assessment of secretion management	No	Yes
Time constraint	Yes	No
View of rapid succession of swallows	Yes	No
Position flexibility	Limited	Yes

Sources: Miller, 2011; Sitton et al., 2011.

Corredor, Fisher-Medina, Cohen, & Rabinowitz, 2001). Aside from a formal diagnosis, SLPs will also want to consider a child's cognitive status, postural ability, respiratory status, gross and fine motor ability, oral motor and sensory skills, and level of fatigue (Morgan, 2010). Related difficulties, such as motor, speech and language, hearing, and vision impairments, will also require an interdisciplinary approach. Documentation is key, so please visit the ASHA website for some examples of templates that may help you organize and document all of the necessary information during assessment.

Treatment Strategies

As you already know, feeding difficulty may result from many different interconnected factors. Because children in an EI classroom will be developing in numerous areas, an SLP can expect to be interacting with individual team members on a variety of issues outside of feeding. Flexibility and creative thinking will be beneficial to maximize therapy time, prioritize goals, and maintain a multidisciplinary approach with your clients.

Aside from being a good team player, the SLP needs an understanding of the fundamentals of normal feeding development, reviewed earlier, to assist a child in achieving appropriate feeding milestones. Although the child's chronological age may imply an expectation of an already established skill, he or she may have experienced difficulty with an earlier stage of feeding, in turn affecting the other stages of feeding. As a result, some of your approaches may seem unforgiving in the presence of missed experience or food refusal and may be met with much resistance. It's helpful to remember that children are making choices that they feel are safe and unthreatening.

We have to gain and retain the trust of our clients and their families in order to obtain the best treatment outcomes. Trust is built through an SLP's manner of interacting with the child and family as well as success in therapy. It's important for families to understand that you are there to help and not to criticize or find fault. As mentioned throughout this text, a more functional intervention approach generalizes to other settings such as home or school. As parents begin to see changes at home, they will begin to trust in your expertise even more.

Continued flexibility and reassessment is needed as the child grows and develops and his or her comforts change. Children are growing and changing even in the presence of a feeding problem, and compensations needed at one time should not be thought of as permanent or static. Chosen treatment strategies can be easily adapted to follow the child through the stages of feeding and swallowing development. For example, the SLP may not want to encourage playing with food beyond a time frame that is developmentally appropriate to do so. Instead, the SLP can choose to use a washcloth or other textured stimulation tool, rather than food, to target sensory integration in therapy when the child is chronologically beyond the stage in which food play is acceptable. The SLP and feeding team should introduce feeding behaviors that will follow the feeding development continuum for a transition to more adult-like patterns. Ultimately, the goal is not to create additional difficulties you will only need to address in the future.

The most important element of your intervention is the caregiver. Not only will caregivers contribute largely to your treatment targets based on their information during the assessment, but without their support therapy cannot be successful. Ideally, the caregiver will learn some of an SLP's skills, such as assessing, treating, and reassessing in relation to his or her child's feeding and swallowing behavior. Most of the work will be done in the home, so the family must be able to identify problem behaviors and apply appropriate strategies to address the feeding difficulty per your guidance. Remember, you will only see the child for a short period of time. Feeding in the home or school occurs several times daily. The success of intervention depends on a caregiver's skill set and willingness to participate.

This information may seem overwhelming, but a thorough assessment will reveal an appropriate path for treatment. Also, you won't be doing this alone. As an SLP, you'll have a team to consult with to assist with setting treatment goals. Below are a few suggestions for key areas to consider in your treatment sessions.

ENVIRONMENT

The environment in which you are working can affect the child's behavior and tolerance of feeding therapy. To determine if this is an important factor, ask the caregiver(s) to describe the child's behavior during meals or, better, observe for yourself. The goal is to make the feeding environment as natural and familiar to the child as possible. This will aid with generalization as long as the environment is not hindering progress in a distracting, counterproductive way. For example, a distracting environment may be detrimental for a child who is hypersensitive, but could be beneficial for a child who is hyposensitive. The opposite is true for a calming environment.

Adapting the sensory system through environmental changes can make a significant difference and can increase the child's participation during intervention sessions. This can be accomplished by considering vestibular, tactile, gustatory (taste), olfactory (smell), visual, and auditory changes. Table 10.6 provides some suggestions regarding environmental adjustments.

Some of the suggestions in Table 10.6 may be difficult to implement in a variety of settings. The SLP may be visiting the child at home or pushing into the classroom during snack time. If the sensory modifications are not possible in every setting, participation by caregivers in the intervention session can provide the tools they need to continue the

TABLE 10.6 **Environmental Suggestions to Improve Mealtime Experience**

CHANNEL	STIMULATION	CALMING
Vestibular	• Rocking/spinning quickly • Sporadic movements • Frequent movement during session	• Rocking/swaying slowly • Rhythmical movements • Weighted vest
Tactile	• Light touch/tickle • Cold stimulation • Frequent texture changes in food and stimulating tools	• Deep, soothing pressure • Warm stimulation • Minimal texture changes
Taste	• Bold, strong flavors	• Bland flavors
Smell	• Foods with strong smells	• Food with dull smells
Visual	• Pictures with bright, bold colors	• Limited colors or cool colors
Auditory	• Exciting music at louder volume • Bubbly speaking rate/volume/intonation	• Soft, soothing music or none • Soft, slow, soothing voice

Sources: Adapted from Morris & Klein, 2000; Swigert, 2010.

feeding program at home or in other settings. With frequent carryover from setting to setting, the new feeding environment can become more natural and familiar to the child.

POSITIONING

If the SLP suspects that a child is frequently aspirating or if the child looks uncomfortable, often repositioning the child will better protect the airway during feeding. In fact, alterations in the feeding position are an easy strategy and a good place to start, especially for children with GERD. Remember, if the child is uncomfortable, sometimes his or her way of telling people is to refuse eating and drinking. A change in position could also provide a stimulating or calming effect. For example, swaddling the child has been shown to support and improve flexor patterns, including oral motor skills and the suck/swallow reflex (Arvedson et al., 2010). To swaddle a child, wrap the infant firmly in a blanket with arms and feet toward midline. Swaddling is illustrated in Figure 10.5.

Positioning options for infants include the caregiver cradling the child in one arm, holding the infant in front (face-to-face), and side lying. Although holding an infant cradled in one arm is the most common position for feeding, if the child becomes fatigued easily, this may not be the best choice as it creates a calming effect. Holding the infant in front while supporting the head, allows for eye contact and limits some of the warm comfort from the cradled position, diminishing sleepiness. Lastly, the side lying position is helpful for infants with a retracted tongue or infants with a cleft palate and/or delayed swallow as it allows food to collect in the cheek before the swallow. These positions are illustrated in Figure 10.6.

For older children, a 90-degree angle at the child's hips, knees, and ankles, is desired. Unfortunately, some children with severe disabilities, such as cerebral palsy, scoliosis, or motor delay, may be unable to sit upright in this position for feeding. In these cases, an occupational therapist or physical therapist should be consulted to assist with positioning

FIGURE 10.5 **Swaddling**

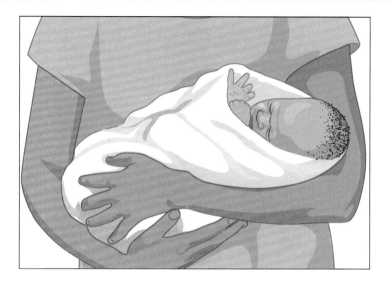

the child and working toward improving motor ability and strength over time (Swigert, 2010). In addition, adaptive equipment such as specialized seating and wheelchairs may be considered.

PACING

Children seeking stimulation, or those who are hyposensitive, may eat and drink very rapidly. Alternatively, children who view eating and drinking as threatening, or those who are hypersensitive, tend to eat very slowly. Much like *Goldilocks and the Three Bears*, the SLP will need to find a pace that's "just right." The argument can be made that these children have chosen a desired pace that is "just right" for them. That said, a fast rate can lead to increased risk of aspiration, and a very slow rate depreciates the caloric benefit of the meal.

There are also instances in which the child is pacing appropriately while bottle drinking, but the flow is inappropriate, or too fast. A few simple changes in pacing and flow may reduce mealtime anxiety for the child and caregiver(s) and eliminate risk for aspiration and poor oral intake. Signs and symptoms include choking, coughing, anterior loss of bolus, and breaks in the suck/swallow/breathe coordination to catch their breath. Simply slowing the flow can help these infants to relax and drink comfortably with no risk of aspiration. Children who are working too hard to drink from the bottle put themselves at risk for burning more calories than they're taking in. In this case, we may need to increase the flow to maintain adequate intake by cross-cutting the nipple (making the opening larger) or using a compressible bottle to assist with fluid flow.

As oral motor sensory skills develop and improve, pacing may adjust itself; otherwise, the SLP and the caregiver will need to control the rate. With older children, an SLP can provide models, cues, and prompts to take small bites and sips. When treating infants, external pacing by an adult may be necessary. Adults can force breaks by removing the bottle or breast or provide tactile cues to start sucking again when appropriate.

TEXTURE CHANGES

It's important to find a way to introduce safe feeding so the child can develop the necessary skills to demonstrate a functional swallow pattern, without sacrificing experience. One way to accomplish this is through changes in the texture of the food ingested. If diet consistency changes, such as thickened liquids, are recommended, a dietitian can assist with assuring adequate caloric intake so as to avoid empty calories.

FIGURE 10.6 **Infant Feeding Positions**

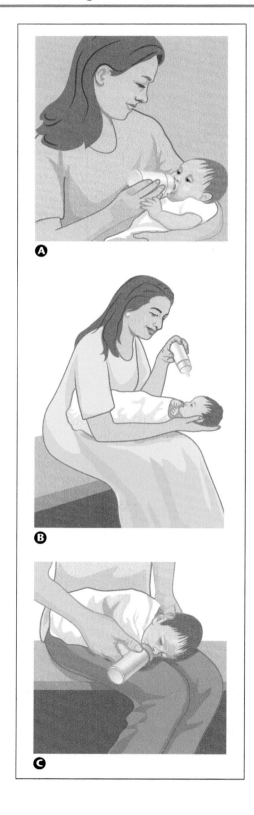

Texture changes can provide additional sensory input, improve oral motor/sensory skills, and allow for additional practice with oral intake. Changes in consistency are not a substitute for oral motor development, which should also continue. We must be cautious, because children with hypersensitivity may find sudden drastic changes in texture to be threatening and unenjoyable. In this case, gradual changes are the best option in making feeding a more pleasant social experience.

Gradual changes may include a decrease in the number of pulses with a blender when transitioning from pureed to solids, or a combination of desired and undesired foods and textures, such as pudding and pieces of banana or graham crackers. Gradual changes are also a good way to gain the trust of your client. Because many of these children have had multiple trips to the doctor's office and hospital, they may be less trusting of health care professionals. You do not want to "trick" the child into alternative feeding experiences.

Texture options for young children include thin, nectar, and honey thick liquids, pureed, chopped (items that require munching), and regular (items that require chewing) textured items. See Table 10.7 for some common textures of children's food items.

Although there is limited evidence to support or reject the use of thickened liquids with children with feeding or swallowing disorders, the practice continues to be used (Gosa, Schooling, & Coleman, 2011), much as in adult dysphagia. Food is sometimes thickened to make it move more slowly and allow the individual to gain better control and avoid aspiration. Thickened liquids or changes to food texture can enable PO feeding and give the child feeding experiences that may have otherwise been lost.

As an SLP, you'll need to be careful, especially with infants, because a large amount of thickener can be considered "empty calories" for the child, and this can result in inadequate nutrition and FTT. Always consult a dietitian. At times, exceptions are made depending on the type of formula. It is important to note that traditional powder thickeners will dissolve quickly in expressed breast milk (milk that has been pumped), causing a return to thin liquid. In this case, gel thickener is more effective.

Of course, safe feeding is always of primary concern, and although helpful, thickened liquids are recommended only as a last resort (Gosa et al., 2011). Traditional therapy approaches should be attempted first to achieve the least restrictive diet texture without the risk of penetration/aspiration. If this is not possible with diet alterations, therapy must continue in an effort to obtain advancement at a later time.

ORAL MOTOR/SENSORY STIMULATION

Earlier we discussed hyper- and hyposensitivity and hyper- and hypotonicity. Sometimes, symptoms can be unclear because a child can demonstrate aspects of more than one simultaneously. One consolation is that, regardless of sensitivity or tonicity, oral motor therapy can yield positive outcomes. In fact, oral motor stimulation has been shown to speed up

TABLE 10.7 **Common Foods for Children per Consistency**

Thin	Nectar	Honey	Pureed	Chopped	Regular
• Water • Formula • Juice • Milk • Jello	• Milkshake • Ice cream • Carbonated beverages • Any of the thin liquids may be thickened to this consistency	• Liquids must be thickened to this consistency	• Baby food • Mashed potatoes • Rice or wheat cereal and oatmeal • Pudding • Yogurt	• Soft cooked vegetables • French fries • Pasta • Dissolvable cookies and crackers • Scrambled eggs	• Meat • Raw vegetables • Raw fruit • Candy • Pizza

the transition from tube feedings to oral feedings in premature infants (Fucile, Gisel, & Lau, 2002). In short, oral motor therapy consists of stimulating and exercising the oral musculature with the presenting deficit.

Oral motor therapy can target any of the relevant oral structures, such as lips, cheeks, tongue, and mandible. This stimulation can be provided using toys, feeding utensils, and/ or gloved hands accompanied with various tastes, temperatures, and textures. Generally, the goals oral motor/sensory stimulation are

- To move toward a more functional sensory response to feeding, and
- To improve motor control and coordination.

Children who demonstrate either hyposensitivity or hypotonicity will participate readily and often seek oral motor stimulation in all forms. In contrast, children who are either hypersensitive or hypertonic may demonstrate defensiveness with this approach. In either case, the child will benefit from a consistent presentation. It can be a challenge, but the SLP's goal is to make this as enjoyable and fun as possible. Remember, feeding should always be a pleasant experience. With the right approach and carryover, the child can enjoy therapy and increase his or her active participation in eating.

There are many tools and games for oral motor therapy designed specifically for children. However, sometimes even the most enjoyable and interactive games won't engage the child who is defensive. In this case, placing a desired food item/texture on an oral motor stimulation tool or gloved finger will increase participation. In addition, a child who is orally defensive may benefit from feeling more in control during the session.

Allowing the child to participate by encouraging his/her oral play in front of a mirror with food items or allowing the child to "play therapist" may help to increase comfort with continued stimulation. For example, the child may enjoy also wearing gloves and touching your face during therapy. Although oral motor stimulation may be a struggle, clinician consistency, support from the caregiver, and carryover to the home/school setting are crucial for decreasing unwanted behavior and increasing wanted behaviors.

Toys and tools designed specifically for oral motor sensory stimulation are plentiful, but you may find you have limited resources or access to a multitude of options. Simply using your hands is also an option. Many SLPs manipulate the muscles of the face and oral cavity with gloved hands by movements such as

- Stroking the inside and outside of the cheeks,
- Running fingers along the outside of the gum line, and
- Stimulating or stretching the lips.

These methods can be easily taught to parents and do not require purchasing additional materials.

All ages can benefit from some form of oral motor stimulation. Although digital manipulation and the use of oral motor therapy games and tools may be beneficial, these methods are not always appropriate for the infant population. Nonnutritive sucking is a form of oral motor sensory stimulation that provides practice and improves strength to mature the suck/swallow pattern (Arvedson et al., 2010). Children with prolonged tube feedings should be receiving oral motor stimulation during their feeds not only to support oral motor/sensory development but to promote a relationship between oral function and sensation and a full tummy. Even a child who is NPO can also benefit from your services, specifically oral motor stimulation. Overall, oral stimulation is a good supplement to feeding treatment (Manno, Fox, Eicher, & Kerwin, 2005). In fact, it is key to their eventual success. By now, you are well aware of the difficulties that can arise from missed oral play and stimulation.

BEHAVIORAL TREATMENT

There will be instances in which sensory integration or stimulation may not yield the greatest benefit and therapies that are more operant based will be more appropriate (Addison et al., 2012). This may be the case for a child with a feeding problem that has a behavioral foundation.

Behavioral feeding disorders usually start as a structural or medical limitation and arise from a lack of experience or prolonged unpleasant experience while ill (Arvedson & Brodsky, 2002). Although some food aversion and refusal of new food items are typical for the young child (Equit et al., 2013), children with behavioral feeding disorders refuse food or have a severe food selectivity to the degree that they are not meeting their nutritional targets (Swigert, 2010). The caregiver may have been advised "He'll eat when he's hungry," but this is not the case with children who have behavioral feeding disorders. These children will not be motivated to eat, and at times supplemental tube feedings are necessary to sustain nutrition (Ernsperger & Stegen-Hanson, 2004).

Behavioral feeding disorders can make for a stressful mealtime experience for the child and caregivers. A power struggle may persist, and parental responses of negotiation, pleading, and scolding are not successful in encouraging a child to eat (Williams, Field, & Seiverling, 2010). In fact, some of these responses may only increase tantruming, crying, throwing food, vomiting, delaying mealtime, and other difficult behaviors. In this section, we'll review a few techniques to address behavioral feeding disorders and still maintain a pleasant feeding environment.

A child needs to feel safe during treatment. As an SLP, you'll need to be aware of the client's medical history, not only regarding feeding development, but emotional status. Sometimes, a negative reaction to feeding is the result of an extensive medical history in which the child who has had many surgical or medical procedures may become fearful as soon as he or she enters a medical environment or comes in contact with a medical professional. For these reasons, when possible, providing therapy in the home setting may be best so the child can feel more comfortable during treatment. If this is not a possibility, again, creating a natural calming environment will be helpful to gain the child's participation and increase his or her willingness to interact with the SLP.

There is strong support for the benefit of behavioral intervention in the professional literature (Sharp, Jaquess, Morton, & Herzinger, 2010). First, the SLP must be in control of the session at all times in order to increase wanted behaviors and decrease unwanted behaviors. Wanted behaviors may include food curiosity or interest, oral motor play, or acceptance of a variety of tastes and textures. Reinforcement strategies are a good way to increase those behaviors. Positive reinforcement, such as praise for good eating behavior, will increase the likelihood of its happening again (Skinner, 1991). This does not need to include a gift or reward, but simply the verbal acknowledgment of a job well done. Alternatively, negative reinforcement allows for the escape from an unwanted situation (Skinner, 1991). For example, if the child eats all of his dinner, he may leave the table. The term "negative reinforcement" is sometimes confused with punishment, but they are very different. Notice that negative reinforcement increases a behavior but punishment has the opposite effect.

Although both types of reinforcement can be used effectively in treatment, the SLP must be cautious so as not to introduce additional unwanted behaviors. Unwanted or inappropriate behaviors may include tantruming, spitting out food, refusing food, kicking, hitting, and vomiting. Negative reinforcement may have the unintended consequence of promoting inappropriate behaviors during meals (Piazza et al., 2003). For example, giving the child desired foods as a reward may teach the child that there are "good" and "bad" foods. He or she may also rush through the targeted taste or texture to get to a preferred taste or texture. The SLP does not want to teach the child that eating/drinking is a negative experience that should be avoided or can be avoided. Sometimes the choice of reinforcement can seem paralyzing. For example, if the child frequently spits out his food, reinforcement, positive or negative, is questionable. It makes sense that the child should not be praised for this action, but the child should also not be permitted to avoid the meal. Negative reinforcement, or removal from the meal, will only reinforce and promote unwanted behaviors.

Extinction, or removal of the opportunity for reinforcement, is an alternative strategy. Using extinction, the SLP would simply continue to offer the food during and after the child's unwanted behaviors (Swigert, 2010). This is used to teach the child that unwanted behaviors do not elicit a different result or provide an escape from the situation. Essentially, you are praising wanted behaviors and ignoring the rest.

Another tactic that avoids eliciting more unwanted behaviors is re-presenting the food. It is used specifically when the child frequently removes food from his or her mouth

(Coe et al., 1997). Spitting out or pocketing food in the cheeks allows the child to avoid the experience of eating, and representing the item consistently may decrease this avoidance behavior, again teaching the child that his or her behavior will not elicit a different result. This technique has been shown to be effective, decreasing expulsion of food, when used in conjunction with a tactile prompt to the chin (Wilkins, Piazza, Groff, & Vaz, 2011).

Lastly, antecedent manipulation is a more preventive strategy that manipulates therapy events to prevent unwanted behaviors from occurring. For example, if the child frequently throws his or her bowl of cereal, simply do not put the bowl within reach. Rather, offer the child a few pieces at a time.

Now that we have discussed a few behavioral strategies, it's important to point out that the child who is defensive or fearful will not respond well to sudden changes. Gradual, small changes are another way to gain the child's and caregiver's trust during treatment. Usually, the goal is the acceptance of an unwanted taste or texture. Simply offering the undesired item may not be the best strategy, resulting in refusal and tantruming, making for an unpleasant experience for the child and therapist. In this case, the SLP may choose to break down a goal into smaller steps or parts (Swigert, 2010). For example, the goal may be that the child will take a small spoonful of a pureed texture. This may be a lot to ask at first if the child is very hypersensitive or fearful. Perhaps, the child begins to tantrum and refuses all PO at the sight of a pureed texture. In this case, the SLP may choose an initial goal of tolerating the texture in the same room or on his or her food tray.

For children who are eating but have very restricted food preferences, again food chaining techniques may also be used to link new foods with colors, shapes, and textures a child already accepts (Cox, Fraker, Walbert, & Fishbein, 2004; Fishbein et al., 2006). For example, if a child eats fish crackers, other foods can be cut into the same shape with a cookie cutter. For more information on food chaining, read the comprehensive text by Fraker, Fishbein, Cox, and Walbert (2007).

When selecting a treatment strategy, the SLP will need to consider the child's cognitive ability to follow directions and ability to understand the changes being made in his or her food and beverage items. In cases where the child has limited awareness or understanding of adaptations to feeding, small gradual changes, a comforting environment, and caregiver support will make feeding less overwhelming for the child.

Caregiver involvement and carryover in the home setting is fundamental for success in treating behavioral feeding disorders. In any type of behavior modification, consistency in adult response is necessary to elicit change in the child. For example, SLP-provided oral stimulation intervention twice weekly in a school setting will not be enough to facilitate change and development. Frequent contact and additional training for the caregivers will be necessary to assure proper technique and participation in goal acquisition.

CULTURAL CONSIDERATIONS

Cultural views will shape the interpretation of recommendations provided by an SLP (Davis-McFarland, 2008). Caregivers are and should be very involved in the therapy process and the establishment of the Individualized Educational Plan (IEP). Communication barriers, such as a difference in language or the team's misunderstanding of the family's culture, could hinder the caregivers' necessary participation in this process. The caregivers may not understand the educational or feeding terminology being used, or they may feel the team doesn't understand their culture as it pertains to feeding. As a result, caregivers are less likely to believe that treatment will be effective (Davis-McFarland, 2008). This may negatively affect their trust of the SLP as well as their participation and carryover of treatment strategies in the home setting.

To better ensure caregiver involvement and participation, the SLP can familiarize himself or herself with the cultural beliefs of the family, including food preferences, health concerns and goals, and beliefs regarding developmental disabilities and treatment (Davis-McFarland, 2008). Alternatively, the SLP must be aware that his or her own cultural beliefs and mores may shape interactions with others, approaches to therapy, and recommendations.

As with any feeding client, the SLP can build a good rapport with the caregivers and gain a better understanding of their specific needs and goals for the child by meeting with the family frequently prior to and during intervention. This will also provide a learning opportunity for the SLP to become more culturally competent to plan the most effective treatment that both individualizes intervention and encourages much-needed family participation. For an excellent review of cultural competence and cultural beliefs about breast-feeding, the introduction of soft solids, and the food varieties offered, read Davis-McFarland (2008).

Conclusion

Feeding and swallowing disorders in the pediatric population require the attention of many health professionals. A team approach is best to address all of the developmental concerns and family needs in regard to medical complications, skill acquisition, and social aspects of feeding. The number of feeding and swallowing cases is growing in both the school setting and in EI services. This is no longer solely the job of an acute care pediatric SLP.

Many professionals in the schools are finding themselves treating children for feeding disorders as a result of an increased survival rate among young children with feeding and swallowing issues. The SLP working with this population may need additional training and coursework to assume competency in the area of dysphagia and feeding disorders. Most importantly, the school or EI SLP needs to advocate for these children to obtain and provide the necessary services that

will further overall development and promote healthy living. In addition, it is the responsibility of the SLP to educate other professionals regarding their role in the treatment of children with feeding disorders to raise awareness.

Lastly, a close interaction with the caregiver(s) will be key to success in treatment. These individuals know the child best, spend the most time with him or her, and will be carrying out your recommendations. Your job as an SLP is ultimately to help caregivers become independent. With this ever-growing field, the education provided to professionals and caregivers will continue to promote the importance of early intervention for children with feeding and swallowing difficulty.

For more information regarding an overview of pediatric feeding disorders, please visit the ASHA website and look for "pediatric dysphagia" under clinical topics in the Practice Portal.

 Click here to gauge your understanding of the concepts in this chapter.

Appendix A
Sample IFSP

IFSP Details

Child's Name: Theo Jones
EIO/D: Sally Smith
Effective Start Date: 10/27/2015
Meeting: Yes
Other:
Parental Consent Obtained: Yes

Currently Assigned SC: Maria Rodriquez
IFSP Type: 2nd Review
End Date: 4/26/2016
IFSP Meeting Date: 10/21/2015
Initial IFSP Date: 4/27/2015
IFSP Status: Active

Number of amendments to this IFSP and its Service Authorizations: 0
Clinically appropriate visits per day must not exceed: 3

Child's Level of Functioning

HEALTH/PHYSICAL DEVELOPMENT

Theo was born at approximately 26 weeks gestational age, weighing 1 lb. 8 oz. He remained in the NICU for three months before being discharged to home. During his stay in the NICU, Theo received his feedings through G-tube and was placed on oxygen. He was diagnosed with bronchopulmonary dysplasia, gastrostomy dependence, GERD, feeding difficulties, and failure to thrive. Nursing was a continuing issue upon release to the home environment.

10/27/2015: There are no hearing or vision concerns at this time although Theo has some difficulty following solely with his eyes. Feeding and communication continue to be concerns.

COGNITIVE DEVELOPMENT

Theo obtained a Cognitive Standard Score of 84, placing him in the below average range.

3/17/2015: Theo has missed some cognitive milestones. He has difficulty attending and focusing on objects and events in his environment.

COMMUNICATION

Theo obtained a total language score of 59, uncorrected for his age prematurity. His babbling consists of canonical syllables with little or no syllable repetition. He will turn-take with sound-making but does not imitate sounds currently in his repertoire, which are limited to /g, k, m, b/. He laughs, gurgles, and makes raspberries. He can protrude his tongue briefly and give kisses.

SELF-CARE ADAPTIVE SKILLS

Theo exhibited a significant feeding aversion with delayed oral preparatory skills due to his limited food acceptance. Although eating a greater variety of foods, calorie intake is a concern.

3/17/2015: Feeding issues continue to be an area of concern. He gags and chokes on lumpy textures.

GROSS/FINE MOTOR DEVELOPMENT

Theo obtained a Standard Score of 87, placing him in the average range. Theo turned his head side to side indicating some difficulty tracking with his eyes. His gross motor quotient is 83, placing him in the 13th percentile compared to peers. Although he attempts to cruise throughout his home, Theo has strength and balance problems. GMQ of 76 on the Peabody Developmental Motor Scales-2.

3/17/2015: Theo can crawl in the home environment, is pulling to a stand, and attempting to cruise. He has a gross motor quotient of 80. He has a lot of motor compensation behaviors and is missing some foundational skills.

SOCIOEMOTIONAL DEVELOPMENT

Socioemotional development continues to be a strength. He laughs and smiles appropriately. Theo's Social-Emotional Standard Score of 103 places him in the average range.

3/17/2015: Adjusting to family routine. Makes eye contact with accompanying sound-making.

Child's Current Setting

Child is at home during the day with his mother.

Family Strength and Resources

The family is very interested in learning methods to help him develop. Mother is very receptive to development ideas and willing to try new methods when suggested.

Family Concerns and Priorities

Finances are a concern, especially given the reduced hours of work for the father. This lack of resources has led to the following concerns:

- Need for transportation to doctors' appointments
- Feeding Theo and other kids at dinner time
- Purchasing a stroller
- Paying the hospital bills

Other concerns include

- Explaining Theo's developmental issues to his grandparents
- Theo's learning to talk
- Obtaining information about infant/toddler stimulation groups

Overall, parents are anxious about what Theo's current status means for the future.

Outcome Statements

Methods to achieve the following goals:

1. Rotate head side to side	Accomplished
2. Focus and attend to objects and people	Accomplished
3. Follow moving object with his eyes alone	Continuing
4. Monitor gross motor skill development	Discontinue
5. Sit and play with both hands above the floor	Accomplished
6. Attend to and complete a task	Continuing
7. Get into a sitting position	Accomplished
8. Crawl	Accomplished
9. Demonstrate balance while standing	Continuing
10. Pull to a stand	Accomplished
11. Cruise	Accomplished
12. Walk unsupported	Continuing
13. Demonstrate improved symmetry	Continuing
14. Run with good patterning	Continuing
15. Tolerate oral/sensory stimulation to face, lips, tongue, and gums	Continuing
16. Tolerate liquid solids by mouth	Accomplished
17. Use a cup	Continuing
18. Tolerate different food textures	Continuing
19. Use simple gestures	Continuing
20. Increase vocal play and babbling	Continuing
21. Imitate sounds	Continuing
22. Say single words	Continuing
23. Identify objects named by pointing	Continuing
24. Follow simple commands	Continuing

Natural Environment

All services are provided in the child's natural environment.

Transportation Needs

Transportation is not needed for services as all services are provided in the home. The caregiver is unable to provide transportation by private vehicle, but the family lives near public transportation.

Non-EI Services Needed

No non-EI services are needed at this time, although the mother has expressed interest in an infant/toddler stimulation group.

Public Programs

Child Health Plus
WIC

Meeting Attendees

10/27/2015: Maria Rodriquez, EISC; Pattie Kim, MD; Fumi Nakamoto, SLP; Ralph Forbes, PT; Sally Jones, parent

IFSP Comments

All findings and recommendations discussed with Theo's mother. Mother also expressed concerns and asked clarifying questions. Mother expressed her pleasure with the level of services so far.

Transition Plans and Services

Transition to CPSE was discussed, but there are currently no firm plans given the child's age.

Service Authorization List

Maria Rodriquez, EISC; Pattie Kim, MD; Fumi Nakamoto, SLP; Ralph Forbes, PT

Family Authorization

We (I) the parent(s)/guardian(s) of _____ hereby certify that we (I) have had the opportunity to participate in the development of our (my) son's/daughter's IFSP. This document accurately reflects our (my) concerns and priorities for our (my) child and family.

We (I) therefore give our (my) permission for this plan to be implemented.

_____ YES _____ NO

_____ _____   _____ _____
Signature of parent/guardian   Date   Signature of parent/guardian   Date

Composite IFSP compiled from several variants.

Special thanks to Colleen Fluman, CCC-SLP, clinical faculty, College of Saint Rose
Other examples of IFSPs are available online. Type "IFSP" into your search engine and several sites will be listed. The Centers for Disease Control and Prevention or "cdc" has several examples for different disorders. The "ifspweb" site has tutorials on writing IFSPs along with examples. The Early Childhood Technical Assistance Center or "ectacenter" offers examples and guidelines by state.

Appendix B
Formal Tests for Young Children

Ages and Stages Questionnaires (ASQ): A Parent-Completed Child-Monitoring System, Second Edition. Bricker, D. D., Squires, J., Mounts, L., Potter, L. Nickel, R., Twombley, E., & Farrell, J. (2003). Baltimore, MD: Paul Brookes.

The *Ages & Stages Questionnaires (ASQ)* is a set of low-cost, reliable, comprehensive parent report tools for screening children for developmental delays. Parents complete the simple questionnaires, which alert SLPs to the need for a more in-depth assessment. As we have noted, parents' observations recorded on survey forms can be very good predictors of developmental delays.

ASQ is a series of 19 questionnaires that screen and monitor a child's development between 4 months and 5 years of age, reflecting developmental milestones for each age group. Questionnaires can be used at a single point in time or at intervals for ongoing monitoring. Each questionnaire consists of 30 items that ask about a child's progress in five developmental areas: communication, gross motor, fine motor, problem-solving, and personal-social skills. The questionnaire takes about 10 to 20 minutes to complete and can be answered in the home, physician's office, school, or other childcare environment.

Assessment, Evaluation, and Programming System: AEPS Measurement for Birth to Three Years (Volume 1), Second Edition. Bricker, D. D. (Ed.). (2002). Baltimore, MD: Paul Brookes.

The AEPS Measurement for Birth to Three Years is part of a comprehensive program of assessment, intervention, and evaluation for children from birth to 6 years who have disabilities or are at risk for developmental delays in six developmental areas: fine motor, gross motor, cognitive, adaptive, social-communication, and social. The entire program consists of the AEPS

- Administration Guide,
- Test for Birth to Three Years and Three to Six Years,
- Curriculum for Birth to Three Years,
- Curriculum for Three to Six Years,
- Child Observation Data Recording Form,
- Child Progress Record, and
- Family Report

For ease of use, the second edition includes AEPS interactive, a web-based electronic management system that automates AEPS's scoring and reporting functions. Additionally, SLPs can compare a child's AEPS test results to cutoff scores that determine or corroborate a child's eligibility for services in most states.

The Birth to Three Years Test, an accurate, reliable, and valid criterion-referenced assessment, can be used to assess single children or groups in home- or center-based settings. Divided into the six developmental areas mentioned, the test can be administered while children and their caregivers engage in everyday activities. SLPs score each item with a 0 (does not pass), 1 (inconsistent performance), or 2 (passes consistently).

The AEPS Curriculum for Birth to Three Years enables SLPs to match the child's goals, identified through testing, with activity-based interventions that correspond to the six areas scored on the AEPS test. Test and intervention items use the same numbering system, so users can easily locate intervention activities that correspond to specific goals and objectives identified with the test.

The Bayley Scales of Infant Development, Second Edition (BSID-2). Bayley, N. (1993). San Antonio, TX: The Psychological Corporation.

The norm-referenced Bayley Scale of Infant Development (BSID-2) is designed for children from 1 to 42 months of age and covers multiple domains of development. It includes three scales:

- Mental Scale, which assesses
  - Memory
  - Habituation
  - Problem-solving
  - Early number concepts
  - Generalization
  - Classification
  - Vocalizations
  - Language and emerging literacy
  - Social skills
- Motor Scale, which assesses control of
  - Gross motor skills such as rolling, crawling, sitting, walking, and jumping
  - Fine motor skills such as imitation of hand movements and drawing
- Behavior Rating Scale, which rates qualitative aspects of a child's behavior during testing sessions, such as engagement with tasks, examiner, and caregiver

Raw scores on the Mental Scale are converted to age-normed Mental Development Index (MDI) scores. Raw scores on the Motor Scale are converted to the age-normed Psychomotor Development Index (PDI).

Test items are administered to the child based on his or her chronological age and take 15–60 minutes depending on the child's age and functioning level. If the child is restless or irritable, the test can be given over two sessions. In addition, testing is shortened by the use of basals and ceilings. Test administration is flexible, and the examiner can readminister earlier items if the child is initially shy or reluctant.

On some items, the examiner elicits the child's response, while on others, the examiner notes having observed the behavior at another point during the assessment. Caregivers may also be asked to attempt eliciting behaviors for certain items.

In general, the BSID-2 is complex to administer and interpret and should not be attempted without some experience and practice. Reliability and validity are high.

Carolina Curriculum for Infants and Toddlers with Special Needs, Third Edition. Johnson-Martin, N. M., Attermeier, S. M., & Hacker, B. J. (2004). Baltimore, MD: Paul Brookes.

The Carolina Curriculum is designed for criterion-referenced assessment of and intervention with infants and toddlers with mild to severe special needs from birth to a 36-month developmental age. The assessment and curriculum are divided into 24 separate teaching sequences covering the five developmental areas of personal-social, cognition, communication, fine motor, and gross motor, and may take several weeks to complete for some difficult-to-test children. If a test item is too difficult for a child, the item can be broken into smaller steps in dynamic assessment style and a successful response is scored as *emerging*. Items scored as unpassed in direct testing may be scored as passed based on parental report.

Once the assessment is complete, professionals can select curricular items that correspond to each child's identified needs. Although a child may have 24 separate intervention goals, each curricular item follows the same format, making the entire program easy to use.

Communication Complexity Scale (CCS; Brady et al., 2012)

Designed by experts in the field of ECI, the CCS focuses specifically on two areas:

- Shifting attention toward the communication partner, and
- Increased variety in forms of communication.

Changes in both contribute to increasingly complex presymbolic communication.

As you might guess, achieving consistent scoring across SLPs is challenging, especially with clients with severe motor and sensory impairments. The CCS uses a 0–11 point scale to try to increase accuracy. These levels of responding include:

- No noticeable response
- Alerting to a stimulus by changing behavior
- Orienting to a single object, event, or person
- Orienting to a single object, event, or person and one potentially communicative behavior (PCB). PCBs include vocalizations, gestures, eye gaze, or AAC switch closures that
  - Appear to be purposeful in response, and
  - Could be considered to be for the purpose of communicating behavior regulation, joint attention, or social interaction.
- Orienting to a single object, event, or person and more than one PCB
- Scanning between objects or events
- Dual orientating between a person and an object or event
- Triadic eye-gazing or dual orientating and one or more PCBs
- Triadic eye-gazing and one PCB
- Triadic eye-gazing and more than one PCB
- One symbol verbalizing, signing, or AAC symbol selection
- Two or more symbol verbalizing, signing, or AAC symbol selection (Brady et al., 2012)

Even when not using the CCS, these levels of performance may offer SLPs a viable way to encode behaviors.

Inter-rater reliability on the CCS is high. In addition, scores significantly correlate with standardized tests of language, indicating high validity. Although the CCS is promising, especially for describing levels of presymbolic and early symbolic communication, further research is still needed. It remains to be seen if the CCS is sensitive to subtle changes in the development of communication.

Some caution is warranted in rating the use of symbols, whether using the CCS or not. First, symbols should be in response to the stimulus and be accompanied by orientation toward the adult. This suggests intentionality. Second, for a behavior to be considered symbolic, it should demonstrate some discrimination by relating to the stimulus. Thus, random symbol selection from an AAC display would not be considered intentional symbolic behavior.

Communication and Symbolic Behavior Scales (1st ed.). Wetherby, A., & Prizant, B. (1993). Chicago: Riverside.

The Communication and Symbolic Behavior Scales (CSBS) is a naturalistic approach to communication for 8- to 30-month-old preverbal to verbal children. The CSBS

- Gathers information about the child's abilities from multiple sources,
- Uses caregivers in multiple roles throughout the assessment process; and
- Measures developmental milestones of critical presymbolic behaviors.

Normed on a sample of more than 300 typically developing American-English-speaking children from 8 to 24 months of age and 30 children with developmental disabilities from 18 to 30 months of age, the CSBS is an appropriate tool to assess and predict the communication development of young children (McCathren, Yoder, & Warren, 2000).

The CSBS Developmental Profile (DP) (Wetherby & Prizant, 2002) is a further adaptation meant to increase the efficacy of early identification. A shortened version of the original CSBS, the CSBS DP consists of three measures of communication:

- An Infant-Toddler Checklist completed by a caregiver,
- A Caregiver Questionnaire (CQ), and
- A Behavior Sample (BS), a face-to-face evaluation of the child interacting with a caregiver present.

The sampling and scoring procedures of both the CSBS and the CSBS DP are based on the social pragmatic model of language acquisition.

The Behavior Sample is an interactive assessment designed to encourage a child to communicate through the use of a series of communication temptations and other opportunities, including presenting a number of interesting toys, books, language comprehension probes, and a play sample. The scoring procedures for the Behavior Sample consist of 20 individual items from which three composites were derived: social, speech, and symbolic. The three composite scores have good concurrent and predictive validity for both children with typical development and those at risk for developmental delays (Wetherby, Allen, Cleary, Kublin, & Goldstein, 2002; Wetherby, Goldstein, Cleary, Allen, & Kublin, 2003; Wetherby & Prizant, 2002). The composite scores also predicted receptive and expressive language outcomes at age 2 (Wetherby et al., 2002).

Studies of the validity and reliability of the three measures found strong correlations between all three and test-retest reliability for all three, although all three measures were also sensitive enough to detect growth over short periods (Wetherby et al., 2002). Moderate to large correlations were found between all of the CSBS DP measures and language outcomes at 2 years of age.

Early Social Communication Scales. Mundy, P., Delgado, C., Block, J., Venezia, M., Hogan, A., & Seibert, J. (2003). University of Miami. A draft can be found online by typing "Early Social Communication Scale ucdavis" into your search engine. I stress that this is a draft and no substitute for the actual tool in print.

The Early Social-Communication Scales (ESCS) is a videotaped structured observation measure of nonverbal communication skills that requires between 15 and 25 minutes to administer. The ESCS was originally designed as a comprehensive clinical measure based on a cognitive, Piagetian, stage-related orientation to early development and a pragmatic-functional orientation (Seibert, Hogan, & Mundy, 1982, 1984). A set of 25 semi-structured eliciting situations were developed to encourage interaction between an adult tester and the child.

The videotape recordings of the ESCS enable observers to classify children's behaviors into one of three mutually exclusive categories of early social communication behaviors:

- Joint Attention Behaviors, or using nonverbal behaviors to share the experience of objects or events with others
- Behavioral Requests, or using nonverbal behaviors to elicit aid in obtaining objects or events
- Social Interaction Behaviors, or engaging in playful, affectively positive, turn-taking interactions with others

Behaviors are also classified as to whether they are child-initiated bids or responses by the child to a tester's bid. A measure of social communication imitation may also be obtained from the ESCS by summing the number of times the child imitates the pointing and/or clapping gestures displayed by the tester.

Infant-Toddler Language Scale. Rossetti, L. (1990). East Moline, IL: LinguiSystem.

Developed for birth to 3 years of age, the Rossetti Infant-Toddler Language Scale assesses the preverbal and verbal skills of children through direct testing, observation, and caregiver report. The comprehensive, easy-to-administer, criterion-referenced scale includes a reproducible parent questionnaire and a test protocol. Although widely viewed by some professionals to be the gold standard in early childhood communication assessment, the Rossetti Scale has not been normed, and there is no statistical information on reliability and validity.

The parent questionnaire, available in English and in Spanish translation and included on the free CD for quick printing, includes questions regarding concerns, interaction, and communication development, and a vocabulary checklist of a child's comprehension and production. Upon completion, the questionnaire can familiarize an SLP with the developmental concerns of the parent and determine the age level at which to begin testing the child. Otherwise, the SLP uses the child's chronological age or suspected developmental level to determine the age interval at which to begin.

Areas assessed in the test at three-month intervals include

- Interaction-Attachment (relationship between the caregiver and the infant),
- Pragmatics (the way language is used to communicate and affect others),
- Gestures,
- Play (both individual and interactive),
- Language Comprehension, and
- Language Expression.

The examiner establishes a baseline and ceiling developmental age in each of the six developmental areas. Items are considered "passed" if the behavior in question is observed (O), elicited (E), or reported (R), giving the SLP flexibility in administration. The manual has tips on how to elicit responses or when and where to look for them.

Language Development Survey. Rescoria, L. (1989). The language development survey: A screening tool for delayed language in toddlers. *Journal of Speech and Hearing Disorders, 54,* 587–599.

The Language Development Survey (LDS) (Rescorla, 1989; Rescorla & Alley, 2001) is a parent report vocabulary checklist and a simple, inexpensive screening tool for identifying language delay. The survey is printed and described in the referenced article. Although it takes only 10 minutes to complete, the LDS has strong reliability and validity against other measures (Klee et al., 1998; Rescorla, 1989; Rescorla & Alley, 2001; Rescorla, Hadicke-Wiley, & Escarce, 1993). Explicitly designed as a screening tool, LDS is shorter and less expensive, and takes less time to complete, than more in-depth measures, but yields information on fewer diverse areas of development.

In a sample of 18- to 35-month-old children, the LDS demonstrated a wide variability within children of the same age (Rescorla, & Achenbach, 2002). In general, SLPs should test further any child of 18 to 23 months of age who receives an LDS vocabulary score at or below the 15th percentile or has 20 words or less. The criterion for a 24- to 29-month-old is fewer than 50 words or no word combinations.

***MacArthur-Bates Communication Development Inventories*, Second Edition.** Fenson, L., Marchman, V. A., Thal, D. J., Dale, P. S., Reznick, S., & Bates, E. (2007). Baltimore: Brookes.

The caregiver report questionnaire format of the MacArthur-Bates Communicative Development Inventories (CDI) is a quick and informative assessment of early comprehension and production vocabularies, including single and combined words, gestures, and imitations, and of early word combinations (Luyster, Qiu, Lopez, & Lord, 2007). The CDI is based on a sample of typically developing children and consists of two portions:

- Words and gestures section designed for children 8–16 months of age, in which caregivers are asked to report whether their child understands each of 28 phrase and 396 vocabulary items. In addition, there are 63 gestures organized into five categories: first communicative gestures, games and routines, actions with objects, pretending to be a parent, and imitating other adult actions.
- A words and sentences portion for children 16–30 months, containing 680 vocabulary items, which are marked only if the child produces the word, and a variety of grammatical items.

The checklist increases the validity of an assessment and provides additional information on children who may provide only a limited sample of language during a face-to-face assessment. Still, one study found that approximately 30 percent of the words produced by children are not on the CDI Words and Gestures Form (Furey, Kosch, & Dunn, 2005).

Results of the CDI have been shown to agree with both standard observational assessments and direct testing (Charman, 2004; Fenson et al., 2006; Miller, Sedey, & Miolo, 1995; Stone & Yoder, 2001). While CDI receptive and expressive language delays and late gestures were predictive at both ages 2 and 3 years, scores at age 3 years were generally more reliable (Charman et al., 2005).

Children with Down syndrome, Williams syndrome, or autism spectrum disorder (ASD) may exhibit specific profiles on the CDI (Caselli, 1998; Mervis & Robinson, 2000; Singer Harris, Bellugi, Bates, Jones, & Rossen, 1997). The CDI may be especially useful with children with ASD because of their often minimal communication behaviors (Charman, Baron-Cohen, et al., 2003; Lord & Bailey, 2002).

A Manual for the Dynamic Assessment of Nonsymbolic Communication.

Snell, M. E., & Loncke, F. T. (2002). Unpublished manuscript, University of Virginia at Charlottesville. A wonderfully informative manual describing the process of dynamic assessment is available by typing "people.virginia.edu" and then typing "snell" in the search box.

This is a wonderful resource that has been updated and tweaked as the authors refine their methods. It includes a description of a dynamic assessment and the tools used for describing nonsymbolic communication via parent/caregiver interview and professional observation of both the child and caregiver. Of most importance are the portions describing the child's present means/form of communication and the "teachability" of the child, which is the dynamic assessment part.

If nothing else, go to the website and download this manual. It is filled with excellent, useful information which can be used as the authors suggest or adapted to your own particular needs.

Maternal Behavior Rating Scale (MBRS).

Mahoney, G. A. & Finger, I. (1986). The Maternal Behavior Rating Scale. *Topics in Early Childhood Special Education, 6,* 44.

Primarily a tool for identifying patterns of maternal behavior that are related to different levels of children's development, the MBRS rates 18 maternal behaviors on a 5-point rating scale and four child behaviors. The MBRS was developed for the purpose of assessing the quality of maternal interactive behavior; it is designed to be used with videotaped home observations of free-play interaction between mother and child. The targeted population is mother-child dyads in which the child has been diagnosed with ID.

Observation of Communicative Interaction (OCI).

Klein, M., & Briggs, M. (1987). Facilitating mother-infant communicative interaction in mothers of high-risk infants. *Journal of Childhood Communication Disorder, 4,* 91.

Developed for use as an informal observational guide, the OCI assesses the communicative interactional strategies used by parents while interacting with their infants. Intended for use as a clinical observation tool, OCI is an informal guide to qualitative assessment of relative strengths and weakness in a caregiver-infant interaction. The data may be used to monitor change over time and to provide guidance in planning individual goals, intervention strategies, and interaction activities. Administered during an observation in which the caregiver and infant engage in a routine interaction, OCI collects data in 10 interaction categories regarding the quality and style of mother-infant interaction, including

- Providing appropriate tactile and kinesthetic stimulation,
- Displaying pleasure,
- Responding to child distress,
- Positioning self for eye-to-eye contact,
- Smiling contingently,
- Varying prosodic features,

- ■ Responding contingently,
- ■ Encouraging conversation,
- ■ Modifying interaction in response to negative cues from the infant, and
- ■ Using communication to teach language.

Preschool Language Scale, Third Edition (PLS-3). Zimmerman, I. L., Steiner, V. G., & Pond, R. E. (1992). San Antonio, TX: The Psychological Corporation.

A standardized and norm referenced evaluative tool, the Preschool Language Scale, Third Edition (PLS-3) is used to assess receptive and expressive language skills in infants and young children ages 2 weeks through 6 years, 11 months of age via direct testing and parent interview. If a language problem exists, the PLS-3 may help in determining if the source of the disorder is auditory, expressive, or an overall problem. The PLS-3 consists of eight receptive and expressive language tasks for each 6-month interval from birth through 4 years, 11 months and eight receptive and expressive tasks for each 12-month interval for 5 and 6 years of age. It also assesses behaviors considered to be language precursors. In addition, the PLS-3 is available in English and a Spanish translation.

The auditory comprehension portion evaluates the child's receptive language skills of attention, semantics (vocabulary and concepts) structure (morphology and syntax) and integrative thinking skills. The expressive portion assesses vocal development, social communication, semantics (vocabulary and concepts), structure (morphology and syntax), and integrative thinking skills. There are three supplemental, optional measures:

- ■ Articulation Screener,
- ■ Language Sample Checklist, and
- ■ Family Information and Suggestions Form.

The PLS-3 also has guidelines for administration to children with severe developmental delays, severe physical impairments, and hearing impairments.

Although administration takes from 15 to 45 minutes, depending on the age of the child, the PLS-3 is not an easy test to give because of the varied tasks involved. As with any evaluative tool, but especially with the PLS-3, practice beforehand is essential. I find it helpful to have someone else score the test while I administer it to a child. In that way, we can keep it moving quickly as I juggle all the parts.

The standardization sample included 1,200 children, ages 2 weeks to 6 years, 11 months, stratified on the basis of parent education level, geographic region, and race/ethnicity according to the 1980 U.S. census. The standardization, which began after June 1991, excluded children with language disorders, those who were more than a month premature, and those who experienced difficulties at birth.

Receptive-Expressive Emergent Language Test, Third Edition (REEL-3). Bzoch, K. R., League, R., & Brown, V. L. (2003). *Receptive-Expressive Emergent Language Test, Third Edition.* Austin, TX: PRO-ED.

A parent interview tool, the Receptive-Expressive Emergent Language Test, Third Edition (REEL-3) is designed to identify infants and toddlers with language impairments or other disabilities that can affect language development. Designed for children birth to age 3 years and taking approximately 20 minutes to administer, the REEL-3 consists of two subtests—receptive and expressive language—and a supplementary Inventory of Vocabulary Words. The REEL-3 is a big improvement over the previous version, especially in the simpler language used in the questions for caregivers.

The REEL-3 is based on current studies of typical development and normed on more than 1,100 infants and toddlers that collectively matched the demographic characteristics of the United States according to the 2000 Census and stratified on the basis of age, gender, race, ethnic group membership, and geographic location.

The reliability for all the test scores is high, and test/retest studies show that the REEL-3 is stable over time. The instrument is also valid when compared to other measures of early childhood language. No items demonstrate a bias based on gender or ethnic identity.

Sequenced Inventory of Communication Development–Revised (SICD-R). Hedrick, D. L., Prather, E. M., & Tobin, A. R. (1984). Los Angeles: Western Psychological Services.

The SICD-R is a standardized measure that screens broad behavioral areas of communication. It evaluates the communication abilities of children at four-month intervals between 4 and 48 months of age. There are two major sections:

- Receptive Scale, which includes behavioral items that test
  - Awareness: Response to speech and sounds other than human vocalization
  - Sound and speech discrimination: Differential response to speech and speech cues
  - Understanding: Response to verbally directed tasks
- Expressive Scale, which includes motor responses, vocal responses, and verbal responses and five factors:
  - Imitating
  - Initiating
  - Responding
  - Verbal Output: Length and grammatical and syntactic structures
  - Articulation for children 2 years and above

All items are sequenced according to the chronological age at which 75 percent or more of children respond. All testing is supplemented by parental reports.

The SICD-R takes 30–75 minutes for administration. A child's attention is engaged through the use of manipulative items. The Receptive Scale is usually administered first, followed by the Expressive. The complete test is not given to a child, but begins where consistent success is anticipated and continues until a ceiling is reached. Both administration and interpretation require fairly extensive practice, and the manual directions are fairly complex.

The test manual reports high validity and reliability. The SICD-R was normed on 252 typically developing children and modified and standardized for Yup'ik Eskimo children, those with ASD and other difficult-to-test children, and children with hearing impairment. There is a Spanish translation. The resulting behavioral/processing profiles can be helpful in developing individualized intervention.

Speech and Language Assessment Scale. Hadley, P. A., & Rice, M. L. (1993). Language Acquisition Preschool Speech and Language Assessment Scale: A resource for assessment and IEP planning. *Seminars in Speech and Language, 14,* 278–288.

The Speech and Language Assessment Scale (SLAS) is a global measure of children's receptive and expressive communicative development, including articulation, in which caregivers or others use a 7-point Likert scale to appraise statements about a child's communication. The statements are global impressions, such as "My child understands language as well as other children."

Transdisciplinary Play-Based Assessment: A functional approach to working with young children (TPBA). Linder, T. (1990). Baltimore, MD: Paul Brookes.

Suitable for arena evaluations, the Transdisciplinary Play-Based Assessment (TPBA) is an assessment tool for children from infancy to 6 years of age. Taking 60–90 minutes to administer, the TPBA assesses cognitive, social-emotional, communication and language, and sensorimotor skills. In addition, the TPBA notes the caregiver-child interaction in both structured and unstructured settings and in a separation-reunion situation. Designed to be used by varying EI professionals and highly individualized and naturalistic, the TPBA results assist with structuring the comprehensive play-based intervention curriculum that is embedded in its overall design. The assessment is designed to be holistic in nature and is both flexible and dynamic.

Using observational and summary worksheets, professionals can give detailed descriptions of a child's abilities in each development a domain. The results are related easily to the suggested intervention program.

Appendix C

Selected Caregiver Questionnaire Examples

In the interest of giving you too much to process all at once, I've selected questions that illustrate how several areas might be addressed in a parent/caregiver questionnaire. These are modified from several questionnaires available online and in professional journals. Please check those sources listed at the end of this appendix. As you read the examples, remember that parents can be very reliable information providers with more structured questions.

Begin with more open-ended questions.

Family Priorities

What is your primary concern?

What are the areas in which you would like more information about your child?

What kinds of information would be most useful to you?

Your Child

What are things your child is really good at doing?

How can we see your child at his or her best?

As more specific information is needed, it may be best to gradually introduce more structured questions. It's not possible to predict all possible answers, so be sure to leave an "Other" option, giving parents and caregivers a little more freedom.

Child's Current Communication

Please tell us how your child lets you know he/she is . . .

Happy? Surprised? Confused? Hungry or thirsty? Sad? Tired? Uncomfortable? Angry?

Please tell us how your child . . .

Asks for information? Comments on people or things in the environment? Directs your attention? Expresses interest in something? Greets others? Indicates that he/she wants to interact? Indicates that he/she does *not* want to interact? Obtains your attention? Requests a "favorite" person? Requests comfort or physical closeness? Requests objects or food? Requests permission? Shows off?

Examples of more structured questions about a child's communication follow.

Does your child (Check those that apply) . . .

_____ Alternate his or her gaze between something he or she wants or is showing and the communication partner?

_____ Change the type (adding gesture or sounds) or quality (louder, with more force) of the signal until the goal is achieved?

_____ Change the type (adding gesture or sounds, replacing one with another) of signal if the partner seems to have misinterpreted the child's meaning?

_____ Persist with these behaviors until his or her goal is attained or failure is obvious? (For example, will he or she continue to reach and make noises until a desired object is obtained?)

_____ Respond positively, such as smiling or calming down when the goal is accomplished?

_____ Stop his or her signal when the goal is accomplished, such as obtaining a desired object or gaining your attention?

_____ Wait expectantly for a response from the partner?

Please check all the other methods your child uses to communicate.

_____ Makes gestures, such as pointing or reaching
_____ Makes manual signs
_____ Uses non-letter symbols, such as Blissymbols or Rhebus pictures
_____ Uses objects
    _____ Actual object, such as a cup to indicate *I'm thirsty*
    _____ Miniature object, such as toy dishes
    _____ Part of a real object to represent object/activity
_____ Uses picture symbols
    _____ Color or black-and-white drawing
    _____ Line drawing, such as Picture Communication Symbols
    _____ Photo
_____ Uses short phrases or sentences
_____ Uses sounds but not words
_____ Uses words or consistent sounds to name objects, actions, or people
_____ Uses written letters or words
_____ Withdraws or turns away from others
_____ Other: (Please specify)

Symbol Use

Please *underline* all the words your child understands.
Please *place a check* (√) before all words your child speaks.
Please *place an X* before all words your child gestures, signs, or conveys in other ways, such as pictures.

airplane/plane	balloon	bike	bottle	bubble
all	banana	bird	bottom/butt	bug
all gone	bath	blanket	bowl	bunny
apple	bathtub	block	boy	bus
arm	bear (teddy)	boat	bread	bye/bye-bye
baby	bed	booboo	breakfast	cake
bad	bee	book	broken	candy
ball	big	boot	brush	car

cat/kitty	feed	key	pig/piggy	sun
catch	feet	kiss	pillow	swing
cereal	finger	knee	pizza	teddy bear
chair	fish	leg	plate	teeth
cheese	fix	light	please	telephone
chicken	flower	little	potty	thank you
chin	food	look	pretty	there
choo-choo	foot	love	pretzel	thirsty
church	French fries	lunch	puppy	throw
clap	girl	mama/mommy	purse	thumb
clean	glasses	man	push	tired
clock	gloves	marker	radio	tissue
coat	go	McDonald's	read	toast
cold	go bed	me	ride	toe
comb	go bye-bye	meat	rock	toothbrush
come	go night-night	milk	run	towel
cookie	go out	mine	school	toy
cough	good	mirror	see	train
cow	Grandma	money	shhhh	tree
cracker	Grandpa	monkey	shirt	truck
crib	grapes	moon	shoe	tummy/belly
cup	gum	more	show (me)	TV
Dada/Daddy	hair	mouth	shut/close	uh-oh
dance	hamburger	nap	sing	under
dark	hand	night-night	sink	up
diaper	happy	no	sit/sit down	walk
dirty	hat	nose	sky	want
doctor	heavy	nugget	sleep	wash
dog/doggie	help	off	slide	water
doll	here	old	snack	wet
don't	hi	on	sneaker	what
done	horse/horsie	open	snow	what's that
done (all done)	hot	orange	so big	woman
down	hot dog	out	soap	wow
dress	house	own name	sock	yes
drink	hug	pajamas/	soda/pop	you
duck	huh?	jammies	soup	yucky
ear	hungry	paper	spaghetti	yum/yummy
eat	I	park	spoon	zoo
egg	ice cream	pattycake	stick	
eye	in	peekaboo	stinky	
face	juice	peepee	stop	
fall down	jump	phone	stove	

Please list other words your child understands or uses.

Partner's Communication Behaviors and Strategies

I talk with my child mostly . . .

_____ For his or her enjoyment. Please give examples.
_____ To complete needed tasks or chores. Please give examples.
_____ To direct his or her behavior. Please give examples.
_____ To discipline him or her. Please give examples.
_____ To teach communication behaviors. Please give examples.

What do you do when you are trying to keep a "conversation" with your child going? (Check all applicable answers. Please circle the one or two that work best.)

____ Add related objects, such as more toys
____ Allow time for my child to initiate or respond
____ Ask questions
____ Do not change my behavior
____ Elaborate on my child's message
____ Focus on a shared object or topic
____ Fulfill my child's requests
____ Imitate my child's message
____ Increase my number of questions
____ Look at my child or the focus of his or her interest
____ Make a spoken or gestural comment about or response to my child's message
____ Move closer
____ Show interest in whatever my child is focusing on
____ Smile at or touch my child
____ Other (Please specify)

How do you create or take advantage of opportunities to communicate with your child? (Check all applicable answers. Please circle the one or two that work best.)

____ Ask questions
____ Be alert to my child's state of alertness as a sign that he/she is ready
____ Become more animated
____ Choose sensory conditions that increase his/her communication (movement, music, touch/no touch, temperature, texture of materials, etc.)
____ Create communication opportunities
____ Do not change my behavior
____ Elaborate on my child's message
____ Engage in communication attempts when I believe he/she is ready
____ Entice my child with interesting objects
____ Identify when my child communicates best
____ Imitate my child
____ Increase my loudness or emphasis
____ Look at my child expectantly
____ Move closer
____ Pick the times, routines, or activities that are most conducive to communication
____ Show interest in whatever my child is focusing on
____ Other (Please specify)

Which styles seem to work best when interacting with your child?

____ Changing the way I talk, such as varying my loudness or pitch
____ Eye contact
____ Facial expression
____ Facing, face-to-face
____ Offering an activity or a choice
____ Speaking directly to my child
____ Speaking in single words or short phrases
____ Speaking in whole sentences as I would with an adult
____ Talking about what my child is interested in
____ Using only gestures
____ Using only signs
____ Using only speech
____ Using speech combined with gestures
____ Using speech combined with pictures or objects
____ Using speech combined with signing
____ Waiting for response
____ Other (Please specify)

Environment

What adults or teens caregivers, including yourself, does your child interact with on a regular basis? Please place a number behind each name indicating the approximate number of hours spent with this person in a typical week.

1. _____ (hrs/wk)   2. _____ (hrs/wk)
3. _____ (hrs/wk)   4. _____ (hrs/wk)
5. _____ (hrs/wk)   6. _____ (hrs/wk)
7. _____ (hrs/wk)   8. _____ (hrs/wk)

In a typical day, how much time in hours or parts of hours does your child spend . . .

____ Awake but playing alone   ____ Directly talking with a teen or adult
____ Looking at books   ____ Playing with an adult
____ Playing with another child   ____ Playing with a group of children
____ Talking with a teen or adult   ____ Watching TV
     to accomplish a task   ____ Other (Please specify)
     (i.e. get dressed)

Concluding Remarks

What are the biggest obstacles to others' understanding your child?
What do you expect from the assessment process?
How would you like to be part of your child's assessment?

____ Answer questions   ____ Assist the other team members
____ Help my child participate   ____ Hold my child
____ Make suggestions   ____ Observe
____ Record results   ____ Other:

Remember, these are only selected examples. These questions were adapted from several existing lists of early communication behaviors (Golinkoff, 1986; Olswang, Bain, & Johnson, 1992; Rossetti, 1990; Shane & Grabowski, 1986; Siegel & Wetherby, 2000; Snell & Loncke, 2002; Wetherby & Prizant, 1990; Wetherby, Alexander, & Prizant, 1998).

Appendix D

Developmental Milestones

Begin at the age that replies to the questionnaire (Appendix A) suggest. There is no set number of responses required to place a child at a certain age. In fact, many children will have behaviors at more than one age level. Several commercially available assessment tools also can be used to accomplish this task.

This list of developmental milestones is a guide, *not* a normed diagnostic tool, and is not a substitute for professional developmental assessments. This list can be used to supplement other assessment indicators. Remember, there's a broad age range even for typically developing children.

1-Month-Old

Does the child . . .

Startle (react to) or show interest in sound?
Appear to recognize your voice by becoming excited if calm or calm if excited?
Quiet down with a soothing voice or when picked up?
Make brief eye contact during feeding?
Cry when upset?
Produce pleasure sounds?
Sucks vigorously, possibly after some initial difficulty?
Prefer bright colors and black/white contrasts?
Enjoy feeling different textures against her skin?

> Cause for concern if child . . .
> Lacks awareness of environment, especially sound
> Lacks responsiveness
> Lacks responsiveness to sound
> Has problems with sucking and swallowing

2-Month-Old

Does the child . . .

Have different cries for different reasons?
Make cooing and gooing pleasure sounds in the back of the throat, such as *g-g-guh* and *k-k-kuh*?
Make noises when not crying, such as grunts and growls or squeaks and squeals?
Pay attention and make eye contact when spoken to in face-to-face communication?
Turn the head toward sounds?
Smile at the sound of mother's voice and/or sight of her face?
Reach for interesting objects?

> Cause for concern if child . . .
>   Does not cry differently when wet, hungry, or tired
>   Does not make pleasure sounds
>   Does not show interest in the human face

3-Month-Old

Does the child . . .

Take turns making sounds with adult?
Produce single syllable cooing ("guh" or "buh")?
Vocalize two syllables together occasionally?
Produce primarily vowel sounds?
Produce several different kinds of sounds?
Make sounds when adult does?
Laugh while playing with adult?
Look directly at adult and watch adult's mouth?
Try to find a speaker who is out of view?
Show more interest in people than in objects?
Signal distress, hunger, and pleasure in consistent ways?

> Cause for concern if child . . .
>   Does not vocalize when face to face with others
>   Does not produce vowel-like sounds
>   Lacks awareness of others

4-Month-Old

Does the child . . .

Respond with distress to an angry voice?
Babble vowels and *g* and *k*, sometimes in consonant-vowel (CV) syllables?
Vocalize in response to your words and sounds?
Vocalize in response to singing?
Make a greater variety of sounds than previously?
Smile or laugh?
Change pitch while producing sounds?
Turn toward familiar sounds?
Show interest in people and objects around him or her?
Reach for and grasp objects?
Anticipate feeding?
Sit propped up for 10 to 15 minutes?
Roll over?
Maintain eye contact with you for a longer time than when he was younger?

> Cause for concern if child . . .
>   Does not search for sounds
>   Is unable to direct attention or focus and is easily overstimulated
>   Does not make some consonant sounds
>   Does not show interest in and reach for objects
>   Does not move by rolling

5-Month-Old

Does the child . . .
  Make sounds while playing with objects?
  Blow raspberries?
  Squeal or whisper?
  Make protest sounds when desired objects removed?
  Initiate "talking" with eye contact and sounds?
  "Talk" to people by making sounds?
  Have more consonant-vowel (CV) syllables when vocalizing?
  Make sounds when alone or with toys?
  Smile and make sounds at his or her own reflection in a mirror?
  Stop crying when sees familiar person, such as mother?
  Smile when playing alone?
  Turn her or his head when name is called?

> Cause for concern if child . . .
>   Does not have variety of sounds
>   Does not make eye contact with familiar people and show recognition
>   Treats people and objects similarly
>   Has catastrophic responses to others' attempts to interact

6-Month-Old

Does the child . . .
  Babble with *more b, p,* and *m* sounds?
  Repeat sounds that he/she hears, such as *ba-ba*?
  Vocalize when playing alone or with others?
  Grunt and growl?
  Make angry sounds of displeasure?
  Initiate babbling to people?
  Vocalize to show displeasure, get attention, or display enthusiasm?
  Recognize some word-action combinations such as *no* (with head shake) and *bye-bye* (with wave)?
  Respond to a pleasant voice with smile or laugh?
  Squeal when excited?
  Respond differently to strangers?
  Seem to know when he or she hears an angry or a pleasant voice?
  Sit and hold up head without support?

> Cause for concern if child . . .
>   Does not display variety of sounds, such as cooing, gurgling, laughing, squealing
>   Does not respond differently to known and unknown others
>   Cannot sit without assistance

7-Month-Old

Does the child . . .
  Babble in three or more syllables, repeating his or her own sounds?
  Make several sounds on one breath?
  Make speech sounds and shout for attention?
  "Talk" to toys by making sounds while playing?
  Look at some family members when their names are mentioned?

Consistently respond to your voice and physical gestures?
Imitate some gestures of others, such as waving bye-bye?
Recognize mother or father on sight?
Inspect, grab, and pull objects and toys?
Sit unsupported?
Sit and use her hands to play or explore?
Hold out her arms to be picked up?

> **Cause for concern if child . . .**
>   Does not babble
>   Has little variety in babbling
>   Has little interest in others and lacks eye contact
>   Does not initiate interactions

8-Month-Old

Does the child . . .
"Sing" along with familiar songs?
Produce nonidentical babbling? (Babbles in which the syllables are not the same, like *beba* or *bada*? Not all babies do this.)
Imitate gestures?
Sound like she's talking and having a conversation?
Understand familiar words, especially when accompanied by gestures?
Recognize his or her name? (She may stop what she's doing to look at you.)
Stop when you say "no"?
Wave bye-bye?
Look at a few common objects when they're named?
Predict that it's time to play a game? (She may become excited, smile, or make eye contact.)
Play pat-a-cake and peek-a-boo?
Respond physically, orally, or with gestures when she sees a familiar person?

> **Cause for concern if child . . .**
>   Does not imitate some gestures, especially within social routines, such as waving bye-bye
>   Does not have some consonants in babbling
>   Does not participate in anticipatory games, such as *I'm gonna get you*
>   Does not raise self up on hands and knees

9-Month-Old

Does the child . . .
Babble with more *b*, *p*, and *m* sounds?
Produce strings of sounds with adult intonation?
Use gestures, such as pointing, head shaking, or reaching?
Mimic sounds and syllables?
Whine when she wants something—either with or without a gesture?
Respond consistently to "no"? (Ignoring you consistently doesn't count.)
Participate in communication games, such as "How big is ____? SO BIG!"?
Look at different pictures for up to one minute? (The important thing is that she notices pictures, not the length of time. As usual, she'll pay attention longer if you talk about the pictures.)
Hand things back and forth?

> Cause for concern if child . . .
>   Does not imitate others physically
>   Does not babble in more than single syllables
>   Does not "show off" for attention

10-Month-Old

Does the child . . .

Use meaningful words that you understand? (Not all children will begin this early, but you may hear "mama," "dada," or "me" used appropriately.)
Say "uh-oh" appropriately?
String together four or more syllables with adult-like intonation?
Gesture and vocalize his intentions?
Imitate sounds, such as coughs, sneezes, or tongue clicks?
Vocalize to call others?
Imitate facial expressions?
Imitate sounds produced by another speaker that he or she has already produced on his or her own?
Use his voice to get attention?
Wave and say "Bye-bye"?
Hand you requested objects?
Pay attention to both a speaker and an object simultaneously?
Look at a person who calls his name?
Crawl?
Sit unsupported for a long time while playing with toys?
Try to "help" with routines like dressing or bathing?
Pull himself up to a stand?
Imitate adult actions like waving?

> Cause for concern if child . . .
>   Does not show objects in his hand
>   Does not transfer gaze from person to object or object to person easily
>   Does not produce some vocalizations that sound like words in structure
>   Does not mimic others' sound-making
>   Lacks a consistent patterns of reduplicative (repetitive) babbling (*ba-ba-ba*)

11-Month-Old

Does the child . . .

Imitate nonspeech sounds?
Imitate speech and gestures?
Point when you ask "Where's X?"
Produce sound sequences that are not real words but are used consistently, such as "aga" to mean *dog*?
Perform a routine activity, such as putting blocks away, when requested?
Initiate "peek-a-boo" and "so big"?

> **Cause for concern if child . . .**
> Does not look at one or two common objects (doggie, Daddy) when they are named
> Does not respond to her name
> Does not indicate a request for object while focusing on object
> Does not have distal gestures, such as pointing or requesting

12-Month-Old

Does the child . . .
Babble when alone?
Listen when others talk?
Respond verbally when you ask him to say something?
Repeat sounds or gestures when you laugh?
Say one or more words consistently? *A child may be in need of intervention if this does not occur by 18 months.*
"Talk" throughout the day to persons and objects?
Vocalize to songs and rhythm play?
Try to follow simple directions?
Identify one or two body parts by name?
Cruise (walking around while holding onto furniture)?
Stand alone?
Drink from a glass with help?
Respond physically to most requests?

> **Cause for concern if child . . .**
> Lacks adult intonation even though words not used
> Babbles only in repeated syllables (*ba-ba*) but not variegated or different ones (*ba-te-ga*)
> Does not babble and gesture concurrently

13-Month-Old

Does the child . . .
Say five or more single words?
Use both sounds and words more during interactions?
Tell what she wants through words, sounds, pointing, and gesturing?
Hand objects to you when you ask for them?
Understand approximately 10 words?
Help with dressing or bathing by holding out her foot or arm?
Look at pictures in book and help turn the pages?
Imitate other children physically and vocally?
Understand words and phrases when gestures are used?
Walk without assistance?

> **Cause for concern if child . . .**
> Seems to understand and respond to fewer than 10 words
> Produces only 3–4 consonant sounds
> Produces only 3–4 vowel sounds

14-Month-Old

Does the child . . .

Shake her head *yes* and *no?*
Imitate some animal sounds?
Imitate most one-syllable words?
Comprehend simple questions? At this age most children understand *what* and *where* questions?
Perform some actions (e.g., *pat, kiss, hug*) with verbal instruction without gestures?
Enjoy acting out routines from home, such as housework?
Explore physically?

> Cause for concern if child . . .
>   Doesn't attempt to imitate some words
>   Does not explore spontaneously

15-Month-Old

Does the child . . .

Gesture and verbalize either simultaneously or in sequence?
Say 10 or more single words?
Identify three or more body parts by name?
Use single words within jargon?
"Sing" independently?
Understand the names of many common objects?
Respond to two-step commands?
Use objects symbolically, creatively, or for a nonintended purpose? (This can be a close call. Random actions don't count. Using a shoe as a doll's car, or a small bottle as a cell phone is the kind of thing we're looking for.)
Point to pictures of things when they're named?
Help turn pages—often more than one at a time—when you share a book?
Scribble with crayons or markers?

> Cause for concern if child . . .
>   Doesn't make sounds and gestures together
>   Doesn't persist in communication when others fail to respond
>   Cannot follow simple commands (i.e., *splash water*)

16-Month-Old

Does the child . . .

Ask "What that?" (Variants include "Wha'," "Tha'," "Dat," and "Wassat.")
Request "More"?
Consistently respond by pointing to the right body parts, especially facial ones, when you name them? (Common body parts include mouth, ear, nose, hand, foot, fingers, and toes.)
Retrieve objects requested by name, not gestures?
Listen as rhymes and songs are repeated a few times?
Try to throw or catch a ball?
Pull a toy as he walks?

> Cause for concern if child . . .
>   Seems to understand and respond to fewer than 20 words
>   Does not engage in play or book "reading" with adults

17-Month-Old

Does the child . . .
>   Use the owner's name to show possession?
>   Say "no" consistently and meaningfully?
>   Say "hi" and "bye" (or other similar words) appropriately?
>   Repeat single words in a conversation?
>   Request assistance from adults?
>   Try to influence the behavior of others?
>   Feed himself (complete with spills)?
>   Walk up stairs with one hand held by adult?

> Cause for concern if child . . .
>   Is over-reliant on gestures with no verbalization

18-Month-Old

Does the child . . .
>   Follow two-step commands with the same object (i.e., "Hug doll, then feed doll")?
>   Understand about 50 single words? *A child may be considered as having a severe speech/language delay when the child has a vocabulary of less than 30 words at 24 months.*
>   Say 20 or more single words?
>   Protest with words, especially "NO"?
>   Use consonants *g, k, b, p, m, w, t, d, n,* and *h*?
>   Talk more and rely on gestures less?
>   Enjoy messy activities such as finger painting and "decorating with food"?
>   Occasionally put two words together?
>   Seldom fall while walking?
>   Walk trying to kick a ball?

> Cause for concern if child . . .
>   Doesn't spontaneously say any recognizable words
>   Seems to understand and respond to fewer than 20 words
>   Lacks vocabulary growth in 6 months
>   Exhibits regression in language or begins echoing phrases of others

19- to 20-Month-Old

Does the child . . .
>   Imitate two- to three-word utterances?
>   Combine two words occasionally? *It is recommended that a child be considered as having a severe speech/language delay when the child has no two-word combinations at 36 months.*
>   Use words during pretend play?
>   Understand and respond to verbal commands, such as *stop that, sit down,* and *come here?*

Imitate environmental noises, such as dogs barking or car horns?
Have 20 or more words in her vocabulary?
Use *mine*, *me*, and *you*?
Enjoy games in which she names things?
Talk for many different purposes, such as asking questions (*Horsie? Where Mommy?*),
     answering questions, greeting, and demanding?
Pretend to "dance"?

> **Cause for concern if child . . .**
>   Produces fewer than 10 words spontaneously
>   Uses words as names exclusively

21- to 22-Month-Old

Does the child . . .
     Mix words and jargon?
     Engage in dialogue with adults?
     Enjoy simple stories?
     Point to appropriate pictures when named?
     Turn book pages one at a time?
     Understand *he*, *she*, and *it*?

> **Cause for concern if child . . .**
>   Produces fewer than 20 words spontaneously
>   Has no word combinations

23- to 24-Month-Old

Does the child . . .
     Refer to herself by name?
     Use some pronouns, such as *me, you, mine, he, she,* and *it*?
     Understand new words quickly?
     Relate personal experiences?
     Use four-word phrases occasionally?
     Understand simple sentences?
     Scribble with a crayon or pencil?
     Draw in a circular motion if shown?

> **Cause for concern if child . . .**
>   Produces fewer than 30 words spontaneously
>   Has largely unintelligible speech
>   Has frequent tantrums in place of speech (Be reasonable here; we are approach-
>   ing the dreaded "terrible twos.")
>   Asks no questions

Sources:
Miller, J. F., & Paul, R. (1995). *The clinical assessment of language comprehension.* Baltimore,
MD: Paul Brookes.

Owens, R. E. (2004). *Help your baby talk.* New York: Perigee.

Owens, R. E. (2008). *Language development: An introduction* (7th Ed.). Boston: Pearson Education.

Appendix E
Interactional Observation

CHILD BEHAVIORS	COMMUNICATION EVENT	TOTAL
Makes no response		
Makes eye contact with object		
Makes eye contact with partner		
Alternates gaze between object and partner		
Touches object		
Touches partner		
Closes distance to partner		
Opens distance to partner		
Turns toward partner		
Turns away from partner		
Pushes partner		
Pulls partner		
Makes facial expression		
Vocalizes		
Uses recognizable gesture		
Exhibits challenging behavior		
Touches pictorial symbol		
Signs		

Verbalizes single word																																	
Verbalizes multiword utterance																																	

PARTNER BEHAVIORS	COMMUNICATION EVENT																																TOTAL
Faces child																																	
Is at child's physical level																																	
Shares joint attention																																	
Speaks directly to child																																	
Makes eye contact with child																																	
Imitates child																																	
Follows child's lead				–																													
Elaborates or extends child's behavior																																	
Fulfills child's intent																																	
Responds in timely manner																																	
Makes no contingent response																																	
Redirects child's behavior																																	
Ignores child's behavior																																	
Cues child to respond with request																																	
Cues child to respond with question																																	
Cues child to respond with sentence completion																																	
Allows time for child to respond																																	
Shows positive affect																																	
Shows negative affect																																	
Persists if misunderstanding occurs																																	
Requests clarification																																	

continued

PARTNER BEHAVIORS	COMMUNICATION EVENT																														TOTAL
Uses appropriate level of communication																															
Vocalizes																															
Gestures or touches child																															
Signs																															
Uses visual pictorial symbol																															
Verbalizes single word																															
Verbalizes multiword utterance																															
COMMUNICATION SUCCESS	COMMUNICATION EVENT																														TOTAL
Successful																															
Unsuccessful																															

Appendix F

Examples of Dynamic Assessment

TABLE F.1 **Dynamic Assessment of One-Word Receptive Language**

Level of Assessment	% of Children by Age	Expected Response	Test Format	Possible Mediated Teaching Format
Joint reference (If child cannot share attention, receptive understanding will be very difficult to assess.)		Look at, move toward, or act as directed	Within a play format, direct child's attention to high-interest objects and activities using *both* words and gestures.	Hold object before child, point to it and say "Look at X." If child does not comply, say "Look at X," and gently touch the child's cheek to turn the child to face the object. Occasionally, children will resist or react negatively to being touched. In these cases, say "Look at X" and move it into the child's field of vision. Make a game of this. When the child is successful without the touch or the object thrust into his field of vision, return to the test mode. Remember, object names are not important here, joint reference is.
Person name and object name	100% at 10–12 mo. & 100% at 13–15 mo	Attention to person or object (Look at, show, get, act on, indicate in another way)	Place several objects on the floor and have family members in the room. Obtain the child's attention. Cue the child by saying "Show me X," "Find X," or "Where's X?" Be careful not to look at or point to the object or person named. Repeat label at least twice.	Simplify the task to two objects or people. Talk about each, then cue the child as before but with only two choices. Because there is a 50% chance of being correct, the task must be performed more than once. If the child is still incorrect, talk about each item again, then cue the child as before but provide a locational prompt with the named item closer to the child. Nonresponse or an incorrect response may indicate that the child does not understand the task. Go to a single item and cue the child again, using a physical assist if needed, then return to the task with a locational prompt. When the child is correct, return to the test mode.
Action name	75% at 16–18 mo.	Behavioral compliance	While playing on the floor, obtain the child's attention. Using object names tested positively above, ask the child to Perform unconventional behaviors, such as handing the child truck and asking him to "Kiss truck"; Perform an action from several possibilities, such as "Sit" or "Doll sit" when has bowl and spoon, toy chair, and ball before child; or Perform action on self, such as "Jump" or "Sit"*	If the child is unsuccessful, check with caregivers to ensure that the child knows the action words being tested. Personally, I prefer the second two test modes. In the several possibilities with toys, reduce the number of toys so only one possibility exists, such as the doll and chair, then cue with "Sit" or "Doll sit." If child does not comply, use a physical prompt along with the verbal cue. Some children find "Action + object" structures easier to comprehend, so it may help to alter the cue to a "Push ball" or "Eat cookie" format. If the child does not comply, perform the action for the child after you give the verbal cue. This method is also helpful when asking the child to perform the action ("Jump") on herself. When the child can perform the action without prompting, return to the test mode.

*Be careful that the child is not required to use as yet undeveloped symbolic play skills. For example, asking a child to "Eat" when a spoon and empty bowl are provided, requires a level of symbolic skills that the child may not possess.

Source: Based on Miller, Chapman, Branston, & Reichle, 1980; Miller & Paul, 1995; Owens, 1982.

TABLE F.2 **Dynamic Semantic Assessment of Multiword Receptive Language within a Play Format**

Type	% of Children by Age	Expected Response	Test Format	Possible Mediated Teaching Format
Possessor + Possessed	83% at 19–21 mos.	Pointing or indicating	Place several similar items before the child, such as several hats belonging to different family members. Ask child "Where's Mommy's X?" It's important that the objects be similar. Otherwise, the child will respond to the object name rather than the possessor plus the object.	Have the possessor take the object and use it, such as putting on the hat. Say "Mommy's hat." Ask "Whose hat? Mommy's hat." Ask child again "Where's Mommy's hat?" If still unsuccessful, try a different cue, such as "Touch Mommy's hat." If unsuccessful, use physical assist to aid point.
Action + Object	67% at 19–21 mos.	Behavioral compliance	Place several items before the child, requiring her to respond to both the action and the object. Ask the child to "Push ball" from a group of objects that might be pushed (truck) or thrown (ball).	Break cue down into two one-word utterances, as in "Ball. Where's ball?" Once child has the object, say "Push." As child attempts say "Yes, push ball." Stop, wait, retry.
Agent + Action	58% at 19–21 mos.	Behavioral compliance	Place several objects before the child, requiring her to respond to both the agent and the action. Direct the child, "Doll eat." Possible choices might include *dog eat, doll sit, dog sit, horse eat*, and so on.	Break cue down into two one-word utterances, as in "Doll. Where's doll?" Once child has the object, say "Doll eat" as you demonstrate the action. Repeat this with various agents, then return to the original cue.
Negative + X		Pointing or indicating	Have two containers, one full, one empty. Say "Show me 'No Juice.'"	Show child full container and say "Juice." Show child empty container and say "No juice. All gone." Present both containers and recue. Try with containers with other contents.

continued

TABLE F.2 **Dynamic Semantic Assessment of Multiword Receptive Language within a Play Format** (*continued*)

Type	% of Children by Age	Expected Response	Test Format	Possible Mediated Teaching Format
Recurrent + X		Pointing or indicating	Place a small quantity of a desirable treat from a full container into a second container and encourage the child to eat it. When the treat is consumed, ask "Where's (Show me) more cookie (Cheerios, chips, etc.)?"	Show child full container and say "More cookie." Show child the empty container and say "No cookie." Ask child to "Show me more cookie." Present both containers and recue. Try with containers with other contents.
X + location		Pointing or indicating	Place identical objects in the same location and ask the child to show you one of them, as in "Show me boy (in) car." Check by asking for the other object, as in "Show me boy (on) chair."	Hold both dolls, place each in a different location, naming the location as you do, such as "Chair. Boy Chair. Car. Boy car." Recue the child. If unsuccessful, have the child help you place the dolls as you comment. Recue.
Attribute + entity		Pointing, indicating or giving	Place two contrasting items (big-little) before the child and ask for one, as in "Show (give) me big ball" or "Where's big ball?" Stay away from colors. They are difficult for many children.	Hold objects in different hands, name each, as in "Ball." Comment on each, as in "Big" and "Little." Recue. If unsuccessful, say "Big ball, little ball, show me big ball."

Note: Only use words previously assessed in single-word utterances or reported by parents.
Source: Based on Miller, Chapman, Branston, & Reichle, 1980; Miller & Paul, 1995; Owens, 1982.

TABLE F.3 Dynamic Assessment of Single-Symbol Expressive Language

Level of Assessment	Expected Response	Test Format	Possible Mediated Teaching Format
Agent	Child says word	Ask child "Who's that?" or "What's that?" (dog, cat) while pointing.	For common associations, try a fill-in-the-blank procedure, as in "Daddy and ___." You might also name the individual and then ask, as in "Mommy" while pointing, "Daddy" while pointing, then back to "Who's this?" If unsuccessful, say the person's name and immediately ask, as in "Mommy! Who's this?" If still unsuccessful, ask the cue followed by the response, as in "Who's this? Say 'Mommy.'"
Action	Child says word	Ask child "What's he doing?" ("What do?") while pointing or "What do you want (to do)?" while poised to perform. You can use a behavior chain interruption strategy in which you stop a popular action and then ask.	If the child indicates that he/she wants to perform or continue to perform an action, say the actions name and recue with "What do you want?" or "What should you make the doll do?" If still unsuccessful, ask the question followed by the answer, and recue the child, as in "What do you want? Jump! What do you want?" If there is no response or an incorrect one, try "What do you want? Say 'Jump.'"
Object	Child says word	Ask child "What's that?" while pointing to an object.	Say the object name and repeat the cue. If unsuccessful, cue, reply, and cue again, as in "What's that? Bike! What's that?" If still unsuccessful, repeat this step but ask the child to imitate the word, as in "What's that? Say 'Bike.'"
Recurrent	Child says word *more* or *'nuther*	Give child a very small snack, such as a few pieces of cereal. When it's consumed, ask the child "What do you want?" ("What want?")	If you get the name of the item instead of more, reply with "More" and give it to the child. Recue. If unsuccessful, reply, "Say 'More.'" Ask again. Repeat with several items and actions, so the word generalizes and is not associated with any one entity.
Negative	Child says word *no*, possible *gone*	Have child search for an item. Ask for the entity in each location. "Doggie?" A variation is to have child consume something, then the adult asks for it. A third variation is to ask "Is this X?" when it clearly is not.	Continue with the activity and model the expected response. Have the child repeat, as in "Is the doggie in the cup? No! Say 'No!", shake your head, "Say 'No!'"
Attribute	Child says word	Offer the child a choice of two desirable but contrasting (big-little) objects and ask "Which one do you want?"	Name the contrast while holding the two objects in different hands, then recue, as in "Big. Little. Which do you want?" If unsuccessful, say "Take one," then comment and recue as in "Take one. You took 'Big' (or 'the big one'), 'Which one?'" If unsuccessful and you know the child's preference or the child has already taken one, you can cue followed by the answer and a request to imitate, as in "Which do you have? Big? Say 'Big.'"
Location	Child says word (usually not *here* or *there*)	Place an object in a location and ask where it is, as in "Where's book?"	Name the location as you place the item and recue, as in "Bed. Where's book?" If unsuccessful, cue, reply, and ask the child to imitate, as in "Where's book. Bed. Say 'Bed.'"

This list is not gospel, and all the semantic functions herein need not be assessed. Rather, the list is suggested.

Be careful that the words asked are in the child's repertoire or are possible given the child's sound and syllable repertoire. Words tested in production should have also been tested previously in reception.

TABLE F.4 Dynamic Assessment of Multisymbol Expressive Language

LEVEL OF ASSESSMENT	EXPECTED RESPONSE	TEST FORMAT	POSSIBLE MEDIATED TEACHING FORMAT
Spontaneous two-word utterance	Child says nonimitated, meaningful two-word utterance	Depending on the semantic structure and the intent, the cue will vary. Suggestions are given below. It is not necessary to test all possible combinations. If the child has previously used some of the structures suggested, you do not need to test.	If unable to get a response from the child, supply the response and cue the child again. If still unsuccessful, cue, say the response. If unsuccessful, cue, say "Say X," and wait. It's possible at this point that the child either does not understand the task or cannot or will not produce a two-word utterance. Have another adult model the desired response, or you can break it into two successive one-word responses and try through a series of single-word imitated response and pointing to get at least one of the words in a non-imitated response. For example, you could say "Say 'Ride'" and when the child responds, point to bike, and hopefully get "Ride bike."

There are multiple ways to elicit different intentions and different semantic-syntactic structures. Below are a few ideas. Be creative. Think about your target, know its parameters, then imagine how you might elicit that. For example, an answer follows a question, a reply follows a statement, a declaration, as I'm defining it, is spontaneous.

TARGET STRUCTURE: TO ELICIT . . .	EXPECTED RESPONSE	SUGGESTED CUES
A greeting	*Hi (Bye), Name.*	"Hi (or bye), Juan!" with wave.
A request containing nomination	*That X.*	"Let's play. I want THAT BABY." Look expectantly toward the child.
An answer containing nomination	*That X.*	"THAT BABY. What's that?"
A reply containing nomination	*That X.*	"Tell me about this?"
A question containing nomination	*What that (this)?*	Play a game in which each of you asks the other what something is. Roger Brown called this "The Original Name Game." Pull an object out of a bag and ask "What's this?" After child's response, say, "Your turn" or "Now you do [it]."
An answer containing negation	*No X.*	Hold up a known object, name it incorrectly. "Is this X?" An alternative is to point to a full cup and say "This juice." Hold an empty cup upside down and say "This juice?"
A reply containing negation	*No X.*	Tell the child "This is X" when it clearly is not. An alternative is to say to the child "Tell me not to [action]." Think of the children's book "Five Little Monkeys Jumping on the Bed." "Tell the monkeys not to jump." Better still, set up a game into which the child can insert "No jump!" spontaneously without any cue. Now we have a negative declaration.
An answer containing an action	*Doggie jump.* *Eat cookie.*	"Doggie jump" is simply an example. The form is "Agent + Action." Likewise, "Eat cookie" is in the form Action + Object." Both forms convey the notion of action. Either can be elicited with "What happened?" Alternatives are "What's happening?" or "What are/is you [or anyone else] doing?" Perform the action or have the child perform it, then ask.

TABLE F.4 **Dynamic Assessment of Multisymbol Expressive Language** (*continued*)

TARGET STRUCTURE: TO ELICIT . . .	EXPECTED RESPONSE	SUGGESTED CUES
A reply containing an action	*Doggie jump.* *Eat cookie.*	Perform an action or have the child or a parent perform the action and then say "Tell me what happened."
A declaration containing an action	*Doggie jump.* *Eat cookie.*	Set up a routine or game in which something happens and is then commented upon. Take your turn, perform the action again or have the child do it, then wait expectantly and possibly nod toward the child, conveying that it is the child's turn.
A request for an action	*Eat cookie.* *Throw ball.*	Engage in an activity the child enjoys, stop, and when the child indicates a desire to continue, say "What do you want?" or "What want?"
A question containing an action	*Throw ball?* *Push car.*	Prepare to perform an action, such as having the ball in your hand or the car on the floor between you and the child. Say "Guess what I'm going to do?"
An answer containing an attribution	*Big ball.*	Hold two objects that differ in very obvious ways (not color). Describe one, as in "Little ball." Ask the child "Which one is this?"
A reply containing an attribute	*Little hat.*	Hold two contrasting objects and say "Tell me about this one."
A declaration containing an attribute	*Big cup.*	Hold two contrasting objects, move one toward the child and say "Little cup." Retract the object, move the other object toward the child and nod, making eye contact with the child.
A request containing an attribute	*Big teddy.*	Place two desirable objects before the child. Say "I want little teddy." Take the little teddy and cuddle it. Put it back and wait. More modeling may be required before the child understands the task.
A question with an attribute	*Little cookie?*	Have several contrasting objects on the table. Name each using the attribute as in "Big cookie." Remove all items, place one in a bag, nod to another adult and ask him/her to guess which one is in the bag. If the guess is incorrect, nod to the child.
An answer containing a recurrent	*More candy.*	Place one item and a pile of similar items before the child. Name the single item, such as "Candy." Ask the child "What's this?" or "What do you see?"
A reply containing a recurrent	*More car.*	Place one item and a pile of similar items before the child. Name the single item, such as "Car." Say to the child "Tell me about these" while pointing to the pile of items.
A declaration containing a recurrent	*More block.*	Place one item and a pile of similar items before the child. Name the single item, such as "Block." Point to the pile and say "More ball." Replace the items by others in the same arrangement and point to the single one saying "Car." Then point to the pile of items and look at the child expectantly.
A request containing a recurrent	*More juice.*	Have another adult model drinking a small amount of juice and asking "More juice." Pour a small amount into the adult's cup. Repeat this procedure with the child.

continued

TABLE F.4 **Dynamic Assessment of Multisymbol Expressive Language** (*continued*)

TARGET STRUCTURE: TO ELICIT . . .	EXPECTED RESPONSE	SUGGESTED CUES
An answer containing possession	*Mommy hat.* *My book.*	Play a game naming owners, as in "Daddy key." You and the parent can model the response following the cue "What's this?" or "Whose is this?"
A reply containing possession	*Daddy key.*	Hold up an object with a readily identifiable owner and say "Tell me about this."
A declaration containing possession	*Mommy book.*	Hold up an object and name the owner and the item, as in "Doggie bowl." Hold up another object, nod toward the child expectantly.
A request containing possession.	*My cup.*	This works especially well if the child has favorite items. Place the object out of reach and await a response. You might also have another adult model the response so the child understands the task. Look at the child expectantly.
A question containing possession	*Mommy coat?* *My shoe?*	Have an item with an easily identifiable owner in a bag. Ask an adult, "Guess what's in the bag." Bring out another bag and cue the child in the same way.
An answer containing a location	*Teddy box.*	Place an object in or on another object. Ask "Where's teddy?"
A reply containing a location	*Shoe chair.*	Place an object in or on another object. Say "Tell me about shoe" or "I can't find shoe" when the location is obvious.
A declaration containing a location	*Ball cup.*	Have two objects in two locations. You or another adult describe one, such as "Key box." Look at child expectantly while glancing at the second object in a different location.
A request containing a location	*Cookie jar.*	Have one desirable object in one location and another in another. Have an adult model ask for one. Then look toward the second object and expectantly toward the child.
A question containing a location	*Doll bed?*	Hide an object and say "Guess where the doll is."

The SLP will want to assess a range of semantic functions and intentions. This will require a variety of cues and consequences, given the variation possible. The methodology above is generic in nature.

You should be assessing at this level only if the child can produce single symbols by speech, sign, or other means, such as pictures or electronics. For some children, the transition to two symbols is difficult, taxing both memory and motor abilities. An intermediate stage may be to use different means, such as saying one word and signing the other.

TABLE F.5 Dynamic Assessment of Joint Attention

LEVEL OF ASSESSMENT	EXPECTED RESPONSE	TEST FORMAT	POSSIBLE MEDIATED TEACHING FORMAT
Responding			
Focusing on a close object	Child orients head and eyes.	Position yourself face to face with the child at his/her eye level. Bring an object of interest, such as a favorite toy or a new, visually interesting toy, into the child's line of vision. Other objects include wind-up or noisemaking toys that the child doesn't know how to operate, or bubbles and puppets.	Respond to any child attention. If none, activate the toy. When the child looks, bring the toy to your face and say the child's name plus "Look!" Hold the toy close to your eyes and shake it to attract the child's attention. If the child looks at the toy, reinforce by activating the toy again.
Following a point	Child orients head and eyes in the direction of the point.	Have very interesting pictures or objects nearby. Call child's name, say "Look," and point to each item with a distal point or a touch of the item. Begin with a distal gesture and if the child does not respond, try the less mature contact one.	Respond to any distant look toward the object by the child, indicated by head turn. If child still does not respond, call the child's name, shake an object in front of child, and verbalize while pointing. If child fails to look at SLP's face, SLP should bring object to face prior to calling child's name, then move it away and point.

Try to make this a fun, playful exchange using eye contact, smiles, facial expression, and verbalizations with lots of inflection. A responsive behavior is all that is needed at this point; however, you may wish to assess the child's initiating behaviors if you feel the child is functioning at a higher level and can initiate intentional gestural communication.

Initiating			
Activated toy	Child looks at the toy and shifts gaze directly from the object to the SLP, gestures to the object while looking at it, or makes a vocalization or verbalization while looking at the object.*	Mechanical remote-operated toy is placed directly in front of the child but out of reach. The SLP activates the toy but does not look at it.	Respond to any child behavior to attract your attention, including reaching toward the toy. If no child behavior occurs, have another person model an attention-getting behavior. Be sure to respond with surprise when you look at the toy.

continued

TABLE F.5 **Dynamic Assessment of Joint Attention** (*continued*)

Level of Assessment	Expected Response	Test Format	Possible Mediated Teaching Format
Book	Child looks at the book and shifts gaze directly from the book to the SLP, gestures to the book while looking at it, or makes a vocalization or verbalization while looking at the object.	Open a book in front of the child, preferably one with several separate pictures per page. Say "What see?" or "What do you see?" Allow the child to look at the book, touch it, or turn the pages. Hold the book open if the child tries to close it.	Respond to any child behavior to attract your attention, including reaching toward the book. If no child behavior is forthcoming, have another person model an attention-getting behavior. Be sure to respond with surprise when you look at the book.
—	—	—	—

Possible objects might include:

Bright clothes	Musical toys
Busy box or kiddie gym	Nonbreakable mirror
Colored balls or objects in a container	Picture books
Favorite foods	Pinwheel or mobile
Flashlight or lighted toy	Pull and push toys
Jack-in-the-box	Puppets and dolls
Keys or other "jingly" toy	Spinning toy such as a top
Kitten or puppy	Stuffed or plush, brightly colored animal
	Wind-up or remotely operated toy

*If child requests assistance in reactivation of toy, behavior should be considered both joint attention and requesting.

Source: Based on MacDonald et al., 2006; Mundy et al., 2003; Owens, 1982.

TABLE F.6 Dynamic Assessment of Motor Imitation

A child's readiness for motor imitation depends on many developmental achievements, not least of which is the ability to move parts of the body independently. For children with neuromotor impairment, such as cerebral palsy, you will have to be very creative. Enlist the help of an occupational therapist to identify possible independent movements. The ability to hold objects, swat at a mobile, or explore toys by bringing them in the mouth are signs that a child may be ready to learn imitation.

As a warm-up activity, the adult might begin with imitation of the child's behavior. This can be repeated with subtle changes to see if the child will imitate in turn.

Remember that we are interested in the ability to imitate on cue and not necessarily in teaching new behaviors. Attempt to get the child to imitate behaviors already in the child's repertoire.

LEVEL OF ASSESSMENT	EXPECTED RESPONSE	TEST FORMAT	POSSIBLE MEDIATED TEACHING FORMAT
Single actions	Child repeats adult's single-action behavior immediately following model.	Call child's name and say "Do this" or name action ("Clap hands") while performing the action.	Respond to any child behavior that approximates an imitation. If the child does not respond or responds in an indiscriminate way, recue the child and gently help the child imitate by hand-over-hand guidance, followed by reinforcement. Some children will have trouble moving from performing with a physical prompt to responding without one. In this case, gradually decrease the prompt to just a gentle touch.
Some children will need more tactile input. For example, perform an action on the child, such as rubbing the child's tummy or touching the child's nose, for more tactile input than the child would get from behaviors such as clap hands.			
Repetitive actions*	Child repeats adult's repetitive behavior immediately following model.	Call child's name and say "Do this" or name action ("Hit table") while performing action twice.	Respond to any child behavior that approximates a dual action imitation. If the child does not respond or responds with a single action, cue the child to imitate a single action immediately followed by a recue for the second while performing each single action. If the child still does not respond correctly, repeat the two single behaviors but give a visual prompt of the initiation of each behavior, such as raising your hands to clap but not clapping, following each request to imitate.
Two different actions	Child imitates adult's different actions in sequence.	Call child's name and say "Do this" while performing two different actions in sequence.	Respond to any child behavior that approximates the two behaviors in the correct sequence. If the child does not respond, responds with only one behavior, or confuses the sequence, modify the behaviors so they are similar but performed in different places, such as pat head and pat tummy. If the child still does not respond correctly, repeat the two different actions but give a visual prompt of the initiation of each behavior, following the request "Do this." If the child is still having difficulty, perform the two different actions, and give a partial physical assist with each action.
—	—	—	—

continued

TABLE F.6 **Dynamic Assessment of Motor Imitation** (*continued*)

LEVEL OF ASSESSMENT	EXPECTED RESPONSE	TEST FORMAT	POSSIBLE MEDIATED TEACHING FORMAT

Possible actions might include:

Clapping your hands	Rolling over
Crawling	Rolling play dough or clay
Dancing, child style	Scribbling with a marker or crayon
Dropping objects into a container	Shaking a rattle or noisemaking object
Jumping	Shaking your head up and down
Opening and closing hand	Stacking blocks into a tower
Patting objects or surfaces	Standing up or lying down
Playing a toy musical instrument	Stretching
Pushing a toy truck or car	Taking a step or marching
Putting on a hat	Tapping a block on the table
Raising or swinging arm	Tapping foot
Ringing a bell	Touching your nose, head, or other facial feature
Rolling or throwing a ball	Waving bye-bye

*Only assess for repetitive actions if the child can imitate single actions.

TABLE F.7 **Dynamic Assessment of Oral Motor Imitation Abilities**

LEVEL OF ASSESSMENT	EXPECTED RESPONSE	TEST FORMAT	POSSIBLE MEDIATED TEACHING FORMAT
Oral imitation	Child follows adult model with immediate repetition.	Call child's name and say "Do this" or name action ("Blow bubbles") while performing the action.	Respond to any child behavior that approximates oral imitation. If the child does not respond or responds in an indiscriminate way, perform the action before a mirror and allow the child to do the same. If the child is still not successful, perform the action with a light touch to the area of the child's mouth prior to imitation.
—	—	—	—

Possible actions might include:

Blowing bubbles or objects on a mobile	Kissing and pouting
Blowing out cheeks	Licking, puckering, or smacking your lips
Closing lips tightly	Opening and closing mouth
Giving raspberries	Smiling
	Sticking out tongue

TABLE F.8 **Dynamic Assessment of Sound-Making Ability**

LEVEL OF ASSESSMENT	EXPECTED RESPONSE	TEST FORMAT	POSSIBLE MEDIATED TEACHING FORMAT
Turn-taking or choral	Child will join adult in simultaneous or alternating vocalizing.	Adult uses contingent vocal imitation to join child's vocalizing.	Respond to any child vocal behavior that continues as simultaneous or alternating vocalizing. If the child does not vocalize spontaneously, ask the family for suggestions of high vocalization activities, such as bouncing on an adult's knee.
Imitation*	Child follows adult single-sound model with immediate vocal imitation.	Call child's name, say "Do this" or "Say X," and say the sound. Begin with sounds already in the child's repertoire of spontaneous sounds. It is not as important to assess ability to learn new sounds as it is to assess the child's ability to imitate.	Initially respond to any vocalization that immediately follows the model. Once the child can perform in this way, try to get a specific sound. Again, try to have the child imitate a sound already in the child's repertoire. If child does not respond with a speech sound, attempt to pair a sound with an action, such as knocking over blocks and saying "Uh-oh" or tasting something sweet and saying "mmmm." Another possibility is to try to get the child to imitate an easy prolonged vowel. If a child seems confused, go back to physical imitation and use a glance, a point, or the passing of an object to indicate the child's turn. Use this device with vocal imitation as well.
Repetitive syllable imitation**	Child follows adult reduplicated vocal model (CVCV reduplicated) with immediate vocal imitation.	Call child's name, say "Do this" or "Say X," and say the model. Use sounds previously imitated by the child or in the child's spontaneous repertoire.	Respond to any child vocal behavior that is two-syllable in nature, and then try to get the specific sounds by breaking the CVCV model into two CV models. If the child does not produce a CVCV imitation, prompt the child with a CVCV model, and when the child produces one CV, prompt the child for the second.
Nonrepetitive syllable imitation***	Child follows adult nonrepetitive multi-syllable (CVCV) vocal model with immediate vocal imitation.	Call child's name, say "Do this" or "Say X," and say the model. Use sounds previously imitated by the child or in the child's spontaneous repertoire.	Respond to any child vocal behavior that is two-syllable in nature, and then try to get the specific sounds by breaking the CVCV model into two CV models. If the child does not produce a CVCV imitation, prompt the child with a CVCV model, and when the child produces one CV, prompt the child for the second.

*I try to get the child to imitate simple CV or VC syllables that can then be used both as words and syllables for building longer CVCV words. Possibilities include the following:

Bye	Da	Eat	Eye	Go	Hi	In	Key	Ma	Me
No	Out	See	Tea	Toy	Up				

**Possibilities that approximate words include *dada, mama, wawa,* and *baba.*
***There are many words that are CVCV in structure, including *Daddy, Mommy, TV, doggie, kitty, bye-bye, cookie, baby,* and *gimme.* In general, words in which the vowel changes but the consonant remains the same, as in *baby* and *cookie,* are easier to produce than those in which the consonant or syllable changes, as in *doggie* and *kitty.*

TABLE F.9   **Dynamic Assessment of Functional Use**

LEVEL OF ASSESSMENT	EXPECTED RESPONSE	TEST FORMAT	POSSIBLE MEDIATED TEACHING FORMAT
Functional play	Child will play with objects in a meaningful way.*	Call child's name, say "Look," and name object(s). Cue child with "Let's play" or "What do you do with this?"	Respond to any child behavior that approximates appropriate play and demonstrates appropriate use of the object. If the child does not respond or responds in an unacceptable or indiscriminate manner, model an action with the object and try to engage the child in play or an interaction. If the child's response is still unacceptable, try to get the child to imitate by performing the action and then prompting the child to do it, as in "Cory, brush hair." After teaching a few actions with the objects, return to each one to see if the child will now demonstrate functional use.

Possible objects include the following:

Airplane	Napkin
Ball	Plate or bowl
Book	Purse and wallet
Bottle	Push/pull toy
Bus and passengers	Puzzle
Child kitchen set	Squeaky toy
Clothes	Stacking toys or blocks
Comb or brush	Stuffed animal
Cup	Sunglasses
Doll with accessories	Toothbrush
Keys	Truck and blocks
Knife, fork, and/or spoon	Trike
Musical instruments	Washcloth and towel

*Be very flexible. There is no one correct way to play with a truck!

TABLE F.10 **Dynamic Assessment of Presymbolic Play**

LEVEL OF ASSESSMENT	EXPECTED RESPONSE	TEST FORMAT	POSSIBLE MEDIATED TEACHING FORMAT
Familiar routines	Child begins game and anticipates outcome.	Using just intonation both with and without words, say the initial line for familiar games in succession, such as "so big," "I'm gonna get you," "This little piggy," and "pat-a-cake."	Practice familiar routines with the child, take a short break, then begin again, using both speech and intonation. If child does not comply by joining game, try again with body movement, such as crouching along with "I'm gonna get you." If child still does not comply, use a physical prompt, such as placing the child in position along with your verbal cue. When the child is successful with two routines, return to the test mode.
Functional play	Child will play with objects in a mean-ingful way.*	Call child's name, say "Look," and name object(s). Cue child with "Let's play" or "What do you do with this?"	Respond to any child behavior that approximates appropriate play and dem-onstrates appropriate use of the object. If the child does not respond or responds in an unacceptable or indiscriminate manner, model an action with the object and try to engage the child in play or an interaction. If the child's response is still unacceptable, try to get the child to imi-tate by performing the action and then prompting the child to do it, as in "Cory, brush hair." After teaching a few actions with the objects, return to each one to see if the child will now demonstrate functional use. See Table F.9.

TABLE F.11 **Dynamic Assessment of Symbolic Play**

LEVEL OF ASSESSMENT	EXPECTED RESPONSE	TEST FORMAT	POSSIBLE MEDIATED TEACHING FORMAT
Object play	Play with object in symbolic manner	Use an object in a symbolic way, such as a shoe for a phone. Say "Hello. Joanie? She's here." Pass the phone to the child. Whatever item you use in a symbolic way, try to get the child to partici-pate. Play and enjoy!	Have an adult model the behavior after you do it and cue the child again. If not successful, try to get the child to imitate your behavior.
Pretend play	Play with nonexistent object	Pretend to play feeding or dressing the baby but have no food or clothes.	Model the behavior for the child. Say "Where food" or "Where clothes?" "No, no food [or no clothes]. Just pretend."

Appendix G

Communication
Stimulation Activities
(Ages are functional not chronological)

The ideas below are for communication stimulation. Activities and ages are based on typically developing children and may need some modification for specific children. Also remember that children develop unevenly and may be at more than one level in communication. In other words, pick your activities carefully to fit the child.

1-Month Level

- Make gentle noises next to the child's ear. This teaches the child about sound production and stimulates hearing, the main pathway for language.
- Attract the child's attention with interesting objects, including your face. Young children love movement and contrasting shades of color, so use brightly colored items, noisemaking objects, or a combination of the two. Shake an object gently in front of the child and then continue to jiggle it while you slowly draw it to your face. When the child looks at you, respond by saying something.

2-Month Level

- Establish a greeting routine whenever you enter the child's vision after being apart for a short time, such as in the morning, after naps, after solitary play, and the like. It will become a routine and the child will learn that the caregiver is predictable.
- Call the child's name and get her attention before interacting, even though at 2 months she isn't yet able to recognize her name. It's still a good place to start.
- Encourage gooing and cooing by making similar pleasure sounds while holding the child against your chest or face.
- Respond to the child's vocalizations with attention and gentle talking.
- Alter your voice or pair it with a stuffed animal, doll, or puppet. Either the toy can talk directly to the child in a different voice or the adult can become a third party and vary his or her voice depending on who's speaking.

3-Month Level

- Incorporate simple games, such as *peek-a-boo* and *I'm gonna get you*, into everyday routines. For example, the adult could begin *I'm gonna get you* after changing a child.

- Accompany the child's movement with talk about different parts involved. Describe what the child is doing as it's done. Although the child won't understand the words, he will begin to make associations, especially as if the words are heard day after day. In addition, you're both focusing on the same thing, just like in a conversation.

4-Month Level

- Broaden imitation of the child's movement and noises to include echoing her speech sounds specifically. After a few imitations, the child may begin to expect your imitation, wait for it, then laugh and smile, and possibly reply with another sound. Don't expect imitation of your sound. What's important is the vocal turn-taking.
- Also imitate in unison. Then vary your performance, sometimes in unison and at other times alternating.
- Encourage smiling and laughing by making big noises with your mouth on the child's tummy, dancing to music, acting surprised, and making funny squeaky noises. Don't be afraid to ham it up.

5-Month Level

- Point out a doll's facial features, body parts, clothes, and actions as you and the child manipulate the doll. Enhance the experience by moving the doll around in front of a mirror.
- Make a knocking noise, show surprise, and then have a toy, puppet, or doll pop up and have a conversation with you and the child. The child will love the element of surprise and the feeling of anticipation as the knock becomes a signal for the toy's appearance.
- Imitate the more varied sounds, squeals, shrieks, and whispers that the child can now make. Don't make any loud or sudden squeals or shrieks. The goal is not to make the child fearful of noisemaking games.
- Follow along when the child starts a "conversation." The child will make eye contact, move around, smile, or make noises to attract attention and signal a readiness to communicate. Respond with enthusiasm and interest.

6-Month Level

- Talk to the child about what he's doing, what you do together, and what he sees you doing. Keep the talk simple and repetitive, and pause after important words.
- Let the child participate and "help" you in your daily activities. Whenever possible, let the child hold and explore objects as you talk.
- Include lots of variations in your own sound-making, such as pitch variations, growls, tongue clicks, whispering, singing, humming, and any other interesting vocal possibilities you can think of. The child will love the variety and just may chime in. If she does, imitate the behavior.
- Reply to *unintended* messages, such as reaching for a toy, as if the child were *intentionally* trying to communicate the message to you ("Oh, Kristin want teddy."). The child is not yet quite able to plan an action to achieve a desired end; she is still *pre-intentional*.
- Sing about what you're doing as you do it, and you may end up in a duet. Use simple, repetitive melodies, such as "Row, row, row your boat," that will attract the child's attention. Adapt the song to whatever you're doing at the time.
- Encourage the child to wave bye-bye in appropriate situations.

7-Month Level

- Sing a CVCV combination song by substituting a CV sound like *ba* for the song lyrics—one sound for each syllable.
- When you or the child points to an interesting object, say the word for the object and talk about it a little.

8-Month Level

- Engage the child in some fun activity like playing patty-cake or bouncing, then stop and wait for the child to vocalize before you continue. If the child's a little slow on the uptake, make a sound first, or just wait until the child makes one by chance, and then continue with your activity. If the child doesn't seem to understand the connection, try to get him to imitate you physically.
- Pick a simple, repetitive song, such as "Old MacDonald," and move (bounce, pick up, raise arms) the child to the music at the same place in each repetition, such as the *e-i-e-i-o* part.
- Pretend play is always fun. For example, pretend to be some sort of animal and make noises. Describe your actions with simple commentary.

9-Month Level

- Have the child imitate sounds she can already make: CV syllables or CV and CVCV words. You can try this with real words, but they should be CV or CVCV in nature. Keep this activity light, easy, and fun. Imitating the child is a way to get the exercise started.
- Showing the child photos of favorite people, animals, or things. Use a photo album, or make a small child-size one with lamination.
- Let the child pretend to use the telephone or, better yet, use it for real and make sounds. This can be fun, but be aware that some kids don't react at all to a disembodied voice.
- Now when the child points, give the child a chance to "name" the item of interest or to babble a comment. Ask "What see? or "What's that?" Respond positively to any vocal or gesture response, then supply the name yourself, as in "Yes, doggie" even if the child said "Ba."

10-Month Level

- Now that the child's on the verge of talking, instead of just presenting visual choices, add names to the objects presented—a big developmental difference.
- The child's already doing things like clapping and waving when you do; now it's time to encourage him to add vocal imitations to the physical ones. Even the most reticent tot can be enticed to mimic sounds when you add action to the mix.
- When the child is playing with something or examining an object as she starts to explore her environment, name the object. After you've told the child the name and thoroughly explored it with her, hold up two objects and say "Show me cup" or "Touch cup." This is a good check.
- At about this time, infants will pretend to cough, hiccup, or sneeze. Play along, or even mimic.
- If you or the child spills something by accident, simply comment "Uh-oh!" It's an easy utterance for a child to imitate and the situation in which it's used is very specific, making it a perfect learning opportunity.

■ Respond to the baby's gestures *only* when they're accompanied by a sound, or a word or word-like noise. If the child makes a gesture out of your direct line of sight, just ignore it for a few seconds to give a chance to attract your attention with a sound. If after ten seconds or so, the child doesn't come up with some sort of vocalization, reply to the gesture by reproducing it and talking about it. Try to prompt it again.

11-Month Level

■ Although you've searched for objects with the child before, you're now going to *ask* him to find them. The teaching emphasis shifts from finding objects to *responding to your question*.

■ As you play with the child, chat about how the toys and objects are *used*. Her early definitions will be based in part on the function of things. As the child begins to talk, she may name a particular food ("Nana") or actually tell you how it's used ("Eat").

■ Up to this point, you've encouraged the child to replicate your actions and sounds. Now we make a qualitative leap. Try to get the child to imitate *very simple words*. Remember the building blocks: CV or VC syllable words, such as *hi, go, out, eat, up, toy, see, ma, da [dad], hi, me, tea, shoe, bye, ear*, etc., are the easiest for 11-month-olds. Also at this age, words only make sense in the appropriate context. Asking the child to say *"Toy"* when there's not one around will only confuse him.

12-Month Level

■ Twelve-month olds love playing dress-up with different hats. Put on different ones, then wave and say "Hello" to each other. Play by a mirror so the child has added stimulation.

■ Create very simple stories with the child as the main character, incorporating familiar environments and routines and recent experiences. The story is interactive and should allow the child to participate. You can use a book with relevant pictures.

■ Ask the child to say particular words, using *"Say X."* Don't overdo it. A few other reminders:
  ▪ Ask for words only in contexts where the words are appropriate, so they make sense to the child.
  ▪ Only request words that refer to things that are visually or audibly present. Pick words that the child has already said or that contain sounds the child can say.
  ▪ Respond in a conversational way.
  ▪ Vary the way you make your request ("Say X," "Tell me X," or say the word then "What's this?", as in "Teddy, what's this?")
  ▪ Only ask for words one at a time.

■ Explore your bodies, supplying words for all the easy-to-say, obvious body parts, and encourage the child to repeat the words after you. Because the child can't see her own face, use a mirror or use your face when you point out and name the parts.

13-Month Level

■ Although it may be difficult for a child to talk to someone she or he can't see, lure her or him into phone-chat by making the other person visible using a cell phone or an extension of your landline while the child uses another phone in the same room. If the child makes sounds, have the phone partner slip out of sight to see if the child continues.

- Continue to play dress-up with hats and add other accessories like gloves and scarves. Imitating each other in front of a mirror adds another dimension along with saying words.
- Use photos in creative ways to elicit language. Play peek-a-boo with photos glued to paper plates or thick cardboard. After showing the child a quick flash of the photo, flip it around to the blank side ask who's on the other side. Get excited when you see who it is.
- Use directions to help the child complete routine tasks like dressing and eating. Don't be too bossy; keep it fun.
- Turn whatever you're doing into a song. It's an excellent way for babies to hear a word over and over in the appropriate situation. Context and real words are key. It's important for the child to hear repetitions of words in relevant situations. Try adapting some classic child tunes, such as "Are you sleeping? (Frere Jacques)," "Here we go 'round the mulberry bush," "London Bridge," or "Twinkle, twinkle, little star." This is a great way to introduce new words and phrases in context and to let the child hear them over and over again without being bored or overwhelmed. Repetition is critical for learning.

14-Month Level

- Have the child perform pretend actions with a favorite teddy bear or doll as the two of you sing about it. Use a familiar melody.
- Using the song "Have you ever seen a lassie" ("Have you ever seen a lassie, a lassie, a lassie; Have you ever seen a lassie go this way and that?"), add variations as in "Did you ever see a kitty sleeping in a hat?" or "Did you ever kiss a fishy while in the bathtub?" Sing the last line as a question, and talk about how silly the words are.
- You will probably be getting a lot of *no's* from the child. The trick is not to take them personally, but respond to them as serious communication attempts. If you continue to get constant negative responses, offer choices. If the child refuses both, then simply move on to the next activity. I believe in real consequences. A consequence of saying "No" to *everything* is that you don't get *anything*. It's also good to have someone else model saying "Yes" and receiving a treat.
- Whenever you and the child are reading or playing with toy animals, be sure to include the appropriate proper animal noises. Ask the child, "What does a cow say?" or "A doggy says . . .?" Because the child can't ask these questions of you, consider pointing to the pictures or toys as a cue for you to make sounds.
- Ask *what* and *where* questions. The child should understand both at this point, and you're teaching names of things and locations, two categories of words that will be useful later when the child is able to speak in longer phrases. Since she's going to try to repeat the name of whatever object you ask for, make sure you request things with names that the child can pronounce. Also encourage the child to ask *what* and *where* questions by showing various objects or by hiding things or pretending not to know where an object is so the child has to ask the location. If the child doesn't ask, have someone else model a question or answer with the wrong location, and hopefully the child will ask again.

15-Month Level

- At this age, children understand limited emotions such as sad, hungry, and tired. As you play with dolls, action figures, and puppets together, talk about how they act, look, and *feel*. Join in with your own facial expressions. *Everybody has Feelings*, by Charles Avery, includes photographs of different emotions on people's faces.

- Finger plays are fun for kids, great for language-learning opportunities and fine motor skills, and extremely portable. The important thing is participating, not getting it all correct.
- We've used songs before to introduce the child to new words. Now, at 15 months, it's the child's turn to join in to a small degree. Use repetitive children's songs and adapt them to things the child knows.

16-Month Level

- Incorporate environmental noises into play and encourage the child to imitate animal noises, car horns, sneezing, coughing, airplanes, trains, and the like. Mimicry requires hearing discrimination.
- Introduce educational toys that are touch and talk. At this point in development, the best ones for language growth are a voice describing a picture, because it provides a context for the words the child hears. Avoid talking toys that just chatter away.
- Ask the child to show you how to do something, as in "Show me how you X," but expand on the action verbs the child already knows by including longer, more specific directions, as in "Show me how you brush your teeth" or "Show me how you eat an ice cream cone." If the child is already using a few action words, let him or her be the one to give you a command.
- Have the child name body parts as you point to them. With increasing memory for words, the child will be able to make the shift from imitating to naming things. If the child doesn't seem to know what to do, demonstrate first.

17-Month Level

- Cut bread into shapes using a cookie cutter, then you and the child can spread peanut butter, marshmallow fluff, or jam on each shape, make faces with raisins, craisins (dried cranberries), chocolate chips, or peanuts. Try for facial expressions of different emotions. Talk about the process and the emotions.
- Give the child a chance to create funny-sounding voices. Show him or her how to talk through a paper towel tube or a hose, and then take turns doing it with him. Try recording your "tube-talk" and playing it back.
- Pile up some things that clearly belong to certain people, then hold up one at a time and say "Whose is this?" or "Whose hat?" This is a more advanced version of the "What's this?" name game.
- Try variations on "Mary Had a Little Lamb" that express possession. Substitute other people and objects as in "Mommy has a little cat." Try to get the child to join in in some way.
- Encourage the child to ask for assistance (*Help, Do, Open*) by presenting challenges that will require help. Try things like difficult buttons or jars that won't open and contain toddler-desirable and visible objects or treats.

18-Month Level

- Draw a happy face on the child's thumb with washable marker. Ask "Thumbkin" simple questions that can be answered with *yes* or *no* or a single word. The child can either verbally reply for his or her thumb or just have Thumbkin move his "head" to signal yes/no.
- Encourage the child to describe the world and to use location names. When looking out the window, say, "Mommy looking out window. What Mommy see? I see . . ." At the end, pause and let the child fill in the blank.

■ While outside, "introduce" the child to inanimate objects. "Hello, tree. I'm Mommy. This is Clarita. Clarita, say 'Hello, tree.'" When Clarita "talks" to the tree (or other objects), reply with a funny tree-like voice.

19- and 20-Month Levels

■ Take photos of the child, put them together in a book, and use it for conversations.

■ Children love to open things and secret things away, and they begin to use the words *in* and *on*. Give the child a little practice by directing her to put her teddy *in* or *on* various things. As the child understands the commands better, you can add more items and make the choices less obvious.

■ Mount pictures on a "Lazy Susan," help the child spin it, then name and talk about the picture that lands the closest to the child. Encourage him to name objects and people in the picture and describe what's going on.

■ Try variations on the song "Oh where, oh where has my little dog gone?" Hide an object, then sing while the child and you search, emphasizing the locations, as in

Oh where, oh, where is rubber duck?
Oh where, oh where is the duck?
Mommy and Suzie look under the chair
Oh where, oh where is the duck?

■ Have make-believe dinners, tea parties, picnics, and shopping expeditions. Take a drive in an imaginary car. And have a conversation about the events. Be creative, and make it fun. You could even ask the child to serve as the "go-between" for you and Teddy. Ask her: "Please ask Teddy what the child wants to eat" or "Ask Teddy what the child wants from market." This type of play is not only fun, but is extremely important for the child's cognitive growth, since imagining and pretending stretches her language.

21- and 22-Month Levels

■ Try variations on children's songs, such as "Old MacDonald" and "Mary Had a Little Lamb," with the child as lead character and everyday items and events. Personalize it, and make it fun. Sing together.

■ Have the child move brightly colored objects *in* and *out* of containers, grocery bags, toy chests, and the like. This is the next stage of the *in* and *on* exercises we did last month. Talk about the locations.

■ Blowing requires muscular strength, the ability to create pressure and release it, and breath control—all important for speech. A few possibilities: blowing bubbles through a straw in clean bathtub water or in a cup of liquid; inflating a collapsed paper bag; and blowing feathers, leaves, dandelion or milkweed fluff, and other lightweight things.

23- and 24-Month Levels

■ When you're talking with a relative or good friend on the phone, have the child talk into the receiver to pass along a very short message, or at least have him say "Hi" or "Bye." Just a quick little chat with someone the child can't actually see will strengthen the child's communication and cognitive skills and stimulate her long-term memory, since the child has to reach into her databank to find the identity of her conversational partner.

■ Have the child lie down on a large piece of paper while you trace her or his body shape with a crayon or marker. When that's done, ask the child to name the parts of his body that are evident in the tracing (arms, legs, hands, head, etc.), and help him find the corresponding parts on the tracing. Color the parts on the tracing together. If you want to take it a step further, trace individual parts in more detail, such as a foot with all the toes, color it, cut it out, then match it to the whole body tracing.

■ Both of you can put on funny hats and silly clothes, or manipulate dolls and puppets, and take turns knocking at the door. First one of you knocks, and when the door is answered, the conversation begins.

■ Storytelling is one of the foundations of good conversational skills. Don't expect plots, character development, or even imaginative or pretend stories yet. The child's stories will be more about the things that make an impression on her—objects, events, and people that are outside the realm of her everyday routines. The tale will be stream of consciousness.

Source: Owens, R. E. (2004). *Help Your Baby Talk*. New York: Perigee.

Expanding Symbols into Different Intentions

Possible Order for Expanding *Negation* into Different Intentions

- *Protesting* with a negative word is something we do all the time when we reject an offered item, as in responding "No" to "Would you like some more coffee?" Notice that the form is an answer, but it is being given to an indirect request in an interrogative form. We can simplify this by simply supplying a nonpreferred or nonrequested item to a child. For example, an adult can ask a child what he or she wants, even if the response is a point, and then hand the child the nonpreferred item.

- *Answering* with a negative can be taught as response to "Is this X?" or "Is the X (filler) in the Y (container)?" The negative response can be taught through imitation. Because the *yes/no* contrast is a difficult concept, I would recommend not asking "Is this X?" when the response is positive. Instead, ask "What's this?" and reserve the "Is this X?" solely for negatives. This strategy has the added advantage of using a specific cue for negation. Make it a game, as in

Adult:	"Is this milk?"
Child:	"No"
Adult:	"No, it's not milk. Is this water?"
Child:	"No."
Adult:	"No, it's not water. What's this?"
Child:	"Juice."
Adult:	"Yes, juice. Want juice?"

- *Replying* can be negative in response to "This is an X (incorrect name)" or "Tell me not to (or "No") X (impossible action)." If the child fails to respond or does so incorrectly, the SLP can use a question such as "Is this an X?" or "Can I X?" to prompt a negative answer.

- *Commenting or declaring* is a spontaneous negative response to the adult's using a known object in an inappropriate manner. If the child fails to respond or does so incorrectly, the SLP can prompt a reply by making an absurd statement ("The shoe is for eating" or "I eat shoe") and awaiting a reply. If all else fails, the SLP can ask a question.

Possible Order for Expanding *Location* into Different Intentions

- *Answering* with a location is a response to "Where's X?" If the child cannot answer this question or is incorrect, the adult can supply the answer, such as "Ball cup," and ask again. If the child is still having difficulty, the adult can reverse the order by ask-ing the question and following it with the answer, as in "Where's ball? Ball cup." This is followed by a nonverbal cue to imitate the adult answer. If all else fails, the adult can say "Where's ball? Say 'cup.'" The adult's answer can gradually be decreased to a whisper so the child does not become dependent on this imitative model.

- *Replying* can be a response to "Tell me where X is" or "I can't find X. I wonder where it is." If the child fails to respond or does so incorrectly, and assuming that the child can answer location questions, the SLP can use a question such as "Where's X?" and then return to the initial cue.

- *Commenting or declaring* can be a response to an object "hidden" in view of the child. The adult can look around as if searching for the object and look at the child quizzically. If the child fails to respond or does so incorrectly, the SLP can use a com-ment to elicit a reply. If searching for the ball, the SLP can state, "I can't find the ball; we can't play" and await a reply.

- *Requesting* can be trained in a game format in which the child directs the adult to place objects or find objects in various places or to perform some action, such as go-ing under the table. If the child fails to respond or does so incorrectly, the SLP can use a question such as "Where is X?" or "What should I do?" These questions can then be faded as the child learns the game.

- *Questioning* can be taught as an attempt to identify a previously hidden object. This works best if a parent or other adult models one-word questions, such as "Cup?" fol-lowed by the SLP or other adult looking in or under a cup. The adult model provides the intonation that demonstrates that the utterance is a question. The child may or may not incorporate the rising intonation. In a variation, also requiring an adult to model the question, the child can hide an object and ask the SLP or other adult "Where?"

Possible Order for Expanding *Nomination* into Different Intentions

- *Answering* with a name is an appropriate response to "What's that?" Although there is a danger in overtraining, it has wide application and can be worked into just about any routine, such as dressing or bathing, in which the child knows the names of ob-jects. If a child cannot name in response to a question, supply the answer first by nam-ing the object and then ask for its identity, as in "Duck. What's this?" If the child still does not respond, reverse the order to enable the child to imitate but in the presence of the question, as in "What's this? Duck." A variation is "What's this? Say 'duck.'" At each level, a second adult or child can model both how to respond and the correct answer. Don't forget to include a point or a nod toward and eye contact with the child to signal that you expect a response. These nonverbal cues can help a child move to spontaneous use of nomination as the adult decreases use of the "What's this?" cue.

- *Replying* can begin in response to a request. Building on answering to "What's this?" the SLP or other adult can request "Tell me what you see" or "Tell me about this." Although the change is subtle, cues such as these do not require a response to the ex-tent that a question cue does. Another strategy that contains a question is "I wonder what's in the box." Notice that "What's in the box" is present but does not include interrogative intonation.

- *Naming or declaring* is a spontaneous behavior that is not in response to a verbal cue. Given its nature, this type of verbalization can be difficult to elicit. On the flip side, the positive aspect of training this intention is the variety of situations in which it can occur. Names can be elicited while pulling objects from a container, riding in the car or on the bus, dressing, bathing, feeding, shopping, or reading together. This is where nonverbal cues become especially important. Other aids include establishing naming routines and modeling by an adult or another child.

- ■ *Calling* familiar people or pets is an important intention to use with nomination. Think how often a young child calls for his or her mother. Calling for household pets can be taught within routines, such as walking the dog or offering a treat. Calling can also be taught within a modified hide-and-seek format in which the child finds family members by following the sound of their voice in response to a call.
- ■ *Requesting* can be taught beginning with the question cue "Do you want yogurt or pudding?" or "What do you want?" Notice that the choice-making cue offers a choice in which both items are named and thus is easier than the second, more open-ended cue.
- ■ *Questioning* is a natural for the "Original Name Game." Adults and young TD children play both parts of the game, naming and responding in turn. Learning to request the name of something is a valuable word-learning tool for a child. Within a routine of pulling object from a container, children can learn to cue the adult with "What's that?" or simply "What?" Initially, the phrase can be taught through imitation.
- ■ *Hypothesizing* when unsure of an object name is a great learning and vocabulary-stretching intention. If questioning is to truly function as a word-learning strategy, the child must be able to test hypotheses about the names of items, as in "Doggie?" when encountering another four-legged animal. This intention can be trained within a guessing game format in which each partner tries to guess something that is hidden. Because potential items form an almost limitless list, adults should confine the game to a few items that are named and shown to the child first. Initially, the adult may need a second adult or child to model the game format for the first child. In a similar fashion, others can model hypothesis-testing with novel items.

Possible Order for Expanding *Attribution* into Different Intentions

- ■ *Answering* is a natural response to questions, such as "Which one is this?" For example, the adult can hold up a ping-pong ball and a beach ball and ask the question. Notice that the contrast between the two is not a subtle one. It's entirely possible that the child will name the object. If the child says "Ball" the adult can respond, "Yes, ball, but which ball is this?" Some children will benefit from moving the one in question closer and cueing again. If the child still responds incorrectly, the adult can say "Ball. Big. Little. Which one is this?" For a child who still does not seem to understand the task, the adult can simply describe the one with the attribute word expected, as in "Ball. Big ball. Big. Which one is this?"
- ■ *Replying* can be taught in response to "Tell me about this one." The child is very likely to say "Ball," so it's important to present both objects of the contrasting pair (*big-little*). Because there is no requirement to reply to a comment as there is following a question, the child may benefit from an adult's modeling the appropriate verbal response. If the child is still unsure of what to do or does not know the desired word, the SLP can present the options, holding each ball forward and saying "Big" and "Little." This is followed by the cue "Tell me about this one." When the child responds with the correct attribution word, the adult can comment further and interact with both the child and the object, as in "Yes, big. Big ball. Here comes the big ball."
- ■ *Commenting or declaring* is a spontaneous behavior that at this point in intervention will be dependent upon nonverbal cues, such as nodding, pointing, and eye contact. The adult can also use the nonverbal cue of moving one of a contrasting pair of objects toward the child. If the child does not respond, the adult can supply the attribute words (*big-little*) and try again. A second adult can model the correct response. If all else fails, the first adult can name the attribute (*big*) and try again. For some children, moving to a spontaneous verbal behavior may be difficult. If so, the adult can go back to replying but with strong emphasis on nonverbal cues.

I have placed much emphasis on the importance of joint attending and the training of pointing as a way to establish this early communication behavior. If a child imitates words, it should be relatively easy to modify a pointing gesture to a point with an accompanying word.

- *Requesting* can be taught in response to the question "Which do you want?" or "Which want?" and offering two desirable items that contrast is some way. If the child names the object but not the contrast, the adult can respond, "Yes, ball, but which one?" If the child responds incorrectly, the adult can name the contrasts, "Big, little," holding each item forward, and ask again. A third option is to ask "Which one do you want? Big? Little?" In order to have the child spontaneously request, the adult can perform a requesting routine but not ask the child the "Which one?" question. Be sure that the child's request is complied with, or the significance of requesting is lost.

  If the child is requesting spontaneously through gestures, it should be relatively easy to get a spontaneous verbal request, assuming the item in question is highly desirable. Another option is to set up a routine, such as saying "Big" to have the larger ball rolled to you by the other person.

- *Questioning* is a form of guessing game, so let's use this milieu. The adult can show the child two contrasting items, hide one and have the child guess which one is hidden. For example, a small or a large ball can be hidden in a large box. If there is an established game routine, such as guessing the name of a hidden object, it should be easy to move to guessing which one of a contrasting pair. If the child has difficulty, the adult can name each contrasting item. It the child only names the item but not the contrast, the adult can respond with "Yes, ball. Which one?" Liberal use of nonverbal cues can be helpful in moving the child from this answering response to a questioning one. It may be helpful to have another person model the questioning behavior.

Possible Order for Expanding *Possession* into Different Intentions

- *Answering* with a possession word can be taught in response to the question "Whose is this?" or "Whose X is this?" There is the danger with the latter that a child who is unsure of the verbal cue may imitate the name of the object. If a child has difficulty naming the owner, the adult and child can explore the object together as the adult names the owner for the child and then cues again with the question. If the child continues to have difficulty, the adult can reverse the order, asking first, then answering, and then cueing the child to imitate the answer.

- *Replying* is a natural response to "Tell me whose X this is" or "I wonder whose X this is." If the child is unsuccessful, the adult can return to a question cue to elicit the correct response. If the child names the object, the adult can respond with the desired response, as in "Yes, Mommy's."

- *Commenting or declaring* can be elicited by an object and a nod. This works best in a routine in which the child and adult are naming owners, such as putting objects away. Believe it or not, young children like to clean up, and the adult can make a game out of it. At first a child may be inclined to use the object name, so the SLP may want to use objects for which the owner is obvious but the child does not possess the object name.

- *Requesting* can be taught as a response to "Whose X do you want?" or "Whose do you want?" There is some danger in naming the object, as in "Whose sock do you want?" Spontaneous requesting can occur within a game format in which each person requests a highly desirable object from another person.

- *Questioning* can be elicited in response to a guessing ownership game or a turn-taking task in which partners ask *whose* questions. The guessing format might go as follows:

Adult: "I have something in the box? Guess whose it is."
Child: [Says nothing]
Adult: "Mommy's? No." [Looks at child]
Child: "Mommy?"
Adult: "No, not Mommy. Try somebody else."
Child: "Sissy?"
Adult: "Yes, Sissy. It's Sissy's hat! Your [or child's name] turn."

- ■ Initially, it may be helpful to have another adult or child model the questioning be-havior. In a similar task, partners can alternately pull objects from a container and ask the other person "Whose?"

Possible Order for Expanding *Recurrent* into Different Intentions

- ■ *Requesting* more is a relatively easy intention to teach. Within feeding, play, or just about any daily routine, the adult can supply a small amount of an edible or an ac-tion and when the item is consumed or after stopping the action, the adult can look quizzically at the child to cue a request for more. If the child does not request, another adult or child can serve as a model. Requesting can become an enjoyable part of the routine. The child can also be prompted with "What do you want?" Remember that the correct response is not the name of the object or action.
- ■ *Answering* can be confused with requesting if the adult is not careful. It might be helpful to make a distinction between *one* and *more than one*, as in "Cracker" and "More." Responses can be cued with a point and "What do you see?" or "Which one is this?"
- ■ *Replying* can be taught in a similar fashion to answering, but the verbal prompt would change subtly to "Tell me what you see."
- ■ *Commenting or declaring* is spontaneous verbalizing that can be taught with the rou-tine of identifying a single object and several or more. The intention can be prompted by a point, eye contact, and an expectant look toward the child.
- ■ *Questioning* can be taught in the form of a game in which one object is presented and named and the child tries to guess if more are hidden in an opaque container. In other words, are more cookies in the box or in the plastic container? The child asks by saying the item name, such as "Ball," and then asks if "More?" is located in the container. This can be fun as the child and adult discover what is hidden in the container.

Possible Order for Expanding *State* into Different Intentions

- ■ *Replying* can be cued within a conversation discussing a doll's, pet's, or other person's state. A book might also be used along with the adult cue, "She looks ____." For ex-ample, if an adult or child is napping, another adult can say, "Daddy's sleeping. He's tired." Initially, this will need to be repeated and may be taught best within doll play in which the situation can be repeated several times.
- ■ *Protesting* may best be served by negative words, but state words can serve as a justifi-cation and then become protest in their own right. The state word can be paired with a negative head shake to indicate not agreement, as when someone asks if you'd like to go out and you respond, "I'm too tired."
- ■ *Answering* can be taught within routines with dolls or puppets in response to "How does dolly [or baby] feel?" Responses can be prompted with yes/no questions, such as "Is doll hungry?" If the child responds, the adult can cue with the original question

again. The adult should make certain that there are obvious signs of the doll's state, such as crying to indicate sadness, laughing to show happiness, or asking for food when hungry. The correct response can be modeled by other children or an adult and feelings discussed with the child.

■ ***Commenting or declaring*** can be taught with a point followed by a description. Expressing state can begin with questions and a scavenger hunt in which the adult and child find the sad doll or picture. Books can also be used, with the adult and child taking turns identifying the state expressed in a picture. If the child fails to initiate a comment, the adult can use the fill-in-the-blank prompt used with replying

■ ***Questioning and hypothesizing*** can be a useful language took for enhancing use of state words. Although it will be difficult for most children at this stage to ask *why* questions or "How does she feel?" a child can use a hypothesis-testing utterance to guess the emotion of a hidden doll or book picture, as in "Hungry?" These questions can be elicited within a guessing routine and turn-taking with others who model the desired behavior.

Possible Order for Expanding *Action* into Different Intentions

■ ***Answering*** can be taught to a variety of question types, depending on the word desired. If the child does not respond or responds incorrectly, the answer can be modeled and the question asked again. A more direct model can be performed with a reverse of these two, asking first and then modeling the correct answer.

> *Agent.* Agent words can be elicited with questions such as "Who (*action*)?" Examples include "Who is jumping?" or "Who threw (the) ball?"
>
> *Action.* If the child is performing the action, the adult can cue the child to answer by asking "What (are) you doing?" If someone else has performed the action, the adult can ask "What happened?" If the child is unsure how to respond, another adult or child can model an answer. An alternative is to name the action and then ask the questions, as in "Let's jump. Jump! Jump! (As you do it) What are you doing?" (or simply "What doing?").
>
> *Object.* Questions that elicit an object word are more awkward. For example, the adult can ask "What are you throwing?" or simply "What throw?" In this case, have a variety of appropriate items so the child does not associate *throw* only with *ball*. Spaghetti in sauce is an all-time favorite!

■ ***Replying*** can be taught in response to "Tell me" or fill-in-the-blank cues. If the child does not respond or responds incorrectly, the adult can use a question prompt with *who* or *what* words or can use a *yes/no* question, as in "Are you rolling?" When the child responds correctly, the adult can comment and return to the original cues, as in "Yes, you are rolling. Tell me." Another alternative is to have another child or adult perform the action and model the correct response. Routines such as naming actions in pictures in a book can also elicit replying.

> *Agent.* As in questions, the adult can cue agent replies with cues such as "Tell me who is dancing."
>
> *Action.* Action words are the easiest to cue, using "Tell me what you're doing" or "Juan is ____" ("Juan ____"). The second form may require some modeling to help the child know what to do.
>
> *Object.* Object words come naturally at the end of an utterance, making it obvious to the child which word is requested. Examples of adult cues include "Tell me what you throw" and "Shawana eat ____."

■ ***Commenting or declaring*** is a spontaneous verbal intention and can be elicited by a pointing gesture, eye contact, and an expectant look while an action is being performed or immediately following the action. Pointing should indicate which type of word the adult desires. If the child does not respond or responds incorrectly, the adult can model a response or return to the cue for replying.

- ■ ***Requesting*** would seem to be limited to asking to perform the action or to obtain the object in order to perform the action. The latter is not unlike nomination requesting, so I won't discuss it here. To get a child to request an action, the adult can show an object that is associated with a particular action and cue with "What do you want to do?" or "What should we do?" A simplified version is "What do?" Once the child is responding reliably, the adult can reduce the cue and attempt to have the child request spontaneously.

- ■ ***Questioning and hypothesizing*** are easiest with simple action words. Cueing for questions about who did the action and what object was used in the action is difficult and somewhat awkward. Action questions consist simply of the word *what*, while hypotheses consist of the action word with rising intonation. These can be taught in a game format in which each partner tries to guess an action being performed out of sight. Another possibility is asking about actions for which the child may not have a name, using "What?" Both forms can be taught through imitation and within routines. Adults can also model the questioning behavior with known words in novel situations.

Feeding Assessment
Interview Questionnaire

- What brought you here today?

- When did this difficulty begin?

- Was it a sudden start or a more gradual start?

- Is there a time of day when the child seems to eat more/less?

- Can you describe his/her behavior during mealtime?

- What are the child's favorite foods/drinks?

- What are the child's least favorite foods/drinks?

- What have you tried to improve his/her eating/drinking?

  - Did it work?

- Is the child currently in any other therapies? (PT, OT, SLP elsewhere)

  - If so, what are their goals?

- What goals would you like to address?

References

CHAPTER 1

Abraham, L. M., Crais, E., Vernon-Feagans, L., & the Family Life Project Phase 1 Key Investigators. (2013). Early maternal language use during book sharing in families from low-income environments. *American Journal of Speech-Language Pathology, 22,* 71–83.

American Speech-Language-Hearing Association (ASHA). (2004c). *Knowledge and skills needed by speech-language pathologists and audiologists to provide culturally and linguistically appropriate services [Knowledge and skills].* Available from www.asha.org/policy/KS2004-00215.htm.

American Speech-Language-Hearing Association (ASHA). (2005a). *Cultural competence [Issues in Ethics].* Available from www.asha.org/policy/ET2005-00174.htm.

American Speech-Language-Hearing Association (ASHA). (2005b). *Roles and responsibilities of speech-language pathologists in service delivery for persons with mental retardation and developmental disabilities: Position statement.* Rockville, MD: Author.

American Speech-Language-Hearing Association (ASHA). (2008a). *Core knowledge and skills in early intervention speech-language pathology practice.* Washington, DC: Author.

American Speech-Language-Hearing Association (ASHA). (2008b). *Roles and responsibilities of speech-language pathologists in early intervention: Guidelines.* Washington, DC: Author.

American Speech-Language-Hearing Association (ASHA). (2008c). *Roles and responsibilities of speech-language pathologists in early intervention: Position statement.* Washington, DC: Author.

American Speech-Language-Hearing Association (ASHA). (2008d). *Roles and responsibilities of speech-language pathologists in early intervention: Technical report.* Washington, DC: Author.

American Speech-Language-Hearing Association (ASHA). (2011). *Cultural competence in professional service delivery [Position statement].* Available from www.asha.org/policy/PS2011-00325.htm.

Applequist, K. L., & Bailey, D. B. (2000). Navajo caregivers' perceptions of early intervention services. *Journal of Early Intervention, 23,* 47–61.

Artiles, A. J., & Ortiz, A. A. (2002). *English language learners with special education needs: Identification, assessment, and instruction.* McHenry, IL: Delta Systems.

Bernstein Ratner, N. (2006). Evidence-based practice: An examination of its ramifications for the practice of speech-language pathology. *Language, Speech, and Hearing Services in Schools, 37,* 257–267.

Bialystok, E. (2001). *Bilingualism in development: Language, literacy, and cognition.* Cambridge, UK: Cambridge University Press.

Bialystok, E., & Craik, F. I. M. (2010). Cognitive and linguistic processing in the bilingual mind. *Current Directions in Psychological Science, 19,* 19–23.

Blue-Banning, M., Summers, J. A., Frankland, H. C., Nelson, L. L., & Beegle, G. (2004). Dimensions of family and professional partnership: Constructive guidelines for collaboration. *Exceptional Children, 70,* 167–184.

Blue-Banning, M., Turnbull, A. P., & Pereira, L. (2000). Group action planning as a support strategy for Hispanic families: Parent and professional perspectives. *Mental Retardation, 38,* 262–275.

Boone, H. A., & Coulter, D. (1995). Achieving family-centered practice in early intervention. *Infant Toddler Intervention, 5*(4), 395–404.

Bruder, M. B., & Dunst, C. J. (2005). Personnel preparation in recommended early intervention practices: Degree of emphasis across disciplines. *Topics in Early Childhood Special Education, 25,* 25–33.

Calandrella, A. M., & Wilcox, J. (2000). Predicting language outcomes for young prelinguistic children with developmental delay. *Journal of Speech, Language, and Hearing Research, 43,* 1061–1071.

Campbell, P. H. (2004). Participation-based services: Promoting children's participation in natural settings. *Young Exceptional Child, 8*(1), 20–29.

Campbell, P. H., & Halbert, J. (2002). Between research and practice: Provider perspective on early intervention. *Topics in Early Childhood Special Education, 22,* 213–226.

Campbell, P. H., & Milbourne, S. A. (2005). Improving the quality of infant-toddler care through professional development. *Topics in Early Childhood Special Education, 25,* 3–14.

Campbell, P. H., & Sawyer, L. B. (2007). Supporting learning opportunities in natural settings through participation-based services. *Journal of Early Intervention, 29*(4), 287–305.

Chao, P., Bryan, T., Burstein, K., & Cevriye, E. (2006). Family-centered intervention for young children at-risk for language and behavior problems. *Early Childhood Education Journal, 34,* 147–153.

Cross, A. F., Traub, E. K., Hutter-Pishgahi, L., & Shelton, G. (2004). Elements of successful inclusion for children with significant disabilities. *Trends in Early Childhood Special Education, 24*(3), 169–183.

Delgado-Gaitan, C. (2004). *Involving Latino families in schools: Raising student achievement through home-school partnerships.* Thousand Oaks, CA: Corwin.

Dunst, C. J. (2002). Family-centered practices: Birth through high school. *Journal of Special Education, 36,* 139–147.

Etscheidt, S. (2006). Least restrictive and natural environments for young children with disabilities: A legal analysis of issues. *Topics in Early Childhood Special Education, 26,* 167–179.

Fair, L., & Louw, B. (1999). Early communication intervention within a community-based intervention model in South Africa. *The South African Journal of Communication Disorders, 46,* 13–23.

Garcia, S. B., Mendez-Perez, A., & Ortiz, A. A. (2000). Mexican American mothers' beliefs about disabilities: Implications for early childhood intervention. *Remedial and Special Education, 21,* 90–100.

Graziano, A. M. (2002). *Developmental disabilities: Introduction to a diverse field.* Boston: Allyn & Bacon.

Gutiérrez-Clellen, V. F. (1999). Language choice in intervention with bilingual children. *American Journal of Speech-Language Pathology, 8,* 291–302.

Gutiérrez-Clellen, V. F., Simon-Cereijido, G., & Wagner, C. (2008). Bilingual children with language impairment: A comparison with monolinguals and second language learners. *Applied Psycholinguistics, 29*, 3–19.

Håkansson, G., Salameh, E.-K., & Nettelbladt, U. (2003). Measuring language development in bilingual children: Swedish-Arabic children with and without language impairment. *Linguistics, 41*, 255–288.

Hamers, J. F., & Blanc, M. H. A. (2000). *Bilinguality and bilingualism* (2nd ed.). Cambridge, UK: Cambridge University Press.

Hanson, M. J., Beckman, P. J., Horn, E., Marquart, J., Sandall, S. R., Grieg, D., et al. (2000). Entering preschool: Family and professional experiences in this transition process. *Journal of Early Intervention, 23*(4), 279–293.

Harbin, G. L., Pelosi, J., Kameny, R., McWilliam, R. A., Kitsul, Y., Fox, E., et al. (2004). *Identifying and predicting successful outcomes of coordinated service delivery*. Chapel Hill: University of North Carolina, FPG Child Development Institute.

Holahan, A., & Costenbader, V. (2000). A comparison of developmental gains for preschool children with disabilities in inclusive and self-contained classrooms. *Topics in Early Childhood Special Education, 20*, 224–235.

Horner, R. H., Carr, E. G., Strain, P. S., Todd, A. W., & Reed, H. K. (2002). Problem behavior interventions for young children with autism: A research synthesis. *Journal of Autism and Developmental Disorders, 32*(5), 423–446.

Hua, Z. (2008). Duelling languages, duelling values: Code-switching in bilingual intergenerational conflict talk in diasporic families. *Journal of Pragmatics, 40*, 1799–1816.

Ijalba, E., Jeffers-Pena, C., & Giraldo, A. (2013, April). *Parent training in the use of focused stimulation with literacy support for Hispanic families of children with autism spectrum disorders (ASD)*. Paper presented at the New York State Speech-Language-Hearing Association Annual Convention, Saratoga Springs.

Individuals with Disabilities Education Improvement Act of 2004, Pub. L. No. 108-446 § 118 Stat. 2647 (2004).

Jacoby, G. P., Lee, L., & Kummer, A. W. (2002). The number of individual treatment units necessary to facilitate functional communication improvements in the speech and language of young children. *American Journal of Speech-Language Pathology, 11*, 370–380.

Joseph, G. E., & Strain, P. S. (2003). Comprehensive evidence-based social-emotional curricula for young children: An analysis of efficacious adoption potential. *Topics in Early Childhood Special Education, 23*, 65–76.

Kalyanpur, M., Harry, B., & Skrtic, T. (2000). Equity and advocacy expectations of culturally diverse families' participation in special education. *International Journal of Disability, Development and Education, 47*(2), 119–136.

Kay-Raining Bird, E., Cleave, P. L., Trudeau, N., Thordardottir, E., Sutton, A., & Thorpe, A. (2005). The language abilities of bilingual children with Down syndrome. *American Journal of Speech-Language Pathology, 1*, 187–199.

Kohnert, K., Yim, D., Nett, K., Kan, P. F., & Duran, L. (2005). Intervention with linguistically diverse preschool children: A focus on developing home language(s). *Language, Speech, and Hearing Services in Schools, 3*, 163–251.

Kritzinger, A. M. (2000). *Early communication intervention in South Africa*. Unpublished thesis, University of Pretoria, South Africa.

Kritzinger, A. M., Louw, B., & Rossetti, L. M. (2001). A transdisciplinary conceptual framework for the early identification of risks for communication disorders in young children. *The South African Journal of Communication Disorders, 48*, 33–44.

Kummerer, S. E., Lopez-Reyna, N. A., & Tejero Hughes, M. (2007). Mexican immigrant mothers' perceptions of their children's communication disabilities, emergent literacy development, and speech-language therapy program. *American Journal of Speech-Language Pathology, 16*, 271–282.

Kupersmidt, J. B., Bryant, D., & Willoughby, M. T. (2000). Prevalence of aggressive behaviors among preschoolers in Head Start and community child care programs. *Behavioral Disorders, 26*(1), 42–52.

Madding, C. C. (2000). Maintaining focus on cultural competence in early intervention services to linguistically and culturally diverse families. *Infant-Toddler Intervention: The Transdisciplinary Journal, 10*(1), 9–18.

McCollum, J. A., Gooler, F., Appl, D. J., & Yates, T. J. (2001). PIWI: Enhancing parent-child interaction as a foundation for early intervention. *Infants and Young Children, 14* (1), 34–45.

McLean, L. K., Brady, N. C., & McLean, J. E. (1996). Reported communication abilities of individuals with severe mental retardation. *American Journal on Mental Retardation, 100*, 580–591.

McWilliam, R. A. (2010). *Routines-based early intervention: Supporting young children and their families*. Baltimore: Brookes.

Mendez-Perez, A. (1998). *Mexican-American mothers' perceptions and beliefs about language acquisition among toddlers with language disabilities*. Unpublished doctoral dissertation, University of Texas at Austin.

Moodley, L., Louw, B., & Hugo, R. (2000). Early identification of at-risk infants and toddlers: A transdisciplinary model of service delivery. *The South African Journal of Communication Disorders, 47*, 25–39.

Odom, S. L. (2000). Preschool inclusion: What we know and where we go from here. *Topics in Early Childhood Special Education, 20*, 20–27.

Paradis, J., Crago, M., Genesee, F., & Rice, M. (2003). French-English bilingual children with SLI: How do they compare with their monolingual peers? *Journal of Speech, Language, and Hearing Research, 46*, 113–127.

Paul, D., Blosser, J., & Jakubowitz, M. (2006). Principles and challenges for forming successful literacy partnerships. *Topics in Language Disorders, 26*(1), 5–23.

Paul-Brown, D., & Caperton, C. J. (2001). Inclusive practices for preschool-age children with specific language impairment. In M. J. Guralnick (Ed.), *Early childhood inclusion: Focus on change* (pp. 433–463). Baltimore: Brookes.

Petitto, L., & Holowka, S. (2002). Evaluating attributions of delay and confusion in young bilinguals: Special insights from infants acquiring a signed and spoken language. *Sign Language Studies, 3*, 4–33.

Polmanteer, K., & Turbiville, V. (2000). Family-responsive individualized family service plans for speech-language pathologists. *Language, Speech, and Hearing Services in Schools, 31*, 4–14.

Portes, A., & Hao, L. (1998). E pluribus unum: Bilingualism and loss of language in the second generation. *Sociology of Education, 71*, 269–294.

Raab, M., & Dunst, C. J. (2004). Early intervention practitioner approaches to natural environment intervention. *Journal of Early Intervention, 27*, 15–26.

Roberts, M. Y., & Kaiser, A. P. (2011). The effectiveness of parent-implemented language interventions: A meta-analysis. *American Journal of Speech-Language Pathology, 20*, 180–199.

Rodriguez, B. L., & Olswang, L. B. (2003). Mexican-American and Anglo-American mothers' beliefs and values about child rearing, education, and language impairment. *American Journal of Speech-Language Pathology, 12*, 452–462.

Rosenkoetter, S. E., Whaley, K. T., Hains, A. H., & Pierce, L. (2001). The evolution of a transition policy for young children with special needs and their families: Past, present, and future. *Topics in Early Childhood Special Education, 21,* 3–15.

Rossetti, L. M. (2001). *Communication intervention: Birth to three* (2nd ed.). Albany, NY: Singular.

Sackett, D. L., Richardson, W. S., Rosenberg, W., & Haynes, R. B. (1997*). Evidence-based medicine: How to practice and teach EBM.* New York: Churchill Livingstone.

Salas-Provance, M. B., Erickson, J. G., & Reed, J. (2002). Disabilities as viewed by four generations of one Hispanic family. *American Journal of Speech-Language Pathology, 11,* 151–162.

Schlosser, R. W. (2002). On the importance of being earnest about treatment integrity. *Augmentative and Alternative Communication, 18,* 36–44.

Schlosser, R. W. (2003). *The efficacy of augmentative and alternative communication: Toward evidence-based practice.* New York: Academic Press.

Schlosser, R. W., & Sigafoos, J. (2002). Selecting graphic symbols for an initial request lexicon: Integrative review. *Augmentative and Alternative Communication, 18,* 102–123.

Seung, H.-K., Siddiqi, S., & Elder, J. H. (2006). Intervention outcomes of a bilingual child with autism. *Journal of Medical Speech-Language Pathology, 1,* 53–63.

Sigafoos, J., & Pennell, D. (1995). Parent and teacher assessment of receptive and expressive language in preschool children with developmental disabilities. *Education and Training in Mental Retardation and Developmental Disabilities, 30,* 329–335.

Smith, S. W., & Daunic, A. P. (2004). Research on preventing behavior problems using a cognitive-behavioral intervention: Preliminary findings, challenges, and future directions. *Behavioral Disorders, 30*(1), 72–76.

Soodak, L. C., Erwin, E. J., Winton, P., Brotherson, M. J., Turnbull, A. P., Hanson, M. J., & Brault, L. M. J. (2002). Implementing inclusive early childhood education: A call for professional empowerment. *Topics in Early Childhood Special Education, 22*(2), 91–102.

Summers, J. A., Steeples, T., Peterson, C., Naig, L., McBride, S., Wall, S., et al. (2001). Policy and management supports for effective service integration in early Head Start and Part C programs. *Topics in Early Childhood Special Education, 21,* 16–30.

Thomas, C. C., Correa, V. I., & Morsink, C. V. (2001). *Interactive teaming: Enhancing programs for students with special needs* (3rd ed.). Upper Saddle River, NJ: Prentice Hall.

Tomlinson, C. A. (2004). Sharing responsibility for differentiated instruction. *Roeper Review, 26*(4), 188–190.

Turnbull, A. P., Turbiville, V. P., & Turnbull, H. R. (2000). Evolution of family-professional partnership models: Collective empowerment as the model for the early 21st century. In S. J. Meisels & J. P. Shonkoff (Eds.), *Handbook of early intervention* (2nd ed., pp. 630–650). New York: Cambridge University Press.

U.S. Department of Education. (2008). *Policy statement on inclusion of children with disabilities in early childhood programs.* Retrieved from http://www2.ed.gov/policy/speced/guid/earlylearning/joint-statement-full-text.pdf

Vakil, S., Freeman, R., & Swim, T. J. (2003). The Reggio Emilia approach and inclusive early childhood programs. *Early Childhood Education Journal, 30*(3), 187–192.

Wilcox, M. J., & Woods, J. (2011). Participation as a basis for developing early intervention outcomes. *Language, Speech, and Hearing Services in Schools, 42,* 365–378.

Wolery, M., & Bailey, D. B. (2002). Early childhood special education research. *Journal of Early Intervention, 25*(2), 88–99.

Wong-Filmore, L. (2000). Loss of family languages: Should educators be concerned? *Theory Into Practice, 39,* 203–210.

World Health Assembly. (2001). Retrieved from http://www.who.int/classifications/icf/wha-en.pdf.

World Health Organization (WHO). (1981). *The international code of marketing of breast-milk substitutes.* Geneva: Author.

CHAPTER 2

Ackerman, J. P., Riggins, T., & Black, M. M. (2010). A review of the effects of prenatal cocaine exposure among school-aged children. *Pediatrics, 125,* 554–565.

Akefeldt, A., Akefeldt, B., & Gillberg, C. (1997). Voice, speech and language characteristics of children with Prader-Willi syndrome. *Journal of Intellectual Disability Research, 41*(4), 302–311.

American College of Obstetricians and Gynecologists. (2002, September). Perinatal care at the threshold of viability. *ACOG Practice Bulletin,* no. 38.

American College of Obstetricians and Gynecologists. (2005, September). Obesity in pregnancy. *ACOG Committee Opinion,* no. 315.

American Psychiatric Association. (2013). *Diagnostic and statistical manual of mental disorders* (5th ed., Text revision). Washington, DC: Author.

American Society for Parenteral and Enteral Nutrition. (2002). Guidelines for the use of parenteral and enteral nutrition in adult and pediatric patients. *Journal of Parenteral and Enteral Nutrition, 26*(1), 1SA–6SA.

American Speech-Language-Hearing Association. (1997–2015). *Definitions of communication disorders and variations.* Retrieved September 20, 2015, from http://www.asha.org/policy/RP1993-00208

American Speech-Language-Hearing Association. (2004). *Cochlear implants: Technical report.* Rockville, MD: Author.

American Speech-Language-Hearing Association. (2006). *Incidence and prevalence of communication disorders and hearing loss in children.* Rockville, MD: Author.

American Speech-Language-Hearing Association. (2008b). *Roles and responsibilities of speech-language pathologists in early intervention: Guidelines.* Washington, DC: Author.

Anday, E. K., Cohen, M. E., Kelley, N. E., & Leitner, D. S. (1989). Effect of in utero cocaine exposure on startle and its modification. *Developmental Pharmacology and Therapeutics, 12,* 137–145.

Anzalone, M., & Williamson, G. (2000). Sensory processing and motor performance in autism spectrum disorders. In A. M. Wetherby & B. M. Prizant (Eds.), *Autism spectrum disorders: A transactional developmental perspective* (pp. 144–166). Baltimore: Brookes.

Aylward, G. P. (2005). Neurodevelopmental outcomes of infants born prematurely. *Journal of Developmental and Behavioral Pediatrics, 26*(6), 427–440.

Bailey, D. S., Hebbeler, K., Spiker, D., Scarborough, A., Mallik, S., & Nelson, L. (2005). Thirty-six-month outcomes for families of children who have disabilities and participated in early intervention. *Pediatrics, 116,* 1346–1352.

Bandstra, E. S., Morrow, C. E., Accornero, V. H., Mansoor, E., Xue, L., & Anthony, J. C. (2011). Estimated effects of in utero cocaine exposure on language development through early adolescence. *Neurotoxicology and Teratology, 33,* 25–35.

Beckett, C., Bredenkamp, D., Castle, C., Groothues, C., O'Connor, T. G., Rutter, M., et al. (2002). Behavior patterns associated with institutional deprivation: A study of children adopted from Romania. *Developmental and Behavioral Pediatrics, 23,* 297–303.

Beeghly, M., Martin, B., Rose-Jacobs, R., Cabral, H., Heeren, T., Augustyn, M., et al. (2006). Prenatal cocaine exposure and children's language functioning at 6 and 9.5 years: Moderating effects of child age, birthweight and gender. *Journal of Pediatric Psychology, 31*, 98–115.

Behrman, R. E. (2004). *Nelson textbook of pediatrics* (17th ed.). Philadelphia: W. B. Saunders.

Bland-Stewart, L. M., Seymour, H. N., Beeghly, M., & Frank, D. A. (1998). Semantic development of African-American children prenatally exposed to cocaine. *Seminars in Speech and Language Disorders, 19*, 167–187.

Brady, N. C., Marquis, J., Fleming, K., & McLean, L. (2004). Prelinguistic predictors of language growth in children with developmental disabilities. *Journal of Speech, Language, and Hearing Research, 47*, 663–677.

Braillion, A., & DuBois, G. (2005). [Letter to the editor]. *The Lancet, 365*, 1387.

Bromberger, P., & Permanente, K. (2004). *Premies.* University of Michigan Health Services. Updated November 30, 2004. Retrieved September 16, 2008, from http://www.med.umich.edu/1libr/pa/pa_premie_hhg.htm

Centers for Disease Control and Prevention (CDC). (2014, November 10). *Autism spectrum disorder: Data and statistics.* Retrieved from http://www.cdc.gov/ncbddd/autism/data.html

Centers for Disease Control and Prevention (CDC). (2016, August 31). *Facts about developmental disabilities.* Retrieved from https://www.cdc.gov/ncbddd/developmentaldisabilities/facts.html

Chakrabarti, S., & Fombonne, E. (2001). Pervasive developmental disorders in preschool children. *Journal of the American Medical Association, 27*, 3093–3099.

Chan, J. B., & Iacono, T. (2001). Gesture and word production in children with Down syndrome. *Augmentative and Alternative Communication, 17*, 73–87.

Chen, W. J., Maier, S. E., Parnell, S. E., & West, J. R. (2004). *Alcohol and the developing brain: Neuroanatomical studies.* Retrieved August 1, 2008, from http://pubs.niaaa.nih.gov/publications/arh27-2/174-180.htm

Cohen, N. J. (2001). *Language impairment and psychopathology in infants, children, and adolescents.* Thousand Oaks, CA: Sage.

Colgan, S., Lanter, E., McComish, C., Watson, L., Crais, E., & Baranek, G. (2006). Analysis of social interaction gestures in infants with autism. *Child Neuropsychology, 12*, 307–319.

Cunningham, M., & Cox, E. O. (2003, February). Hearing assessment in infants and children: Recommendations beyond neonatal screening. *Pediatrics, 111*(2), 436-440.

Curfs, L. M., Wiegers, A. M., Sommers, J. R., Borghgraef, M., & Fryns, J. P. (1991). Strengths and weaknesses in the cognitive profile of youngsters with Prader-Willi syndrome. *Clinical Genetics, 40*, 430–434.

Darnall, R. A., Ariagno, R. L., & Kinney, H. C. (2006). The late preterm infant and the control of breathing, sleep, and brainstem development: A review. *Clinical Perinatology, 33*(4), 883–914.

Dawson, M., Soulières, I., Gernsbacher, M. A., & Mottron, L. (2007). The level and nature of autistic intelligence. *Psychological Science, 18*, 657–662.

Devescovi, A., Caselli, M. C., Marchione, D., Pasqualetti, P., Reilly, J., & Bates, E. (2005). A crosslinguistic study of the relationship between grammar and lexical development. *Journal of Child Language, 32*, 759–786.

Dhossche, D. M., & Rout, U. (2006). Are autistic and catatonic regression related? A few working hypotheses involving GABA, purkinje cell survival, neurogenesis, and ECT. *International Review of Neurobiology, 72*, 55–79.

Dow-Edwards, D. L., Benveniste, H., Behnke, M., Bandstra, E. S., Singer, L. T., Hurd, Y. L., et al. (2006). Neuroimaging of prenatal drug exposure. *Neurotoxicology and Teratology, 28*, 386–402.

Downey, D. A., & Knutson, C. L. (1995). Speech and language issues. In L. R. Greenswag & R. C. Alexander (Eds.), *Management of Prader-Willi syndrome* (2nd ed.). New York: Springer-Verlag.

Dykens, E. M., Hodapp, R. M., Walsh, K., & Nash, L. J. (1992). Profiles, correlates, and trajectories of intelligence in Prader-Willi syndrome. *Journal of the American Academy of Child & Adolescent Psychiatry, 31*, 1125–1130.

Esposito, G., & Venuti, P. (2009). Comparative analysis of crying in children with autism, developmental delays, and typical development. *Focus on Autism and Other Developmental Disabilities, 24*, 240–247.

Evans, G. W., & English, K. (2002). The environment of poverty: Multiple stressor exposure, psychophysiological stress, and socioemotional adjustment. *Child Development, 73*, 1238–1248.

Feldman, H. M., Dollaghan, C. A., Campbell, T. F., Kurs-Lasky, M., Janosky, J. E., & Paradise, J. L. (2000). Measurement properties of the MacArthur Communicative Development Inventories at ages one and two years. *Child Development, 71*, 310–322.

Finer, N. N., Higgins, R., Kattwinkel, J., & Martin, R. J. (2006). Summary proceedings from the apnea-of-prematurity group. *Pediatrics, 117*(3, Pt 2), S47–51.

Fombonne, E. (2003a). Modern views of autism. *Canadian Journal of Psychiatry, 48*, 503–505.

Fombonne, E. (2003b). The prevalence of autism. *Journal of the American Medical Association, 289*, 87–89.

Fombonne, E., & Chakrabarti, S. (2001). No evidence for a new variant of measles-mumps-rubella-induced autism. *Pediatrics, 108*, E58.

Geers, A., Tobey, E., Moog, J., & Brenner, C. (2008). Long-term outcomes of cochlear implantation in the preschool years: From elementary grades to high school. *International Journal of Audiology, 47*(Suppl 2), 21–30.

Gernsbacher, M. A., Sauer, E., Geye, H., Schweigert, E., & Goldsmith, H. H. (2008). Infant and toddler oral- and manual-motor skills predict later speech fluency in autism. *Journal of Child Psychology and Psychiatry, 49*, 43–50.

Glennen, S. L., & Masters, M. G. (2002). Typical and atypical language development in infants and toddlers adopted from Eastern Europe. *American Journal of Speech-Language Pathology, 11*, 417–433.

Gogate, L. J., Maganti, M., & Perenyi, A. (2014). Preterm and term infants' perception of temporally coordinated syllable–object pairings: Implications for lexical development. *Journal of Speech, Language, and Hearing Research, 57*, 187–198.

Goldenberg, R. L., Andrews, W. W., Faye-Petersen, O., Cliver, S. P., Goepfert, A., & Hauth J. C. (2006). The Alabama preterm birth project: Placental histology in recurrent spontaneous and indicated preterm birth. *American Journal of Obstetrics and Gynecology, 195*, 792–796.

Goldenberg, R. L., Culhane, J. F., Iams, J. D., & Romero, R. (2008). Epidemiology and causes of preterm birth. *Lancet, 5*(371), 75–84.

Hahn, L. J., Zimmer, B. J., Brady, N. C., Swinburne Romine, R. E., & Fleming, K. K. (2014). Role of maternal gesture use in speech use by children with fragile X syndrome. *American Journal of Speech-Language Pathology, 23*, 146–159.

Halpern, R. (2000). Early childhood intervention for low-income children and families. In J. P. Shonkoff & S. J. Meisels (Eds.), *Handbook of early childhood intervention* (2nd ed., pp. 361–386). Cambridge, UK: Cambridge University Press.

Harvey, J. A. (2004). Cocaine effects on the developing brain: Current status. *Neuroscience Biobehavioral Review, 27*, 751–764.

Hernandez, D. J. (2004). *Demographic change and the life circumstances of immigrant families*. Albany: State University of New York Press.

Holte, L., Glidden Prickett, J., Van Dyke, D. C., Olson, R. J., Lubrica, P., Knutson, C. J. L., et al. (2006). Issues in the management of infants and young children who are deaf-blind. *Infants & Young Children, 19*, 323–337.

Hooper, S. J., Roberts, J. E., Zeisel, S. A., & Poe, M. (2003). Core language predictors of behavioral functioning in early elementary school children: Concurrent and longitudinal findings. *Behavioral Disorders, 29*(1), 10–21.

Horwitz, S. M., Irwin, J. R., Briggs-Gowan, M. J., Heenan, J. M. B., Mendoza, J., & Carter, A. S. (2003). Language delay in a community cohort of young children. *Journal of the American Academy of Child & Adolescent Psychiatry, 42*, 932–940.

Howlin, P. (2005). Outcomes in autism spectrum disorders. In F. R. Volkmar, R. Paul, A. Klin, & D. Cohen (Eds.), *Handbook of autism and pervasive developmental disorders: Diagnosis, development, neurobiology, and behavior* (3rd ed., Vol. 1). Hoboken, NJ: Wiley.

Howlin, P., Mahood, L., & Rutter, M. (2000). Autism and developmental receptive language disorder—A follow-up comparison in early adult life: Social, behavioral, and psychiatric outcomes. *Journal of Child Psychology and Psychiatry, 41*, 561–578.

Hwa-Froelich, D. A., Matsuo, H., & Becker, J. C. (2014). Emotion identification from facial expressions in children adopted internationally. *American Journal of Speech-Language Pathology, 23*, 641–654.

Iams, J. D. (2003). The epidemiology of preterm birth. *Clinics in Perinatology, 30*, 651–654.

Irwin, J., Carter, A., & Briggs-Gowan, M. (2002). The social-emotional development of late-talking toddlers. *Journal of the American Academy of Child & Adolescent Psychiatry, 41*, 1324–1332.

Jaycox, L. H., Zoellner, L., & Foa, E. B. (2002). Cognitive-behavior therapy for PTSD in rape survivors. *Journal of Clinical Psychology, 58*, 891–906.

Johnson, D. E. (2000). Medical and developmental sequelae of early childhood institutionalization in Eastern European adoptees. In C. A. Nelson (Ed.), *The Minnesota Symposia on Child Psychology: The Effects of Early Adversity on Neurobehavioral Development* (Vol. 31, pp. 113–162). Minneapolis: University of Minnesota Press.

Kemper, A. R., & Downs, S. M. (2000, May). A cost-effectiveness analysis of newborn hearing screening strategies. *Archives of Pediatric and Adolescent Medicine, 154*(5), 484–488.

Kirk, K. I., Miyamoto, R. T., Lento, C. L., Ying, E., O'Neill, T., & Fears, T. (2002). Effects of age of implantation in young children. *Annals of Otology, Rhinology and Laryngology, 111*, 69–73.

Kover, S. T., & Ellis Weismer, S. (2013). Lexical characteristics of expressive vocabulary in toddlers with autism spectrum disorder. *Journal of Speech, Language, and Hearing Research, 57*, 1428–1441.

Krakow, R., Mastriano, B., & Reese, L. (2005). *Early intervention and international adoption*. Paper presented at the annual convention of the American Speech-Language-Hearing Association, San Diego.

Larroque, B., Ancel, P. Y., Marret, S., Marchand, L., André, M., Arnaud, C., et al. (2008). Neurodevelopmental disabilities and special care of 5-year-old children born before 33 weeks of gestation (the EPIPAGE study): A longitudinal cohort study. *Lancet, 371*(9615), 813–820.

Laucht, M., Esser, G., Baving, L., Gerhold, M., Hoesch, I., Ihle, W., et al. (2000). Behavioral sequelae of perinatal insults and early family adversity at 8 years of age. *Journal of the American Academy of Child & Adolescent Psychiatry, 39*, 1229–1237.

Leddy, M., Rosin, P., & Miller, J. F. (2003, November 13). *Improving the speech intelligibility of young children with Down syndrome*. Two-hour seminar, ASHA Convention, Chicago.

Levy, S. E., & Hyman, S. L. (2002). Alternative/complementary approaches to treatment of children with autistic spectrum disorders. *Infants and Young Children, 14*(3), 33–42.

Lewis, B. A., Freebairn, L., Heeger, S., & Cassidy, S. B. (2002). Speech and language skills of individuals with Prader-Willi syndrome. *American Journal of Speech-Language Pathology, 11*, 285–294.

Lewis, B. A., Kirchner, H. L., Short, E. J., Minnes, S., Weishampel, P., Satayathum, S., et al. (2007). Prenatal cocaine and tobacco effects on children's language trajectories. *Pediatrics, 120*, e78–e85.

Lewis, B. A., Minnes, S., Short, E. J., Min, M. O., Wu, M., Lang, A., et al. (2013). Language outcomes at 12 years for children exposed prenatally to cocaine. *Journal of Speech, Language, and Hearing Research, 56*, 1662–1676.

Lewis, B. A., Minnes, S., Short, E. J., Weishampel, P., Satayathum, S., Min, M. O., et al. (2011). The effects of prenatal cocaine exposure on language at 10 years of age. *Neurotoxicology and Teratology, 33*, 17–24.

Lingam, R., Simmons, A., Andrews, N., Miller, E., Stowe, J., & Taylor, B. (2003). Prevalence of autism and parentally reported triggers in a north east London population. *Archives of Disease in Childhood, 88*, 666–670.

Liss, M., Harel, B., Fein, D., Allen, D., Dunn, M., Feinstein, C., et al. (2001). Predictors and correlates of adaptive functioning in children with developmental disorders. *Journal of Autism and Developmental Disorders, 31*, 219–230.

Locke, J. (2011). *Duels and duets*. New York: Cambridge University Press.

Loocke, C., Conry, J., Cook, J. L., Chudley, A. E., & Rosales, T. (2005). Identifying fetal alcohol spectrum disorder in primary care. *Canadian Medical Association Journal, 172*, 628–630.

Lord, C., Risi, S., & Pickles, A. (2004). Trajectory of language development in autistic spectrum disorders. In M. L. Rice & S. F. Warren (Eds.), *Developmental language disorders: From phenotypes to etiologies* (pp. 1–38). Mahwah, NJ: Erlbaum.

Luckasson, R., Borthwick-Duffy, S., Buntinx, W. H., Coulter, D. L., Craig, E. M., Reeve, A., et al. (2002). *Mental retardation: Definition, classification, and systems of supports* (10th ed.). Washington, DC: American Association on Mental Retardation.

Lum, J. A. G., Powell, M., Timms, L., & Snow, P. (2015). A meta-analysis of cross sectional studies investigating language in maltreated children. *Journal of Speech, Language, and Hearing Research, 58*, 961–976.

Madison, C. L., Johnson, J. L., Seikel, J. A., Arnold, M., & Schultheis, L. (1998). Comparative study of the phonology of preschool children prenatally exposed to cocaine and multiple drugs and nonexposed children. *Journal of Communication Disorders, 31*, 231–243.

Malakoff, M. E., Mayes, L. C., Schottenfeld, R. S., & Howell, S. (1999). Language production in 24-month-old inner-city children of cocaine-and-other-drug-using mothers. *Journal of Applied Developmental Psychology, 20*, 159–180.

Malloy, M. H. (2008). Impact of cesarean section on neonatal mortality rates among very preterm infants in the United States, 2000–2003. *Pediatrics, 122*(2), 285–292.

Mandell, D. S., Listerud, J., Levy, S. E., & Pino-Martin, J. A. (2002). Race differences at the age of diagnosis among Medicaid-eligible children with autism. *Journal of American Academy of Child and Adolescent Psychiatry, 41*, 1447–1453.

Mansoor, E., Morrow, C. E., Accornero, V. H., Xue, L., Johnson, A. L., Anthony, J. C., et al.. (2012). Longitudinal effects of prenatal cocaine use on mother-child interactions at 3 and 5 years. *Journal of Developmental and Behavioral Pediatrics, 33*, 32–41.

March of Dimes. (2007). Premature birth. Updated February 2007. Retrieved September 15, 2008, from http://www.march-ofdimes.com/prematurity/21326_1157.asp

Marchman, V. A., Martínez-Sussmann, C., & Dale, P. S. (2004). The language-specific nature of grammatical development: Evidence from bilingual language learners. *Developmental Science, 7*, 212–224.

Marquardt, T. (2000). Dysarthria. In R. Gillam, T. Marquardt, & F. Martin (Eds.), *Communication sciences and disorders: From science to clinical practice.* San Diego: Singular.

Marschik, P. B., Einspieler, C., Garzarolli, B., & Prechtl, H. F. R. (2007). Events at early development: Are they associated with early word production and neurodevelopmental abilities at the preschool age? *Early Human Development, 83*, 107–114.

Martin, J. A., Hamilton, B. E., Sutton, P. D., Ventura, S. J., Menacker, F., & Kirmeyer, S. (2006). *Births: Final data for 2004.* Hyattsville, MD: National Center for Health Statistics.

Matson, J. L., & Boisjoli, J. A. (2008). Strategies for assessing Asperger's syndrome: A critical review of data based methods. *Research in Autism Spectrum Disorders, 2*, 237–248.

Matson, J. L., & Wilkins, J. (2008). Nosology and diagnosis of Asperger's syndrome. *Research in Autism Spectrum Disorders, 2*, 288–300.

Matson, J. L., Wilkins, J., & Fodstad, J. C. (2010). Children with autism spectrum disorders: A comparison of those who regress versus those who do not. *Developmental Neurorehabilitation, 13*, 37–45.

Maulik, P. K., Mascarenhas, M. N., Mathers, C. D., Dua, T., & Saxena, S. (2011). Corrigendum to "Prevalence of intellectual disability: A meta-analysis of population-based studies." *Research in Developmental Disabilities, 32*(2), 419–436.

Mawhood, L., Howlin, P., & Rutter, M. (2000). Autism and developmental receptive language disorder—A comparative follow-up in early adult life: I. Cognitive and language outcomes. *Journal of Child Psychology and Psychiatry and Allied Disciplines, 41*, 547–559.

Meis, P. J., Klebanoff, M., Thom, E., Dombrowski, M. P., Sibai, B., Moawad, A. H., et al. (2003). Prevention of recurrent preterm delivery by 17 alpha-hydroxyprogesterone caproate. *New England Journal of Medicine, 348*, 2379–2385.

Mentis, M., & Lundgren, K. (1995). Effects of prenatal exposure to cocaine and associated risk factors on language development. *Journal of Speech and Hearing Research, 38*, 1303–1318.

Mercer, B. M., Goldenberg, R. L., Meis, P. J., Moawad, A. H., Shellhaas, C., Das, A., et al. (2000). The preterm prediction study: Prediction of preterm premature rupture of membranes through clinical findings and ancillary testing. *American Journal of Obstetrics and Gynecology, 183*, 738–745.

Mercer, B. M., Goldenberg, R. L., Moawad, A. H., Meis, P. J., Iams, J. D., Das, A. F., et al. (1999). The preterm prediction study: Effect of gestational age and cause of preterm birth on subsequent obstetric outcome. National Institute of Child Health and Human Development Maternal-Fetal Medicine Units Network. *American Journal of Obstetrics and Gynecology, 181*, 1216–1221.

Miller, L., & Hendric, N. (2000). Health of children adopted from China. *Pediatrics, 105*(6). Retrieved from http://www.pediatrics.org/cgi/content/full/105/6/e76

Minnes, S., Singer, L. T., Arendt, R., Farkas, K., & Kirchner, H. L. (2005). Effects of cocaine/poly drug use on maternal-infant feeding interaction over the first year of life. *Journal of Developmental and Behavioral Pediatrics, 26*, 194–200.

Moretti, P., Peters, S. U., Del Gaudio, D., Sahoo, T., Hyland, K., Bottiglieri, T., et al. (2008). Brief report: Autistic symptoms, developmental regression, mental retardation, epilepsy, and dyskinesias in CNS folate deficiency. *Journal of Autism and Developmental Disorders, 38*, 1170–1177.

Morrow, C. E., Bandstra, E. S., Anthony, J. C., Ofir, A. Y., Xue, L., & Reyes, M. B. (2003). Influence of prenatal cocaine exposure on early language development: Longitudinal findings from four months to three years of age. *Developmental and Behavioral Pediatrics, 24*, 39–50.

National Academy of Sciences. (2013). Preterm birth: Causes, consequences, and prevention. *Institute of Medicine.* Updated July 2006. Retrieved July 3, 2013, from http://books.nap.edu/openbook.php?record_id=11622&page=398

National Institute on Deafness and Other Communication Disorders. (2014). *Usher syndrome.* National Institutes of Health. Retrieved September 18, 2015, from http://www.nidcd.nih.gov/health/hearing/pages/usher.aspx

National Institutes of Health. (2014). *Prader-Willi syndrome (PWS): Condition information.* Retrieved September 26, 2015, from http://www.nichd.nih.gov/health/topics/prader-Willi/conditioninfo/Pages/default.aspx

Neish, S. R. (2006). *Patent ductus arteriosus. eMedicine.* Article last updated July 10, 2006. Retrieved September 25, 2008, from http://www.emedicine.com/ped/topic1747.htm

Newson, E. (2001). The pragmatics of language: Remediating the central deficit for autistic 2–3 year olds. In J. Richer & S. Coates (Eds.), *Autism: The search for coherence.* London: Jessica Kingsley.

Oslejsková, H., Dusek, L., Makovská, Z., Pejcochová, J., Autrata, R., & Slapák, I. (2008). Complicated relationship between autism with regression and epilepsy. *Neuroendocrinology Letters, 29*, 558–570.

Owens, R. E. (2004). *Help your baby talk.* New York: Penguin Putnam.

Ozonoff, S., Macari, S., Young, G. S., Goldring, S., Thompson, M., & Rogers, S. J. (2008). Atypical object exploration at 12 months of age is associated with autism in a prospective sample. *Autism, 12*, 457–472.

Ozonoff, S., Williams, B. J., & Landa, R. (2005). Parental report of the early development of children with regressive autism. *Autism, 9*, 461–486.

Pan, B. A., Rowe, M. L., Singer, J. D., & Snow, C. E. (2005). Maternal correlates of growth in toddler vocabulary production in low-income families. *Child Development, 76*, 763–782.

Paparella, T., Goods, K. S., Freeman, S., & Kasari, C. (2011). The emergence of nonverbal joint attention and requesting skills in young children with autism. *Journal of Communication Disorders, 44*, 569–583.

Paul, R. (2000). Predicting outcomes of early expressive delay: Ethical implications. In D. V. M. Bishop & L. B. Leonard (Eds.), *Speech and language impairments in children: Causes, characteristics, intervention and outcome* (pp. 195–209). Hove, East Sussex, UK: Psychology Press.

Paul, R., & Roth, F. B. (2011a). Characterizing and predicting outcomes of communication delays in infants and toddlers: Implications for clinical practice. *Language, Speech, and Hearing Services in Schools, 42*, 331–340.

Pollak, S., & Bechner, A. (2000). *Wisconsin international adoption research project: A study of our children's development.* Unpublished manuscript, University of Wisconsin at Madison.

Potter, S. M., Zelazo, P. R., Stack, D. M., & Papageorgiou, A. N. (2000). Adverse effects of fetal cocaine exposure on neonatal auditory information processing. *Pediatrics, 105,* e40.

Prizant, B. M., Schuler, A. L., Wetherby, A. M., & Rydell, P. (1997). Enhancing language and communication: Language approaches. In D. Cohen & F. Volkmar (Eds.), *Handbook of autism and pervasive developmental disorders* (2nd ed.). New York: Wiley

Provost, B., Lopez, B., & Heimerl, S. (2007) A comparison of motor delays in young children: Autism spectrum disorder, developmental delay, and developmental concerns. *Journal of Autism and Developmental Disorders, 37,* 321–328.

Pry, R., Petersen, A. F., & Baghdadli, A. (2009). Developmental changes of expressive language and interactive competences in children with autism. *Research in Autism Spectrum Disorders, 3,* 98–112.

Raju, T. N., Higgins, R. D., Stark, A. R., & Leveno, K. J. (2006). Optimizing care and outcome for late-preterm (near-term) infants: A summary of the workshop sponsored by the National Institute of Child Health and Human Development. *Pediatrics, 118*(3), 1207–1214.

Redmond, S. M., & Rice, M. L. (2002). Stability of behavioral ratings of children with SLI. *Journal of Speech, Language, and Hearing Research, 45,* 190–201.

Reichman, N. E. (2005). Low birth weight and school readiness. *The Future of Children, 15,* 91–116.

Rescorla, L. A. (2002). Language and reading outcomes to age 9 in late-talking toddlers. *Journal of Speech, Language, and Hearing Research, 45,* 360–371.

Rescorla, L. A. (2005). Age 13 language and reading outcomes in late-talking toddlers. *Journal of Speech, Language, and Hearing Research, 48,* 459–472.

Rescorla, L. A., & Achenbach, T. M. (2002). Use of the Language Development Survey in a national probability sample of children aged 18–35 months. *Journal of Speech, Language, and Hearing Research, 45,* 733–743.

Rescorla, L. A., & Alley, A. (2001). Validation of the Language Development Survey (LDS): A parent report tool for identifying language delay in toddlers. *Journal of Speech, Language, and Hearing Research, 44,* 434–445.

Rescorla, L. A., Bernstein Ratner, N., Jusczyk, P., & Jusczyk, A. M. (2005). Concurrent validity of the Language Development Survey: Associations with the MacArthur-Bates Communicative Development Inventories: Words and Sentences. *American Journal of Speech-Language Pathology, 14,* 156–163.

Rescorla, L. A., Dahlsgaard, K., & Roberts, J. (2000). Late-talking toddlers: MLU and IPSyn outcomes at 3;0 and 4;0. *Journal of Child Language, 27,* 643–664.

Rescorla, L. A., Ross, G. S., & McClure, S. (2007). Language delay and behavioral/emotional problems in toddlers: Findings from two developmental clinics. *Journal of Speech, Language, and Hearing Research, 50,* 1063–1078.

Resnick, M. B., Gomatam, S. V., Carter, R. L., Ariel, M., Roth, J., Kilgore, K. L., et al. (1998). Educational disabilities of neonatal intensive care graduates. *Pediatrics, 102,* 308–314.

Rice, M. L., Spitz, R. V., & O'Brien, M. (1999). Semantic and morphosyntactic language outcomes in biologically at-risk children. *Journal of Neurolinguistics, 12,* 213–234.

Rivkees, S. A. (2001). Mechanisms and clinical significance of circadian rhythms in children. *Current Opinion in Pediatrics, 13,* 352–357.

Roberts, D., & Dalziel, S. (2006, July 19). Antenatal corticosteroids for accelerating fetal lung maturation for women at risk of preterm birth. *Cochrane Database System Review, 3,* CD004454.

Roberts, J. E., Mirrett, P., Anderson, K., Burchinal, M., & Neebe, E. (2002). Early communication, symbolic behavior, and social profiles of young males with fragile X syndrome. *American Journal of Speech-Language Pathology, 11,* 295–304.

Rogers, S. J. (2006). Evidence-based intervention for language development in young children with autism. In T. W. C. Stone (Ed.), *Social and communication development in autism spectrum disorders: Early identification, diagnosis, and intervention.* New York: Guilford Press.

Rogers-Adkinson, D., & Rinaldi, (2006). Collaborative Services: Children Experiencing Neglect and the Side Effects of Prenatal Alcohol Exposure.

Rosenberg, S. A., Zhang, D., & Robinson, C. C. (2008). Prevalence of developmental delays and participation in early intervention services for young children. *Pediatrics, 121,* 1503–1509.

Rutter, M. (1998). Developmental catch-up and deficit following adoption after severe global early privation. *Journal of Child Psychology and Psychiatry, 39,* 465–476.

Rutter, M. (2005). Aetiology of autism: Findings and questions. *Journal of Intellectual Disability Research, 49,* 231–238.

Rutter, M. L., Kreppner, J. M., & O'Connor, T. G. (2001). Specificity and heterogeneity in children's responses to profound institutional privation. *British Journal of Psychiatry, 179,* 97–103.

Schalock, R. L., Luckasson, R. A., Shogren, K. A., Borthwick-Duffy, S., Bradley, B., Buntinx, W. H., et al. (2007). The renaming of *mental retardation*: Understanding the change to the term *intellectual disability*. *Intellectual and Developmental Disabilities, 45*(2), 116–124.

Schopler, E., Reichler, R. J., & Renner, B. R. (2010). *The Childhood Autism Rating Scale—2nd Edition.* Los Angeles: Western Psychological Services.

Sheinkopf, S., Mundy, P., Oller, D. K., & Steffens, M. (2000). Vocal atypicalities of preverbal autistic children. *Journal of Autism and Developmental Disorders, 30*(4), 345–354.

Shprintzen, R. J. (1999) *Syndrome identification for speech-language pathology: An illustrated pocketbook.* Independence, KY: Cengage Learning.

Siefer, R., LaGasse, L. L., Lester, B., Bauer, C. R., Shankaran, S., Bada, H. S., et al. (2004). Attachment status in children prenatally exposed to cocaine and other substances. *Child Development, 75,* 850–868.

Singer, L. T., Arendt, R., Minnes, S., Salvator, A., Siegel, C., & Lewis, B. A. (2001). Developing language skills of cocaine-exposed infants. *Pediatrics, 107,* 1057–1064.

Singer, L. T., Nelson, S., Short, E., Min, M. O., Lewis, B., Russ, S., et al. (2008). Prenatal cocaine exposure: Drug and environmental effects at 9 years. *Journal of Pediatrics, 153,* 105–111.

Smith, J. M., DeThorne, L. S., Logan, J. A., Channell, R. W., & Petrill, S. A. (2014). Impact of prematurity on language skills at school age. *Journal of Speech, Language, and Hearing Research, 57,* 901–916.

Smith, L. K., Draper, E. S., Manktelow, B. N., Dorling, J. S., & Field, D. J. (2007). Socioeconomic inequalities in very preterm birth rates. *Archives Disease in Childhood, Education and Practice, 92,* F11–F14.

Smith, T., Groen, A. D., & Wynn, J. W. (2000). Randomized trial of intensive early intervention for children with pervasive developmental disorder. *American Journal of Mental Retardation, 105,* 269–285.

Sokol, R. J., Delaney-Black, V., & Nordstrom, B. (2003). Clinician corner: Fetal alcohol spectrum disorder. *Journal of the American Medical Association, 290*(22), 2996–2999.

Spiker, M., Lin, C. E., Van Dyke, M., & Wood, J. (2012). Restricted interests and anxiety in children with autism. *Autism: The International Journal of Research and Practice, 16,* 306–320.

Springer, S. C., & Annibale, D. J. (2007). Necrotizing enterocolitis. *eMedicine*. Last updated December 11, 2007. Retrieved September 24, 2008, from http://www.emedicine.com/ped/topic2601.htm

Stanton-Chapman, T. L., Chapman, D. A., Kaiser, A. P., & Hancock, T. B. (2004). Cumulative risk and low-income children's language development. *Topics in Early Childhood Special Education, 24*, 227–238.

Stevens, M., Fein, D., Dunn, M., Allen, D., Waterhouse, L., Feinstein, C., et al. (2000). Subgroups of children with autism by cluster analysis: A longitudinal examination. *Journal of the American Academy of Child and Adolescent Psychiatry, 39*, 346–352.

Stone, W. L., & Yoder, P. J. (2001). Predicting spoken language level in children with autism spectrum disorders. *Autism, 5*, 341–361.

Sullivan, P. M., & Knutson, J. E. (2000). Maltreatment and disabilities: A population-based epidemiological study. *Child Abuse & Neglect, 24*, 1257–1274.

Svirsky, M. A., Robbins, A. M., Kirk, K. I., Pisoni, D. B., & Miyamoto, R. T. (2000). Language development in profoundly deaf children with cochlear implants. *Psychological Science, 11*, 153–158.

Tager-Flusberg, H., Paul, R., & Lord, C. E. (2005). Language and communication in autism. In F. Volkmar, R. Paul, A. Klin, & D. J. Cohen (Eds.), *Handbook of autism and pervasive developmental disorder* (3rd ed., Vol. 1, pp. 335–364). New York: Wiley

Takarae, Y., Luna, B., Minshew, N. J., & Sweeney, J. A. (2008). Patterns of visual sensory and sensorimotor abnormalities in autism vary in relation to history of early language delay. *Journal of the International Neuropsychological Society, 14*, 980–989.

Tanne, J. H. (2006). Report demands investigation into rise in preterm births. *British Medical Journal, 333*(7560), 169.

Task Force on Newborn and Infant Hearing. (1999, February). Newborn and infant hearing loss: Detection and intervention. *Pediatrics, 103*(2), 527–530.

Thiemann-Bourque, K. S., Warren, S. F., Brady, N., Gilkerson, J., & Richards, J. A. (2014). Vocal interaction between children with Down syndrome and their parents. *American Journal of Speech-Language Pathology, 23*, 474–485.

Thompson, J. M., Irgens, I. M., Rasmussen, S., & Daltveit, A. K. (2006). Secular trends in socio-economic status and the implications for preterm birth. *Paediatric Perinatal Epidemiology, 20*, 182–187.

Tomblin, J. B., Smith, E., & Zhang, X. (1997). Epidemiology of specific language impairment: Prenatal and perinatal risk factors. *Journal of Communication Disorders, 30*(4), 325–343.

Tucker, J., & McGuire, W. (2004). *Epidemiology of preterm birth.* London: BMJ.

Uhlhorn, D. S., Messinger, D. S., & Bauer, C. R. (2005). Cocaine exposure and mother-toddler play. *Infant Behavior and Development, 28*, 62–73.

United Nations Children's Fund and World Health Organization. (2004). *Low birth weight: Country, regional and global estimates.* Geneva: WHO Publications. Retrieved July 23, 2013, from http://whqlibdoc.who.int/publications/2004/9280638327.pdf

U.S. Department of Health and Human Services, Health Resources and Services Administration, Maternal and Child Health Bureau. (2013). *Child health USA 2013.* Rockville, MD: U.S. Department of Health and Human Services.

U.S. Department of Health and Human Services, Substance Abuse and Mental Health Administration. (2008). *Fetal alcohol spectrum disorders.* Retrieved August 1, 2008, from http://www.fascenter.samhsa.gov

U.S. Department of State. (2012). *FY 2012 annual report on intercountry adoption.* Retrieved June 26, 2013, from http://adoption.state.gov/content/pdf/fy2012_annual_report.pdf

U.S. National Library of Medicine. (2010, December 15). *Mental retardation.* U.S. Department of Health and Human Services, National Institutes of Health. Retrieved January 2, 2011, from http://www.nlm.nih.gov/medlineplus/ency/article/001523.htm

Wachtel, K., & Carter, A. S. (2008). Reaction to diagnosis and parenting styles among mothers of young children with ASDs. *Autism, 12*, 575–594.

Wattendorf, D. J., & Muenke, M. (2005). Fetal alcohol spectrum disorders. *American Family Physician, 72*(2), 279–283.

Westerlund, M., Berglund, E., & Eriksson, M. (2006). Can severely language delayed 3-year-olds be identified at 18 months? Evaluation of a screening version of the MacArthur-Bates Communicative Development Inventories. *Journal of Speech, Language, and Hearing Research, 49*, 237–247.

Wetherby, A. M., Prizant, B. M., & Schuler, A. L. (2000). Understanding the nature of communication and language impairments. In A. M. Wetherby & B. M. Prizant (Eds.), *Autism spectrum disorders: A transactional developmental perspective* (pp. 109–141). Baltimore: Brookes.

Windsor, J., Glaze, L. E., & Koga, S. F. (2007). Language acquisition with limited input: Romanian institution and foster care. *Journal of Speech, Language, and Hearing Research, 50*, 1365–1381.

World Health Organization. (2010). *Mental retardation: From knowledge to action.* Retrieved January 2, 2011, from http://www.searo.who.int/en/Section1174/Section1199/Section1567/Section1825_8090.htm

Yoshinaga-Itano, C. (2003). From screening to early identification and intervention: Discovering predictors of successful outcomes for children with significant hearing loss. *Journal of Deaf Studies and Deaf Education, 8*, 11–30.

Young, R. L., Brewer, N., & Pattison C. (2003). Parental identification of early behavioural abnormalities in children with autistic disorder. *Autism, 7*, 125–143.

Zahaka, K. G., & Patel, C. R. (2002). Congenital defects. In A. A. Fanaroff & R. J. Martin (Eds.), *Neonatal-perinatal medicine: Diseases of the fetus and infant* (7th ed., pp. 1120–1139). St. Louis: Mosby.

Zipes, D. P., Libby, P., Bonow, R. O., Braunwald, E. (2007). *Braunwald's heart disease: A textbook of cardiovascular medicine* (8th ed.). St. Louis: W. B. Saunders.

Zubrick, S. R., Taylor, C. L., Rice, M. L., & Slegers, D. W. (2007). Late language emergence at 24 months: An epidemiological study of prevalence, predictors, and covariates. *Journal of Speech, Language, and Hearing Research, 50*, 1562–1592.

Zwaigenbaum, L., Bryson, S.E., Rogers, T., Roberts, W., Brian, J., & Szatmari, P. (2005). Behavioural manifestations of autism in the first year of life. *International Journal of Developmental Neuroscience, 23*, 143-152.

Zwaigenbaum, L., Thurm, A., Stone, W., Baranek, G., Bryson, S., Iverson, J., et al. (2007). Studying the emergence of autism spectrum disorders in high risk infants: Methodological and practical issues. *Journal of Autism and Developmental Disorders, 37*, 466-480.

CHAPTER 3

Abbeduto, L., & Short-Meyerson, K. (2002). Linguistic influences on social interaction. In H. Goldstein, L. Kaczmarek, & K. English (Eds.), *Promoting social interaction* (pp. 27–54). Baltimore: Brookes.

Alston, E., & St. James-Roberts, I. (2005). Home environments of 10-month-old infants selected by the WILSTAAR screen for pre-language difficulties. *International Journal of Language & Communication Disorders, 40,* 123–136.

American Speech-Language-Hearing Association (ASHA). (2008b). *Roles and responsibilities of speech-language pathologists in early intervention: Guidelines.* Washington, DC: American Speech-Language-Hearing Association.

Angelman, H. (1965). "Puppet" children: A report of three cases. *Developmental Medicine & Child Neurology, 7,* 681–688.

Bailey, D. B., Hebbeler, K., Scarborough, A., Spiker, D., & Mallik, S. (2004). First experiences with early intervention: A national perspective. *Pediatrics, 113,* 887–896.

Bibby, P., Eikeseth, S., Martin, N., Mudford, O., & Reeves, D. (2001). Progress and outcomes for children with autism receiving parent-managed intensive interventions. *Research in Developmental Disabilities, 22,* 425–447.

Boone, H., & Crais, E. (2001). Strategies for achieving family-driven assessment and intervention planning. In *Young Exceptional Children Monograph Series, No. 3.* Missoula, MT: Division for Early Childhood of the Council for Exceptional Children.

Bowen, M. (1978). *Family therapy in clinical practice.* New York and London: Jason Aronson.

Brady, N. C., & Halle, J. W. (2002). Breakdowns and repairs in conversations between beginning AAC users and their partners. In J. Reichle, D. R. Beukelman, & J. C. Light (Eds.), *Exemplary practices for beginning communicators: Implications for AAC* (pp. 323–351). Baltimore: Brookes.

Brady, N. C., Marquis, J., Fleming, K., & McLean, L. (2004). Prelinguistic predictors of language growth in children with developmental disabilities. *Journal of Speech, Language, and Hearing Research, 47,* 663–677.

Brady, N. C., Steeples, T., & Fleming, K. (2005). Effects of prelinguistic communication levels on initiation and repair of communication in children with disabilities. *Journal of Speech, Language, and Hearing Research, 48,* 1098–1113.

Bronfenbrenner, U. (1979). *The Ecology of human development: Experiments by nature and design.* Cambridge, MA: Harvard University Press.

Brown, W. H., Odom, S. L., & Conroy, M. A. (2001). An intervention hierarchy for promoting young children's peer interactions in natural environments. *Topics in Early Childhood Special Education, 21,* 162–176.

Buysse, V., & Wesley, P. (2005). *Consultation in early childhood settings.* Baltimore: Brookes.

Calandrella, A. M., & Wilcox, J. (2000). Predicting language outcomes for young prelinguistic children with developmental delays. *Journal of Speech, Language, and Hearing Research, 43,* 1061–1071.

Calculator, S. N. (2002). Use of enhanced natural gestures to foster interactions between children with Angelman syndrome and their parents. *American Journal of Speech-Language Pathology, 11,* 340–355.

Campbell, P. H., & Sawyer, L. B. (2007). Supporting learning opportunities in natural settings through participation-based services. *Journal of Early Intervention, 29,* 287–305.

Carpenter, M., & Tomasello, M. (2000). Joint attention, cultural learning, and language acquisition: Implications for children with autism. In A. M. Wetherby & B. M. Prizant (Eds.), *Autism spectrum disorders: A transactional developmental perspective* (pp. 31–54). Baltimore: Brookes.

Cole, K. N., Mills, P. E., Dale, P. S., & Jenkins, J. R. (1996). Preschool language facilitation methods and child characteristics. *Journal of Early Intervention, 20,* 113–131.

Crais, E. R., Boone, H., Harrison, M., Freund, P., Downing, K., & West, T. (2004). Interdisciplinary personnel preparation: Graduates' use of targeted practices. *Infants & Young Children, 17,* 82–92.

Davis, P. S., & Malone, D. M. (2001). Family assessment. In D. J. O'Shea, L. J. O'Shea, R. Algozzine, & D. Hammitte (Eds.), *Families and teachers of individuals with disabilities: Collaborative orientations and responsive practice* (pp. 102–126). Needham Heights, MA: Allyn & Bacon.

Doherty, G., Lero, D., Goelman, H., Tougas, J., & LaGrange, A. (2000). *You bet I care: Key findings and their implications.* Guelph, Ontario: The Centre for Families, Work and Well-Being.

Dunst, C. J. (2001). Participation of young children with disabilities in community learning activities. In M. J. Guralnick (Ed.), *Early childhood inclusion: Focus on change* (pp. 307–336). Baltimore: Brookes.

Dunst, C. J. (2004). Revisiting "Rethinking Early Intervention." In M. A. Feldman (Ed.), *Early intervention: The essential readings* (pp. 262–283). Oxford, UK: Blackwell.

Dunst, C. J., & Bruder, M. B. (2002). Valued outcomes of service coordination, early intervention, and natural environments. *Exceptional Children, 68,* 361–375.

Dunst, C. J., Bruder, M. B., Trivette, C. M., Hamby, D., Raab, M., & McLean, M. (2001). Characteristics and consequences of everyday natural learning opportunities. *Topics in Early Childhood Special Education, 21*(2), 68–92.

Dunst, C. J., Hamby, D., Trivette, C. M., Raab, M., & Bruder, M. B. (2000). Everyday family and community life and children's naturally occurring learning opportunities. *Journal of Early Intervention, 23*(3), 156–159.

Dunst, C. J., & Trivette, C. M. (2009a). Let's be PALS: An evidence-based approach to professional development. *Infants and Young Children, 22,* 164–176.

English, K., Goldstein, H., Shafer, K., & Kaczmarek, L. (1997). Promoting interactions among preschoolers with and without disabilities: Effects of a buddy skills-training program. *Exceptional Children, 63,* 229–243.

Fey, M. E., Warren, S. F., Brady, N., Finestack, L. H., Bredin-Oja, S. L., Fairchild, M., et al. (2006). Early effects of responsivity education/prelinguistic milieu teaching for children with developmental delays and their parents. *Journal of Speech, Language, and Hearing Research, 49,* 526–547.

Fixsen, D. L., Naoom, S. F., Blasé, K. A., Friedman, R. M., & Wallace, F. (2005). *Implementation research: A synthesis of the literature.* Tampa: Florida Mental Health Institute, University of South Florida.

Girolametto, L. E., Hoaken, L., Weitzman, E., & van Lieshout, R. (2000). Patterns of adult-child linguistic interaction in integrated day care groups. *Language, Speech, and Hearing Services in Schools, 31,* 155–168.

Girolametto, L. E., & Weitzman, E. (2002). Responsiveness of child care providers in interactions with toddlers and preschoolers. *Language, Speech, and Hearing Services in Schools, 33,* 268–281.

Girolametto, L. E., Weitzman, E., & Greenberg, J. (2003). Training day care staff to facilitate children's language. *American Journal of Speech-Language Pathology, 12,* 299–311.

Girolametto, L. E., Weitzman, E., & Greenberg, J. (2004). The effects of verbal support strategies on small-group peer interactions. *Language, Speech, and Hearing Services in Schools, 35,* 254–268.

Goldstein, H., English, K., Shafer, K., & Kaczmarek, L. (1997). Interaction among preschoolers with and without disabilities: Effects of across-the-day peer intervention. *Journal of Speech and Hearing Research, 40,* 33–48.

Goldstein, H., Walker, D., & Fey, M. (2005, November). *Comparing strategies for promoting communication of infants and toddlers.* Seminar presented at the annual convention of the American Speech-Language-Hearing Association, San Diego, CA.

Hammer, C., Tomblin, B., Zhang, X., & Weiss, A. (2001). Relationships between parenting behaviors and specific language impairment in children. *International Journal of Language & Communication Disorders, 36,* 185–205.

Hancock, T. B., & Kaiser, A. P. (2002). The effects of trainer-implemented enhanced milieu teaching on the social communication of children who have autism. *Topics in Early Childhood Special Education, 22,* 39–54.

Hancock, T. B., & Kaiser, A. P. (2006). Enhanced milieu teaching. In McCauley, R., & Fey, M. (Eds.), *Treatment of language disorders in children: Communication and language intervention series* (pp. 203–236). Baltimore: Brookes.

Hanft, B. E., Rush, D. D., & Sheldon, M. L. (2004). *Coaching families and colleagues in early childhood.* Baltimore: Brookes.

Hoff, E., & Naigles, L. (2002). How children use input to acquire a lexicon. *Child Development, 73,* 418–433.

Iverson, J. M, & Goldin-Meadow, S. (2005). Gesture paves the way for language development. *Psychological Science, 16*(5), 367–371.

Kaiser, A. P., & Delaney, E. (2001). Responsive conversations: Creating opportunities for naturalistic language teaching. In S. Sandall & M. Ostrosky (Eds.), *Young Exceptional Children Monograph Series, No. 3* (pp. 13–23). Washington, DC: Division for Early Childhood of the Council for Exceptional Children.

Kaiser, A. P., Hancock, T., & Neitfield, J. P. (2000). The effects of parent-implemented enhanced milieu teaching on social communication of children who have autism [Special issue]. *Journal of Early Education and Development, 4,* 423–446.

Kashinath, S. (2006). Enhancing generalized teaching strategy use in daily routines by parents of children with autism. *Journal of Speech, Language, and Hearing Research, 49,* 466–485.

Kelly, J., & Barnard, K. (2000). Assessment of parent-child interaction: Implications for early intervention. In J. Shonkoff & S. Meisels (Eds.), *Handbook of early childhood intervention* (2nd ed., pp. 258–289). Cambridge, UK: Cambridge University Press.

Knowles, M. S., Holton, E. F., & Swanson, R. A. (2005). *The adult learner: The definitive classic in adult education and human resource development* (6th ed.). London: Elsevier.

Koegel, L. K. (2000). Interventions to facilitate communication in autism. *Journal of Autism and Developmental Disorders, 30,* 383–391.

Kohler, F. W., Greteman, C., Raschke, D., & Highnam, C. (2007). Using a buddy skills package to increase the social interactions between a preschooler with autism and her peers. *Topics in Early Childhood Education, 27,* 155–164.

Kohler, F. W., Strain, P. S., & Goldstein, H. (2005). The effectiveness of peer-mediated intervention for young children with autism. In E. Hibbs & P. Jenson (Eds.), *Psychosocial treatments for child and adolescent disorders* (pp. 659–688). Washington, DC: American Psychological Association.

Kupetz, B. (2008). Do you see what I see? Appreciating diversity in early childhood settings. *Early Childhood News.* Retrieved April 26, 2016, from http://www.earlychildhoodnews.com/earlychildhood/article_view.aspx?ArticleID=147

Levitch, A., & Gable, S. (2015, December 2). *Reducing stereotyping in the preschool classroom.* Human Environmental Sciences Extension, University of Missouri Extension. Retrieved April 26, 2016, from http://extension.missouri.edu/hes/childcare/reducestereotype.htm

McCollum, J. A., Gooler, F., Appl, D. J., & Yates, T. J. (2001). PIWI: Enhancing parent-child interaction as a foundation for early intervention. *Infants and Young Children, 14*(1), 34–45.

McConnell, S. R. (2002). Interventions to facilitate social interaction for young children with autism: Review of available research and recommendations for educational interventions and future research. *Journal of Autism and Developmental Disorders, 12,* 351–372.

McLean, L. K. & Woods-Cripe, J. (1997). The effectiveness of early intervention for children with communication disorders. In M. J. Guralnick (Ed.), The effectiveness of early intervention: Second generation research (pp. 349–428). Baltimore: Brookes.

McWilliam, R. A. (2000). It's only natural . . . to have early intervention in the environments where it's needed. In S. Sandall & M. Ostrosky (Eds.), *Young Exceptional Children Monograph Series, No. 2* (pp. 17–26). Denver: Division for Early Childhood of the Council for Exceptional Children.

Mellon, A., & Winton, P. (2003). Interdisciplinary collaboration among early intervention faculty members. *Journal of Early Intervention, 25,* 173–188.

Mize, J. (1995). Coaching preschool children in social skills: A cognitive-social learning curriculum. In G. Carteledge, & J. F. Milbum (Eds.), *Teaching social skills to children and youth: Innovative approaches* (3rd ed., pp. 237–261). Boston: Allyn & Bacon.

Mize, J., & Ladd, G. W. (1990). A cognitive-social learning approach to social skill training with low-status preschool children. *Developmental Psychology, 26,* 388–397.

Mobayed, K., Collins, B., Strangis, D., Schuster, J., & Hemmeter, M. (2000). Teaching parents to employ Mand-model procedures to teach their children requesting. *Journal of Early Intervention, 23,* 165–179.

Odom, S. L., Brown, W. H., Frey, T, Karasu, N., Smith-Canter, L. L., & Strain, P. S. (2003). Evidence-based practices for young children with autism: Contributions for single-subject design research. *Focus on Autism and Other Developmental Disabilities, 18,* 166–175.

Odom, S. L., Zercher, C., Li, S., Marquart, J., Sandall, S., & Wolfberg, P. (2001). *Social relationships of children with disabilities and their peers in inclusive preschool classrooms.* Manuscript submitted for publication.

Owens, R. E. (2004). *Help your baby talk.* New York: Penguin Putnam.

Owens, R. E. (2014). *Language disorders: A functional approach to assessment and intervention* (6th ed.). Boston: Allyn & Bacon.

Paul-Brown, D., & Caperton, C. J. (2001). Inclusive practices for preschool-age children with specific language impairment. In M. J. Guralnick (Ed.), *Early childhood inclusion: Focus on change* (pp. 433–463). Baltimore: Brookes.

Pepper, J., & Weitzman, E. (2004). *It Takes Two to Talk®: A practical guide for parents of children with language delays* (2nd ed.). Toronto: The Hanen Centre.

Peterson, C. A., Luze, G. J., Eshbaugh, E. M., Jeon, H., & Kantz, K. R. (2007). Enhancing parent-child interactions through home visiting: Promising practice or unfulfilled promise? *Journal of Early Intervention, 29,* 119–140.

Pino, O. (2000). The effect of context on mother's interaction style with Down's syndrome and typically developing children. *Research in Developmental Disabilities, 21*(5), 329–346.

Polmanteer, K., & Turbiville, V. (2000). Family-responsive individualized family service plans for speech-language pathologists. *Language, Speech, and Hearing Services in Schools, 31,* 4–14.

Raab, M., & Dunst, C. J. (2007). Influence of child interests on variations in child behavior and functioning. In *Winterberry Research Syntheses* (Vol. 1, no. 21). Asheville, NC: Winterberry Press.

Roberts, M. Y., & Kaiser, A. P. (2011). The effectiveness of parent-implemented language interventions: A meta-analysis. *American Journal of Speech-Language Pathology, 20*, 180–199.

Roberts, M. Y., Kaiser, A. P., & Wright, C. (2010). *Parent training: Specific strategies beyond "Try this at home."* Paper presented at the annual convention of the American Speech-Language-Hearing Association, Philadelphia.

Rogers-Adkinson, D. L., & Stuart, S. K. (2007). Collaborative services: Children experiencing neglect and the side effects of prenatal alcohol exposure. *Language, Speech, and Hearing Services in Schools, 38*, 149–156.

Rollins, P. R. (2003). Caregivers' contingent comments to 9-month-old infants: Relationships with later language. *Applied Psycholinguistics, 24*, 221–234.

Roper, N., & Dunst, C. J. (2003). Communication intervention in natural environments. *Infants & Young Children, 16*, 215–225.

Roth, F. P., & Baden, B. (2001). Investing in emergent literacy intervention: A key role for speech-language pathologists. *Seminars in Speech and Language, 22*, 163–174.

Rowe, M. (2008). Child-directed speech: Relation to socioeconomic status, knowledge of child development and child vocabulary skill. *Journal of Child Language, 35*, 185–205.

Sandall, S., Hemmeter, M. L., Smith, B. J., & McLean, M. E. (2005). *DEC recommended practices: A comprehensive guide for practical application in early intervention/early childhood special education.* Longmont, CO: Sopris West Education Services.

Smith, J., Warren, S., Yoder, P., & Feurer, I. (2004). Teachers' use of naturalistic communication intervention practices. *Journal of Early Intervention, 27*(1), 1–14.

Smith, V., Mirenda, P., & Zaidman-Zait, A. (2007). Predictors of expressive vocabulary growth in children with autism. *Journal of Speech, Language, and Hearing Research, 50*, 149–160.

Tomasello, M. (2001). Perceiving intentions and learning words in the second year of life. In M. Bowerman & S. Levinson (Eds.), *Language acquisition and conceptual development* (pp. 133–158). New York: Cambridge University Press.

Trivette, C., & Dunst, C. (2007). Capacity-building family-centered help-giving practices. *Winterberry Research Syntheses* (Vol. 1, no. 1). Asheville, NC: Winterberry Press.

Trivette, C., Dunst, C., Hamby, D., & O'Herin, C. (2009). Characteristics and consequences of adult learning methods and strategies. *Winterberry Research Syntheses* (Vol. 2, no. 2). Asheville, NC: Winterberry Press.

U.S. Census Bureau. (2013). Population estimates. Retrieved July 9, 2013, from http://factfinder2.census.gov/faces/tableservices/jsf/pages/productview.xhtml?src=bkmk

Vigil, D., Hodges, J., & Klee, T. (2005). Quantity and quality of parental language input to late-talking toddlers during play. *Child Language Teaching and Therapy, 21*, 107–122.

Watt, N., Wetherby, A., & Shumway, S. (2006). Prelinguistic predictors of language outcome at 3 years of age. *Journal of Speech, Language, and Hearing Research, 49*, 1224–1237.

Weiss, R. S. (1981). INREAL intervention for language handicapped and bilingual children. *Journal of Early Intervention, 4*(1), 40–51.

Weitzman, E. (1992). *Learning language and loving it: A guide to promoting children's social and language development in early childhood settings.* Toronto: The Hanen Centre.

Weitzman, E. (1994). The Hanen Program® for early childhood educators: Inservice training for child care providers on how to facilitate children's social, language, and literacy development. *Infant-Toddler Intervention: The Transdisciplinary Journal, 4*, 173–202.

Weitzman, E. (2005). *Routines: Powerful ways to foster interaction and language learning.* Paper presented at the annual convention of the American Speech-Language-Hearing Association, San Diego, CA.

Weizman, Z., & Snow, C. (2001). Lexical input as related to children's vocabulary acquisition: Effects of sophisticated exposure and support for meaning. *Developmental Psychology, 37*, 265–279.

Wetherby, A. M., & Woods, J. J. (2006). Early social interaction project for children with autism spectrum disorders beginning in the second year of life: A preliminary study. *Topics in Early Childhood Special Education, 26*, 67–82.

Wilcox, M. J., Bacon, C. K., & Greer, D. C. (2005). *Evidence-based early language intervention: Caregiver verbal responsivity training.* Retrieved June 23, 2010, from http://www.asu.edu/clas/icrp/research/presentations/p1/pdf2.pdf

Wilcox, M. J., Guimond, A. B., & Kim, S. J. (2010, February). *The relationship between home visiting practices focused on teaching caregivers and children's outcomes.* Poster presented at the biannual meeting of the Conference on Research Innovations in Early Intervention, San Diego.

Wilcox, M. J., & Woods, J. (2011). Participation as a basis for developing early intervention outcomes. *Language, Speech, and Hearing Services in Schools, 42*, 365–378.

Woods, J. J., Kashinath, S., & Goldstein, H. (2004). Effects of embedding caregiver-implemented teaching strategies in daily routines on children's communication outcomes. *Journal of Early Intervention, 26*, 175–193.

Woods, J. J., & Lindeman, D. P. (2008). Gathering and giving information with families. *Infants and Young Children, 21*, 272–284.

Woods, J. J., Wilcox, M. J., Friedman, M., & Murch, T. (2011). Collaborative consultation in natural environments: Strategies to enhance family-centered supports and services. *Language, Speech, and Hearing Services in Schools, 42*, 379–392.

Yoder, P., McCathren, R., Warren, S., & Watson, A. (2001). Important distinctions in measuring maternal responses to communication in prelinguistic children with disabilities. *Communication Disorders Quarterly, 22*, 135–147.

Yoder, P. J., & Warren, S. F. (2001b). Relative treatment effects of two prelinguistic communication interventions on language development in toddlers with developmental delays vary by maternal characteristics. *Journal of Speech, Language, and Hearing Research, 44*, 224–237.

Yoder, P. J., & Warren, S. F. (2002). Effects of prelinguistic milieu reaching and parent responsivity education on dyads involving children with intellectual disabilities. *Journal of Speech, Language, and Hearing Research, 45*, 1158–1174.

CHAPTER 4

Abbeduto, L., & Boudreau, D. (2004). Theoretical influences in research on language development and intervention in individuals with mental retardation. *Mental Retardation and Developmental Disabilities Research Reviews, 10*, 184–192.

American Academy of Pediatrics. (2012). Patient- and family-centered care and the pediatrician's role. *Pediatrics, 29*(2), 394–404.

American Speech-Language-Hearing Association (ASHA). (1996, April). Discrepancy models and the discrepancy between policy and evidence. In N. W. Nelson (Ed.), *Newsletter of Special Interest Division 1, Language Learning and Education* (Vol. 3, Issue 1). Rockville, MD: Author.

American Speech-Language-Hearing Association (ASHA). (1999). *Guidelines for the roles and responsibilities of the school-based speech-language pathologist.* Rockville, MD: Author.

American Speech-Language-Hearing Association (ASHA). (2000, July). Cognitive referencing. In P. M. Rhyner (Ed.), *Newsletter of Special Interest Division 1, Language Learning and Education* (Vol. 7, Issue 1). Rockville, MD: Author.

American Speech-Language-Hearing Association (ASHA). (2004a). Admission/discharge criteria in speech-language pathology. *ASHA Supplement, 24,* 65–70.

American Speech-Language-Hearing Association. (2008b). *Roles and responsibilities of speech-language pathologists in early intervention: Guidelines.* Washington, DC: Author.

Anzalone, M., & Williamson, G. (2000). Sensory processing and motor performance in autism spectrum disorders. In A. M. Wetherby & B. M. Prizant (Eds.), *Autism spectrum disorders: A transactional developmental perspective* (pp. 144–166). Baltimore: Brookes.

Applequist, K. L., & Bailey, D. B. (2000). Navajo caregivers' perceptions of early intervention services. *Journal of Early Intervention, 23,* 47–61.

Bailey, D. B., (2004). Assessing family resources, priorities, and concerns. In M. McLean, M. Wolery, & D. Baile (Eds.), *Assessing infants and preschoolers with special needs* (3rd ed., pp. 172–203). Upper Saddle River, NJ: Pearson/Merrill/Prentice Hall.

Bailey, D. B., Jr., Hatton, D. D., Skinner, M., & Mesibov, G. (2001). Autistic behavior, FMR1 protein, and developmental trajectories in young males with fragile X syndrome. *Journal of Autism and Developmental Disorders, 31,* 165–174.

Barrera, I., & Corso, R. (2002). Cultural competency as skilled dialogue. *Topics in Early Childhood Special Education, 22*(20), 103–113.

Bates, E., & Dick, F. (2002). Language, gesture, and the developing brain. *Developmental Psychobiology, 40,* 293–310.

Bayley, N. (1993). *Bayley Scales of Infant Development, Second Edition.* San Antonio, TX: The Psychological Corporation.

Bedore, L. M., Peña, E. D., García, M., & Cortez, C. (2005). Clinical forum: Conceptual versus monolingual scoring: When does it make a difference? *Language, Speech, and Hearing Services in Schools, 36,* 188–200.

Beuker, K., Rommelse, N., Donders, R., & Buitelaar, J. (2013). Development of early communication skills in the first two years of life. *Infant Behavior and Development, 36,* 71–83.

Bialystok, E., & Feng, X. (2011). Language proficiency and its implications for monolingual and bilingual children. In A. Y. Durgunoglu & C. Goldenberg (Eds.), *Dual-language learners: The development and assessment of oral and written language.* New York: Guilford Press.

Blake, J. (2000). *Routes to child language: Evolutionary and developmental precursors.* New York: Cambridge University Press.

Bodfish, J., Symons, F., Parker, D., & Lewis, M. (2000) Varieties of repetitive behavior in autism: Comparisons to mental retardation. *Journal of Autism and Developmental Disorders, 30,* 237–243.

Bono, M. A., Daley, T., & Sigman, M. (2004). Relations among joint attention, amount of intervention and language gain in autism. *Journal of Autism and Developmental Disorders, 34,* 495–505.

Bono, M. A., & Sigman, M. (2004). Relations among joint attention, amount of intervention and language gain in autism. *Journal of Autism and Developmental Disorders, 34,* 495–505.

Bopp, K. D., Brown, K. E., & Mirenda, P. (2004). Speech-language pathologists' roles in the delivery of positive behavior support for individuals with developmental disabilities. *American Journal of Speech-Language Pathology, 13,* 5–19.

Brady, N. C., & Halle, J. W. (2002). Breakdowns and repairs in conversations between beginning AAC users and their partners. In J. Reichle, D. R. Beukelman, & J. C. Light (Eds.), *Exemplary practices for beginning communicators: Implications for AAC* (pp. 323–351). Baltimore: Brookes.

Brady, N. C., Marquis, J., Fleming, K., & McLean, L. (2004). Prelinguistic predictors of language growth in children with developmental disabilities. *Journal of Speech, Language, and Hearing Research, 47,* 663–677.

Brady, N. C., Skinner, D., Roberts, J., & Hennon, E. (2006). Communication in young children with fragile X syndrome: A qualitative study of mothers' perspectives. *American Journal of Speech-Language Pathology, 15,* 353–364.

Brian, J., Bryson, S. E., Garon, N., Roberts, W., Smith, I. M., Szatmari, P., et al. (2008). Clinical assessment of autism in high-risk 18-month-olds. *Autism, 12,* 433–456.

Bricker, D. (Ed.). (2002). *AEPS: Assessment, evaluation, and programming system for infants and children* (2nd ed.). Baltimore: Brookes.

Bruder, M. B. (2000). Family-centered early intervention: Clarifying our values for the new millennium. *Topics in Early Childhood Special Education, 20,* 105–115.

Bryson, S. E., Zwaigenbaum, L., Brian, J., Roberts, W., Szatmari, P., Rombough, V., et al. (2007). A prospective case series of high-risk infants who developed autism. *Journal of Autism and Developmental Disorders, 37,* 12–24.

Calandrella, A. M., & Wilcox, J. (2000). Predicting language outcomes for young prelinguistic children with developmental delays. *Journal of Speech, Language, and Hearing Research, 43,* 1061–1071.

Capone, N. C. (2007). Tapping toddlers' evolving semantic representation via gesture. *Journal of Speech, Language, and Hearing Research, 50,* 732–745.

Capone, N. C., & McGregor, K. K. (2004). Gesture development: A review for clinical and research practices. *Journal of Speech, Language, and Hearing Research, 47,* 173–186.

Carpenter, R. L. (1987). Play Scale. In L. Olswang, C. Stoel-Gammon, T. Coggins, & R. L. Carpenter (Eds.), *Assessing prelinguistic and early behaviors in developmentally young children* (pp. 44–77). Seattle: University of Washington Press.

Carr, E. (1988). Functional equivalence as a mechanism of response generalization. In R. Horner, R. Koegel, & G. Dunlap (Eds.), *Generalization and maintenance: Life-style changes in applied settings* (pp. 221–241). Baltimore: Brookes.

Carr, D., & Felice, D. (2000). Application of stimuli equivalence to language intervention with severe linguistic disabilities. *Journal of Intellectual and Developmental Disability, 25,* 181–205.

Carruth, B. R., & Skinner, J. D. (2002). Feeding behaviors and other motor development in healthy children (2–24 months). *Journal of the American College of Nutrition, 21*(2), 88–96.

Carruth, B. R., Ziegler, P. J., Gordon, A., et al. (2004). Developmental milestones and self-feeding behaviors in infants and toddlers. *Journal of the American Dietetic Association, 104*(1 Suppl 1), s51–56.

Carson, C. P., Klee, T., Carson, D. K., & Hime, L. K. (2003). Phonological profiles of 2-year-olds with delayed language development: Predicting clinical outcomes at age 3. *American Journal of Speech-Language Pathology, 12,* 28–39.

Casby, M. W. (2003). Developmental assessment of play: A model for early intervention. *Communication Disorders Quarterly, 24*, 175-183.

Chakrabarti, S., & Fombonne, E. (2005). Pervasive developmental disorders in preschool children: Confirmation of high prevalence. *American Journal of Psychiatry, 162*, 1133-1141.

Chan, J. B., & Iacono, T. (2001). Gesture and word production in children with Down syndrome. *Augmentative and Alternative Communication, 17*, 73-87.

Chapman, R., Seung, H., Schwartz, S., & Bird, E. (2000). Predicting language production in children and adolescents with Down syndrome: The role of comprehension. *Journal of Speech, Language, and Hearing Research, 43*, 340-350.

Charman, T. R., Baron-Cohen, S., Swettenham, J., Baird, G., Drew, A., & Cox, A. (2003). Predicting language outcome in infants with autism and pervasive developmental disorder. *International Journal of Language and Communication Disorders, 38*, 265-285.

Charman, T. R., Swettenham, B. S., Cox, A., Baird, G., & Drew, A. (1998). An experimental investigation of social-cognitive abilities in infants with autism: Clinical implications. *Infant Mental Health Journal, 19*, 260-275.

Chen, Y., & McCollum, J. (2001). Taiwanese mothers' perspectives of parent-infant interaction with children with Down syndrome. *Journal of Early Intervention, 24*, 252-265.

Chiat, S., & Roy, P. (2008). Early phonological and sociocognitive skills as predictors of later language and social communication outcomes. *Journal of Child Psychology and Psychiatry, 49*, 635-645.

Colgan, S., Lanter, E., McComish, C., Watson, L., Crais, E., & Baranek, G. (2006). Analysis of social interaction gestures in infants with autism. *Child Neuropsychology, 12*, 307-319.

Conboy, B. T., & Thal, D. J. (2006). Ties between the lexicon and grammar: Cross-sectional and longitudinal studies of bilingual toddlers. *Child Development, 77*, 712-735.

Core, C., Hoff, E., Rumiche, R., & Seño, M. (2013). Total and conceptual vocabulary in Spanish-English bilinguals from 22 to 30 months: Implications for assessment. *Journal of Speech, Language, and Hearing Research, 56*, 1637-1649.

Crais, E. R., & Belardi, C. (1999). Family participation in child assessment: Perceptions of families and professionals. *Infant-Toddler Intervention: The Transdisciplinary Journal, 9*, 209-238.

Crais, E. R., Douglas, D., & Campbell, C. (2004). The intersection of the development of gestures and intentionality. *Journal of Speech, Language, and Hearing Research, 47*, 678-694.

Crais, E., & Roberts, J. (2004). Assessing communication skills. In M. McLean, M. Wolery, & D. Bailey (Eds.), *Assessing infants and preschoolers with special needs* (3rd ed., pp. 345-411). Upper Saddle River, NJ: Pearson/Merrill/Prentice Hall.

Crais, E. R., Roy, V. P., & Free, K. (2006). Parents' and professionals' perceptions of the implementation of family-centered practices in child assessments. *American Journal of Speech-Language Pathology, 15*, 365-377.

Dale, P. S., Price, T. S., Bishop, D. V. M., & Plomin, R. (2003). Outcomes of early language delay: I. Predicting persistent and transient language difficulties at 3 and 4 years. *Journal of Speech, Language, and Hearing Research, 46*, 544-560.

Dawson, G., Osterling, J., Meltzoff, A., & Kuhl, P. (2000). Case study of the development of an infant with autism from birth to two years of age. *Journal of Applied Developmental Psychology, 21*, 299-313.

Dawson, G., Toth, K., Abbott, R., Osterling, J., Munson, J., Estes, A., & Liaw, J. (2004). Early social attention impairments in autism: Social orienting, joint attention, and attention to distress. *Developmental Psychology, 40*, 271-283.

Dawson, G., & Watling, R. (2000) Interventions to facilitate auditory, visual, and motor integration in autism: A review of the evidence. *Journal of Autism and Developmental Disorders, 30*, 415-421.

DeGangi, G. (2000). *Pediatric disorders of regulation in affect and behavior: A therapist's guide to assessment and treatment.* San Diego, CA: Academic Press.

Dempsey, I., & Dunst, C. (2004). Helpgiving styles and parent empowerment in families with a young child with a disability. *Journal of Intellectual and Developmental Disability, 29*(1), 40-51.

DeVeney, S. L., Hoffman, L., & Cress, C. J. (2012). Communication-based assessment of developmental age for young children with developmental disabilities. *Journal of Speech, Language, and Hearing Research, 55*, 695-709.

Dore, J. (1975). Holophrases, speech acts and language universals. *Journal of Child Language, 2*, 20-40.

Duchesne, L., Sutton, A., & Trudeau, N. (2005). *Semantic relations in toddlers' gesture-speech combinations.* Paper presented at the annual convention of the American Speech-Language-Hearing Association, San Diego.

Dunst, C. J. (2002). Family-centered practices: Birth through high school. *Journal of Special Education, 36*, 139-147.

Durand, V. M., & Merges, E. (2001). Functional communication training: A contemporary behavior analytic technique for problem behavior. *Focus on Autism and Other Developmental Disabilities, 16*, 110-119.

Dziuk, M., Gidley, J., Larson, J., Apostu, A., Mahone, E., Denckla, M., & Mostofsky, S. (2007). Dyspraxia in autism: Association with motor, social, and communicative deficits. *Developmental Medicine & Child Neurology, 49*, 734-739.

Eicher, P. (2002). Feeding. In M. L. Batshaw (Ed.), *Children with disabilities* (5th ed., pp. 549-566). Baltimore: Brookes.

Evans, J. A., Alibali, M. W., & McNeil, N. M. (2001). Divergence of verbal expression and embodied knowledge: Evidence from speech and gesture in children with specific language impairment. *Language and Cognitive Processes, 16*, 309-331.

Fenson, L., Marchman, V., Thal, D., Dale, P., Reznick, S., & Bates, E. (2006). *The MacArthur-Bates Communicative Development Inventories: User's guide and technical manual* (2nd ed.). Baltimore: Brookes.

Flagler S. (1996). *The Infant-Preschool Play Assessment Scale.* Chapel Hill, NC: Chapel Hill Training-Outreach Project, Inc.

Fox, L., Dunlap, G., & Buschbacher, P. (2000). Understanding and intervening with children's challenging behavior: A comprehensive approach. In S. F. Warren & J. Reichle (Series Eds.) & A. M. Wetherby A. M. Wetherby & B. M. Prizant (Vol. Eds.), *Communication and language intervention series: Vol. 9. Autism spectrum disorders: A transactional developmental perspective* (pp. 307-331). Baltimore: Brookes.

Gisel, E. G. (1991). Effect of food texture on the development of chewing of children between six months and two years of age. *Developmental Medicine & Child Neurology, 33*(1), 69-79.

Gogate, L. J., Maganti, M., & Perenyi, A. (2014). Preterm and term infants' perception of temporally coordinated syllable-object pairings: Implications for lexical development. *Journal of Speech, Language, and Hearing Research, 57*, 187-198.

Gogate, L. J., Prince, C. G., & Matatyaho, D. (2009). Two-month-old infants' sensitivity to syllable-object pairings: The role of temporal synchrony. *Journal of Experimental Psychology: Human Perception and Performance, 35*, 508-519.

Goldin-Meadow, S., & Butcher, C. (2003). Pointing toward two-word speech in young children. In S. Kita (Ed.), *Pointing: Where language, culture, and cognition meet* (pp. 85–107). Mahwah, NJ: Erlbaum.

Goodwyn, S. W., Acredolo, L. P., & Brown, C. A. (2000). Impact of symbolic gesturing on early language development. *Journal of Nonverbal Behavior, 24,* 81–103.

Hadley, P. A. (2006). Assessing the emergence of grammar in toddlers at-risk for specific language impairment. *Seminars in Speech and Language, 27,* 173–186.

Hadley, P. A., & Holt, J. (2006). Individual differences in the onset of tense marking: A growth curve analysis. *Journal of Speech, Language, and Hearing Research, 49,* 984–1000.

Hadley, P. A., & Short, H. (2005). The onset of tense marking in children at risk for specific language impairment. *Journal of Speech, Language, and Hearing Research, 48,* 1344–1362.

Halle, J., Brady, N., & Drasgow, E. (2004). Enhancing socially adaptive communicative repairs of beginning communicators with disabilities. *American Journal of Speech-Language Pathology, 13,* 43–54.

Halle, J. W., & Drasgow, E. (2003). Response classes: Don Baer's contribution to understanding their structure and function. In K. S. Budd & T. Stokes (Eds.), *A small matter of proof: The legacy of Donald M. Baer* (pp. 113–124). Reno, NV: Context Press.

Hanson, R., & Olswang, L. (2005). *Prelinguistic signals of requesting and repair strategies.* Paper presented at the annual convention of the American Speech-Language-Hearing Association, San Diego.

Harris, S., & Handleman, J. (2000). Age and IQ at intake as predictors of placement for young children with autism: A four- to six-year follow-up. *Journal of Autism and Developmental Disorders, 30,* 137–142.

Hawdon, J., Beauregard, N., Slattery, J., & Kennedy, G. (2000). Identification of neonates at risk of developing problems in infancy. *Developmental Medicine and Child Neurology, 42,* 235–239.

Hoff, E., Core, C., Place, S., Rumiche, R., Señor, M., & Parra, M. (2012). Dual language exposure and early bilingual development. *Journal of Child Language, 39,* 1–27.

Hollich, G., Hirsh-Pasek, K., & Golinkoff, R. (2000). Breaking the language barrier: An emergentist coalition model for the origins of word learning. *Monographs of the Society for Research in Child Development, 65*(3, Serial No. 262).

Ingersoll, B. (2008). The effect of context on imitation skills in children with autism. *Research in Autism Spectrum Disorders, 2,* 332–340.

Institute of Medicine. (2001). *Crossing the Quality Chasm: A New Health System for the 21st Century.* Washington, DC: National Academy Press.

Iverson, J. M., & Goldin-Meadow, S. (2005). Gesture paves the way for language development. *Psychological Science, 16*(5), 367–371.

Iyer, S., & Ertmer, D. J. (2014). Relationships between vocalization forms and functions in infancy: Preliminary implications for early communicative assessment and intervention. *American Journal of Speech-Language Pathology, 23,* 587–598.

Johnson, C. P., & Myers, S. M. (2007). Identification and evaluation of children with autism spectrum disorders. *Pediatrics, 120,* 1183–1215.

Johnson, C. P., Myers, S. M., & The Council on Children with Disabilities. (2007). *Identification and evaluation of children with autism spectrum disorders.* Elk Grove, IL: American Academy of Pediatrics.

Johnson-Martin, N. M., Attermeier, S. M., & Hacker, B. J. (2004). *The Carolina Curriculum for Infants & Toddlers With Special Needs, Third Edition.* Baltimore: Brookes.

Junker, D. A., & Stockman, I. J. (2002). Expressive vocabulary of German-English bilingual toddlers. *American Journal of Speech-Language Pathology, 11,* 381–394.

Keen, D. (2003). Communication repair strategies and problem behaviours of children with autism. *International Journal of Disability Development and Education, 50*(1), 53–64.

Keen, D., Sigafoos, J., & Woodyatt, G. (2001). Replacing prelinguistic behaviors with functional communication. *Journal of Autism and Developmental Disorder, 31,* 385–398.

Kelly-Vance, L., Needelman, H., Troia, K., & Ryalls, B. (1999). Early childhood assessment: A comparison of the Bayley Scales of Infant Development and play-based assessment in two-year-old at-risk children. *Developmental Disabilities Bulletin, 27*(1), 1–15.

Kent, R., & Vorperian, H. (2007). In the mouths of babes: Anatomic, motor, and sensory foundations of speech development in children. In R. Paul (Ed.), *Language disorders from a developmental perspective* (pp. 55–82). Mahwah, NJ: Erlbaum.

Klee, T., Gavin, W., & Letts, C. (2002, June). *Development of a reference profile of children's grammatical development.* Poster presented at the International Congress for the Study of Child Language/Symposium for Research on Child Language Disorders, Madison, WI.

Kuhl, P. K., Coffey-Corina, S., Padden, D., & Dawson, G. (2005). Links between social and linguistic processing of speech in preschool children with autism: Behavioral and electrophysiological measures. *Developmental Science, 8*(1), F1–F12.

Landry, R., & Bryson, S. E. (2004). Impaired disengagement of attention in young children with autism. *Journal of Child Psychology and Psychiatry, 45,* 1115–1122.

Lee, J. (2011). Size matters: Early vocabulary as a predictor of language and literacy competence. *Applied Psycholinguistics, 32,* 69–92.

Leekam, S. R., Lopez, B., & Moore, C. (2000). Attention and joint attention in preschool children with autism. *Developmental Psychology, 36,* 261–273.

Leonard, L. B., Camarata, S., Brown, B., & Camarata, M. (2004). Tense and agreement in the speech of children with specific language impairment: Patterns of generalization through intervention. *Journal of Speech, Language, and Hearing Research, 47,* 1363–1379.

Light, J. C., Parsons, A., & Drager, K. D. (2002). "There's more to life than cookies": Developing interactions for social closeness with beginning communicators who use AAC. In J. Reichle, D. Beukelman, & J. Light (Eds.), *Exemplary practices for beginning communicators: Implications for AAC* (pp. 187–218). Baltimore: Brookes.

Linder, T. (1993). *Transdisciplinary play-based assessment: A functional approach to working with young children (TPBA).* Baltimore: Brookes.

Liss, M., Saulnier, C., Fein, D., & Kinsbourne, M. (2006). Sensory and attention abnormalities in autistic spectrum disorders. *Autism, 10,* 155–172.

Loh, A., Soman, T., Brian, J., Bryson, S., Roberts, W., Szatmari, P., et al. (2007). Stereotyped motor behaviours associated with autism in high-risk infants: A pilot videotape analysis of a sibling sample. *Journal of Autism and Developmental Disorders, 37,* 25–36.

Lord, C., & Risi, C. (2000). Diagnosis of autism spectrum disorders in young children. In A. Wetherby & B. Prizant (Eds.), *Autism spectrum disorders* (pp. 11–30). Baltimore: Brookes.

Lowe, M., & Costello, A. J. (1988). *Symbolic play test* (2nd ed.). Oxford, UK: NFER-Nelson.

Lyytinen, P., Poikkeus, A.-M., Laakso, M.-L., Eklund, K., & Lyytinen, H. (2001). Language development and symbolic play in children with and without familial risk for dyslexia. *Journal of Speech, Language, and Hearing Research, 44*, 873–885.

Määttä, S., Laakso, M.-L., Tolvanen, A., Ahonen, T., & Aro, T. (2012). Developmental trajectories of early communication skills. *Journal of Speech, Language, and Hearing Research, 55*, 1083–1096.

Mandell, D. S., Novak, M., & Zubritsky, C. (2005). Factors associated with age of diagnosis among children with autism spectrum disorders. *Pediatrics, 116*, 1480–1486.

Marchman, V. A., Martínez-Sussmann, C., & Dale, P. S. (2004). The language-specific structure of grammatical development: Evidence from bilingual language learners. *Developmental Science, 7*, 212–224.

Masur, E. F., & Eichorst, D. L. (2002). Infants' spontaneous imitation of novel versus familiar words: Relations to observational and maternal report measures of their lexicons. *Merrill-Palmer Quarterly, 48*, 405–426.

Matson, J. L., Wilkins, J., & Gonzalez, M. (2008). Early identification and diagnosis in autism spectrum disorders in young children and infants: How early is too early? *Research in Autism Spectrum Disorders, 2*, 75–84.

McCathren, R. B., Yoder, P. J., & Warren, S. F. (2000). Testing predictive validity of the communication composite of the Communication and Symbolic Behavior Scales. *Journal of Early Intervention, 23*(3), 36–46.

McCune, L. (1995). A normative study of representational play at the transition to language. *Developmental Psychology, 31*, 200–211.

McGregor, K., & Capone, N. (2001, December). *Contributions of genetic, environmental, and health-related factors to the acquisition of early gestures and words: A longitudinal case study of quadruplets.* Poster presented at the Early Lexicon Acquisition Conference, Lyon, France.

McNeil, N. M., Alibali, M. W., & Evans, J. (2000). The role of gesture in children's comprehension of spoken language: Now they need it, now they don't. *Journal of Nonverbal Behavior, 24*(2), 131–149.

McWilliam, R. A., Synder, P., Harbin, G., Porter, P., & Munn, D. (2000). Professionals' and families' perceptions of family-centered practices in infant-toddler services. *Early Education and Development, 11*(4), 519–538.

Meadan, H., Halle, J. W., Watkins, R. V., & Chadsey, J. G. (2006). Examining communication repairs of two young children with autism spectrum disorder: The influence of the environment. *American Journal of Speech-Language Pathology, 15*(1), 57–71.

Mirenda, P., Smith, V., Fawcett, S., & Johnston, J. (2003, November). *Language and communication intervention outcomes for young children with autism.* Paper presented at the American Speech-Language-Hearing Association Annual Conference, Chicago.

Moeller, M. P. (2000). Early intervention and language development in children who are deaf and hard-of-hearing. *Pediatrics, 106*, 43–61.

Morales, M., Mundy, P., Delgado, C., Yale, M., Messinger, D., Neal, R., & Schwartz, H. (2000). Responding to joint attention across the 6- through 24-month age period and early language acquisition. *Journal of Applied Developmental Psychology, 21*, 283–298.

Morris, S. (1982). *Pre-Speech Assessment Scale.* Clifton, NJ: Preston.

Mundy, P., & Acra, C. (2006). Joint attention, social engagement, and the development of social competence. In P. Marshall & N. Fox (Eds.), *The development of social neurobiological perspectives* (pp. 81–117). New York: Oxford University Press.

Mundy, P., Block, J., Delgado, C., Pomaes, Y., Van Hecke, A. V., & Parlade, M. V. (2007). Individual differences and the development of joint attention in infancy. *Child Development, 78*, 938–954.

Mundy, P., & Newell, L. (2007). Attention, joint attention, and social cognition. *Current Directions in Psychological Science, 16*, 269–274.

Namy, L. L., Acredolo, L., & Goodwyn, S. (2000). Verbal labels and gestural routines in parental communication with young children. *Journal of Nonverbal Behavior, 24*(2), 63–79.

Nathani, S., Ertmer, D. J., & Stark, R. E. (2006). Assessing vocal development in infants and toddlers. *Clinical Linguistics & Phonetics, 20*, 351–369.

Neitzel, J. L., Watson, R., Crais, E., Baranek, G., Dysinger, A., Wood, S., & Barry, S. (2003, April). *Gesture use in infants with autism at 9–12 and 15–18 months.* Paper presented at the Biennial Meeting of the Society for Research and Child Development, Tampa, FL.

Newborg, J., Stock, J. R., Wnek, L., Guidubaldi, J., & Svinicki, J. (2005). *Battelle Developmental Inventory* (2nd ed.). Chicago: Riverside.

Nobrega, L., Borion, M., Henrot, A., & Saliba, E. (2004). Acoustic study of swallowing behavior in premature infants during tube-bottle feeding and bottle feeding period. *Early Human Development, 78*, 53–60.

Oller, D. K. (2000). *The emergence of the speech capacity.* Mahwah, NJ: Erlbaum.

O'Neill, D. K. (2007). The language use inventory for young children: A parent-report measure of pragmatic language development for 18- to 47-month-old children. *Journal of Speech, Language, and Hearing Research, 50*, 214–228.

Osterling, J. A., Dawson, G., & Munson, J. A. (2002). Early recognition of 1-year-old infants with autism spectrum disorder versus mental retardation. *Development and Psychopathology, 14*, 239–251.

Owens, R. (1978). *Speech acts in the early language of non-delayed and retarded children: A taxonomy and distributional study.* Unpublished doctoral dissertation, The Ohio State University.

Özçalişkan, S., & Goldin-Meadow, S. (2005). Gesture is at the cutting edge of early language development. *Cognition, 96*, B101–B113.

Parra, M., Hoff, E., & Core, C. (2011). Relations among language exposure, phonological memory, and language development in Spanish-English bilingually-developing two-year-olds. *Journal of Experimental Child Psychology, 108*, 113–125.

Patten, E., & Watson, L. R. (2011). Interventions targeting attention in young children with autism. *American Journal of Speech-Language Pathology, 20*, 60–69.

Paul, R. (2000). Predicting outcomes of early expressive delay: Ethical implications. In D. V. M. Bishop & L. B. Leonard (Eds.), *Speech and language impairments in children: Causes, characteristics, intervention and outcome* (pp. 195–209). Hove, East Sussex, UK: Psychology Press.

Paul, R. (2007). *Language disorders from infancy through adolescence: Assessment and intervention* (3rd ed.). St. Louis, MO: Mosby.

Paul, R., Chawarska, K., Fowler, C., Cicchetti, D., & Volkmar, F. (2007). "Listen my children and you shall hear": Auditory preferences in toddlers with autism spectrum disorders. *Journal of Speech, Language, and Hearing Research, 50*, 1350–1364.

Plumb, A. M., & Wetherby, A. M. (2013). Vocalization development in toddlers with autism spectrum disorder. *Journal of Speech, Language, and Hearing Research, 56*, 721–734.

Prizant, B. M., Wetherby, A. M., Rubin, E., & Laurent, A. C. (2003). The SCERTS model: A transactional, family-centered approach to enhancing communication and socioemotional abilities of children with autism spectrum disorder. *Infants and Young Children, 16*, 296–316.

Prizant, B. M., Wetherby, A. M., & Rydell, P. J. (2000). Communication intervention issues for children with autism spectrum disorders. In A. M. Wetherby & B. M. Prizant (Eds.), *Autism spectrum disorders: A transactional developmental perspective* (Vol. 9, pp. 193–224). Baltimore: Brookes.

Renner, P., Klinger, L. G., & Klinger, M. R. (2006). Exogenous and endogenous attention orienting in autism spectrum disorders. *Child Neuropsychology, 12*, 361–382.

Rescorla, L. (2002). Language and reading outcomes to age 9 in late-talking toddlers. *Journal of Speech, Language, and Hearing Research, 45*, 360–371.

Rispoli, M., & Hadley, P. (2005, June). *The acquisition and automaticity of finiteness marking.* Poster presented at the Symposium on Research in Child Language Disorders, Madison, WI.

Robinson, L. A., & Owens, R. E. (1995). Clinical notes: Functional augmentative communication and positive behavior change. *Augmentative and Alternative Communication, 11*, 207–211.

Rogers, S. J., Hepburn, S. L., Stackhouse, T., & Wehner, E. (2003). Imitation performance in toddlers with autism and those with other developmental disorders. *Journal of Child Psychology and Psychiatry, 44*, 763–781.

Ross, B., & Cress, C. J. (2006). Comparison of standardized assessments for cognitive and receptive communication skills in young children with complex communication needs. *Augmentative and Alternative Communication, 22*, 100–111.

Rossetti, L. M. (1990). *Rossetti Infant Toddler Language Scale.* East Moline, IL: LinguaSystems.

Selley, W., Parrot, L., Lethbridge, P., Flack, F., Ellis, R., Johnston, K., et al. (2001). Objective measures of dysphagia complexity in children related to suckle feeding histories, gestational ages, and classification of their cerebral palsy. *Dysphagia, 16*, 200–207.

Sheinkopf, S. J., Mundy, P., Oller, D. K., & Steffens, M. (2000). Vocal atypicalities of preverbal autistic children. *Journal of Autism and Developmental Disorders, 30*, 345–354.

Sheppard, J. J. (1987). Assessment of oral motor behaviors in cerebral palsy. In E. D. Mysak (Ed.), *Current methods of assessing and treating communication disorders of the cerebral palsied* [*Seminars in Speech and Language, 8*] (pp. 57–70). New York: Theime-Stratton.

Shriberg, L. D., Campbell, T., Karlsson, B., Brown, R., McSweeny, J., & Nadler, C. (2003). A diagnostic marker for childhood apraxia of speech: The lexical stress ratio. *Clinical Linguistics & Phonetics, 17*, 549–556.

Siegel, E., & Wetherby, A. (2000). Nonsymbolic communication. In M. E. Snell & F. Brown (Eds.), *Instruction of students with severe disabilities* (5th ed., pp. 409–451). Upper Saddle River, NJ: Merrill/Prentice-Hall.

Sigafoos, J., & Mirenda, P. (2002). Strengthening communicative behaviors for gaining access to desired items and activities. In J. Reichle, D. Beukelman, & J. Light (Eds.), *Exemplary practices for beginning communicators: Implications for AAC* (pp. 123–156). Baltimore: Brookes.

Sigafoos, J., O'Reilly, M., Drasgow, E., & Reichle, J. (2002). Strategies to achieve socially acceptable escape and avoidance. In J. Reichle, D. Buekelman, & J. Light (Eds.), *Exemplary practices for*

beginning communicators: Implications for AAC (pp. 157–186). Baltimore: Brookes.

Siller, M., & Sigman, M. (2002). The behaviors of parents of children with autism predict the subsequent development of their children's communication. *Journal of Autism and Developmental Disorders, 32*, 77–89.

Simpson, R. L. (2005). Evidence-based practices and students with autism spectrum disorders. *Focus on Autism and Other Developmental Disabilities, 20*, 140–149.

Skarakis-Doyle, E., Campbell, W., & Dempsey, L. (2009). Identification of children with language impairment: Investigating the classification accuracy of the MacArthur-Bates Communicative Development Inventories, Level III. *American Journal of Speech-Language Pathology, 18*(3), 277–288.

Sleight, M., & Niman, C. (1984). *Gross motor and oral motor development in children with Down syndrome: Birth through age three years.* St. Louis, MO: St. Louis Association for Retarded Citizens.

Smith, V., Mirenda, P., & Zaidman-Zait, A. (2007). Predictors of expressive vocabulary growth in children with autism. *Journal of Speech, Language, and Hearing Research, 50*, 149–160.

Snell, M. E., & Loncke, F. T. (2002). *A manual for the dynamic assessment of nonsymbolic communication.* Unpublished manuscript, University of Virginia at Charlottesville. Retrieved November 10, 2008, from http://people.virginia.edu/~mes5l/manual9-02.pdf

Steeples, T. (2002, February). *Communication breakdowns in mother-child dyads.* Paper presented as part of a conference to the Kansas Division of Early Childhood, Wichita.

Stone, W. L., Conrood, E., & Ousley, O. Y. (1999). Brief report: Can autism be diagnosed accurately in children under three years? *Journal of Child Psychology and Psychiatry, 40*, 219–226.

Stone, W. L. & Yoder, P. J. (2001). Predicting spoken language level in children with autism spectrum disorders. *Autism, 5*, 341–361.

Swettenham, J., Baron-Cohen, S., Charman, T., Cox, A., Baird, G., Drew, A., et al. (1998). The frequency and distribution of spontaneous attention shifts between social and nonsocial stimuli in autistic, typically developing, and nonautistic developmentally delayed infants. *Journal of Child Psychology and Psychiatry, 39*, 747–753.

Thal, D., Tobias, S., & Morrison, D. (1991). Language and gesture in late talkers: A 1-year follow-up. *Journal of Speech and Hearing Research, 34*, 604–612.

Thordardottir, E., Rothenberg, A., Rivard, M. E., & Naves, R. (2006). Bilingual assessment: Can overall proficiency be estimated from separate measurement of two languages? *Journal of Multilingual Communication Disorders, 4*, 1–21.

Tomasello, M. (1988). The role of joint attentional process in early language development. *Language Sciences, 10*, 69–88.

Tomasello, M. (2001). Perceiving intentions and learning words in the second year of life. In M. Bowerman & S. Levinson (Eds.), *Language acquisition and conceptual development* (pp. 133–158). New York: Cambridge University Press.

Tomasello, M. (2003). *Constructing a language: A usage based theory of language acquisition.* Cambridge, MA: Harvard University Press.

Vagh, S. B., Pan, B.A., & Mancilla-Martínez, J. (2009). Measuring growth in bilingual and monolingual children's English productive vocabulary development: The utility of combining parent and teacher report. *Child Development, 80*, 1545–1563.

Wang, X. L., Bernas, R., & Eberhard, P. (2001). Effects of teachers' verbal and non-verbal scaffolding on everyday classroom performances of students with Down syndrome. *International Journal of Early Years Education, 9*(1), 71–80.

Watson, L., Baranek, G., & Crais, E. (2005, March). *Gesture development in infants with autism spectrum disorders.* Paper presented at Gatlinburg Conference on Theory and Research in Intellectual and Developmental Disabilities, Annapolis, MD.

Watson, L. R., Crais, E. R., Baranek, G. T., Dykstra, J. R., & Wilson, K. P. (2013). Communicative gesture use in infants with and without autism: A retrospective home video study. *American Journal of Speech-Language Pathology, 22,* 25–39.

Watt, N., Wetherby, A. M., Barber, A., & Morgan, L. (in press). Repetitive and stereotyped behaviors in children with autism spectrum disorders in the second year of life. *Journal of Autism and Developmental Disorders.*

Watt, N., Wetherby, A., & Shumway, S. (2006). Prelinguistic predictors of language outcome at 3 years of age. *Journal of Speech, Language, and Hearing Research, 49,* 1224–1237.

Wells, G. (1985). *Language at home and at school: Vol. 2. Language development in the pre-school years.* Cambridge, UK: Cambridge University Press.

Werner, E., Dawson, G., Osterling, J., & Dinno, N. (2000). Recognition of autism spectrum disorder before one year of age: A retrospective study based on home videotapes. *Journal of Autism and Developmental Disorders, 30,* 157–162.

Wetherby, A. M., Allen, L., Cleary, J., Kublin, K., & Goldstein, H. (2002). Validity and reliability of the Communication and Symbolic Behavior Scales Developmental Profile with very young children. *Journal of Speech, Language, and Hearing Research, 45,* 1202–1218.

Wetherby, A. M., Goldstein, H., Cleary, J., Allen, L., & Kublin, K. (2003). Early identification of children with communication disorders: Concurrent and predictive validity of the CSBS Developmental Profile. *Infants and Young Children, 16,* 161–174.

Wetherby, A., & Prizant, B. (1993). *Communication and Symbolic Behavior Scales–Normed Edition.* Chicago: Applied Symbolix.

Wetherby, A. M., & Prizant, B. M. (2002). *Communication and Symbolic Behavior Scales Developmental Profile: First Normed Edition.* Baltimore: Brookes.

Wetherby, A. M., Prizant, B. M., & Schuler, A. L. (2000). Understanding the nature of communication and language impairments. In A. M. Wetherby & B. M. Prizant (Eds.), *Autism spectrum disorders: A transactional developmental perspective* (pp. 109–141). Baltimore: Brookes.

Wetherby, A. M., Woods, J., Allen, L., Cleary, J., Dickinson, H., & Lord, C. (2004). Early indicators of autism spectrum disorders in the 2nd year of life. *Journal of Autism & Developmental Disorders, 34,* 473–493.

Wiggins, L. D., Baio, J., & Rice, C. (2006). Examination of the time between first evaluation and first autism spectrum diagnosis in a population-based sample. *Developmental and Behavioral Pediatrics, 27,* S79–S87.

Wiggins, L. D., Robins, D. L., Bakeman, R., & Adamson, L. B. (2009). Brief report: Sensory abnormalities as distinguishing symptoms of autism spectrum disorders in young children. *Journal of Autism and Developmental Disorders, 40,* 1087–1092.

Wilson, E. M., & Green, J. R. (2009). The development of jaw motion for mastication. *Early Human Development, 85*(5), 303–311

Wilson, E. M., Green, J. R., & Weismer, G. (2012). A kinematic description of the temporal characteristics of jaw motion for early chewing: preliminary findings. *Journal of Speech, Language and Hearing Research, 55,* 626– 638

Winton, P. J., Brotherson, M. J., & Summers, J. A. (2008). Learning from the field of early intervention about partnering with families. In M. M. Cornish (Ed.), *Promising practices for partnering with families in the early years* (pp. 21–20). Charlotte, NC: Information Age.

Woods, J. J., & Wetherby, A. M. (2003). Early identification of and intervention for infants and toddlers who are at risk for autism spectrum disorder. *Language, Speech and Hearing Services in Schools, 34,* 180–193.

Yoder, P. J., & Stone, W. L. (2006a). A randomized comparison of the effect of two prelinguistic communication interventions on the acquisition of spoken communication in preschoolers with ASD. *Journal of Speech, Language, and Hearing Research, 49,* 698–711.

Yoder, P. J., & Warren, S. F. (2001b). Relative treatment effects of two prelinguistic communication interventions on language development in toddlers with developmental delays vary by maternal characteristics. *Journal of Speech, Language, and Hearing Research, 44,* 224–237.

Zangl, R., & Mills, D. L. (2007). Increased brain activity to infant-directed speech in 6- and 13-month-old infants. *Infancy, 11,* 31–62.

Zwaigenbaum, L., Bryson, S. E., Rogers, T., Roberts, W., Brian, J., & Szatmari, P. (2005). Behavioural manifestations of autism in the first year of life. *International Journal of Developmental Neuroscience, 23,* 143–152.

CHAPTER 5

Accardo, P. J., & Capute, A. J. (2005). *The Capute Scales: Cognitive Adaptive Test/Clinical Linguistic and Auditory Milestone Scale (CAT/CLAMS).* Baltimore: Brookes.

Achenbach, T., & Rescorla, L. (2000). *Child Behavior Checklist for Ages 1½–5.* Burlington: ASEBA, University of Vermont.

American Guidance Service, Inc. (1984). *Vineland Adaptive Behavior Scales.* Circle Pines, MN: Author.

American Guidance Service, Inc. (1992). *BASC: Behavior Assessment System for Children.* Circle Pines, MN: Author.

American Speech-Language-Hearing Association. (2004c). *Knowledge and skills needed by speech-language pathologists and audiologists to provide culturally and linguistically appropriate services [Knowledge and skills].* Retrieved from www.asha.org/policy/KS2004-00215.htm

American Speech-Language-Hearing Association. (2008b). *Roles and responsibilities of speech-language pathologists in early intervention: Guidelines.* Washington, DC: Author.

Ammer, J. J., & Bangs, T. (2000). *Birth to Three Assessment and Intervention Model.* Austin, TX: Pro-Ed.

Baird, G., Charman, T., Baron-Cohen, S., Cox, A., Swettenham, J., Wheelwright, S., et al. (2000). A screening instrument for autism at 18 months of age: A 6-year follow-up study. *Journal of the American Academy of Child & Adolescent Psychiatry, 39,* 694–702.

Baron-Cohen, S., Allen, J., & Gillberg, C. (1992). Can autism be detected at 18 months? The needle, the haystack, and the CHAT. *British Journal of Psychiatry, 161,* 839–843.

Baron-Cohen, S., Cox, A., Baird, G., Swettenham, J., Nightingale, N., Morgan, K., et al. (1996). Psychological markers in the detection of autism in infancy in a large population. *British Journal of Psychiatry, 168,* 158–163.

Barrera, I., & Corso, R. (2002). Cultural competency as skilled dialogue. *Topics in Early Childhood Special Education, 22*(20), 103–113.

Bernheimer, L., & Weismer, T. (2007). "Let me tell you what I do all day . . .": The family story at the center of intervention research and practice. *Infants and Young Children, 20*(3), 192–201.

Bliss, L. S., & Allen, D. V. (1983). *Screening Kit of Language Development (SKOLD)*. Baltimore: University Park Press.

Boone, H., & Crais, E. (2001). Strategies for achieving family-driven assessment and intervention planning. In *Young Exceptional Children Monograph Series, No. 3*. Missoula, MT: Division for Early Childhood of the Council for Exceptional Children.

Bornstein, M. H., Painter, K. M., & Park, J. (2002). Naturalistic language sampling in typically developing children. *Journal of Child Language, 29*, 687–699.

Brady, N. C. (2003, March). *Communication repair strategies by young children with developmental disabilities*. Paper presented at the 36th annual Gatlinburg Conference on Research and Theory in Intellectual and Developmental Disabilities, Annapolis, MD.

Bryson, S. E., Zwaigenbaum, L., McDermott, C., Rombough, V., & Brian, J. (2008). The Autism Observation Scale for Infants: Scale development and reliability data. *Journal of Autism and Developmental Disorders, 38*, 731–738.

Buschbacher, P. W., & Fox, L. (2003). Understanding and intervening with the challenging behavior of young children with autism spectrum disorder. *Language, Speech, and Hearing Services in Schools, 34*, 217–227.

Campbell, P. H., Milbourne, S. A., & Wilcox, M. J. (2008). Using assistive technology as an intervention to promote participation in everyday activities and routines. *Infants and Young Children, 21*, 94–106.

Carter, M., & Iacono, T. (2002) Professional judgments of the intentionality of communicative acts. *Augmentative and Alternative Communication, 18*, 177–191.

Chan, J. B., & Iacono, T. (2001). Gesture and word production in children with Down syndrome. *Augmentative and Alternative Communication, 17*, 73–87.

Cherney, J. D., Kelly-Vance, L., Glover, K. G., Ruane, A., & Ryalls, B. O. (2003). The effects of stereotyped toys and gender on play assessment in children aged 18–47 months. *Educational Psychology, 23*(1), 95–106.

Coplan, J. (1993). *The Early Language Milestone Scale, Second Edition (ELM-2)*. Austin, TX: Pro-Ed.

Coplan, J., Gleason, J. R., Ryan, R., Burke, M. G., & Williams, M. L. (1982). Validation of an early language milestone scale in a high-risk population. *Pediatrics, 70*(5), 677–683.

Crais, E. (1994). Moving from "parent involvement" to family-centered services. *Hearsay: Journal of the Ohio Speech and Hearing Association, 9*(2), 12–15.

Crais, E. R. (2011). Testing and beyond: Strategies and tools for evaluating and assessing infants and toddlers. *Language, Speech, and Hearing Services in Schools, 42*, 341–364.

Crais, E. R., Roy, V. P., & Free, K. (2006). Parents' and professionals' perceptions of the implementation of family-centered practices in child assessments. *American Journal of Speech-Language Pathology, 15*, 365–377.

Dietz, C., Swinkels, S., Daalen, E., Engeland, H., & Buitelaar, J. (2006). Screening for autistic spectrum disorders in children aged 14–15 months: II. Population screening with the Early Screening of Autistic Traits Questionnaire (ESAT): Design and general findings. *Journal of Autism and Developmental Disorders, 36*, 713–722.

Dunst, C. J., & Trivette, C. M. (2009a). Let's be PALS: An evidence-based approach to professional development. *Infants and Young Children, 22*, 164–176.

Fenson, L., Marchman, V., Thal, D., Dale, P., Reznick, S., & Bates, E. (2006). *The MacArthur-Bates Communicative Development Inventories: User's guide and technical manual* (2nd ed.). Baltimore: Brookes.

Feuerstein, R., Feuerstein, R. S., & Falik, L. (2010). *Beyond smarter: Mediated learning and the brain's capacity for change*. New York: Teachers College Press.

Filipek, P. A., Accardo, P. J., Baranek, G. T., Cook, E. H., Dawson, G., Gordon, B., et al. (1999). The screening and diagnosis of autistic spectrum disorders. *Journal of Autism and Developmental Disorders, 29*, 439–484.

Fitzgerald, C. E., Hadley, P. A., & Rispoli, M. (2013). Are some parents' interaction styles associated with richer grammatical input? *American Journal of Speech-Language Pathology, 22*, 476–488.

Frankenburg, W. K., & Bresnick, B. (1998). *DENVER II Prescreening Questionnaire (PDQ II)*. Denver: Denver Developmental Materials.

Frankenburg, W. K., & Dodds, J. B. (1990). *Denver Developmental Screening Test II (DDST-II)*. Denver: Denver Developmental Materials.

Furey, J. E. (2011). Production and maternal report of 16- and 18-month-olds' vocabulary in low- and middle-income families. *American Journal of Speech-Language Pathology, 20*, 38–46.

Glascoe, F. (1993). The usefulness of the Batelle Developmental Inventory Screening Test. *Clinical Pediatrics, 32*, 273–280.

Glascoe, F. P., Byrne, K. E., Ashford, L. G., Johnson, K. L., Chang, B., & Strickland, B. (1992). Accuracy of the Denver-II in developmental screening. *Pediatrics, 89*(6, Pt 2), 1221–1225.

Glennen, S. (2002). Language development and delay in international adoption: A review. *American Journal of Speech Language Pathology, 11*, 333–339.

Guiberson, M., Rodríguez, B. L., & Dale, P. S. (2011). Classification accuracy of brief parent report measures of language development in Spanish-speaking toddlers. *Language, Speech, and Hearing Services in Schools, 42*, 536–549.

Gutiérrez-Clellen, V. F. (2000). Dynamic assessment: An approach to assessing children's language-learning potential. *Seminars in Speech and Language, 21*, 215–222.

Haebig, E., McDuffie, A., & Ellis Weismer, S. (2013). The contribution of two categories of parent verbal responsiveness to later language for toddlers and preschoolers on the autism spectrum. *American Journal of Speech-Language Pathology, 22*, 57–70.

Hagopian, L. P., Long, E. S., & Rush, K. S. (2004). Preference assessment procedures for individuals with developmental disabilities. *Behavior Modification, 28*(5), 668–677.

Halle, J., Brady, N., & Drasgow, E. (2004). Enhancing socially adaptive communicative repairs of beginning communicators with disabilities. *American Journal of Speech-Language Pathology, 13*, 43–54.

Halle, J. W., & Meadan, H. (2007). A protocol for assessing early communication of young children with autism and other developmental disabilities. *Topics in Early Childhood Special Education, 27*, 49–62.

Halle, J. W., Phillips, B., & Carey, Y. (1999, December). *Examining communicative repairs in young children who lack language*. Paper presented at the International Conference of the Association for Persons With Severe Handicaps, Chicago.

Hanft, B. E., Rush, D. D., & Sheldon, M. L. (2004). *Coaching families and colleagues in early childhood*. Baltimore: Brookes.

Harrison, P. L., Kaufman, A. S., Kaufman, N. L., Bruininks, R. H., Bruininks, R. H., Ilmer, S., Rynders, J., et al. (1990). *Early screening profiles*. Circle Pines, MN: American Guidance Service.

Harrower, J. K., Fox, L., Dunlap, G., & Kincaid, D. (2000). Functional assessment and comprehensive early intervention. *Exceptionality, 8*(3), 189–204.

Horner, R. H., Carr, E. G., Strain, P. S., Todd, A. W., & Reed, H. K. (2002). Problem behavior interventions for young children with autism: A research synthesis. *Journal of Autism and Developmental Disorders, 32*(5), 423–446.

Jackson-Maldonado, D., Bates, E., & Thal, D. (1992). *Fundación MacArthur: Inventario del desarrollo de habilidades comunicativas.* San Diego, CA: San Diego State University.

Jackson-Maldonado, D., Thal, D. J., Fenson, L., Marchman, V. A., Newton, T., & Conboy, B. (2003). *MacArthur Inventarios del Desarrollo de Habilidades Comunicativas user's guide and technical manual.* Baltimore, MD: Brookes.

Johnson, L. J., Cook, M. J., & Kullman, A. J. (1992). An examination of the concurrent validity of the Battelle Developmental Inventory as compared with the Vineland Adaptive Scales and the Bayley Scales of Infant Development. *Journal of Early Intervention, 16,* 353–359.

Jung, L. (2007). Writing individualized family service plan strategies that fit into the routine. *Young Exceptional Children, 10*(3), 2–9.

Kaufman, N. R. (2007). *Kaufman Speech Praxis Test for Children.* Austin, TX: Pro-Ed.

Klee, T. (1992). Developmental and diagnostic characteristics of quantitative measures of children's language production. *Topics in Language Disorders, 12,* 28–41.

Klee, T., Carson, D. K., Gavin, W. J., Hall, L., Kent, A., & Reece, S. (1998). Concurrent and predictive validity of an early language screening program. *Journal of Speech, Language, and Hearing Research, 41,* 627–641.

Kleinman, J., Robins, D., Ventola, P., Pandey, J., Boorstein, H., Esser, E., et al. (in press). The Modified Checklist for Autism in Toddlers: A follow-up study investigating the early detection of autism spectrum disorders. *Journal of Autism and Developmental Disorders.*

Kummerer, S. E., Lopez-Reyna, N. A., & Tejero Hughes, M. (2007). Mexican immigrant mothers' perceptions of their children's communication disabilities, emergent literacy development, and speech-language therapy program. *American Journal of Speech-Language Pathology, 16,* 271–282.

Lichtert, G. (2003). Assessing intentional communication in deaf toddlers. *Journal of Deaf Studies and Deaf Education, 8*(1), 43–56.

Lord, C., Risi, S., Lambrecht, L., Cook, E. H., Leventhal, B. L., DiLavore, P. C., et al. (2000). The Autism Diagnostic Observation Schedule–Generic: A standard measure of social and communication deficits associated with the spectrum of autism. *Journal of Autism and Developmental Disorders, 30*(3), 205–223.

Lynch, E. W., & Hanson, M. J. (Eds.). (2004). *Developing cross-cultural competence: A guide for working with children and their families* (3rd ed.). Baltimore: Brookes.

MacDonald, R., Anderson, J., Dube, W. V., Geckeler, A., Green, G., Holcomb, W., et al. (2006). Behavioral assessment of joint attention: A methodological report. *Research in Developmental Disabilities, 27,* 138–150.

McLaughlin, D. M., & Carr, E. G. (2005). Quality of rapport as a setting event for problem behavior: Assessment and intervention. *Journal of Positive Behavioral Interventions, 7,* 68–91.

McLean, M., McCormick K., Bruder, M. B., & Burdg, N. B. (1987). An investigation of the validity and reliability of the Battelle Developmental Inventory with a population of children younger than 30 months with identified handicapping conditions. *Journal of the Division for Early Childhood, 11,* 238–246.

McWilliam, R. A. (2000). It's only natural . . . to have early intervention in the environments where it's needed. In S. Sandall & M. Ostrosky (Eds.), *Young Exceptional Children Monograph Series, No. 2* (pp. 17–26). Denver, CO: Division for Early Childhood of the Council for Exceptional Children.

Meadan, H., Halle, J. W., & Dragsow, E. (2003, December). *Examining communication repairs of young children with disabilities who are nonverbal.* Paper presented at the International Conference of the Association for Persons With Severe Handicaps, Chicago.

Miller, J. F., Chapman, R., Branston, M. L., & Riechle, J. (1980). Language comprehension in sensorimotor stages V and VI. *Journal of Speech and Hearing Research, 23,* 284–311.

Miller, J.F., & Paul, R. (1995). *The clinical assessment of language comprehension.* Baltimore: Brookes.

Moore, S. M., & Pérez-Méndez, C. (2006). Working with linguistically diverse families in early intervention: Misconceptions and missed opportunities. *Seminars in Speech & Language, 27*(3), 187–198.

Morris, S. R. (2010). Clinical application of the mean babbling level and syllable structure level. *Language, Speech, and Hearing Services in Schools, 41,* 223–230.

Mullen, E. M. (1995). *Mullen Scales of Early Learning* (AGS ed.). Circle Pines, MN: American Guidance Service Inc.

Mundy, P., Delgado, C., Block, J., Venezia, M., Hogan, A., & Seibert, J. (2003). A manual for the Abridged Early Social Communication Scales (ESCS). Retrieved from the University of California, Davis, at http://www.ucdmc.ucdavis.edu/mindinstitute/ourteam/faculty_staff/mundy.html

Neisworth, J. T., & Bagnato, S. J. (2004). The mismeasure of young children. *Infants & Young Children, 17*(3), 198–212.

Newborg, J. (2005). *Batelle Developmental Inventory, Second Edition.* Itasca, IL: Riverside Publishing.

Newmeyer, A. J., Grether, S., Grasha, C., White, J., Akers, R., Aylward, C., et al. (2007). Fine motor function and oral-motor imitation skills in preschool-age children with speech-sound disorders. *Clinical Pediatrics, 46,* 604–611.

Ogletree, B. T., Pierce, K., Harn, W. E., & Fischer, M. A. (2002). Assessment of communication and language in classical autism: Issues and practices. *Assessment for Effective Intervention, 21,* 61–71.

Olswang, L. B., Feuerstein, J. L., Pinder, G. L., & Dowden, P. (2013). Validating dynamic assessment of triadic gaze for young children with severe disabilities. *American Journal of Speech-Language Pathology, 22,* 449–462.

Olswang, L., Stoel-Gammon, C., Coggins, T., & Carpenter, R. (Eds.). (1987). *Assessing prelinguistic and early linguistic behaviors in developmentally young children* (p. 122). Seattle: University of Washington Press.

Oosterling, I. J., Swinkels, S. H., van der Gaag, R. J., Visser, J. C., Dietz, C., & Buitelaar, J. K. (2009). Comparative analysis of three screening instruments for autism spectrum disorder in toddlers at high risk. *Journal of Autism and Developmental Disorders, 39,* 897–909.

Owens, R. E. (1982). *Program for the Acquisition of Language with the Severely Impaired (PALS).* Columbus, OH: Merrill.

Owens, R.E. (2014). *Language disorders: A functional approach to assessment and intervention* (6th ed.). Boston: Allyn & Bacon.

Owens, R. E. (2016). *Language development: An introduction.* Boston: Pearson Education.

Paul, R. (2007). *Language disorders from infancy through adolescence: Assessment and intervention* (3rd ed.). St. Louis, MO: Mosby.

Paul, R., & Jennings, P. (1992). Phonological behavior in toddlers with slow expressive language development. *Journal of Speech and Hearing Research, 35,* 99–107.

Pharr, A. B., Ratner, N. B., & Rescorla, L. (2000). Syllable structure development of toddlers with expressive specific language impairment. *Applied Psycholinguistics, 21,* 429–449.

Rescorla, L. (1989). The Language Development Survey: A screening tool for delayed language in toddlers. *Journal of Speech and Hearing Disorders, 54,* 587–599.

Rescorla, L., Ratner, N., Jusczyk, P., & Jusczyk, A. M. (2005). Concurrent validity of the Language Development Survey: Associations with the MacArthur-Bates Communicative Development Inventories: Words and Sentences. *American Journal of Speech-Language Pathology, 14,* 156–163.

Reznick, J. S., Baranek, G. T., Reavis, S., Watson, L. R., & Crais, E. R. (2007). A parent-report instrument for identifying one-year-olds at risk for an eventual diagnosis of autism: The first year inventory. *Journal of Autism and Developmental Disorders, 37,* 1691–1710.

Robins, D. L., & Dumont-Mathieu, T. M. (2006). Early screening for autism spectrum disorders: Update on the Modified Checklist for Autism in Toddlers and other measures. *Developmental and Behavioral Pediatrics, 27,* S111–S119.

Robins, D. L., Fein, D., Barton, M., & Green, J. A. (2001). The Modified Checklist for Autism in Toddlers: An initial study investigating the early detection of autism and pervasive developmental disorders. *Journal of Autism and Developmental Disorders, 31,* 131–151.

Siegel, E., & Wetherby, A. (2000). Nonsymbolic communication. In M. E. Snell & F. Brown (Eds.), *Instruction of students with severe disabilities* (5th ed., pp. 409–451). Upper Saddle River, NJ: Merrill/Prentice-Hall.

Snell, M. E. (2002). Using dynamic assessment with learners who communicate nonsymbolically. *Augmentative and Alternative Communication, 18,* 163–176.

Snell, M. E., & Loncke, F. T. (2002). *A manual for the dynamic assessment of nonsymbolic communication.* Unpublished manuscript, University of Virginia at Charlottesville. Retrieved November 10, 2008, from http://people.virginia.edu/~mes5l/manual9-02.pdf

Stott, D., Merricks, M., Bolton, P., & Goodyer, I. (2002). Screening for speech and language disorders: The reliability, validity and accuracy of the General Language Screen. *International Journal of Language and Communication Disorders, 36,* 117–132.

Tzuriel, D. (2000). Dynamic assessment of young children: Educational and intervention perspectives. *Educational Psychology Review, 12*(4), 385–435.

Vygotsky, L. (1978). *Mind in society: The development of higher psychological processes.* Cambridge, MA: Harvard University Press.

Westby, C. E. (1998). Social-emotional bases of communication development. In W. Haynes & B. Shulman (Eds.), *Communication development: Foundations, processes, and clinical applications* (2nd ed., pp. 165–204). Baltimore: Williams & Wilkins.

Westby, C. E. (2000). A scale for assessing development of children's play. In K. Gitlin-Weiner, A. Sandgrund, & C. E. Schaefer (Eds.), *Play diagnosis and assessment* (2nd ed., pp. 15–57). New York: Wiley.

Wetherby, A. M., Woods, J., Allen, L., Cleary, J., Dickinson, H., & Lord, C. (2004). Early indicators of autism spectrum disorders in the 2nd year of life. *Journal of Autism & Developmental Disorders, 34,* 473–493.

Wetherby, A., & Prizant, B. (1989). *The Expression of Communicative Intent: Assessment Issues.* Seminars in Speech and Language, 10, 77–91.

Wetherby, A. & Prizant, B. (1993). *Communication and Symbolic Behavior Scales,* Normed Edition. Chicago, IL: Applied Symbolix.

Wetherby, A., & Prizant, B. (2002). *Communication and Symbolic Behavior Scales Developmental Profile.* Baltimore: Brookes.

Wetherby, A. M., & Woods, J. J. (2006). Early social interaction project for children with autism spectrum disorders beginning in the second year of life: A preliminary study. *Topics in Early Childhood Special Education, 26,* 67–82.

Wilcox, M. J., & Woods, J. (2011). Participation as a basis for developing early intervention outcomes. *Language, Speech, and Hearing Services in Schools, 42,* 365–378.

Yoder, P. J. (2006). Predicting lexical density growth rate in young children with autism spectrum disorders. *American Journal of Speech-Language Pathology, 15,* 378–388.

Zimmerman, I. L., Steiner, V. G., & Pond, R. E. (2002). *Preschool Language Scale, Fourth Edition, Spanish Edition.* San Antonio, TX: Harcourt Assessment.

Zwaigenbaum, L., Bryson, S. E., Rogers, T., Roberts, W., Brian, J., & Szatmari, P. (2005). Behavioural manifestations of autism in the first year of life. *International Journal of Developmental Neuroscience, 23,* 143–152.

CHAPTER 6

American Speech-Language-Hearing Association. (2008b). *Roles and responsibilities of speech-language pathologists in early intervention: Guidelines.* Washington, DC: Author.

Arntson, R. (2009). *A systematic but flexible therapy format in early intervention.* Paper presented at the annual convention of the American Speech-Language-Hearing Association, New Orleans.

Bleile, K. (2004). *Manual of articulation and phonological disorders: Infancy through adulthood* (2nd ed.). Clifton Park, NY: Delmar Cengage Learning.

Bopp, K. D., Brown, K. E., & Mirenda, P. (2004). Speech-language pathologists' roles in the delivery of positive behavior support for individuals with developmental disabilities. *American Journal of Speech-Language Pathology, 13,* 5–19.

Bricker, D., & Cripe, J. J. W. (1992). An activity-based approach to early intervention. Baltimore: Brookes.

Bruder, M. B. (2001). Inclusion of infants and toddlers. In M. J. Guralnick (Ed.), *Early childhood inclusion: Focus on change* (pp. 203–228). Baltimore: Brookes.

Buschbacher, P. W., & Fox, L. (2003). Understanding and intervening with the challenging behavior of young children with autism spectrum disorder. *Language, Speech, and Hearing Services in Schools, 34,* 217–227.

Calculator, S. N. (2002). Use of enhanced natural gestures to foster interactions between children with Angelman syndrome and their parents. *American Journal of Speech-Language Pathology, 11,* 340–355.

Carpenter, M., Tomasello, M., & Striano, T. (2005). Role reversal imitation and language in typically-developing infants and children with autism. *Infancy, 8,* 253–278.

Carr, E. G., Dunlap, G., Horner, R. H., Koegel, R. L., Turnbull, A. P., Sailor, W., et al. (2002). Positive behavior support: Evolution of an applied science. *Journal of Positive Behavior Intervention, 4,* 4–16.

Carter, M., & Grunsell, J. (2001). The behavior chain interruption strategy: A review of research and discussion of future directions. *Journal of the Association for Persons with Severe Handicaps, 26,* 37–49.

Crais, E. R., Watson, L. R., & Baranek, G. T. (2009). Use of gesture development in profiling children's prelinguistic communication skills. *American Journal of Speech Language Pathology, 18,* 95–108.

Cress, C. J. (2001). *A communication "tool'" model for AAC intervention with early communicators.* Proceedings of the 24th Annual RESNA Conference, Reno, NV.

Cress, C. J. (2002). Expanding children's early augmented behaviors to support symbolic development. In J. Reichle, D. Beukelman, & J. Light (Eds.), *Implementing an augmentative communication system: Exemplary strategies for beginning communicators* (pp. 219–272). Baltimore: Brookes.

DeThorne, L. S., Johnson, C. J., Walder, L., & Mahurin-Smith, J. (2009). When "Simon Says" doesn't work: Alternatives to imitation for facilitating early speech development. *American Journal of Speech-Language Pathology, 18,* 133–145.

Duker, P. C., Didden, R., & Sigafoos, J. (2004). *One-to-one training: Instructional procedures for learners with developmental disabilities.* Austin, TX: Pro-Ed.

Dunst, C. J., Hamby, D., Trivette, C. M., Raab, M., & Bruder, M. B. (2000). Everyday family and community life and children's naturally occurring learning opportunities. *Journal of Early Intervention, 23*(3), 151–164.

Dyches, T. T., Wilder, L. K., Sudweeks, R. R., Obiakor, F. E., & Algozzine, B. (2004). Multicultural issues in autism. *Journal of Autism and Developmental Disorders, 34,* 211–222.

Fey, M. E., Warren, S. F., Brady, N., Finestack, L. H., Bredin-Oja, S. L., Fairchild, M., et al. (2006). Early effects of responsivity education/prelinguistic milieu teaching for children with developmental delays and their parents. *Journal of Speech, Language, and Hearing Research, 49,* 526–547.

Field, T., Field, T., Sanders, C., & Nadel, J. (2001). Children with autism display more social behaviors after repeated imitation sessions. *Autism, 5,* 317–323.

Fisher, W., Thompson, R., Hagopian, L., Bowman, L., & Krug, A. (2000). Facilitating tolerance of delayed reinforcement during functional communication training. *Behavior Modification, 24,* 3–29.

Fox, L., Dunlap, G., & Buschbacher, P. (2000). Understanding and intervening with children's challenging behavior: A comprehensive approach. In S. F. Warren & J. Reichle (Series Eds.) & A. M. Wetherby & B. M. Prizant (Vol. Eds.), *Communication and language intervention series: Vol. 9. Autism spectrum disorders: A transactional developmental perspective* (pp. 307–331). Baltimore: Brookes.

Goldin-Meadow, S., Goodrich, W., Sauer, E., & Iverson, J. (2007). Young children use their hands to tell their mothers what to say. *Developmental Science, 10,* 778–785.

Goodwyn, S. W., Acredolo, L. P., & Brown, C. A. (2000). Impact of symbolic gesturing on early language development. *Journal of Nonverbal Behavior, 24,* 81–103.

Gros-Louis, J., West, M. J., Goldstein, M. H., & King, A. P. (2006). Mothers provide differential feedback to infants' prelinguistic sounds. *International Journal of Behavioral Development, 30,* 509–516.

Hambly, C., & Fombonne, E. (2012). The impact of bilingual environments on language development in children with autism spectrum disorders. *Journal of Autism and Developmental Disorders, 42,* 1342–1352.

Hancock, T. B., & Kaiser, A. P. (2006). Enhanced milieu teaching. In R. McCauley & M. Fey (Eds.), *Treatment of language disorders in children: Communication and language intervention series* (pp. 203–236). Baltimore: Brookes.

Hanft, B., & Feinberg, E. (1997). Toward a new paradigm for determining the frequency and intensity of early intervention services. *Infants and Young Children. 9*(1), 27–37.

Hardy, L., Mullen, R., & Martin, N. (2001). Effect of task-relevant cues and state anxiety on motor performance. *Perceptual and Motor Skills, 92,* 943–946.

Hebbler, K., Zercher, C., Mallik, S., Spiker, D., & Levin, J. (2003). *The national early intervention longitudinal study: Service and provider characteristics and expenditures.* Arlington, VA: Division for Early Childhood of the Council for Exceptional Children.

Heimann, M., Laberg, K. E., & Nordøen, B. (2006). Imitative interaction increases social interest and elicited imitation in non-verbal children with autism. *Infant & Child Development, 15,* 297–309.

Horner R. H. (2000). Positive behavior supports. Focus on Autism and Other Developmental Disabilities, 15, 97–105.

Iacoboni, M. (2005). Neural mechanisms of imitation. *Current Opinion in Neurobiology, 15,* 632–637.

Iacoboni, M., & Wilson, S. M. (2006). Beyond a single area: Motor control and language within a neural architecture encompassing Broca's area. *Cortex, 42,* 503–506.

Johnston, S., Evans, J., and Reichle, M. (2004). Supporting augmentative and alternative communication use by beginning communicators with severe disabilities. *American Journal of Speech-Language Pathology, 13,* 20-30.

Jones, E. A., & Carr, E. G. (2004). Joint attention in children with autism: Theory and intervention. *Focus on Autism and Other Developmental Disabilities, 19,* 13–26.

Kaiser, A. P., & Delaney, E. (2001). Responsive conversations: Creating opportunities for naturalistic language teaching. In S. Sandall & M. Ostrosky (Eds.), *Young Exceptional Children Monograph Series, No. 3* (pp. 13–23). Washington, DC: Division for Early Childhood of the Council for Exceptional Children.

Kaiser, A. P., Hancock, T., & Neitfield, J. P. (2000). The effects of parent-implemented enhanced milieu teaching on social communication of children who have autism [Special issue]. *Journal of Early Education and Development, 4,* 423–446.

Kennedy, C. H., Meyer, K. A., Knowles, T., & Shulka, S. (2000). Analyzing the multiple functions of stereotypical behavior for students with autism: Implications for assessment and treatment. *Journal of Applied Behavior Analysis, 33,* 559–571.

Koegel, L. K., Steibel, D., & Koegel, R. L. (1998). Reducing aggression in children with autism toward infant or toddler siblings. *Journal of the Association for Persons with Severe Handicaps, 23,* 111–118.

Kouri, T. A. (2005). Lexical training through modeling and elicitation procedures with late talkers who have specific language impairment and developmental delays. *Journal of Speech, Language, and Hearing Research, 48,* 157–171.

Kremer-Sadlik, T. (2004). To be or not to be bilingual: Autistic children from multilingual families. *Proceedings of the Fourth International Symposium on Bilingualism* (pp. 1225–1234). Somerville, MA: Cascadilla Press.

Law, J., Garrett, Z., & Nye, C. (2004). The efficacy of treatment for children with developmental speech and language delay/disorder: A meta-analysis. *Journal of Speech, Language, and Hearing Research, 47,* 924–943.

Lof, G. L. (2003). Oral motor exercises and treatment outcome. *Perspectives on Language Learning and Education, 10,* 7–11.

Lof, G. L. (2006, November). *Logic, theory and evidence against the use of non-speech oral motor exercises to change speech sound productions.* Paper presented at the Annual Convention of the American Speech-Language-Hearing Association, Miami, FL.

Lucyshyn, J. M., Kayser, A. T., Irvin, L. K., & Blumberg, E. R. (2002). Functional assessment and positive behavior support at home with families: Designing effective and contextually appropriate behavior support plans. In J. M. Lucyshyn, G. Dunlap, & R. W. Albin (Eds.), *Families & positive behavior support: Addressing problem behavior in family contexts* (pp. 97–132). Baltimore: Brookes.

Mahoney, G., & Perales, F. (2005). Relationship-focused early intervention with children with pervasive developmental disorders and other disabilities: A comparative study. *Developmental and Behavioral Pediatrics, 26*, 77–85.

Masur, E. F., & Eichorst, D. L. (2002). Infants' spontaneous imitation of novel versus familiar words: Relations to observational and maternal report measures of their lexicons. *Merrill-Palmer Quarterly, 48*, 405–426.

Masur, E., Flynn, V., & Eichorst, D. (2005). Maternal responsive and directive behaviours and utterances as predictors of children's lexical development. *Journal of Child Language, 32*, 63–91.

McWilliam, R. A. (2005). DEC recommended practices: Interdisciplinary models. In S. Sandall, M. L. Hemmeter, B. Smith, & M. E. McLean (Eds.), *DEC recommended practices: A comprehensive guide for practical application in early intervention/early childhood special education* (pp. 127–132). Longmont, CO: Sopris West.

Millar, D. C., Light, J. C., & Schlosser, R. W. (2006). The impact of augmentative and alternative communication intervention on the speech production of individuals with developmental disabilities: A research review. *Journal of Speech, Language, and Hearing Research, 49*, 248–264.

Mundy, P., & Thorp, D. (2006). The neural basis of early joint attention behavior. In T. Charman & W. L. Stone (Eds.), *Social and communication development in autism spectrum disorders: Early identification, diagnosis, and intervention* (pp. 296–336). New York: Guilford Press.

National Research Council, Committee on Educational Interventions for Children with Autism, Division of Behavioral and Social Sciences and Education. (2001). *Educating children with autism*. Washington, DC: National Academy Press.

Oberman, L. M., & Ramachandran, V. S. (2007). The simulating social mind: The role of the mirror neuron system and simulation in the social and communicative deficits of autism spectrum disorders. *Psychological Bulletin, 133*, 310–327.

Ohashi, J. K., Mirenda, P., Marinova-Todd, S., Hambly, C., Fombonne, E., Szatmari, P., et al. (2012). Comparing early language development in monolingual- and bilingual-exposed young children with autism spectrum disorders. *Research in Autism Spectrum Disorders, 6*, 890–897.

Owens, R. E. (2004). *Help your baby talk*. New York: Penguin Putnam.

Paul-Brown, D., & Caperton, C. J. (2001). Inclusive practices for preschool-age children with specific language impairment. In M. J. Guralnick (Ed.), *Early childhood inclusion: Focus on change* (pp. 433–463). Baltimore: Brookes.

Peck Peterson, S., Derby, K., Harding, J., Weddle, T., & Barretto, A. (2002). Behavioral support for school-age children with developmental disabilities and problem behavior. In J. M. Lucyshyn, G. Dunlap, & R. W. Albin (Eds.), *Families & positive behavior support: Addressing problem behavior in family contexts* (pp. 287–304). Baltimore: Brookes.

Perry, A. C., & Fisher, W. W. (2001). Behavioral economic influences on treatments designed to decrease destructive behavior. *Journal of Applied Behavior Analysis, 34*, 211–215.

Petersen, J. M., Marinova-Todd, S. H., & Mirenda, P (2012). Brief report: An exploratory study of lexical skills in bilingual children with autism spectrum disorder. *Journal of Autism and Developmental Disorders, 42*, 1499–1503.

Raab, M. (2005). *Supporting children with challenging behaviors: Teaching research assistant to childcare providers (TRAC)*. Monmouth, OR: The Teaching Research Institute.

Raab, M., & Dunst, C. J. (2004). Early intervention practitioner approaches to natural environment intervention. *Journal of Early Intervention, 27*, 15–26.

Richman, D. M., Wacker, D. P., & Winborn, L. (2001). Response efficiency during functional communication training: Effects of effort and response allocation. *Journal of Applied Behavior Analysis, 34*, 73–76.

Rossetti, L. M. (2001). *Communication intervention: Birth to three* (2nd ed.). Albany, NY: Singular.

Sandall, S., McLean, M. E., & Smith, B. J. (Eds.). (2000). *DEC recommended practices in early intervention/early childhood special education*. Longmont, CO: Sopris West.

Sandall, S., Hemmeter, M. L., Smith, B. J., & McLean, M. E. (2005). *DEC recommended practices: A comprehensive guide for practical application in early intervention/early childhood special education*. Longmont, CO: Sopris West Education Services.

Sigafoos, J., Arthur, M., & O'Reilly, M. (2003). *Challenging behavior and developmental disability*. London: Whurr.

Sigafoos, J., Drasgow, E., Reichle, J., O'Reilly, M., Green, V. A., & Tait, K. (2004). Tutorial: Teaching communicative rejecting to children with severe disabilities. *American Journal of Speech-Language Pathology, 13*, 31–42.

Sigafoos, J., O'Reilly, M., Drasgow, E., & Reichle, J. (2002). Strategies to achieve socially acceptable escape and avoidance. In J. Reichle, D. Buekelman, & J. Light (Eds.), *Exemplary practices for beginning communicators: Implications for AAC* (pp. 157–186). Baltimore: Brookes.

Smith, B. J., Strain, P. A., Snyder, P., Sandall, S., McLean, M. E., Ramsey, A. B., & Sumi, W. C. (2002). DEC recommended practices: A review of nine years of EI/ECSE research literature. *Journal of Early Intervention, 25*(2), 108–119.

Smith, J., Warren, S., Yoder, P., & Feurer, I. (2004). Teachers' use of naturalistic communication intervention practices. *Journal of Early Intervention, 27*(1), 1–14.

Smith, T., Buch, G. A., & Gamby, T. E. (2000). Parent-directed, intensive early intervention for children with pervasive developmental disorder. *Research in Developmental Disabilities, 21*(4), 297–309.

Stowe, M. J., & Turnbull, H. R. (2001). Legal considerations of inclusion for infants and toddlers and for preschool-age children. In M. J. Guralnick (Ed.), *Early childhood inclusion: Focus on change* (pp. 69–100). Baltimore: Brookes.

Tamis-LeMonda, C., Bornstein, M., & Baumwell, L. (2001). Maternal responsiveness and children's achievement of language milestones. *Child Development, 72*, 748–767.

U.S. Department of Education. (2003). *Twenty-fifth annual report to Congress on the implementation of the Individuals with Disabilities Education Act*. Retrieved from www.ed.gov/about/reports/annual/osep/2003/index.html

van Kleeck, A., Schwarz, A. L., Fey, M. E., Kaiser, A. P., Miller, J., & Weitzman, E. (2010). Should we use telegraphic or grammatical input in the early stages of language development with children who have language impairments? A meta-analysis of the research and expert opinion. *American Journal of Speech-Language Pathology, 19*, 3–21.

Velleman, S. (2006, November). *Childhood apraxia of speech: Assessment/treatment for the school-aged child*. Paper presented at the Annual Convention of the American Speech-Language-Hearing Association, Miami, FL.

Warren, S. E., & Yoder, P. J. (1998). Facilitating the transition from preintentional to intentional communication. In A. Wetherby, S. Warren, & J. Reichle (Eds.), *Transitions in prelinguistic communication* (pp. 365–384). Baltimore: Brookes.

Wharton, R. H., Levine, K., Miller, E., Breslau, J., & Greenspan, S. I. (2000). Children with special needs in bilingual families:

A developmental approach to language recommendations. In S. I. Greenspan & S. Wieder, *The Interdisciplinary Council on Developmental and Learning Disorders clinical practice guidelines* (pp. 141–151). Bethesda, MD: The Interdisciplinary Council on Developmental and Learning Disorders.

Wilcox, M. J., & Shannon, M. S. (1996). Integrated early intervention practices in speech-language pathology. In McWilliam, R. A. (Ed.), Rethinking pull-out services in early intervention (pp. 218–241). Baltimore: Brookes.

Wilcox, M. J., & Shannon, M. S. (1998). Facilitating the transition from prelinguistic to linguistic communication. In A. M. Wetherby, S. F. Warren, & J. Reichle (Eds.), *Communication and Language Intervention Series Volume 5: Transitions in prelinguistic communication* (pp. 385–416). Baltimore: Brookes.

Wing, C., Kohnert, K., Pham, G., Cordero, K. N., Ebert, K. D., Kan, P. F., & Blaiser, K. (2007). Culturally consistent treatment for late talkers. *Communication Disorders Quarterly, 29*(1), 20–27.

Wolery, M. (2004). Monitoring children's progress and intervention implementation. In M. McLean, M. Wolery, & D. Bailey (Eds.), *Assessing infants and preschoolers with special needs* (pp. 545–584). Baltimore: Brookes.

Woods, J. J., Kashinath, S., & Goldstein, H. (2004). Effects of embedding caregiver implemented teaching strategies in daily routines on children's communication outcomes. *Journal of Early Intervention, 26*, 175–193.

Woynaroski, T., Yoder, P. J., Fey, M. E., & Warren, S. F. (2014). A transactional model of spoken vocabulary variation in toddlers with intellectual disabilities. *Journal of Speech, Language, and Hearing Research, 57*, 1754–1763.

Yoder, P. J., & Munson, L. J. (1995). The social correlates of coordinated attention to adult and objects in mother-infant interaction. *First Language, 15*, 219–230.

Yoder, P. J., & Stone, W. L. (2006a). A randomized comparison of the effect of two prelinguistic communication interventions on the acquisition of spoken communication in preschoolers with ASD. *Journal of Speech, Language, and Hearing Research, 49*, 698–711.

Yoder, P. J., & Stone, W. L. (2006b). Randomized comparison of two communication interventions for preschoolers with autism spectrum disorders. *Journal of Counseling and Clinical Psychology, 74*, 426–435.

Yoder, P. J., & Warren, S. F. (2002). Effects of prelinguistic milieu reaching and parent responsivity education on dyads involving children with intellectual disabilities. *Journal of Speech, Language, and Hearing Research, 45*, 1158–1174.

Yu, B. (2013). Issues in bilingualism and heritage language maintenance: Perspectives of minority-language mothers of children with autism spectrum disorders. *American Journal of Speech-Language Pathology, 22*, 10–24.

CHAPTER 7

Abbeduto, L. (2003). *International review of research in mental retardation: Language and communication.* New York: Academic Press.

American Speech-Language-Hearing Association (ASHA). (2008b). *Roles and responsibilities of speech-language pathologists in early intervention: Guidelines.* Washington, DC: Author.

American Speech-Language-Hearing Association (ASHA). (2015). *Relation of age to service eligibility: Services in birth-to-3.* Retrieved December 22, 2015, from http://www.asha.org/NJC/Relation-of-Age-to-Service-Eligibility

Angelo, D. H. (2000). Impact of augmentative and alternative communication devices on families. *Augmentative and Alternative Communication, 16*, 37–47.

Axmear, E., Reichle, J., Alamsaputra, M., Kohnert, K., Drager, K., & Sellnow, K. (2005). Synthesized speech intelligibility in sentences: A comparison of monolingual English speaking and bilingual children. *Language, Speech, and Hearing Services in Schools, 36*, 244–250.

Barton, A., Sevcik, R. A., & Romski, M. A. (2006). Exploring visual-graphic symbol acquisition by pre-school age children with developmental and language delays. *Augmentative and Alternative Communication, 22*, 10–20.

Beck, A. R., Bock, S., Thompson, J., & Kosuwan, K. (2002). Influence of communicative competence and augmentative and alternative communication technique on children's attitudes toward a peer who uses AAC. *Augmentative and Alternative Communication, 18*, 217–227.

Beck, A. R., Fritz, H., Keller, A., & Dennis, M. (2000). Attitudes of school-aged children toward their peers who use augmentative and alternative communication. *Augmentative and Alternative Communication, 16*, 13–26.

Beukelman, D. R., & Mirenda, P. (2005). *Augmentative and alternative communication: Supporting children and adults with complex communication needs* (3rd ed.). Baltimore: Brookes.

Binger, C., Kent-Walsh, J., Berens, J., Del Campo, S., & Rivera, D. (2008). Teaching Latino parents to support the multi-symbol message productions of their children who require AAC. *Augmentative and Alternative Communication, 24*, 323–338.

Binger, C., & Light, J. (2006). Demographics of preschoolers who require augmentative and alternative communication. *Language Speech and Hearing Services in Schools, 37*, 200–208.

Binger, C., & Light, J. (2007). The effect of aided AAC modeling on the expression of multi-symbol messages by preschoolers who use AAC. *Augmentative and Alternative Communication, 23*, 30–43.

Blischak, D. M. (2003). Use of speech-generating devices: In support of natural speech. *Augmentative and Alternative Communication, 19*, 29–35.

Bondy, A. S., & Frost, L. A. (1998). The picture exchange communication system. *Seminars in Speech and Language, 19*, 373–389.

Bondy, A. S., & Frost, L. A. (2001). *A picture's worth: PECS and other visual communication strategies in autism.* Bethesda, MD: Woodbine.

Brady, N. C. (2000). Improved comprehension of object names following voice output communication aid use: Two case studies. *Augmentative and Alternative Communication, 16*, 197–204.

Brady, N. C., Thiemann-Bourque, K., Fleming, K., & Matthews, K. (2013). Predicting language outcomes for children learning augmentative and alternative communication: Child and environmental factors. *Journal of Speech, Language, and Hearing Research, 56*, 1595–1612.

Campbell, P. H., Milbourne, S. A., Dugan, L. M., & Wilcox, M. J. (2006). A review of evidence on practices for teaching young children to use assistive technology devices. *Topics in Early Childhood Special Education, 26*, 3–14.

Campbell, P. H., Milbourne, S. A., & Wilcox, M. J. (2008). Using assistive technology as an intervention to promote participation in everyday activities and routines. *Infants and Young Children, 21*, 94–106.

Cress, C. J. (2001). *A communication "tool" model for AAC intervention with early communicators.* Proceedings of the 24th Annual RESNA Conference, Reno, NV.

Cress, C. J. (2002). Expanding children's early augmented behaviors to support symbolic development. In J. Reichle, D. Beukelman, & J. Light (Eds.), *Implementing an augmentative communication system: Exemplary strategies for beginning communicators* (pp. 219–272). Baltimore: Brookes.

Cress, C. J. (2003). Responding to a common early AAC question: "Will my child talk?" *Perspectives on Augmentative and Alternative Communication, 12*, 10–11.

Cress, C. J., & Marvin, C. A. (2003). Common questions about AAC services in early intervention. *Augmentative and Alternative Communication, 19*, 254–272.

Da Fonte, M. A., & Taber-Doughty, T. (2007, November). *Augmentative and Alternative Communication: How early can we start?* Paper presented at the American Speech-Language Hearing Association Annual Convention, Boston.

Dowden, P. A., & Cook, A. M. (2002). Choosing effective selection techniques for beginning communicators. In J. Reichle, D. R. Beukelman, & J. C. Light (Eds.), *Exemplary practices for beginning communicators* (pp. 395–429). Baltimore: Brookes.

Drager, K. D., Clark-Serpentine, E. A., Johnson, K. E., & Roeser, J. L. (2006). Accuracy of repetition of digitized and synthesized speech for young children in background noise. *American Journal of Speech-Language Pathology, 15*, 155–164.

Drager, K. D., Ende, E., Harper, E., Iapalucci, M., & Rentschler, K. (2004). *Using digitized speech output for young children who require AAC.* Poster presented at the annual conference of the American Speech Language Hearing Association, Philadelphia.

Drager, K. D., Light, J. C., Carlson, R., D'Silva, K., Larsson, B., Pitkin, L., & Stopper, G. (2004). Learning of dynamic display AAC technologies by typically developing 3-year-olds: Effect of different layouts and menu approaches. *Journal of Speech, Language, and Hearing Research, 47*, 1133–1148.

Drager, K. D., Light, J., Speltz, K., Fallon, L., & Jeffries, K. (2003). The performance of typically developing 2½-year-olds on dynamic display AAC technologies with different system layouts and language organizations. *Journal of Speech, Language, and Hearing Research, 46*, 298–312.

Dropik, P. L., & Reichle, J. (2008). Comparison of accuracy and efficiency of directed scanning and group-item scanning for augmentative communication selection techniques with typically developing preschoolers. *American Journal of Speech-Language Pathology, 17*, 35–47.

Fallon, K., Light, J., & Achenbach, A. (2000, December). *The semantic organization patterns of young children: Implications for AAC.* Paper presented at the biennial conference of the International Society for Augmentative and Alternative Communication, Taipei.

Fallon, K. A., Light, J., & Achenbach, A. (2003). The semantic organization patterns of young children: Implications for augmentative and alternative communication. *Augmentative and Alternative Communication, 19*, 74–85.

Fenson, L., Marchman, V. A., Thal, D. J., Dale, P. S., Reznick, J. S., & Bates, E. (2006). *McArthur-Bates Communicative Development Inventories.* Baltimore: Brookes.

Frea, W. D., Arnold, C. L., & Vittimberga, G. L. (2001). A demonstration of the effects of augmentative communication on the extreme aggressive behavior of a child with autism within an integrated preschool setting. *Journal of Positive Behavior Interventions, 3*, 194–198.

Frost, L., & Bondy, A. (2002). *PECS: The picture exchange communication system training manual* (2nd ed.). Cherry Hill, NJ: Pyramid Educational Consultants.

Goldbart, J., & Marshall, J. (2004). "Pushes and pulls" on the parents of children who use AAC. *Augmentative and Alternative Communication, 20*, 194–208.

Grodzicki, L., Jones, J., Panek, E., & Parkin, E. (2006). Re-designing scanning to reduce learning demands: The performance of typically developing 2-year-olds. *Augmentative and Alternative Communication, 22*, 269–283.

Hochstein, D. D., McDaniel, M. A., Nettleton, S., & Hannah Neufeld, K. (2003). The fruitfulness of a nomothetic approach to investigating AAC: Comparing two speech encoding schemes across cerebral palsied and nondisabled children. *American Journal of Speech-Language Pathology, 12*, 110–120.

Hustad, K. C. (2001). Unfamiliar listeners' evaluation of speech supplementation strategies for improving the effectiveness of severely dysarthric speech. *Augmentative and Alternative Communication, 17*, 213–220.

Hustad, K. C., Morehouse, T. B., & Gutmann, M. (2002). AAC strategies for enhancing the usefulness of natural speech in children with severe intelligibility challenges. In J. Reichle, D. Beukelman, & J. Light (Eds.), *Implementing an augmentative communication system: Exemplary strategies for beginning communicators* (pp. 433–452). Baltimore: Brookes.

Light, J. C., & Drager, K. D. (2000). *Improving the design of AAC technologies for young children.* Presentation at the International Society for Augmentative and Alternative Communication Conference, Washington, DC.

Light, J. C., & Drager, K. D. (2002). Improving the design of augmentative and alternative communication technologies for young children. *Assistive Technology, 14*, 17–32.

Light, J. C., & Drager, K. D. (2005). *Maximizing language development with young children who require AAC.* Paper presented at the annual convention of the American Speech-Language-Hearing Association, San Diego.

Light, J. C., & Drager, K. D. (2007). AAC technologies for young children with complex communication needs: State of the science and future research directions. *Augmentative and Alternative Communication, 23*, 204–216.

Light, J. C., Drager, K., McCarthy, J., Mellott, S., Millar, D., Parrish, C., Parsons, A., Rhoads, S., Ward, M., & Welliver, M. (2004). Performance of typically developing four- and five-year-old children with AAC systems using different language organization techniques. *Augmentative and Alternative Communication, 20*, 63–88.

Light, J. C., Roberts, B., Dimarco, R., & Greiner, N. (1998). Augmentative and alternative communication to support receptive and expressive communication for people with autism. *Journal of Communication Disorders, 31*, 153–180.

Light, J., Worah, S., Drager, K., Burki, B., D'Silva, K., Kristiansen, L., et al. (2007). *Graphic representations of early emerging language concepts by young children from different cultural backgrounds: Implications for AAC symbols.* Manuscript in preparation.

Lilienfeld, M., & Alant, E. (2002). Attitudes of children toward an unfamiliar peer using an AAC device with and without voice output. *Augmentative and Alternative Communication, 18*, 91–101.

Long, T., Huang, L., Woodbridge, M., Woolverton, M., & Minkel, J. (2003). Integrating assistive technology into an outcome-drive model of service delivery. *Infants and Young Children, 16*, 272–283.

McCarthy, J., Light, J., Drager, K. D., McNaughton, D., Grodzicki, L., Jones, J., Panek, E., & Parkin, E. (2006). Re-designing scanning to reduce learning demands: The performance of typically developing 2-year-olds. *Augmentative and Alternative Communication, 22*, 269–283.

Millar, D. C., Light, J. C., & Schlosser, R. W. (2000). The impact of AAC on natural speech development: A meta-analysis. In *Proceedings of the 9th biennial conference of the International Society for Augmentative and Alternative Communication* (pp. 740–741). Washington, DC: ISAAC.

Millar, D. C., Light, J. C., & Schlosser, R. W. (2006). The impact of augmentative and alternative communication intervention on the speech production of individuals with developmental disabilities: A research review. *Journal of Speech, Language, and Hearing Research, 49,* 248–264.

Mirenda, P. (2003). Toward functional augmentative and alternative communication for students with autism: Manual signs, graphic symbols, and voice output communication aids. *Language, Speech, and Hearing Services in Schools, 34,* 203–216.

Mirenda, P., & Bopp, M. (2003). Playing the game: Strategic competence in AAC. In J. Light, D. Beukelman, & J. Reichle (Eds.), *Communicative competence for individuals who use AAC* (pp. 401–440). Baltimore: Brookes.

Mirenda, P., & Erickson, K. (2000). Augmentative communication and literacy. In A. Wetherby & B. Prizant (Eds.), *Autism spectrum disorders: A transactional developmental perspective* (pp. 333–367). Baltimore: Brookes.

Mistrett, S. (2001). *Synthesis on the use of assistive technology with infants and toddlers (birth through age two)* (Contract No. HS97017002 Task Order No. 14). Washington, DC: U.S. Department of Education, Office of Special Education Programs, Division of Research to Practice.

Mistrett, S. (2004). Assistive technology helps young children with disabilities participate in daily activities. *Technology in Action, 3*(4), 1–8.

Namy, L. L., Campbell, A. L., & Tomasello, M. (2004). The changing role of iconicity in nonverbal symbol learning: A U-shaped trajectory in the acquisition of arbitrary gestures. *Journal of Cognition and Development, 5*(1), 37–57.

National Research Council. (2001) *Educating children with autism.* Committee on Educational Interventions for Children with Autism, Division of Behavioral and Social Sciences and Education. Washington, DC: National Academy Press.

Nigam, R., Schlosser, R., & Lloyd, L. (2006). Concomitant use of the matrix strategy and the mand-model procedure in teaching graphic symbol combinations. *Augmentative and Alternative Communication, 22,* 160–177.

Olin, A. R., Reichle, J., Johnson, L., & Monn, E. (2010). Examining dynamic visual scene displays: Implications for arranging and teaching symbol selection. *American Journal of Speech-Language Pathology, 19,* 284–297.

Oller, D. K., Eilers, R. E., Neal, A. R., & Cobo-Lewis, A. B. (1998). Late onset canonical babbling: A possible early marker of abnormal development. *American Journal on Mental Retardation, 103,* 249–263.

Oxley, J., & Norris, J. (2000). Children's use of memory strategies: Relevance to voice output communication aid use. *Augmentative and Alternative Communication, 16,* 79–94.

Petersen, K., Reichle, J., & Johnston, S. S. (2000). Examining preschoolers' performance in linear and row-column scanning techniques. *Augmentative and Alternative Communication, 16,* 27–36.

Pinkoski-Ball, C. L., Reichle, J., & Munson, B. (2012). Synthesized speech intelligibility and early preschool-age children: Comparing accuracy for single-word repetition with repeated exposure. *American Journal of Speech-Language Pathology, 21,* 293–301.

Reichle, J., Buekelman, D., & Light, J. (2002). *Exemplary practices for beginning communicators: Implications for AAC.* Baltimore: Brookes.

Reichle, J., Dettling, E. E., Drager, K. D., & Leiter, A. (2000). A comparison of correct responses and response latency for fixed and dynamic displays: Performance of a learner with severe developmental disabilities. *Augmentative and Alternative Communication, 16,* 154–163.

Richman, D. M., Wacker, D. P., & Winborn, L. (2001). Response efficiency during functional communication training: Effects of effort and response allocation. *Journal of Applied Behavior Analysis, 34,* 73–76.

Robinson, L. A., & Owens, R. E. (1995). Clinical notes: Functional augmentative communication and positive behavior change. *Augmentative and Alternative Communication, 11,* 207–211.

Romski, M. A., & Sevcik, R. A. (2005) Augmentative communication and early intervention: Myths and realities. *Infants and Young Children, 18,* 174–185.

Romski, M. A., Sevcik, R. A., & Adamson, L. (1999). Communication patterns of youth with mental retardation with and without their speech-output communication devices. *American Journal of Mental Retardation, 104,* 249–259.

Romski, M., Sevcik, R. A., Adamson, L. B., Smith, A., Cheslock, M., & Bakeman, R. (2011). Parent perceptions of the language development of toddlers with developmental delays before and after participation in parent-coached language interventions. *American Journal of Speech-Language Pathology, 20,* 111–118.

Romski, M. A., Sevcik, R. A., Cheslock, M., & Barton, A. (2006). The system for augmenting language. In R. McCauley & M. Fey (Eds.), *Treatment of language disorders in children* (pp. 123–148). Baltimore: Brookes.

Romski, M. A., Sevcik, R. A., & Forrest, S. (2001). Assistive technology and augmentative communication in early childhood inclusion. In M. J. Guralnick (Ed.), *Early childhood inclusion: Focus on change* (pp. 465–479). Baltimore: Brookes.

Romski, M. A., Sevcik, R. A., Hyatt, A., & Cheslock, M. B. (2002). Enhancing communication competence in beginning communicators: Identifying a continuum of AAC language intervention strategies. In J. Reichle, D. Beukelman, & J. Light (Eds.), *Implementing an augmentative communication system: Exemplary strategies for beginning communicators* (pp. 1–23). Baltimore: Brookes.

Ross, B., & Cress, C. J. (2006). Comparison of standardized assessments for cognitive and receptive communication skills in young children with complex communication needs. *Augmentative and Alternative Communication, 22,* 100–111.

Rowland, C., & Schweigert, P. (1989). Tangible symbols: Symbolic communication for individuals with multisensory impairments. *Augmentative and Alternative Communication, 5,* 226–234.

Rowland, C., & Schweigert, P. (1990). *Tangible symbol systems.* Tucson, AZ: Communication Skill Builders.

Rowland, C., & Schweigert, P. (2000). Tangible symbols, tangible outcomes. *Augmentative and Alternative Communication, 16,* 61–78.

Scally, C. (2001). Visual design: Implications for developing dynamic display systems. *Perspectives on Augmentative and Alternative Communication, 10*(4), 16–19.

Schlosser, R. W., & Lee, D. L. (2000). Promoting generalization and maintenance in augmentative and alternative communication: A meta-analysis of 20 years of effectiveness research. *Augmentative and Alternative Communication, 16,* 208–226.

Schlosser, R. W., & Raghavendra, P. (2004). Evidence-based practice in augmentative and alternative communication. *Augmentative and Alternative Communication, 20*, 1–21.

Schlosser, R. W., & Sigafoos, J. (2002). Selecting graphic symbols for an initial request lexicon: Integrative review. *Augmentative and Alternative Communication, 18*, 102–123.

Shane, H. C. (2006). Using visual scene displays to improve communication and communication instruction in persons with autism spectrum disorders. *Perspectives in Augmentative and Alternative Communication, 15*(1), 8–13.

Shane, H. C., & Weiss-Kapp, S. (2007). *Visual language in autism.* San Diego, CA: Plural.

Sigafoos, J., & Drasgow, E. (2001). Conditional use of aided and unaided AAC: A review and clinical case demonstration. *Focus on Autism and Other Developmental Disabilities, 16*, 152–161.

Smith, M. M., & Grove, N. (2003). Asymmetry in input and output for individuals who use AAC. In J. Light, D. Beukelman, & J. Reichle (Eds.), *Communicative competence for individuals who use augmentative and alternative communication: From research to effective practice* (pp. 163–195). Baltimore: Brookes.

Stephenson, J. (2007). The effect of color on the recognition and use of line drawings by children with severe intellectual disabilities. *Augmentative and Alternative Communication, 23*, 44–55.

Sundberg, M., & Michael, J. (2001). The benefits of Skinner's analysis of verbal behavior for children with autism. *Behavior Modification, 25*, 698–724.

Thistle, J. J., & Wilkinson, K. (2009). The effects of color cues on typically developing preschoolers' speed of locating a target line drawing: Implications for augmentative and alternative communication display design. *American Journal of Speech-Language Pathology, 18*, 231–240.

Wilkinson, K. M., Carlin, M., & Jagaroo, V. (2006). Preschoolers' speed of locating a target symbol under different color conditions. *Augmentative and Alternative Communication, 22*, 123–133.

Wilkinson, K. M., Carlin, M., & Thistle, J. (2008). The role of color cues in facilitating accurate and rapid location of aided symbols by children with and without Down syndrome. *American Journal of Speech-Language Pathology, 17*, 179–193.

Wilkinson, K. M., & Hennig, S. (2007). The state of research and practice in augmentative and alternative communication for children with developmental/intellectual disabilities. *Mental Retardation and Developmental Disabilities Research Reviews, 13*, 58–69.

Yoder, P. J., Warren, S. F., & McCathren, R. B. (1998). Determining spoken language prognosis in children with developmental disabilities. *American Journal of Speech Language Pathology, 7*, 77–87.

CHAPTER 8

Angelo, D. H. (2000). Impact of augmentative and alternative communication devices on families. *Augmentative and Alternative Communication, 16*, 37–47.

Banajee, M., Dicarlo, C., & Stricklin, S. (2003). Core vocabulary determination for toddlers. *Augmentative and Alternative Communication, 19*, 67–73.

Bartman, S., & Freeman, N. (2003). Teaching language to a two-year-old with autism. *Developmental Disabilities, 10*, 47–53.

Beck, A. R., & Fritz-Verticchio, H. (2003). The influence of information and role-playing experiences on children's attitudes toward peers who use AAC. *American Journal of Speech-Language Pathology, 12*, 51–60.

Beukelman, D. R., & Mirenda, P. (2005). *Augmentative and alternative communication: Supporting children and adults with complex communication needs* (3rd ed.). Baltimore: Brookes.

Binger, C., & Light, J. (2006). Demographics of preschoolers who require augmentative and alternative communication. *Language Speech and Hearing Services in Schools, 37*, 200–208.

Binger, C., & Light, J. (2007). The effect of aided AAC modeling on the expression of multi-symbol messages by preschoolers who use AAC. *Augmentative and Alternative Communication, 23*, 30–43.

Blackstone, S. W., & Hunt-Berg, M. (2003) *Social networks: An assessment and intervention planning inventory for individuals with complex communication needs and their communication partners.* Monterey, CA: Augmentative and Alternative Communication.

Bondy, A. S., & Frost, L. A. (1998), Picture Exchange Communication System. *Topics in Language Disorders, 19*, 373–390.

Bondy, A. S., & Frost, L. A. (2001). *A picture's worth: PECS and other visual communication strategies in autism.* Bethesda, MD: Woodbine.

Brady, N. C. (2000). Improved comprehension of object names following voice output communication aid use: Two case studies. *Augmentative and Alternative Communication, 16*, 197–204.

Brady, N. C., Thiemann-Bourque, K., Fleming, K., & Matthews, K. (2013). Predicting language outcomes for children learning augmentative and alternative communication: Child and environmental factors. *Journal of Speech, Language, and Hearing Research, 56*, 1595–1612.

Broderick, A., & Kasa-Hendrickson, C. (2001). "SAY JUST ONE WORD AT FIRST": The emergence of reliable speech in a student labeled with autism. *Journal of the Association for Persons with Severe Handicaps, 26*, 13–24.

Cafiero, J. (2001) The effect of an augmentative communication intervention on the communication, behavior, and academic program of an adolescent with autism. *Focus on Autism and Other Developmental Disabilities, 16*, 179–189.

Campbell, P. H. & Sawyer, L. B. (2007) Supporting learning opportunities in natural settings through participation-based services. *Journal of Early Intervention, 29*, 287–305.

Capilouto, G. J. (2005). *Evidence-based decision making in AAC.* Paper presented at the American Speech-Language-Hearing Association Convention, San Diego.

Charlop-Christy, M. H., Carpenter, M., Le, L., LeBlanc, L. A., & Kellet, K. (2002). Using the Picture Exchange Communication System (PECS) with children with autism: Assessment of PECS acquisition, speech, social communicative behavior, and problem behavior. *Journal of Applied Behavior Analysis, 35*, 213–231.

Chiang, H.-M. (2009). Differences between spontaneous and elicited expressive communication in children with autism. *Research in Autism Spectrum Disorders, 3*, 214–222.

Clarke, M., & Kirton, A. (2003) Patterns of interaction between children with physical disabilities using augmentative and alternative communication systems and their peers. *Child Language Teaching and Therapy, 19*, 135–151.

Cress, C. J. (2002). Expanding children's early augmented behaviors to support symbolic development. In J. Reichle, D. Beukelman, & J. Light (Eds.), *Implementing an augmentative communication system: Exemplary strategies for beginning communicators* (pp. 219–272). Baltimore: Brookes.

Cress, C. J., & Marvin, C. A. (2003). Common questions about AAC services in early intervention. *Augmentative and Alternative Communication, 19*, 254–272.

Cress, C. J., Shapley, K., Linke, M., Clark, J., Elliott, J., Bartels, K., Aaron, E. (2000) *Characteristics of intentional communication in young children with physical impairments*. Presentation at the 9th Biennial ISAAC International Conference on AAC, Washington, DC.

DeRuyter, F., McNaughton, D., Caves, K., Bryen, D. N., & Williams, M. B. (2007). Enhancing AAC connections with the world. *Augmentative and Alternative Communication, 23*, 258–270.

Drager, K. D., Postal, V., Carrolus, L., Castellano, M., Gagliano, C., & Glynn, J. (2006) The effect of aided language modeling on symbol comprehension and production in 2 preschoolers with autism. *American Journal of Speech-Language Pathology, 15*, 112–125.

Dunst, C. J., & Lowe, L. W. (1986). From reflex to symbol: Describing, explaining and fostering communicative competence. *Augmentative and Alternative Communication, 2*, 11–18.

Fager, S., Hux, K., Beukelman, D., & Karantounis, R. (2006). Augmentative and alternative communication use and acceptance by adults with traumatic brain injury. *Augmentative and Alternative Communication, 22*, 37–47.

Fallon, K. A., Light, J., & Achenbach, A. (2003). The semantic organization patterns of young children: Implications for augmentative and alternative communication. *Augmentative and Alternative Communication, 19*, 74–85.

Fallon, K. A., Light, J. C., & Paige, T. (2001). Enhancing vocabulary selection for preschoolers who require augmentative and alternative communication (AAC). *American Journal of Speech-Language Pathology, 10*, 81–94.

Ferm, U., Ahlsén, E., & Björck-Åkesson, E. (2005). Conversational topics between a child with complex communication needs and her caregiver at mealtime. *Augmentative and Alternative Communication, 21*, 19–41.

Flippin, M., Reszka, S., & Watson, L. R. (2010). Effectiveness of the Picture Exchange Communication System (PECS) on communication and speech for children with autism spectrum disorders: A meta-analysis. *American Journal of Speech-Language Pathology, 19*, 178–195.

Frost, L., & Bondy, A. (2002). *PECS: The picture exchange communication system training manual* (2nd ed.). Cherry Hill, NJ: Pyramid Educational Consultants.

Ganz, J. B., Sigafoos, J., Simpson, R. L., & Cook, K. E. (2008). Generalization of a pictorial alternative communication system across trainers and distance. *Augmentative and Alternative Communication*.

Ganz, J. B., Simpson, R. L., & Corbin-Newsome, J. (2008). The impact of the Picture Exchange Communication System on requesting and speech development in preschoolers with autism spectrum disorders and similar characteristics. *Research in Autism Spectrum Disorders, 2*, 157–169.

Garrett, K. L., & Kimelman, M. D. Z. (2000). AAC and aphasia: Cognitive-linguistic considerations. In D. R. Beukelman, K. M. Yorkston, & J. Reichle (Eds.), *Augmentative and alternative communication for adults with acquired neurologic disorders*. Baltimore: Brookes.

Goldbart, J., & Marshall, J. (2004). "Pushes and Pulls" on the parents of children who use AAC. *Augmentative and Alternative Communication, 20*, 194–208.

Granlund, M., Björck-Åkesson, E., Wilder, J., & Ylven, R. (2008). AAC interventions for children in a family environment: Implementing evidence in practice. *Augmentative and Alternative Communication, 24*, 207–219.

Grodzicki, L., Jones, J., Panek, E., & Parkin, E. (2006). Re-designing scanning to reduce learning demands: The performance of typically developing 2-year-olds. *Augmentative and Alternative Communication, 22*, 269–283.

Grove, N., & Dockrell, J. (2000). Multisign combinations by children with intellectual impairments: An analysis of language skills. *Journal of Speech, Language and Hearing Research, 43*, 309–323.

Guralnick, M. J. (2001) A framework for change in early childhood education. In M. J. Guralnick (Ed.), *Early childhood inclusion: Focus on change* (pp. 3–35). Baltimore: Brookes.

Hamm, B., & Mirenda, P. (2006). Post-school quality of life for individuals with developmental disabilities who use AAC. *Augmentative and Alternative Communication, 22*, 134–146.

Harper, L. V., & McCluskey, K. S. (2002) Caregiver and peer responses to children with language and motor disabilities in inclusive preschool programs. *Early Childhood Research Quarterly, 17*, 148–166.

Harris, M. D., & Reichle, J. (2004). The impact of aided language stimulation on symbol comprehension and production in children with moderate cognitive disabilities. *American Journal of Speech-Language Pathology, 13*, 155–167.

Hurd, R. (2007). AAC from a parent's perspective. *SIG 12 Perspectives on Augmentative and Alternative Communication, 16*, 12–14.

Hustad, K. C., Berg, A., Bauer, D., Keppner, K., Schanz, A., & Gamradt, J. (2005). *AAC interventions for toddlers and preschoolers: Who, what, when, why*. Miniseminar presented at the annual convention of the American Speech Language Hearing Association, San Diego.

Hutchins, P. (1990). New York: MacMillan. Good-Night Owl.

Johnston, S., McDonnell, A. P., Nelson, C., & Magnavito, A. (2003). Teaching functional communication skills using augmentative and alternative communication in inclusive settings. *Journal of Early Intervention, 25*, 263–280.

Johnston, S., Nelson, C., Evans, J., & Palazolo, K. (2003). The use of visual supports in teaching young children with autism spectrum disorder to initiate interactions. *Augmentative and Alternative Communication, 19*, 86–103.

Johnston, S., Reichle, J., & Evans, J. (2004). Supporting augmentative and alternative communication use by beginning communicators with severe disabilities. *American Journal of Speech Language Pathology. 13*(1), 20–30.

Joseph, N., & Alant, E. (2000). Strangers in the house? Communication between mother and their children who are hearing impaired. *South African Journal of Communication Disorders, 47*, 15–24.

Justice, L. (2006). *Clinical approaches to emergent literacy intervention*. San Diego, CA: Plural.

Kaiser, A. P., & Hancock, T. B. (2003). Teaching parents new skills to support their young children's development. *Infants and Young Children, 16*, 9–21.

Keen, D., Sigafoos, J., & Woodyatt, G. (2001). Replacing prelinguistic behaviors with functional communication. *Journal of Autism and Developmental Disorder, 31*, 385–398.

Kent-Walsh, J. (2003). *The effects of an educational assistant instructional program on the communicative turns of students who use augmentative and alternative communication during book-reading activities*. Unpublished doctoral dissertation, Penn State University, University Park, PA.

Kent-Walsh J., Binger, C., & Hasham, Z. (2010). Effects of parent instruction on the symbolic communication of children using augmentative and alternative communication during storybook reading. *American Journal of Speech-Language Pathology, 19,* 97–107.

Kent-Walsh, J., & Light, J. (2003). *Communication partner training in AAC: A literature review.* Paper presented at the Pennsylvania Speech-Language-Hearing Association annual convention, Harrisburg, PA.

Kent-Walsh, J., & McNaughton, D. (2005). Communication partner instruction in AAC: Present practices and future directions. *Augmentative and Alternative Communication, 21,* 195–204.

Kravits, T. R., Kamps, D. M., Kemmerer, K., & Potucek, J. (2002). Brief report: Increasing communication skills for an elementary-aged student with autism using the Picture Exchange Communication System. *Journal of Autism and Developmental Disorders, 32,* 225–230.

Light, J. (1997). "Communication is the essence of human life": Reflections on communicative competence. *Augmentative and Alternative Communication, 13,* 61–70.

Light, J., Binger, C., & Kelford Smith, A. (1994). Story reading interactions between preschoolers who use AAC and their mothers. *Augmentative and Alternative Communication, 10,* 255–268.

Light, J. C., & Drager, K. D. (2002). Improving the design of augmentative and alternative communication technologies for young children. *Assistive Technology, 14,* 17–32.

Light, J. C., & Drager, K. D. (2005). *Maximizing language development with young children who require AAC.* Paper presented at the annual convention of the American Speech-Language-Hearing Association, San Diego.

Light, J. C., & Drager, K. D. (2007). AAC technologies for young children with complex communication needs: State of the science and future research directions. *Augmentative and Alternative Communication, 23,* 204–216.

Light, J. C., Drager, K., & Nemser, J. (2004). Enhancing the appeal of AAC technologies for young children: Lessons from the toy manufacturers. *Augmentative and Alternative Communication, 20,* 137–149.

Light, J. C., Page, R., Curran, J., & Pitkin, L. (2007). Children's ideas for the design of assistive technologies for young children with complex communication needs. *Augmentative and Alternative Communication, 23,* 274–287.

Light, J. C., Parsons, A., & Drager, K. D. (2002). "There's more to life than cookies": Developing interactions for social closeness with beginning communicators who use AAC. In J. Reichle, D. Beukelman, & J. Light (Eds.), *Exemplary practices for beginning communicators: Implications for AAC* (pp. 187–218). Baltimore: Brookes.

Loncke, F. J., Clibbens, J. P., Arvidson, H. H. & Lloyd, L. L. (Eds.) (1999). Augmentative and Alternative Communication: New directions in research and practice. London: Whurr Publishers.

Lund, S., & Light, J. (2006). Long-term outcomes for individuals who use augmentative and alternative communication: Part I. What is a good outcome? *Augmentative and Alternative Communication, 22,* 284–299.

Magiati, I., & Howlin, P. (2003). A pilot evaluation study of the Picture Exchange Communication System (PECS) for children with autistic spectrum disorders. *Autism, 7,* 297–320.

Magiati, I., & Howlin, P. (2003). A pilot evaluation study of the Picture Exchange Communication System (PECS) for children with autistic spectrum disorders. *Autism, 7,* 297–320.

Marvin, C., Beukelman, D., Bilyeu, D. (1994). "Vocabulary-Use Patterns in Preschool Children: Effects of Context and Time Sampling." AAC, Vol. 10, No. 4.

McNaughton, D., Rackensperger, T., Benedek-Wood, E., Krezman, C., Williams, M., & Light, L. (2008). "A child needs to be given a chance to succeed": Parents of individuals who use AAC to describe the benefits and challenges of learning. *Augmentative and Alternative Communication, 24,* 43–55.

Mirenda, P. (2001). Autism, augmentative communication, and assistive technology: What do we really know? *Focus on Autism and Other Developmental Disabilities, 16,* 141–151.

Mirenda, P. (2003). Toward functional augmentative and alternative communication for students with autism: Manual signs, graphic symbols, and voice output communication aids. *Language, Speech, and Hearing Services in Schools, 34,* 203–216.

Mirenda, P. (2005). *AAC for individuals with autism: From symbol wars to EBP.* Short course presented at the annual convention of the American Speech Language Hearing Association, San Diego.

Mirenda, P. (2008). "A back door approach to autism and AAC." *Augmentative and Alternative Communication, 24,* 219–233.

Mirenda, P., Wilk, D., & Carson, P. (2000). A retrospective analysis of technology use patterns in students with autism over a five-year period. *Journal of Special Education Technology, 15,* 5–16.

Moeller, M. P. (2000). Early intervention and language development in children who are deaf and hard-of-hearing. *Pediatrics, 106,* 43–61.

Moes, D., & Frea, W. (2002). Contextualized behavioral support in early intervention for children with autism and their families. *Journal of Autism and Developmental Disorders, 32,* 519–533.

Mulvihill, B. A., Shearer, D., & Van Horn, M. L. (2002). Training, experience and child care providers' perceptions of inclusion. *Early Childhood Research Quarterly, 17,* 197–215.

National Research Council. (2001). *Educating children with autism.* Committee on Educational Interventions for Children with Autism, Division of Behavioral and Social Sciences and Education. Washington, DC: National Academy Press.

Owens, R. (2012). *Language development: An introduction* (8th ed.). New York: Pearson Education.

Parette, H. P., Huer, M. B., & Brotherson, M. J. (2001). Related service personnel perceptions of team AAC decision-making across cultures. *Education and Training in Mental Retardation and Developmental Disabilities, 36,* 69–82.

Preston, D., & Carter, M. (2009). A review of the efficacy of the picture exchange communication system intervention. *Journal of Autism and Developmental Disorders, 39,* 1471–1486.

Romski, M. A., & Sevcik, R. A. (1996). Breaking the speech barrier: Language development through augmented means. Baltimore: Brookes.

Romski, M. A., & Sevcik, R. A. (2005) Augmentative communication and early intervention: Myths and realities. *Infants and Young Children, 18,* 174–185.

Romski, M. A., Sevcik, R., Adamson, L. B., Cheslock, M. Toddlers, parent implemented augmented language interventions, and communication development. Paper presented at the biennial conference of the International Society for Augmentative and Alternative Communication, Dusseldorf Germany, 2006.

Rowland, C., & Schweigert, P. D. (2000). Tangible symbols, tangible outcomes. *Augmentative and Alternative Communication, 16,* 61–78.

Rudd, H., Grove, N., & Pring, T. (2007). Teaching productive sign modifications to children with intellectual disabilities. *Augmentative and Alternative Communication, 23,* 154–163.

Rycroft-Malone, J. (2004). The PARIHS framework: A framework for guiding the implementation of evidence-based practice. *Journal of Nursing Care Quality, 19*, 297–304.

Rycroft-Malone, J., Seers, K., Titchen, A., Harvey, G., Kitson, A., & McCormack, B. (2004). What counts as evidence in evidence-based practice? *Journal of Advanced Nursing, 47*, 81–90.

Schepis, M., Reid, D., Behrmann, M., & Sutton, K. (1998). Increasing communicative interactions of young children with autism using a voice output communication aid and naturalistic teaching. *Journal of Applied Behavior Analysis, 31*, 561–578.

Schlosser, R.W., & Lee, D. L. (2000). Promoting generalization and maintenance in augmentative and alternative communication: A meta-analysis of 20 years of effectiveness research. *Augmentative and Alternative Communication, 16*, 208–226.

Schreibman, L. (2006). *The science and fiction of autism.* Cambridge, MA: Harvard University Press.

Schwartz, J. B., & Nye, C. (2006). Improving communication for children with autism: Does sign language work? *EBP Briefs, 1*(2), 1–17.

Sevcik, R. A., Romski, M. A., Watkins, R. V., & Deffebach, K. P. (1995). Adult partner-augmented communication input to youth with mental retardation using the System for Augmenting Language (SAL). *Journal of Speech and Hearing Research, 38*, 902–912.

Sigafoos, J. (1998). Assessing conditional use of graphic mode requesting in a young boy with autism. *Journal of Developmental and Physical Disabilities, 10*(2), 133–151.

Sigafoos, J., Arthur-Kelly, M., & Butterfield, N. (2006). *Enhancing everyday communication for children with disabilities.* Baltimore: Brookes.

Sigafoos, J., Woodyatt, G., Keen, D., Tait, K., Tucker, M., & Roberts-Pennell, D. (2000). Identifying potential communicative acts in children with developmental and physical disabilities. *Communication Disorders Quarterly, 21*, 77–86.

Sigafoos, J., Didden, R., & O'Reilly, M. (2003). Effects of speech output on maintenance of requesting and frequency of vocalizations in three children with developmental disabilities. *Augmentative and Alternative Communication, 19*, 37–47.

Sigafoos, J., & Drasgow, E. (2001). Conditional use of aided and unaided AAC: A review and clinical case demonstration. *Focus on Autism and Other Developmental Disabilities, 16*, 152–161.

Sigafoos, J., Drasgow, E., Reichle, J., O'Reilly, M., Green, V. A., & Tait, K. (2004). Tutorial: Teaching communicative rejecting to children with severe disabilities. *American Journal of Speech-Language Pathology, 13*, 31–42.

Smith, A. L., & Hustad, K. C. (2015). AAC and early intervention for children with cerebral palsy: Parent perceptions and child risk factors. *Augmentative and Alternative Communication, 31*, 336–350.

Smith, M. M. (2003). Environmental influences on aided language development: The role of partner adaptation. In S. von Tetzchner, & N. Grove (Eds.), *Augmentative and alternative communication: Developmental issues* (pp. 155–175). London: Whurr.

Smith, M. M., & Grove, N. (2003). Asymmetry in input and output for individuals who use AAC. In J. Light, D. Beukelman, & J. Reichle (Eds.), *Communicative competence for individuals who use augmentative and alternative communication: From research to effective practice* (pp. 163–195). Baltimore: Brookes.

Stiebel, D. (1999). Promoting augmentative communication during daily routines: A parent problem-solving intervention. *Journal of Positive Behavior Interventions, 1*, 159–169.

Stoner, J. B., Beck, A. R., Bock, S. J., Hickey, K., Kosuwan, K., & Thompson, J. R. (2006). The effectiveness of the Picture Exchange Communication System with nonspeaking adults. *Remedial and Special Education, 27*, 154–165.

Stremel, K. (2000). *Communication Module I-III what to teach.* Monmouth: Western Oregon University, Teaching Research Division.

Sutton, A. E., Soto, G., & Blockberger, S. (2002). Grammatical issues in graphic symbol communication. *Augmentative and Alternative Communication, 18*, 192–204.

van Kleeck, A., Stahl, S. A., & Bauer, E. B. (2003). *On reading books to children: Parents and teachers.* Mahwah, NJ: Erlbaum.

von Tetzchner, S., & Grove, N. (2003). The development of alternative language forms. In S. von Tetzchner, & N. Grove (Eds.), *Augmentative and alternative communication: Developmental issues* (pp. 1–27). London: Whurr.

von Tetzchner, S., Brekke, K., Sjøthun, B., & Grindheim, E. (2005). Constructing preschool communities of learners that afford alternative language development. *Augmentative and Alternative Communication, 21*, 82–100.

Wendt, O., Schlosser, R., & Lloyd, L. L. (2006) *The effectiveness of AAC in autism spectrum disorders: A quantitative research synthesis.* Paper presented at the 12th biennial conference of the International Society for Augmentative and Alternative Communication, Dusseldorf, Germany.

Wilder, J., & Granlund, M. (2015). Stability and change in sustainability of daily routines and social networks in families of children with profound intellectual and multiple disabilities. *Journal of Applied Research in Intellectual Disability, 28* (2), 133–144.

Yoder, P. J., & Munson, L. J. (1995). The social correlates of coordinated attention to adult and objects in mother-infant interaction. *First Language, 15*, 219–230.

Yoder, P. J., & Stone, W. L. (2006a). A randomized comparison of the effect of two prelinguistic communication interventions on the acquisition of spoken communication in preschoolers with ASD. *Journal of Speech, Language, and Hearing Research, 49*, 698–711.

Yoder, P. J., & Stone, W. L. (2006b). Randomized comparison of two communication interventions for preschoolers with autism spectrum disorders. *Journal of Counseling and Clinical Psychology, 74*, 426–435.

Yoder, P. J., & Warren, S. F. (2001a). Intentional communication elicits language-facilitating maternal responses. *American Journal of Mental Retardation, 4*, 327–335.

Yoder, P. J., & Warren, S. F. (2001b). Relative treatment effects of two prelinguistic communication interventions on language development in toddlers with developmental delays varies by maternal characteristics. *Journal of Speech, Language, Hearing Research, 44*, 224–237.

Yoon, S.-Y., & Bennett, G. (2000). Effects of stimulus-stimulus pairing procedure on conditioning vocal sounds as reinforcers. *Analysis of Verbal Behavior, 17*, 75–88.

CHAPTER 9

American Speech-Language-Hearing Association. (2008b). *Roles and responsibilities of speech-language pathologists in early intervention: Guidelines.* Washington, DC: Author.

Arntson, R. (2009). *A systematic but flexible therapy format in early intervention*. Paper presented at the annual convention of the American Speech-Language-Hearing Association, New Orleans.

Brown, R. (1973). A First Language. Cambridge, MA: Harvard University Press.

Cameron-Faulkner, T., Lieven, E., & Tomasello, M. (2003). A Construction Based Analysis of Child Directed Speech. *Cognitive Science, 27*, 843–873.

Carpenter, M., Tomasello, M., & Striano, T. (2005). Role reversal imitation and language in typically developing infants and children with autism. *Infancy, 8*, 253–278.

Cleave, P. L., Becker, S. D., Curran, M. K., Van Horne, A. J., & Fey, M. E. (2015). The efficacy of recasts in language intervention: A systematic review and meta-analysis. *American Journal of Speech-Language Pathology, 24*, 237–255.

Cole, K., Maddox, M., & Lim, Y. Language is the key: Constructive interactions around books and play. In: McCauley, R., & Fey, M., editors. Treatment of language disorders in children. Baltimore: Brookes; 2006. (pp. 149–173).

Fey, M. E., Long, S. H., Finestack, L.H. (2003). Ten principles of grammatical intervention for children with specific language impairments. *American Journal of Speech-Language Pathology*, 12: 3–15.

Fey, M. E., Warren, S. F., Brady, N., Finestack, L. H., Bredin-Oja, S. L., Fairchild, M., et al. (2006). Early effects of responsivity education/prelinguistic milieu teaching for children with developmental delays and their parents. *Journal of Speech, Language, and Hearing Research, 49*, 526–547.

Flax, J. F., Realpe-Bonilla, T., Roesler, C., Choudhury, N., & Benasich, A. (2009). Using early standardized language measures to predict later language and early reading outcomes in children at high risk for language-learning impairments. *Journal of Learning Disabilities, 62*, 61–75.

Gibbard, D., Coglan, L., & McDonald, J. (2004). Cost-effectiveness analysis of current practice and parent intervention for children under 3 years presenting with expressive language delay. *International Journal of Communication Disorders, 39*, 229–244.

Girolametto, L., & Weitzman, E. (2006). The Hanen Program for parents. In R. J. McCauley & M. E. Fey (Eds.), *Treatment of language disorders in children* (pp. 77–103). Baltimore: Brookes.

Glogowska, M., Roulstone, S., Enderby, P., & Peters, T. (2000). Randomised controlled trial of community based speech and language therapy in preschool children. *British Medical Journal, 321*, 923–926.

Golinkoff, R., Hirsh-Pasek, K. & Schweisguth, M. (2001). A reappraisal of young children's knowledge of grammatical morphemes. In J. Weissenborn & B. Hoele (Eds.), Approaches to bootstrapping: Phonological, syntactic and neurological aspects of early language acquisition. Amsterdam, Philadelphia: John Benjamins. 167–189.

Hargrave, A. C., & Sénéchal, M. (2000). A book reading intervention with preschool children who have limited vocabularies: The benefits of regular reading and dialogic reading. *Early Childhood Research Quarterly, 15*, 75–90.

Höhle, B., & Weissenborn, J. (2003). German-learning infants' ability to detect unstressed closed-class elements in continuous speech. *Developmental Science, 6*, 122–127.

Hutchins, P. (1990). Good Night Owl. New York: MacMillan,

Ingersoll, B., Meyer, K., Bonter, N., & Jelinek, S. (2012). A comparison of developmental social-pragmatic and naturalistic behavioral interventions on language use and social engagement in children with autism. *Journal of Speech, Language, and Hearing Research, 55,* 1301–1313.

Justice, L. M., & Kaderavek, J. (2002). Using shared storybook reading to promote emergent literacy. *Council for Exceptional Children, 34*(4), 8–13.

Kaiser, A. P., Hancock, T. B., & Trent, J. A. (2007). Teaching parents communication strategies. *Early Childhood Services: An Interdisciplinary Journal of Effectiveness, 1*, 107–136.

Kaiser, A. P., & Roberts, M. Y. (2013). Parent-implemented Enhanced Milieu Teaching with preschool children who have intellectual disabilities. *Journal of Speech, Language, and Hearing Research, 56,* 295–309.

Law, J., Garrett, Z., & Nye, C. (2004). The efficacy of treatment for children with developmental speech and language delay/disorder: A meta-analysis. *Journal of Speech, Language, and Hearing Research, 47*, 924–943.

Mahoney, G., & Perales, F. (2005). Relationship-focused early intervention with children with pervasive developmental disorders and other disabilities: A comparative study. *Developmental and Behavioral Pediatrics, 26*, 77–85.

Manolson, A. (1992). *It takes two to talk: A parent's guide to helping children communicate* (2nd ed.). Toronto: The Hanen Centre.

Pepper, J., & Weitzman, E. (2004). It Takes Two to Talk®: A practical guide for parents of children with language delays (2nd ed.). Toronto: The Hanen Centre.

Plante, E., Ogilvie, T., Vance, R., Aguilar, J. M., Dailey, N. S., Meyers, C., et al. (2014). Variability in the language input to children enhances learning in a treatment context. *American Journal of Speech-Language Pathology, 23*, 530–545.

Proctor-Williams, K., Fey, M., & Loeb, D. (2001). Parental recasts and production of copulas and articles by children with specific language impairment and typical development. *American Journal of Speech-Language Pathology, 10*, 155–168.

Roberts, M. Y., & Kaiser, A. P. (2012). Assessing the effects of a parent-implemented language intervention for children with language impairments using empirical benchmarks: A pilot study. *Journal of Speech, Language, and Hearing Research, 55*, 1655–1670.

Saxton, M. (2005). "Recast" in a new light: Insights for practice from typical language studies. *Child Language Teaching and Therapy, 21*(1), 23–38.

Tomasello, M. (2003). *Constructing a language: A usage-based theory of language acquisition*. Cambridge, MA: Harvard University Press.

van Kleeck, A., Schwarz, A. L., Fey, M. E., Kaiser, A. P., Miller, J., & Weitzman, E. (2010). Should we use telegraphic or grammatical input in the early stages of language development with children who have language impairments? A meta-analysis of the research and expert opinion. *American Journal of Speech-Language Pathology, 19*, 3–21.

Warren, S. F., Bredin-Oja, S. L., Fairchild, M., Finestack, L. H., Fey, M. E., & Brady, N. C. (2006). Responsivity education/Prelinguistic milieu teaching. In R. J. McCauley & M. E. Fey (Eds.), *Treatment of language disorders in children* (pp. 47–76). Baltimore: Brookes.

Wilcox, M. J., Bacon, C. K., & Greer, D. C. (2005). *Evidence-based early language intervention: Caregiver verbal responsivity training*. Retrieved June 23, 2010, from http://www.asu.edu/clas/icrp/research/presentations/p1/pdf2.pdf

Williams, L. (1968). The little old lady who wasn't afraid of anything. New York: Harper Trophy.

Yoder P. J. & Stone, W. (2006b). Randomized comparison of two communication interventions for preschoolers with autism spectrum disorders. *Journal of Consulting and Clinical Psychology, 74*, 426–435.

Yoder, P. J., & Warren, S. F. (1998). Maternal responsivity predicts the prelinguistic communication intervention that facilitates generalized intentional communication. *Journal of Speech, Language, and Hearing Research, 41*, 1207–1219.

Yoder, P. J., & Warren, S. F. (1999a). Maternal responsivity mediates the relationship between prelinguistic intentional communication and later language. *Journal of Early Intervention, 22*, 126–136.

Yoder, P. J. & Warren, S. F. (2001a). Relative treatment effects of two prelinguistic communication interventions on language development in toddlers with developmental delays varies by maternal characteristics. *Journal of Speech, Language, Hearing Research, 44*, 224–237.

Yoder, P. J., & Warren, S. F. (2001b). Relative treatment effects of two prelinguistic communication interventions on language development in toddlers with developmental delays vary by maternal characteristics. *Journal of Speech, Language, and Hearing Research, 44*, 224–237.

Yoder, P. J., & Warren, S. F. (2002). Effects of prelinguistic milieu reaching and parent responsivity education on dyads involving children with intellectual disabilities. *Journal of Speech, Language, and Hearing Research, 45*, 1158–1174.

Yoder, P. J., & Warren, S. F. (2004). Early predictors of language in children with and without Down syndrome. *American Journal on Mental Retardation, 109*, 285–300.

Yoder, P. J., Spruytenburg, H., Edwards, A., & Davies, B.(1995). Effect of verbal routine contexts and expansions on gains in the mean length of utterance in children with developmental delays. *Language, Speech, Hearing Services in Schools, 26*, 21–32.

CHAPTER 10

Addison, L. R., Piazza, C. C., Patel, M. R., Bachmeyer, M. H., Rivas, K. M., Milnes, M., & Oddo, J. (2012). A comparison of sensory integrative and behavioral therapies as treatment for pediatric feeding disorders. *Journal of Applied Behavioral Analysis, 45*(3), 455–471.

American Heart Association. (2015). *About congenital heart defects.* Available from http://www.heart.org/HEARTORG/Conditions/CongenitalHeartDefects/AboutCongenitalHeartDefects/About-Congenital-Heart-Defects_UCM_001217_Article.jsp

American Speech-Language-Hearing Association. (2001). *Roles of speech-language pathologists in swallowing and feeding disorders: technical report* [Technical Report]. Available from www.asha.org/policy

American Speech-Language-Hearing Association (ASHA). (2002). *Knowledge and skills needed by speech-language pathologists providing services to individuals with swallowing and/or feeding disorders* [Knowledge and Skills]. Available from www.asha.org/policy.

American Speech-Language-Hearing Association. (2013a). Pediatric Dysphagia. Retrieved from http://www.asha.org/PRPSpecificTopic.aspx?folderid=8589934965&section=Incidence_and_Prevalence

American Speech-Language-Hearing Association. (2013b). *Swallowing disorders (dysphagia) in adults.* Retrieved from http://www.asha.org/public/speech/swallowing/Swallowing-Disorders-in-Adults/#causes

American Speech-Language-Hearing Association (ASHA). (2014). *Roles of speech-language pathologists in swallowing and feeding disorders* [Position Statement]. Available from www.asha.org/policy

Arvedson, J. C. (2008). Assessment of pediatric dysphagia and feeding disorders: Clinical and instrumental approaches. *Developmental Disabilities Research Reviews, 14*, 118–127.

Arvedson, J. C., & Brodsky, L. (2002). *Pediatric swallowing and feeding: Assessment and management* (2nd ed.). Clifton Park, NY: Delmar Cengage Learning.

Arvedson, J., Clark, H., Lazarus, C., Schooling, T., & Frymark, T. (2010). Evidence-based systematic review: Effects of oral motor interventions on feeding and swallowing in preterm infants. *American Journal of Speech-Language Pathology, 19*, 321–340.

Bingham, P. M. (2009). Deprivation and dysphagia in premature infants. *Journal of Child Neurology, 24*(6), 743–749.

Burklow, K. A., Phelps, A. N., Schultz, J. R., McConnell, K., & Rudolph, C. (1998). Classifying complex pediatric feeding disorders. *Journal of Pediatric Gastroenterology & Nutrition, 27*(2), 143–147.

Coe, D. A., Babbitt, R. L., Williams, K. E., Hajimihalis, C., Snyder, A. M., Ballard, C., & Efron, L. A. (1997). Use of extinction and reinforcement to increase food consumption and reduce expulsion. *Journal of Applied Behavioral Analysis, 30*(3), 581–583.

Cox, S. Y., Fraker, C., Walbert, L., & Fishbein, M. (2004). Food chaining: A systematic approach for the treatment of children with eating aversion. *Journal of Pediatric Gastroenterology & Nutrition, 39*, S1-S583, S1-518.

da Silva, A. P., Lubianca Neto, J. F., & Santoro, P. P. (2010). Comparison between videofluoroscopy and endoscopic evaluation of swallowing for the diagnosis of dysphagia in children. *Otolaryngology-Head and Neck Surgery, 143*(2), 204–209.

Davis-McFarland, E. (2008). Family and cultural issues in a school swallowing and feeding program. *Language, Speech, and Hearing Services in Schools, 39*, 199–213.

Delaney, A. L., & Arvedson, J. C. (2008). Development of swallowing and feeding: Prenatal through first year of life. *Developmental Disabilities Research Reviews, 14*, 105–117.

Equit, M., Palmke, M., Becker, N., Moritz, A., Becker, S., & von Gontard, A. (2013). Eating problems in young children: A population-based study. *Acta Paediatrica, 102*, 149–155.

Ernsperger, L., & Stegen-Hanson, T. (2004). *Just take a bite: Easy, effective answers to food aversions and eating challenges!* Arlington, TX: Future Horizons, Inc.

Fishbein, M., Cox, S., Swenny, C., Mogren, C., Walbert, L., & Fraker, C. (2006). Food chaining: A systematic approach for the treatment of children with feeding aversion. *Nutrition in Clinical Practice, 21*(2), 182–184.

Fraker, C., Fishbein, M., Cox, S., & Walbert, L. (2007). *Food chaining: The proven 6-step plan to stop picky eating, solve feeding problems, and expand your child's diet.* Cambridge, MA: Da Capo Press.

Fucile, S., Gisel, E., & Lau, C. (2002). Oral stimulation accelerates the transition from tube to oral feeding in preterm infants. *Journal of Pediatrics, 141*(2), 230–236.

Gosa, M., Schooling, T., & Coleman, J. (2011). Thickened liquids as a treatment for children with dysphagia and associated adverse effects: A systematic review. *ICAN: Infant, Children, & Adolescent Nutrition, 3*(6), 344–350.

Hamilton, B. E., Minino, A. M., Martin, J. A., Kochanek, K. D., Strobino, D. M., & Guyer, B. (2007). Annual summary of vital statistics: 2005. *Pediatrics, 119*, 345–360.

International Craniofacial Institute. (2014). Retrieved July 18, 2014, from http://www.craniofacial.net/syndromes-down

Joseph, R. A. (2011). Tracheostomy in infants: Parent education for home care. *Neonatal Network, 20*(4), 231–242.

Kersten, H. B., & Bennett, D. (2012). A multidisciplinary team experience with food insecurity & failure to thrive. *Journal of Applied Research on Children: Informing Policy for Children at Risk, 3*(1), Article 6.

Kohr, L. M., Dargan, M., Hague, A., Nelson, S. P., Duffy E., Backer, C. L., & Mavroudis, C. (2003). The incidence of dysphagia in pediatric patients after open heart procedures with transesophageal echocardiography. *Annals of Thoracic Surgery, 76*, 1450–1456.

Kummer, A. W. (2014). *Cleft palate and craniofacial anomalies: Effects on speech and resonance* (3rd ed.). Clifton Park, NY: Delmar Cengage Learning.

Kuperminc, M. N., & Stevenson, R. D. (2008). Growth and nutrition disorders in children with cerebral palsy. *Developmental Disabilities Research Review, 14*(2), 137–146.

Laya, B. F., & Lee, E. Y. (2012). Congenital causes of upper airway obstruction in pediatric patients: Updated imaging techniques and review of imaging findings. *Semin Roentgenol, 47*(2), 147–158.

Lewis, E., & Kritzinger, A. (2004). Parental experiences of feeding problems in their infants with Down syndrome. *Down Syndrome Research and Practice, 9*(2), 45–52.

Loots, C., van Herwaarden, M. Y., Benninga, M. A., VanderZee, D. C., van Wijk, M. P., & Omari, T. I. (2013). Gastroesophageal reflux, esophageal function, gastric emptying, and the relationship to dysphagia before and after antireflux surgery in children. *Journal of Pediatrics, 162*(3), 566–573.

Manno, C. J., Fox, C., Eicher, P. S., & Kerwin, M. E. (2005). Early oral-motor interventions for pediatric feeding problems: What, when and how. *Journal of Early and Intensive Behavior Intervention, 2*(3), 145–159.

Miller, C. (2011). Aspiration and swallowing dysfunction in pediatric patients. *Infant, Child, & Adolescent Nutrition, 3*(6), 336–343.

Morgan, A. (2010). Dysphagia in childhood traumatic brain injury: A reflection on the evidence and its implications for practice. *Developmental Neurorehabilitation, 13*(3), 192–203.

Morgan, A., Ward, E., Murdoch, B., Kennedy, B., & Murison, R. (2003). Incidence, characteristics, and predictive factors for dysphagia after pediatric traumatic brain injury. *Journal of Head Trauma Rehabilitation, 18*(3), 239–251.

Morris, S. E., & Klein, M. D. (2000). *Pre-feeding skills: A comprehensive resource for mealtime development* (2nd ed.). Austin, TX: Pro-Ed, Inc.

Nancarrow, S. A., Booth, A., Ariss, S., Smith, T., Enderby, P., & Roots, A. (2013). Ten principles of good interdisciplinary team work. *Human Resources for Health, 11*(19).

Norman, V., Louw, B., & Kritzinger, A. (2007). Incidence and description of dysphagia in infants and toddlers with tracheostomies: A retrospective review. *International Journal of Pediatric Otorhinolaryngology, 71*, 1087–1092.

O'Donoghue, C. R. & Dean-Claytor, A. (2008). Training and self-reported confidence for dysphagia management among speech-language pathologists in the schools. *Language, Speech, and Hearing Services in Schools, 39*, 192–198.

Piazza, C. C., Fisher, W. W., Brown, K. A., Shore, B. A., Patel, M. R., Katz, R. M., et al. (2003). Functional analysis of inappropriate mealtime behaviors. *Journal of Applied Behavior Analysis, 36*(2), 187–204.

Prasse, J. E., & Kikano, G. E. (2009). An overview of pediatric dysphagia. *Clinical Pediatrics, 48*(3), 247–251.

Rogers, B. (2004). Feeding method and health outcomes of children with cerebral palsy. *Journal of Pediatrics, 145*, S28–S32.

Rudolf, C. D., Mazur, L. J., Liptak, G. S., Baker, R. D., Boyle, J. T., Colletti, R. B., et al. (2001). Guidelines for evaluation and treatment of gastroesophageal reflux in infants and children: Recommendations of the North American Society for Pediatric Gastroenterology and Nutrition. *Journal of Pediatric Gastroenterology & Nutrition, 32*, S1–S31.

Schwarz, S. M., Corredor, J., Fisher-Medina, J., Cohen, J., & Rabinowitz, S. (2001). Diagnosis and treatment of feeding disorders in children with developmental disabilities. *Pediatrics, 108*(3), 671–676.

Sharp, W. G., Jaquess, D. L., Morton, J. F., & Herzinger, C. V. (2010). Pediatric feeding disorders: A quantitative synthesis of treatment outcomes. *Clinical Child and Family Psychology Review, 13*(4), 348–365.

Shprintzen, R. J. (2008). Velo-cardio-facial syndrome: 30 years of study. *Developmental Disabilities Research Reviews, 14*(1), 3–10.

Sitton, M., Arvedson, J., Visotcky, A., Braun, N., Kerschner, J., Tarima, S., & Brown, D. (2011). Fiberoptic endoscopic evaluation of swallowing in children: Feeding outcomes related to diagnostic groups and endoscopic findings. *International Journal of Pediatric Otorhinolaryngology, 75*, 1024–1031.

Skinner, B.F. (1991). *The behavior of organisms.* Cambridge, MA: B.F. Skinner Foundation.

Swigert, N. (2010). *The source for pediatric dysphagia* (2nd ed.). East Moline, IL: LinguiSystems, Inc.

Wilkins, J. W., Piazza, C. C., Groff, R. A., & Vaz, P. C. (2011). Chin prompt plus representation as treatment for expulsion in children with feeding disorders. *Journal of Applied Behavioral Analysis, 44*(3), 513–522.

Williams, K. E., Field, D. G., & Seiverling, L. (2010). Food refusal in children: A review of the literature. *Research in Developmental Disabilities, 31*, 625–633.

APPENDIX B

Caselli, M. C. (1998). Gestures and words in early development of children with Down syndrome. *Journal of Speech, Language, and Hearing Research, 41*, 1125–1135.

Charman, T. R. (2004). Matching preschool children with autism spectrum disorders and comparison children for language ability: Methodological challenges. *Journal of Autism and Developmental Disorders, 34*, 59–64.

Charman, T. R., Baron-Cohen, S., Swettenham, J., Baird, G., Drew, A., & Cox, A. (2003). Predicting language outcome in infants with autism and pervasive developmental disorder. *International Journal of Language and Communication Disorders, 38*, 265–285.

Charman, T. R., Taylor, E., Drew, A., Cockerill, H., Brown, J., & Baird, G. (2005). Outcome at 7 years of children diagnosed with autism at age 2: Predictive validity of assessments conducted at 2 and 3 years of age and pattern of symptom change over time. *Journal of Child Psychology and Psychiatry, 46*, 500–513.

Fenson, L., Marchman, V. A., Thal, D. J., Dale, P. S., Reznick, J. S., & Bates, E. (2006). MacArthur-Bates Communicative Development Inventories. Baltimore, MD: Brookes.

Furey, J. E., Kosch, B., & Dunn, N. (2005). *Production and maternal-report of Vocabulary in low- and middle-income families.* Poster presented at the American Speech-Language-Hearing Association Convention, San Diego.

Klee, T., Carson, D. K., Gavin, W. J., Hall, L., Kent, A., & Reece, S. (1998). Concurrent and predictive validity of an early language screening program. *Journal of Speech, Language, and Hearing Research, 41*, 627–641.

Lord, C., & Bailey, A. (2002). Autism spectrum disorders. In M. Rutter & E. Taylor (Eds.), *Child and adolescent psychiatry* (4th ed., pp. 636–663). Oxford, England: Blackwell.

McCathren, R. B., Yoder, P. J., & Warren, S. F. (2000). Testing predictive validity of the communication composite of the Communication and Symbolic Behavior Scales. *Journal of Early Intervention, 23*(3), 36–46.

Mervis, C., & Robinson, B. (2000). Expressive vocabulary ability of toddlers with Williams syndrome or Down syndrome. *Developmental Neuropsychology, 17*, 111–126.

Miller, J. F., Sedey, A. L., & Miolo, G. (1995). Validity of parent report measures of vocabulary development for children with Down syndrome. *Journal of Speech and Hearing Research, 38*, 1037–1044.

Rescorla, L. A. (1989). The Language Development Survey: A screening tool for delayed language in toddlers. *The Journal of speech and hearing disorders, 54*, 587–599.

Rescorla, L. A., & Achenbach, T. M. (2002). Use of the Language Development Survey in a national probability sample of children aged 18–35 months. *Journal of Speech, Language, and Hearing Research, 45*, 733–743.

Rescorla, L. A., & Alley, A. (2001). Validation of the Language Development Survey (LDS): A parent report tool for identifying language delay in toddlers. *Journal of Speech, Language, and Hearing Research, 44*, 434–445.

Rescorla, L., Hadicke-Wiley, M., & Escarce, E. (1993). Epidemiological investigation of expressive language delay at age two. *First Language, 13*, 5–22.

Seibert, J. M., Hogan, A. E., & Mundy, P. C. (1982). Assessing interactional competencies: The Early Social-Communication Scales. *Infant Mental Health Journal, 3*, 244–245.

Seibert, J. M., Hogan, A. E., & Mundy, P. C. (1984). Mental age and cognitive stage in young handicapped and at-risk children. *Intelligence, 8*(1), 11–29.

Singer Harris, N. G., Bellugi, U., Bates, E., Jones, W., & Rossen, M. (1997). Contrasting Profiles of Language Development in Children with Williams and Down Syndromes. *Developmental Neuropsychology, 13*, 345–370.

Stone, W. L. & Yoder, P. J. (2001). Predicting spoken language level in children with autism spectrum disorders. *Autism, 5*, 341–361.

Wetherby, A. M., Allen, L., Cleary, J., Kublin, K., & Goldstein, H. (2002). Validity and reliability of the Communication and Symbolic Behavior Scales Developmental Profile with very young children. *Journal of Speech, Language, and Hearing Research, 45*, 1202–1218.

Wetherby, A. M., Goldstein, H., Cleary, J., Allen, L., & Kublin, K. (2003). Early identification of children with communication disorders: Concurrent and predictive validity of the CSBS Developmental Profile. *Infants and Young Children, 16*, 161–174.

Wetherby, A., & Prizant, B. (2002). *Communication and Symbolic Behavior Scales Developmental Profile.* Baltimore: MD Brookes.

APPENDIX C

Golinkoff, R. M. (1986). I beg your pardon?: The preverbal negotiation of failed messages. Journal of Child Language, 13(3), 455–476. doi:10.1017/S0305000900006826

Olswang, L. B., Bain, B. A., & Johnson, G. A. (1992). The zone of proximal development: Dynamic assessment of language disordered children. In Warren, S. & Reichle, J. (Eds.) *Perspectives on communication and language intervention: Development, assessment, and remediation* (pp. 187–216). Baltimore, MD: Paul H. Brooks Publishing Co.

Rossetti, L. M. (1990). *Rossetti Infant Toddler Language Scale.* East Moline, IL: LinguaSystems.

Shane, H. & Grabowski, K. (1986) Communication profile for the severely speech impaired. Unpublished manuscript.

Siegel, E., & Wetherby, A. (2000). Nonsymbolic communication. In M. E. Snell & F. Brown (Eds.), *Instruction of students with severe disabilities* (5th ed.) (pp. 409–451). Upper Saddle River, NJ: Merrill/Prentice-Hall.

Snell, M. E., & Loncke, F. T. (2002). *A manual for the dynamic assessment of nonsymbolic communication.* Unpublished manuscript, University of Virginia at Charlottesville. Retrieved on November 10, 2008. http://people.virginia.edu/~mes5l/manual9-02.pdf

Wetherby, A., & Prizant, B. (2002). *Communication and Symbolic Behavior Scales.* Baltimore: Brookes.

Wetherby, A. M., Alexander, D. G., & Prizant, B. M. (1998). The ontogeny and role of repair strategies. In A. M. Wetherby, S. F. Warren, & J. Reichle (Eds.), *Transitions in prelinguistic communication* (pp. 135–159). Baltimore: Brookes.

APPENDIX F

MacDonald, R., Anderson, J., Dube, W. V., Geckeler, A., Green, G., Holcomb, W., et al. (2006). Behavioral assessment of joint attention: A methodological report. *Research in Developmental Disabilities, 27*, 138–150.

Miller, J. F., Chapman, R. S., Branston, M. B., & Reichle, J. (1980). Language comprehension in sensorimotor stages V and VI. *Journal of Speech and Hearing Research, 23*, 284–311.

Miller, J., & Paul, R. (1995). The Clinical Assessment of Language Comprehension. Baltimore: Brookes.

Mundy, P., Delgado, C., Block, J., Venezia, M., Hogan, A., & Seibert, J. A manual for the Abridged Early Social Communication Scales (ESCS) 2003. Davis: University of California, MIND.

Owens, R. E. (1982). *Program for the Acquisition of Language with the Severely Impaired (PALS).* Columbus, OH: Merrill.

Glossary

AAC system An integrated group of components used by an individual to enhance communication.

Aided AAC Communication that incorporates the use of communication devices in addition to the user's body

American Indian Hand Talk (Amer-Ind) A form of gestural communication consisting of 250 conceptual signals, most of which can be performed with one hand.

Anemia Condition occurring in nearly every preterm infant during the first 2 months of life in which they do not have enough red blood cells.

Apgar score Newborn or neonatal screening tool used to rapidly assess overall health.

Apnea Cessation of breathing for 20 seconds or more, resulting from immaturity and/or depression of the central respiratory drive in the brain.

Arena assessment A transdisciplinary communication assessment in which parents and professionals observe the entire evaluation and simultaneously assess the child.

ASL American Sign Language, a non-English sign communication method used by many people with deafness in the U.S.

Assistive technology Adaptations and devices that enable an individual to function more independently.

At-risk In this broad category of children served by early intervention programs, there is the potential for both biological and environmental factors to interfere with a child's ability to interact in a typical way with the environment and to develop typically.

Attention-following The ability to change the direction of head and eyes in response to adult focus.

Augmentative and alternative communication (AAC) A form of assistive technology and an intervention approach that uses other-than-speech means to complement or supplement a child's communication abilities.

Autism spectrum disorder (ASD) One of a group of developmental disorders collectively called pervasive developmental disorder (PDD) that is characterized by hyper- and hyposensitivity to external stimuli; relational difficulties with other humans; motor deficits, including motor speech problems; challenging behaviors, such as self-injury and self-stimulation; and communication disorders, including lack of intent.

Automatic scanning A preset type of scanning in which the indicator moves in a predictable, predetermined pattern that is controlled by the electronic scanning device, and a child activates a switch to select an item when it is highlighted by the cursor.

Behavior chain interruption A method to accomplish initial communication in which a favorable activity, such as rocking together, listening to music, or eating a treat, is interrupted and does not resume until the child signals for this to happen.

Bronchopulmonary dysplasia (BPD) Oxygen dependence involving abnormal development of lung tissue—more specifically, inflammation and scarring in the lungs—that results primarily from pressured ventilation and excess oxygen intake by a newborn but can also arise from other conditions, such as lung trauma, pneumonia, and other infections.

Canonical syllables A consonant and vowel sequence that is produced with adult-like speech timing.

Centering Related to scanning, the scanning indicator automatically returns to the center of the scanner display after each selection.

Cerebral palsy (CP) A group of chronic brain disorders that affect movement, muscle tone, and muscle coordination due to damage to one or more motor areas of the brain that disrupts the brain's ability to control movement and posture because of the faulty signals sent to the muscles.

Circular scanning This is the simplest of the scanning patterns, in which the individual items are displayed in a circle and are electronically scanned, one at a time, until the AAC user stops the scanner and selects an item.

Communication breakdown A situation in which a child's attempt to communicate does not result in their intended outcome.

Communication impairment (CI) A significant disability in young children, characterized by difficulty receiving, sending, processing, and comprehending concepts or verbal and nonverbal communication and evidenced in any or all modes of communication and social interaction.

Communication temptations Minor challenges to the expected occurrence of events in familiar situations that are likely to result in a child attempting to communicate.

Contextual fit Congruence between an intervention and variables, such as the child and caregivers characteristics and needs.

Contingent caregiver response An environmental response based on the perceived intent of the child and thus one that is related to the child's behavior.

Continuous positive airway pressure (CPAP) A technique used with preterm infants that delivers slightly pressurized, warm, moist oxygen in varying concentrations through the nose and can help keep the airways open.

Cultural competence A dynamic, ongoing process of attaining knowledge, skills, attitudes, behaviors, and practices that enable professionals to work effectively in cross-cultural settings.

Deafness A profound hearing loss of 90 dB or greater.

Developmental disability A severe, chronic disability of an individual 5 years of age or older that is attributable to mental or physical impairment or a combination of impairments; is manifested before the age of 22 years; is likely to continue indefinitely; results in substantial functional limitations in three or more areas of life activity; and reflects the individual's need for a combination and sequence of special, interdisciplinary, or generic services, individualized supports, or other forms of assistance that are of lifelong or extended duration.

Direct selection A child indicates his or her selection by pointing.

Directed scanning The scanning pattern is under the control of the user. By using multiple switches, the user can move the scanning indicator up, down, left, right, or diagonally, directing it toward a target.

Disability An inability or lack of ability to perform particular tasks, functions, or skills.

Dynamic assessment Procedure designed to describe a child's optimal level of functioning and can help identify a child's potential and the amount of external support needed.

Dynamic display Aided AAC design in which selection results in a new array of graphic symbols.

Early communication intervention (ECI) An intervention approach primarily focused on a young child's speech, language, and/or feeding difficulties.

Early intervention (EI) An educational approach for young children who have or are at risk of developing a handicapping condition or other special need that may affect their development, providing both remediation and prevention services focused on both the child and the family.

EI assessment An ongoing process of identifying a child's unique needs; the family's priorities, concerns, and resources; and the nature and extent of the EI services needed by both.

EI evaluation Used to determine a child's eligibility for services and requiring identification of a child's level of developmental functioning in a manner that is comprehensive, nondiscriminatory, and conducted by qualified personnel.

Enhanced natural gestures Intentional behaviors that are present in a child's motor repertoire or can be easily taught based on a child's motor skills and are easily recognizable and interpretable.

Environmental sabotage Manipulation of the environment in such a way so that a child's access to a desired object or activity is prohibited, thus creating an opportunity for communication.

Established risk In this broad category of children served by early intervention programs, there is a strong relationship between the condition and developmental difficulties.

Evidence-based practice Process of clinical decision-making informed by a combination of scientific evidence, clinical experience, and client needs.

Expectant delays An opportunity and a reason for a child to use communication behaviors by environmental arrangement so that a child will require assistance.

Fading Elimination of a teaching prompt entirely, enabling the child to perform the behavior independently.

Family systems theory Suggests that individuals, such as children, cannot be understood in isolation but should be considered as part of an emotional unit, known as the family, a system of interconnected and interdependent individuals in which each member has a role to play and rules to follow.

Fetal alcohol spectrum disorder (FASD) Condition resulting from prenatal exposure to alcohol because of maternal alcoholism or heavy drinking, including episodic or "binge" drinking during pregnancy.

Functional communication Communication that "works" or functions for a child to accomplish her or his goals, often through the mediation of a listener or communication partner, typically a parent.

Functional equivalence When two behaviors have the same effect on the environment.

General case programming The use of strategies, such as caregiver cuing and responding, and the selection and sequencing of teaching to build generalized responding across contexts.

Handicap Social consequences of disability or impairment that prevent an individual from realizing her or his potential.

Hyper-reactivity A heightened state of arousal and emotion and a limited ability to learn and interact resulting from a low threshold for physiological stimuli and from emotional reactivity.

Hypo-reactivity Under-arousal, the result of high thresholds for physiological and emotional reactivity resulting in passivity, lethargy, and an inability to process social and environmental experiences.

Impairment An abnormality in function or structure.

Incidental teaching A naturalistic child-directed intervention strategy used during unstructured activities that occurs when a child has shown an interest in something and an adult or peer mediates the situation.

Individualized Family Service Plan (IFSP) An intervention plan that addresses both child and family needs that affect the child's development and includes the child and family's current status, the recommended services and expected outcomes, and a projection of the duration of service delivery.

Intellectual disability (ID) Limitation in general intellectual ability, originating before the age of 18, that is characterized by significant limitations in intellectual functioning and significant limitations in adaptive behavior as expressed in conceptual, social, and practical adaptive skills.

Intentional communication Any child gesture and/or vocalization that is either conventional or symbolic in form and produced in combination with a behavior that demonstrates coordinated attention to both an object or event and a person simultaneously.

Intraventricular hemorrhage (IVH) Usually occurs in the first three days of life and is the most common variety of neonatal intracranial or brain hemorrhage. In severe IVH, the fluid-filled structures in the brain called ventricles expand rapidly, causing pressure on the brain that can lead to brain damage.

Inverse scanning An AAC selection method in which a child holds down a switch that highlights items sequentially until an item is reached and then the child releases the switch to select the highlighted item.

Item-based constructions A Constructionist step in building multiword combinations in which children seem to be following word-order rules with specific words..

Jaundice A condition of newborns marked by a yellowish color to skin and eyes and caused by immature livers that cannot effectively remove bilirubin from the blood.

Joint attention The ability to coordinate attention between people and objects for social purposes.

Legal blindness A visual acuity of 20/200 or less in the better eye with the best possible correction as compared to 20/20 for typical vision.

Lexical density A measure of vocabulary is typically derived from the number of different non-imitative words used within a time period.

Linear scanning AAC selection method in which items are presented sequentially one at a time in a row or rows as the cursor moves through the display.

Low birth weight Below 2500 grams or 5.5 pounds at birth.

Maltreatment "Physical and mental injury, sexual abuse, negligent treatment, or maltreatment of a child under the age of 18 . . . perpetrated by a person who is responsible for the child's welfare under circumstances which indicate that the child's health or welfare is harmed or threatened" (Keeping Children and Families Safe Act of 2003, P.L. 108-36).

Mand-model A communication elicitation and teaching model in which an adult waits until the child shows interest and then "mands" or requests that the child communicate. If the child does not respond or responds inappropriately, the desired communication behavior is modeled for the child.

Mediated assistance A dynamic assessment method in which an adult provides the amount and type of individualized guidance needed for a child to be successful.

Morbidity Illness or disability.

Necrotizing enterocolitis (NEC) A serious and potentially dangerous intestinal problem found in some preterm infants, usually two to three weeks after birth, characterized by temporary or permanent *necrosis* or death of intestinal tissue.

Neglect Failure to provide for the basic needs of a child.

Patent ductus arteriosis (PDA) A congenital heart defect common in premature infants, caused by an abnormal circulation of blood between two major arteries near the heart.

Pivot schemes A Constructionist step in building multiword utterances in which one word or phrase, such as *want* or *more*, acts as a carrier phrase for other words.

Preterm Delivery before 37 completed weeks' gestation.

Proto-declarative A gestural and/or vocal initiative behaviors that indicates a desire to share attention with a partner.

Recognitory gestures Play schemes in which an object is used for its intended function.

Reinforcing combinations Gesture-word combinations in which both convey matching information.

Representational gestures Object-related gestures that signify some feature of the referent, such as a cupped hand to mouth to represent *drinking*.

Representative symbol systems Pictures, photos, line drawings and miniature objects that represent or stand for the object.

Respiratory distress syndrome (RDS) Condition of preterm infants caused by immature lungs and a lack of surfactant; symptoms may include a bluish color to the skin and mucus membranes, brief stoppage of breathing, and struggling breathing.

Retinopathy of prematurity (ROP) An abnormal growth of blood vessels in the eye.

Row-column scanning An AAC selection method in which the cursor systematically advances or steps through groups of symbols until the user selects the group containing the target symbol and then the cursor presents each item sequentially within the selected group.

Scaffolding The use of both verbal and nonverbal prompts to "frame" a behavior.

Scanning An indirect method of accessing a computer or a voice output device. It requires an individual to activate a switch and make a succession of choices that lead to the desired input. These choices are usually made via a switch or switches, some other type of keyboard emulator, or voice. See also Centering; Circular scanning; Directed scanning; Preset scanning; Step scanning.

SEE₁ A signing system in which morphemes are usually formed as separate signs and there are well over 100 obligatory affixes.

SEE₂ A signing system that is an offshoot of SEE₁, is intended for use with young children and contains approximately 70 affixes to be used with primarily ASL signs plus additional signs for pronouns, plurals, possession, and the verb *BE*.

Signed English A signing system developed at Gallaudet University and widely used that is simpler to learn than the SEEs, because, although it follows English word order, a child does not need to include the 16 optional morphological endings. Although most signs were taken from ASL, many were simplified for young hands.

Speech generating device An AAC system (SGD) that provides a spoken model of a child's messages that may, in turn, enhance his or her language learning.

Step scanning This scanning technique allows the user to advance one step at a time for each activation of the switch. There is a one-to-one correspondence between cursor movement and switch activation.

Supplemental combinations Gesture-word combinations that convey different cross-modality information, such as the representational gesture of holding a cup up and saying "Juice" to convey "Want juice."

Tangible symbols An aided AAC system that uses three-dimensional objects and two-dimensional photographs and line drawings.

Task analysis Breaking a teaching goal into steps which take a child from his or her present functioning level to the goal.

Telegraphic speech An early term characterizing children's earliest word combinations as sounding like old telegrams in which some components of grammar are omitted.

Total blindness A complete lack of form and visual light perception.

Total parenteral nutrition (TPN) A method of feeding for infants who cannot feed orally that bypasses the gastrointestinal tract through an IV line that is placed into a vein in the infant's hand, foot, or scalp or an umbilical vein.

Transactional model An interactional model of typical communication and language development, in which the parent and child are both contributing partners.

Transdisciplinary team An assessment and intervention unit consisting of family members and facilitators from multiple disciplines who share responsibility for planning and implementing intervention, contributing their own unique expertise in a fully integrated manner that leads to a consensual service plan and its delivery.

Unaided AAC An AAC system that uses the body's own devices to communicate and include signs and gestures in addition to vocalizations and verbalizations.

Vertical structuring Using prompts and questions to build a longer utterance from its parts.

Voice output communication aids Another name for a speech-generating device.

Word combinations A Constructionist step in building multi-word utterances in which roughly equivalent words are paired in combination but are not combined with other words.

Zone of proximal development Term coined by Vygotsky's which recognizes that we all learn best things that differ only slightly from (are *proximal* or close to) what we already know.

Index

Page numbers followed by *f* indicate a figure and those followed by *t* indicate a table.